Movement Disorder Genetics

Susanne A. Schneider • José M. Tomás Brás
Editors

Movement Disorder Genetics

Springer

Editors
Susanne A. Schneider
Department of Neurology
University Hospital Kiel
Kiel
Germany

José M. Tomás Brás
Department of Molecular Neuroscience
University College London,
Institute of Neurology
London
UK

ISBN 978-3-319-17222-4 ISBN 978-3-319-17223-1 (eBook)
DOI 10.1007/978-3-319-17223-1

Library of Congress Control Number: 2015940324

Springer Cham Heidelberg New York Dordrecht London

Printed on acid-free paper

Springer International Publishing AG Switzerland is part of Springer Science+Business Media (www.springer.com)

To Holger and Julius and to my dear parents,
in loving memory of Barbara

Susanne A. Schneider

To Eduardo, Maria Joaquina, Martinha
and especially to Rita

Jose Bras

This book is also dedicated to our mentors
in acknowledgement of their continuous
support.

Preface

Recent years have seen fascinating developments in the field of genetics. New technologies have, and continue to, enter the market; new genes have been and continue to be identified. In 2012 and in the USA alone, the genetic testing market was estimated to be around US$6 billion and predicted to rapidly increase by a factor of 3–4 until the year 2021. Neurogenetics is a part of this rapidly evolving field. Here, too, new methods and wider applications have led to the identification of novel genes associated with both Mendelian and/or complex inheritance.

While this has provided valuable insights into neurological conditions, at the same time it poses new challenges for clinicians. As the list of differential molecular diagnoses has grown, so has the difficulty in diagnosing patients with an obviously positive family history. In fact, this also holds true for patients with a negative family history, since it has become clear that heritable factors underlie a much larger proportion of patients than previously anticipated. Thus, even in these "sporadic" cases, genetic mutations should be considered and molecular testing may, in some cases, enable confirmation of a precise diagnosis. De novo mutations are an example of a previously underappreciated type of mutation that we now know are responsible for a significant proportion of early-onset sporadic disease. This, of course, has led to an increasing number of genetic tests becoming commercially available (with gene panels being the current trend at a continuously decreasing cost) requiring knowledge of how to best select the right test.

In parallel, the molecular genetic revolution has also changed the daily work of many scientists whose job is to understand the complexity of heritable diseases. Pathways are disentangled; complex puzzles of gene and protein interactions are unravelled. Yet the broader pathophysiology of the disease entities remains poorly understood; and we have only just begun to get a grasp on the roles of genes, the environment, and their interplay on the brain. Currently, treatment of the majority of heritable neurological disorders remains symptomatic, and knowledge of a molecular diagnosis has no direct consequence on therapeutic strategies. However, improved scientific understanding will, in the future, hopefully allow for the development of specific and perhaps even curative therapies.

This special edition is dedicated to movement disorders genetics and ties together up-to-date clinico-genetic knowledge, reviews on latest technologies as well as critical treatises about adjacent aspects, including ethical and legal considerations of genetic testing and contractual obligations in the context of health and life insurances. Indeed, with access to genetic testing becoming easier (because costs are dropping and because direct-to-consumer testing allows bypassing clinical services), there is a call for clear guidelines for genetic counselling and genetic testing. Because of this, we chose to dedicate separate chapters for a thoughtful and sensible discussion of these topics.

Putting this volume together has been an exciting journey, and we are grateful to all those who have contributed with their expertise and knowledge, with their time and other input. We are grateful to our patients who teach us valuable lessons and we are grateful to our own families who support us in what we do – every day.

Kiel, Germany Susanne A. Schneider
London, England, UK José M. Tomás Brás

Contents

Contributors

Mathieu Anheim, MD, PhD Movement Disorders Unit, Department of Neurology, University Hospital of Strasbourg, Strasbourg, France

Robin L. Bennett, MS, LGC, ScD Hon Division of Medical Genetics, Department of Medicine, University of Washington Medical Center, Seattle, WA, USA

Kailash P. Bhatia, MD, DM, FRCP Sobell Department, University College London/Institute of Neurology, London, UK

Saskia Biskup, MD, PhD Executive board, CeGaT GmbH, Tuebingen, Germany

Pascal Borry, PhD Department of Public Health and Primary Care, KU Leuven, Leuven, Belgium

José M. Tomás Brás, PhD Department of Molecular Neuroscience, Institute of Neurology, University College London, London, England, UK

Knut Brockmann, MD Interdisciplinary Pediatric Center for Children with Developmental Disabilities and Severe Chronic Disorders, University Medical Center, Georg August University Göttingen, Göttingen, Germany

Davit Chokoshvili, MA, MSc Department of Public Health and Primary Care, KU Leuven, Leuven, Belgium

Gianfilippo Coppola, PhD Child Study Center, Yale School of Medicine, New Haven, CT, USA

Petr Dusek, MD, PhD Department of Neurology and Center of Clinical Neuroscience, Charles University, Prague, Czech Republic

1st Faculty of Medicine, General University Hospital, Prague, Czech Republic

Thomas V. Fernandez, MD Child Study Center & Psychiatry, Yale University School of Medicine, New Haven, CT, USA

Ida Ngueng Feze, BA, JD, LLM Faculty of Medicine, Department of Human Genetics, Centre of Genomics and Policy, McGill University, Montreal, Canada

Josef Finsterer, MD, PhD Neurological Department, Krankenanstalt Rudolfstiftung (KAR), Vienna, Austria

Dirk Hadaschik, PhD Tumor Diagnostics, CeGaT GmbH, Tuebingen, Germany

Orla Hardiman, BSc, MD Academic Unit of Neurology, Trinity College Dublin, Trinity Biomedical Sciences Institute, Dublin, Ireland

Sasja Heetveld, MSc Genome Biology of Neurodegenerative Diseases, Tübingen, Germany

Eberhard Karls University, Tübingen, Germany

Dena G. Hernandez, MS Laboratory of Neurogenetics, Genomic Technologies Group, National Institute on Aging, National Institutes of Health, Bethesda, MD, USA

Peter Heutink, MSc, PhD Genome Biology of Neurodegenerative Diseases, Tübingen, Germany

Eberhard Karls University, Tübingen, Germany

Henry Houlden, MD, MRCP, PhD Department of Molecular Neuroscience, Institute of Neurology, University College London, London, UK

Heidi Carmen Howard, PhD Department of Public Health and Caring Sciences, Centre for Research Ethics and Bioethic, Uppsala University, Uppsala, Sweden

Yann Joly, DCL (PhD) Faculty of Medicine, Department of Human Genetics, Centre of Genomics and Policy, McGill University, Montreal, Canada

Louiza Kalokairinou, LLM, MSc Department of Public Health and Primary Care, KU Leuven, Leuven, Belgium

Kevin Patrick Kenna, BSc PhD Ocular Genetics Unit, Smurfit Institute of Genetics, Trinity College Dublin, College Green, Dublin 2, Ireland

Stephan Klebe, MD Department of Neurology, University Hospital Würzburg, Würzburg, Germany

Gregor Kuhlenbäumer, MD, PhD Department of Neurology, University Hospital Schleswig Holstein, Kiel, Kiel, Germany

Jessica B. Lennington, PhD Child Study Center, Yale University School of Medicine, New Haven, CT, USA

Suzanne Lesage, PhD INSERM U M27, Pitié-Salpêtrière hospital, Brain and Spinal Cord Institute (ICM), Paris, France

Mario Manto, MD, PhD Neurologie, ULB-Erasme, Bruxelles, Belgium

Russell L. Margolis, MD Department of Psychiatry, Johns Hopkins University School of Medicine, Baltimore, MD, USA

Daniele Marmolino, PhD Parkinson Disease Area, UCB Pharma S.A., Braine-l'Alleud, Belgium

Russell Lewis McLaughlin, BSc, HDip, PhD Population Genetics Laboratory, Smurfit Institute of Genetics, Trinity College Dublin, College Green, Dublin 2, Ireland

Emilia Niemiec, MSc Erasmus Mundus Joint International Doctoral Fellow in Law, Science and Technology, Brussels, Belgium

Department of Law, University of Turin, Italy

Centre for Ethics and Law in the Life Sciences, Leibniz University Hannover, Germany

Patrizia Rizzu, PhD Applied Genomics of Neurodegenerative Diseases, Tübingen, Germany

Hendrik Rosewich, MD Division of Pediatric Neurology, Department of Pediatrics and Adolescent Medicine, University Medical Center Göttingen, Georg August University, Göttingen, Germany

Department of Pediatrics of Pediatric NeurologyUniversity Medical Center Göttingen, Georg August University, Göttingen, Germany

Dobrila D. Rudnicki, PhD Department of Psychiatry, Johns Hopkins University, Baltimore, MD, USA

Shahad Salman, LLB, JD Faculty of Medicine, Department of Human Genetics, Centre of Genomcis and Policy, McGill University, Montreal, Canada

Susanne A. Schneider, MD, PhD Department of Neurology, University Hospital Kiel, Kiel, Germany

Ludger Schöls, MD Department of Neurology and Hertie Institute for Clinical Brain Research, University Hospital Tübingen, Tübingen, Germany

Rebecca Schüle, MD Department of Neurodegenerative Disease – Movement Disorder Genomics, Center for Neurology, Tübingen, Germany

Eva C. Schulte, MD, PhD Neurologische Klinik und Poliklinik, Klinikum rechts der Isar, Technische Universität München, Munich, Germany

Neurologische Klinik und Poliklinik, Institut für Humangenetik, Helmholtz Zentrum München, Munich, Germany

Yasmin Singh, PhD Project management, CeGaT GmbH, Tuebingen, Germany

Andrew B. Singleton, PhD Laboratory of Neurogenetics, National Institute on Aging, National Institutes of Health, Bethesda, MD, USA

Maria Stamelou, MD, PhD Department of Neurology, Philipps-University Marburg, Marburg, Germany

Second Department of Neurology, National and Kapodistrian University of Athens, Athens, Greece

Ronald J. Trent, PhD, MBBS, DPhil, FRACP, FRCPA Department of Medical Genomics and Sydney Medical School, Royal Prince Alfred Hospital B65L6, University of Sydney, Camperdown, NSW, Australia

Danya F. Vears, BS, MS School of Population and Global Health, Centre for Health Equity, University of Melbourne, Parkville, Australia

Salma Majid Wakil, PhD Department of Genetics, King Faisal Specialist Hospital and Research Center, Riyadh, Saudi Arabia

Ruth H. Walker, MB, ChB, PhD Department of Neurology, James J. Peters Veterans Affairs Medical Center, Bronx, NY, USA

Sarah Wiethoff, MD Department of Molecular Neuroscience, Institute of Neurology, University College London, London, UK

Juliane Winkelmann, MD Department of Neurology, Stanford University, Palo Alto, CA, Country

Daniela Zahorakova, RNDr, PhD Department of Pediatrics and Adolescent Medicine, General University Hospital, Prague, Czech Republic

First Faculty of Medicine, Charles University, Prague, Czech Republic

Part I
Clinical Aspects

Chapter 1
Genetics of Mendelian Forms of Parkinson's Disease

Suzanne Lesage

Abstract Over the past decade, genetic causes of parkinsonism have been elucidated but in less than 10 % of the cases. Since the discovery of the first gene responsible for Parkinson's disease (PD), *SCNA* encoding α-synuclein, linkage mapping, and positional cloning have identified autosomal dominantly or recessively inherited PD-causing mutations in the genes encoding *Parkin*, PTEN-induced kinase 1 (*PINK1*), *DJ-1*, leucine-rich repeat kinase 2 (*LRRK2*), and *ATP13A2*, indicating that PD has a highly heterogeneous etiology. With the introduction of next-generation sequencing, rare mutations in *DNAJC6*, *SYNJ1*, *VPS35*, and *DNAJC13* were then discovered to cause inherited parkinsonism. In addition, polymorphic variants in *SNCA* and *LRRK2* and heterozygous mutations in the genes encoding β-glucocerebrosidase (*GBA*) and guanosine triphosphate cyclohydrolase 1 (*GCH1*) appear to contribute to sporadic PD in several populations. These mutations have been linked to mitochondrial dysfunction, accumulation of abnormal and misfolded proteins, impaired protein clearance, defective recycling of synaptic vesicles, and oxidative stress. Identification of other Mendelian forms of PD will be the main challenge for the next decade.

Keywords Parkinson' disease • Parkinsonism • Mendelian forms • Autosomal dominant inheritance • Autosomal recessive inheritance • Next-generation sequencing

Introduction

Intense genetic research during the past 15 years, in particular the mapping and cloning of genes, has led to the identification of at least 18 loci (designated as PARK1 to PARK18) and 13 genes associated with inherited forms of parkinsonism (Fig. 1.1). Two of these genes [*SNCA* and leucine-rich repeat kinase 2 (*LRRK2*)] have been conclusively associated with autosomal dominant forms of PD and 4 genes [*parkin*,

S. Lesage, PhD
INSERM U M27, Pitié-Salpêtrière Hospital, Brain and Spinal Cord Institute (ICM), Paris 75013, France
e-mail: suzanne.lesage@upmc.fr

S.A. Schneider, J.M.T. Brás (eds.), *Movement Disorder Genetics*,
DOI 10.1007/978-3-319-17223-1_1

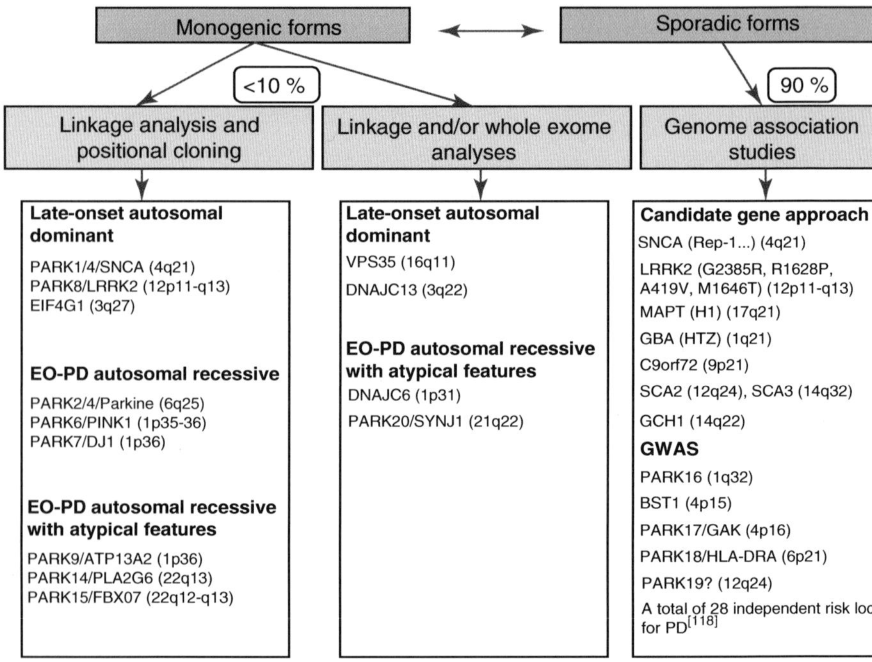

Fig. 1.1 Schematic representation of defined loci and genes for PD, including Mendelian genes and loci identified by association studies. The loci, gene symbols, and chromosomal position are indicated. *EO-PD* early-onset Parkinson's disease, *GWAS* genome-wide association studies

PTEN-induced kinase 1 (*PINK1*), *DJ-1*, *ATP13A2*] with autosomal recessive forms of the disease. In addition, with the advent of promising next-generation sequencing (NGS) technologies, two new dominant, vacuolar protein sorting 35 homolog (*VPS35*) and *DNAJC13*, and two new recessive, *DNAJC6* and *SYNJ1*, PD-associated genes were recently identified. Except for an early age at onset in most patients with monogenic PD, no other specific clinical signs or syndromes seem to distinguish familial from sporadic forms of the disease. Although alterations in the genes identified so far account for less than 10 % of familial forms, there is some evidence that these genes may play a role in the much more common sporadic forms of PD. A large amount of research has also focused on genetic variability that confers susceptibility to PD and will help to create a risk profile for disease in the general population.

This review focuses on the genes which have been conclusively associated with Mendelian forms of the disease, highlighting the most recent advances in this field of research.

Autosomal Dominant Forms of Mendelian PD

The two autosomal dominant genes, *SNCA* and *LRRK2*, which confer a gain of function that is neurotoxic for dopaminergic neurons, are now known to be of major importance in the pathogenesis of both familial and sporadic PD. *VPS35* and

EIF4G1 were identified only recently, and the role they play remains unknown. Other disease-causing genes, such as repeat expansions in ataxin-2 (*ATXN2*) and ataxin-3 (*ATXN3*), which cause spinocerebellar ataxias; guanosine triphosphate cyclohydrolase 1 (*GCH1*), which causes dopa-responsive dystonia; hexanucleotide expansions in *C9orf72*, which cause frontotemporal dementia (FTD)/amyotrophic lateral sclerosis (ALS); and heterozygous mutations in the β-glucocerebrosidase (*GBA*) gene, which are responsible for a recessive disorder, Gaucher's disease, have been associated with typical parkinsonism.

LRRK2

Mutations in *LRRK2* are the most common cause of dominantly inherited PD and explain up to ~10 % of all familial forms of the disease with clearly dominant inheritance [1, 2]. The *LRRK2* gene, which spans a genomic region of 144 kb containing 51 exons, encodes a large 2,527-amino-acid protein with two enzymatic domains (GTPase and kinase) and multiple protein-protein interaction domains [3]. About 80 different *LRRK2* variants have been reported worldwide. Only 7 of these *LRRK2* mutations (N1437H, R1441G/C/H, Y1699C, G2019S, and I2020T), which appear to be clustered in functionally important regions that are highly conserved through evolution, have been proven to be pathogenic on the basis of co-segregation with the disease and their absence or rarity in specific control populations [4]. Some of them are strikingly population specific. The most common G2019S mutation in the kinase domain of the protein is particularly enriched in Arab patients from North Africa (30–40 %) [5] and in Ashkenazi Jewish PD patients (10–30 %) [6] and probably arose from a common ancestor in the Middle East [7]. The R1441G substitution in the ROC GTPase domain appears to be geographically restricted to Northern Spain, particularly the Basque population, in which it is responsible for ~20 % of familial PD [1, 8, 9]; however, the same mutation was recently reported on a different haplotype in a Japanese family [10]. I2020T was originally identified in a Japanese kindred [11]. The most recently identified mutation, N1437H, was originally described in two Norwegian families [12] and a Swedish PD patient [13]. Common polymorphisms in *LRRK2*, such as G2385R, R1628P [14], and, more recently, A419V [4], may be strong risk factors for sporadic PD in Asian populations. In contrast, the *LRRK2* M1646T mutation seems to be a common polymorphism that is specifically associated with PD in Caucasian populations [4]. In both Asian and Caucasian populations, genome-wide association studies (GWAS) identified risk factors in the 5′ region of the *LRRK2* gene in sporadic PD [15, 16].

Penetrance of the most common G2019S mutation, which is incomplete and age-dependent, ranges from ~25 to 70 % at age 80 years [17–19], explaining the frequency of its occurrence in sporadic PD patients [20], in families with apparently autosomal recessive inheritance [21], and in healthy mutation carriers over 80 years of age [22]. Homozygous G2019S mutation carriers were also identified among healthy elderly subjects [23].

The clinical features of patients with the G2019S mutation are surprisingly uniform and resemble those of patients with typical late-onset PD. The mean age at onset is close to 60 years, with unilateral tremor as the initial sign of disease, a good response to treatment, and slow progression [17]. Atypical features, such as amyotrophy, dystonia, supranuclear gaze palsy, primary progressive aphasia, or corticobasal syndrome, have also been reported [24–26]. Some homozygous mutation carriers, mostly among North African Arabs, are clinically similar to those with heterozygous mutations [23, 27], indicating an absence of gene dosage. In contrast to the clinical homogeneity of patients with *LRRK2* mutations, the associated pathology is remarkably variable, even within a given family. Most patients with the G2019S mutation have neuronal loss in the *substantia nigra* and α-synuclein-positive Lewy bodies as in typical PD; in some cases, nigral degeneration without Lewy bodies, diffuse Lewy body disease, and tau pathology have been observed [25, 28–31].

LRRK2 is a ubiquitous protein of unknown function. Many studies have focused on its GTPase and kinase activities and have shown that mutations in the kinase domain (G2019S, I2020T) increase kinase activity, whereas those in the ROC GTPase domain decrease GTPase activity [32]. Because of the increase in kinase activity associated with *LRRK2* mutations, LRRK2 kinase inhibitors have been developed as a potential treatment for PD [33]. LRRK2 plays a role in multiple cell functions, including intracellular trafficking, cytoskeletal dynamics, mitochondrial function, autophagy regulation, and, recently, a cellular pathway related to the immune system and regulation of neuroinflammation [34].

α-synuclein

SNCA mutations are the second most common cause of dominantly inherited PD; genomic duplications have been detected in ~1–2 % of the PD families with autosomal dominant inheritance [35, 36]. Other *SNCA* mutations are extremely rare and include whole-locus triplications [37] and point mutations; A53T was identified in a few families of Greek ancestry and also in families and apparently sporadic cases of European and Asian origin [38–43]. A30P and E46K were each identified in a single family of German and Spanish origin, respectively [44, 45]. Very recently, five new rare missense variants (A18T, A29S, H50Q, G51D, and A53E) were identified in PD patients. H50Q was found in one isolated case of English origin who had pathologically confirmed PD [46] and one Canadian case of English/Welsh origin who had a family history of parkinsonism and dementia [47]; the mutation arose from a common ancestor. G51D cosegregated with the disease in two independent families of French and English origin [48, 49] and in an isolated case of Japanese origin with family history of parkinsonism and dementia [50]. A53E was found in a Finnish family associated with atypical multiple system atrophy and PD [51]. A18T and A29S were detected in single patients of Polish origin presenting with a typical late-onset sporadic PD phenotype, but their pathogenicity has not been proven [52].

Postmortem examination of brains from patients with *SNCA* mutations revealed consistent neuronal loss and an abundance of α-synuclein-positive Lewy bodies and neurites in the *substantia nigra* and *locus ceruleus*, but limbic and glial abnormalities are also observed; pathologies associated with both PD and multiple system atrophy (MSA) may overlap [48, 49, 51, 53]. In contrast, the associated clinical spectrum is broad, ranging from typical late-onset PD, generally observed in patients with genomic duplications as well as those with H50Q mutations, to atypical PD, characterized by more severe features, including an earlier age at onset (<40 years), myoclonus, more rapid progression, and a high prevalence of dementia and autonomic dysfunction, observed in patients with rare genomic triplications and A53T/E, E46K, or G51D missense mutations. In view of the overlapping clinical features, it has been proposed that PD, parkinsonism with dementia, dementia with Lewy bodies, and MSA are causally related and are collectively referred to as "synucleinopathy" disorders.

Common variants in *SNCA* that may influence the expression of the disease [54, 55] have been found to be the most consistent and robust risk factors in large, population-based, multiethnic sporadic PD in all GWAS conducted so far, as well as in subsequent meta-analyses [56–60].

α-Synuclein is a 140-residue natively unfolded protein that is abundantly expressed in presynaptic nerve terminals [61]. It consists of three domains: an amino-terminal lipid-binding α-helix characterized by seven imperfect repeats (KTKEGV), a non-amyloidogenic core (NAC) domain, and an unstructured carboxy-terminus. Interestingly, most of *SNCA* mutations are clustered in the amphipathic alpha helical domain, suggesting a mutational hotspot. Although its physiological function is not fully known, it appears to be particularly prone to rapid conformational changes and has been implicated in the regulation of synaptic transmission and dopamine biosynthesis. The aggregation dynamics of mutant SNCA has been reported to be faster or slower than wild-type SNCA, suggesting that the process of aggregation is related to SNCA-induced neurotoxicity [62].

Recently Identified Genes Causing Autosomal Dominant PD

Recently, three new genes were reported to cause autosomal dominant PD. *VPS35* was the first PD-causing gene identified by exome sequencing. The same D620N mutation was originally reported, by two independent groups, to segregate in two large kindreds of Swiss and Austrian origin, respectively [63, 64]. Subsequent studies in multiple ethnic groups, including a large multicenter study [65, 66], indicated that the *VPS35* D620N mutation rarely causes autosomal dominant PD; the frequency ranges from 0.1 to 1 %, with an overall frequency lower than 0.1 % (24/22,612). It was absent from >16,000 healthy controls [67]. Like *LRRK2* mutations, the *VPS35* D620N mutation was found in rare sporadic cases [68] and unaffected individuals over 80 years of age [63], indicating reduced penetrance. Haplotype analyses suggest that this mutation arose independently by recurrent mutational events [63]. Mutational screening of the entire coding regions has not revealed any other variants with unequivocal pathogenicity [64, 66, 69]. Patients with *VPS35* mutations have typical levodopa-responsive PD but with a slightly earlier age at onset (on the average in the fifth decade of life) [67]. The *VPS35* gene encodes a subunit of the retromer complex involved in endosomal-lysosomal trafficking and recycling of synaptic vesicles and proteins. Mutations in *VPS35* may result in impaired cargo recognition and binding and thus defective receptor recycling.

Exome sequencing was recently used to identify a new N855S mutation in receptor-mediated endocytosis 8/RME-8 (*DNAJC13*); it segregated with the disease in a multi-generation Mennonite family of 118 family members in which 13 affected individuals were sampled [70]. This mutation was subsequently found in two small families and two isolated cases with a common ancestral haplotype but was not identified in >2,600 controls. The phenotype was consistent with a late-onset asymmetric PD, although rare cases had dementia and neuropathology consistent with brainstem or transitional Lewy body disease. However, due to incomplete penetrance and the presence of phenocopies in the large family and the lack of further studies on *DNAJC13* mutations, proof that *DNAJC13* causes PD is still lacking. DNAJC13 plays a role in endosomal trafficking by regulating the dynamics of clathrin coats on early endosomes. Preliminary functional analyses showed that the *DNAJC13* N855S mutation confers a toxic gain of function that impairs endosomal transport.

A traditional linkage study in a large French family in which an R1502H mutation in EIF4G1 segregated with the disease identified eukaryotic translation initiation factor 4 gamma 1 (*EIF4G1*) to be another new cause of dominantly inherited PD [71]. The same R1502H mutation and another missense variation, A502V, were found in a few small families of European and North African descent with mutation frequencies of 0.2 and 0.02 %, respectively, as were additional single variants, G686C, S1164R, and R1197W. However, most subsequent studies failed to replicate these findings, and some found the two most common *EIF4G1* mutations in healthy controls [72, 73]. The associated phenotype was late-onset PD with a good response to levodopa and neuropathology consistent with brainstem Lewy body disease [71]. The encoded protein, EIF4G1, is a central component of the eIF4F complex that regulates mRNA translation and might be involved in the stress response. Functional analyses demonstrated that the two most frequent *EIF4G1* variants, R1502H and A502V, impair formation of the multi-subunit complex, compatible with a dominant-negative mechanism of action [71].

SCA/Ataxins, GBA, GCH1, c9orf72: *Risk Factors or Dominant Causal Genes?*

Trinucleotide expansions in *SCAs/ataxins* cause autosomal dominant spinocerebellar ataxias with a broad phenotype that often includes parkinsonism; however, the parkinsonism may also be pure, particularly in *SCA2* or *SCA3* carriers. The frequency of *SCA2* mutations in familial parkinsonism ranges from 1.5 to ~10 %, and seems to be particularly high in patients of Asian origin [74–77]. In these patients, parkinsonism may range from typical levodopa-responsive PD to Parkinson-plus phenotypes. The configuration of the *SCA2* repeat expansion has recently been shown to play an important role in phenotypic variability. Whereas uninterrupted CAG repeat expansions are associated with ataxia, shorter expansions interrupted by CAA triplets are associated with parkinsonism [75, 78]. More rarely, repeat expansions in *SCA3* have also been associated with a phenotype resembling pure parkinsonism without prominent ataxia [79].

Candidate gene association studies identified heterozygous mutations in *GBA* as solid risk factors for PD although, in the homozygous or compound heterozygous state, the same gene causes Gaucher's disease (GD), a recessive lysosomal storage disorder. Historically, the occurrence of parkinsonism and Lewy body pathology in patients with GD and their relatives and the identification of *GBA* mutations in patients with PD indicated that there was a link between GD and PD [80]. *GBA* mutations cause an ethnic group-dependent increase in the risk of developing PD, accounting for ~7 % of Caucasian PD patients and up to 8 % in patients with family history of PD [81]; they are found in only ~1 % of control subjects. The frequency is much higher in Ashkenazi Jews, reaching ~20 % in PD patients versus 4 % in controls [82]. The clinical phenotype resembles that of typical late-onset PD with widespread and abundant α-synuclein pathology and prominent diffuse neocortical Lewy body pathology [83]. However, the greater the family history of PD, the earlier the disease begins and the more severe the non-motor symptoms, including more marked and rapid cognitive impairment [81, 82, 84] and a relatively high penetrance of PD among *GBA* mutation carriers [85]; this suggest that *GBA* could be a dominant causal gene with reduced penetrance rather than a risk factor. The mechanisms by which *GBA* mutations exert their pathogenic effects or act as risk factors for PD are not yet understood. Effects on lysosome function, ceramide metabolism, the ubiquitin-proteasome system, or lipid metabolism have been postulated in relation with α-synuclein clearance [86].

Mutations in the candidate gene, guanosine triphosphate cyclohydrolase 1 (*GCH1*), are the most common cause of levodopa-responsive dystonia (DYT5) [87], a rare movement disorder starting in childhood with sustained response to small doses of levodopa, but also cause adult-onset parkinsonism in the absence of dystonia [88]. A recent multicenter study identified rare *GCH1* variants as risk factors for PD (odds ratio (OR) 7.5, confidence intervals (CIs) 2.4–25.3) [89].

Parkinsonism has been described in some individuals with hexanucleotide repeat expansions in *C9orf72* that are now recognized as the most frequent cause of frontotemporal lobar degeneration (FTLD)/amyotrophic lateral sclerosis (ALS) [90, 91]. Parkinsonism related to this mutation may present as typical idiopathic PD without any signs of dementia [92].

Autosomal Recessive Forms of Mendelian PD

One of the most important findings of these last years was the relatively high proportion of patients with early-onset parkinsonism caused by recessively inherited mutations in numerous genes: *parkin*/PARK2, *PINK1*/PARK6, and *DJ-1*/PARK7. More recessive genes were recently identified in a few patients with early-onset atypical parkinsonism: *ATP13A2*/PARK9, *PLA2G6*/PARK14, *FBXO7*/PARK15, *DNAJC6*, and *SYNJ1*/PARK20.

Parkin

Homozygous exon deletions in the *parkin* gene at the PARK2 locus were first described, in 1998, in consanguineous Japanese families with a syndrome previously known as autosomal recessive juvenile parkinsonism, which is characterized by young onset (<20 years) in most cases, a good response to levodopa, and the frequent occurrence of levodopa-induced dyskinesias [93]. Subsequent screening of this large gene, which spans 1.3 Mb of genomic DNA, for both point mutations and exonic rearrangements showed that homozygous and compound heterozygous mutations in the *parkin* gene are the most common cause of early-onset PD (<45 years) in populations of all ethnic origins; it accounts for ~50 % of recessive familial forms with onset before age 25 years and ~15 % of isolated cases in European populations. Interestingly, the frequency of *parkin* mutations decreases as the age at onset increases; *parkin* mutations are therefore uncommon in patients with late-onset PD. More than 100 different mutations have been identified throughout the gene; they comprise large deletions or duplications and triplications of one or more exons in more than 50 % of the reported cases, but small deletions/insertions, nonsense, and missense mutations are also found. In addition, heterozygous *parkin* mutations have been reported in sporadic, late-onset PD and may constitute genetic risk factors.

Clinically, PD patients with *parkin* mutations have classical PD but, compared to patients without *parkin* mutations, earlier and more symmetrical onset, usually with dystonia, hyperreflexia, slower disease progression, sleep benefit, and a better response to low doses of levodopa, complicated by early motor fluctuations, the development of dyskinesias, and, in rare cases, atypical features, such as psychiatric manifestations [94]. In contrast to patients with typical forms of PD, PD patients with *parkin* mutations have a severe loss of dopaminergic neurons in the *substantia nigra* and *locus ceruleus* and gliosis but, in general, no Lewy bodies. Thus, nigral cell loss in PD patients with *parkin* mutations appears to be caused by a loss of function of the protein. The *parkin* gene encodes a cytosolic 465-amino-acid protein containing an ubiquitin-like (UBL) N-terminal domain, followed by three RING (really interesting new gene) finger motifs separated by an IBR (In-Between-Ring) domain in the C terminus. Parkin is an E3 ubiquitin ligase responsible for the transfer of activated ubiquitin molecules to a protein substrate [95], a signal for proteosomal degradation of the protein. Mutations in *parkin* were reported to impair the E3 ubiquitin ligase activity of Parkin, resulting in insufficient protein clearance and the subsequent formation of protein aggregates [95].

PTEN-Induced Kinase 1 (*PINK1*)

PINK1 was first mapped at the PARK6 locus, in 2004, in three consanguineous families with autosomal recessive early-onset PD [96]. Following these findings, more than 50 homozygous and compound heterozygous mutations have been found in the *PINK1* gene, ranging from frameshift, truncating, and splice site point mutations to deletion of the entire *PINK1* gene. *PINK1* is, therefore, the second most frequent known cause of autosomal recessive early-onset parkinsonism after *parkin* (1–8 % mutation frequency). *PINK1* mutations are also a rare cause of sporadic early-onset PD [97].

The clinical phenotype of *PINK1*-related disease appears broadly similar to that of *parkin*-related disease but usually with a later age at onset; there may also be a higher prevalence of psychiatric disturbances [98]. The neuropathological manifestations in a single patient with compound heterozygous mutations in *PINK1* resemble Lewy body and Lewy neurite pathology [99]. The *PINK1* gene encodes a 581-amino-acid protein, containing a 34-amino-acid mitochondrial targeting motif and a highly conserved protein kinase domain that has homologies with the calcium/calmodulin family of serine/threonine kinases [96]. Most of the described mutations lie near or within the functional serine/threonine kinase domain of PINK1. These mutations reduce or impair kinase activity, accelerate degradation, or induce misfolding of the protein.

DJ-1

The third locus for autosomal recessive early-onset parkinsonism, PARK7, was mapped in a Dutch family [100]; the PD-causing gene was identified, in 2003, as the oncogene DJ-1. A *DJ-1* missense mutation (L166P) and large exonic deletions were first identified in two European families with early-onset PD [101]. A number of other pathogenic mutations causing familial PD were later identified but are responsible for the disease in less than 1 % of early-onset PD patients. Clinically, onset of PD in patients with *DJ-1* mutations occurs in the third decade, with asymmetric symptoms, slow disease progression, and a sustained response to levodopa treatment. No neuropathological studies of *DJ-1* patients have as yet been reported. The *DJ-1* gene encodes a highly conserved 189-amino-acid protein of the ThiJ/Pfp1 family of molecular chaperones that are induced during oxidative stress.

Other Forms of Early-Onset Recessively Inherited Atypical Parkinsonism

Mutations in the neuronal lysosomal P-type ATPase (*ATP13A2*) in the PARK9 locus, calcium-independent phospholipase A2, group VI (*PLA2G6*) in PARK14, and F-box only protein 7 (*FBXO7*) in PARK15 cause recessively inherited forms of atypical parkinsonism characterized by juvenile to early-onset, poor response to levodopa and variable combinations of additional clinical signs: dystonia, cognitive impairment, neurobehavioural abnormalities, pyramidal disturbances, ophthalmoparesis, and autonomic dysfunction. Of note, mutations in *ATP13A2* are associated with Kufor-Rakeb syndrome (KRS), a form of recessively inherited, juvenile, multisystemic parkinsonism, characterized by rapid disease progression, pyramidal signs, dementia, and supranuclear gaze palsy [102]. Recessive mutations in *PLA2G6* are also associated with other childhood or young adult-onset syndromes, including infantile neuroaxonal dystrophy (INAD) [103], idiopathic neurodegeneration with brain iron accumulation (NBIA) [104], and adult-onset parkinsonism with dystonia and pyramidal involvement [105]. Mutations in *FBXO7* cause a complex combination of pyramidal and extrapyramidal syndromes, predominantly characterized by childhood-onset dystonia [106]. The *ATP13A2* gene encodes a large transmembrane protein with putative ATPase activity located in lysosomes, further linking abnormal function of these organelles to neurodegeneration. *PLA2G6* encoding a group VI calcium-independent A2 phospholipase, which catalyzes fatty acid release from phospholipids, may be implicated in inflammatory responses and apoptosis [107]. The *FBXO7* gene encodes a member of the F-box family of proteins, which play a role in the ubiquitin-proteasome protein degradation pathway. Very recently, recessive mutations in *DNAJC6* and *SYNJ1* were shown, by homozygosity mapping and exome sequencing, then subsequent replication in other studies, to cause autosomal recessive juvenile parkinsonism in rare families [108–112]. *DNAJC6* encodes auxilin, a clathrin-associated protein and *SYNJ1* encodes synaptojanin 1, both of which may be implicated in the recycling of synaptic vesicles.

Conclusion

The discovery of mutations [38] and, later, gene multiplications in *SWCA* [37], which cause dominant forms of PD, triggered 15 years of gene discoveries and new efforts to model parkinsonian neurodegeneration. Although, Mendelian forms of PD account for only a small proportion of PD cases, it is now clear that the genetic component of PD plays a much more important role in the pathogenesis of PD than previously thought. Notably, studies of PD-linked genes in some heritable forms of PD have brought to light several molecular abnormalities in the *substantia nigra* that are associated with neuronal death: protein aggregation, defects in the ubiquitin-proteasome pathway, impaired defenses against oxidative stress, abnormal protein phosphorylation, mitochondrial and lysosomal dysfunction, apoptosis, and now defective post-endocytic recycling of synaptic vesicles, thus improving our understanding of the more common sporadic form of the disease. An illustration is offered by *LRRK2* and *SNCA* that contain both rare, highly penetrant variants and common, weakly penetrant variants, suggesting that Mendelian forms of PD might also explain common non-Mendelian forms of PD, and vice versa.

Genetic studies are now moving forward with the discovery that most of the products of PD-causing genes function in shared or overlapping networks or pathways involved in the pathogenesis of the disease. An illustration is provided by the role of recessive gene products such as Parkin, PINK1, FBXO7, and DJ-1 centered on mitochondrial functions, such as mitogenesis, mitophagy, mitochondrial homeostasis, and transport. Studies in Drosophila models of *PINK1*-associated PD have suggested that PINK1 acts upstream of Parkin in a common biochemical pathway centered on maintenance of mitochondrial function and regulation of mitochondrial remodeling (fusion and fission) [113]. Notably, the kinase activity of PINK1 is necessary for recruitment of Parkin to the mitochondrial membrane [114], leading to the ubiquitination of several targets including mitofusins, which are mitochondrial fusion proteins [115]. In the same pathway, FBXO7, which acts downstream of PINK, participates in the recruitment of Parkin to depolarized mitochondria. DJ-1, which is a potent antioxidant, is known to translocate to the mitochondrial membrane where it is thought to play a role in neuroprotection [116]. Furthermore, it associates with Parkin during oxidative stress, suggesting that these proteins might work together in a neuroprotective mechanism.

Many more genetic factors, those responsible for monogenic disease as well as susceptibility loci, will most likely be uncovered in the near future with the development of new technologies, such as whole exome or whole genome sequencing, meta-analysis of genome-wide association studies associated with analyses of gene-gene or gene-environment interactions, and molecular pathways. As an example, a recent analysis of GWAS data associated with a pathway-based approach implicated the immune response in the development of PD [117].

Acknowledgments The author is grateful to Dr. Merle Ruberg for critical reading of the manuscript. This work was supported by the National Research Funding Agency (ANR-08-NEUR-004-01) in association with ERA-NET NEURON, the France-Parkinson Association, and the French program "Investissements d'avenir" (ANR-10-IAIHU-06).

References

1. Paisan-Ruiz C, Jain S, Evans EW, et al. Cloning of the gene containing mutations that cause PARK8-linked Parkinson's disease. Neuron. 2004;44:595–600.
2. Zimprich A, Biskup S, Leitner P, et al. Mutations in LRRK2 cause autosomal-dominant parkinsonism with pleomorphic pathology. Neuron. 2004;44:601–7.
3. Mata IF, Wedemeyer WJ, Farrer MJ, Taylor JP, Gallo KA. LRRK2 in Parkinson's disease: protein domains and functional insights. Trends Neurosci. 2006;29:286–93.
4. Ross OA, Soto-Ortolaza AI, Heckman MG, et al. Association of LRRK2 exonic variants with susceptibility to Parkinson's disease: a case-control study. Lancet Neurol. 2011;10: 898–908.
5. Lesage S, Durr A, Tazir M, et al. LRRK2 G2019S as a cause of Parkinson's disease in North African Arabs. N Engl J Med. 2006;26(354):422–3.
6. Ozelius LJ, Senthil G, Saunders-Pullman R, et al. LRRK2 G2019S as a cause of Parkinson's disease in Ashkenazi Jews. N Engl J Med. 2006;354:424–5.
7. Lesage S, Patin E, Condroyer C, et al. Parkinson's disease-related LRRK2 G2019S mutation results from independent mutational events in humans. Hum Mol Genet. 2010;15(19): 1998–2004.
8. Simon-Sanchez J, Marti-Masso JF, Sanchez-Mut JV, et al. Parkinson's disease due to the R1441G mutation in Dardarin: a founder effect in the Basques. Mov Disord. 2006;21: 1954–9.
9. Mata IF, Hutter CM, Gonzalez-Fernandez MC, et al. Lrrk2 R1441G-related Parkinson's disease: evidence of a common founding event in the seventh century in Northern Spain. Neurogenetics. 2009;10:347–53.

10. Hatano T, Funayama M, Kubo SI, et al. Identification of a Japanese family with LRRK2 p.R1441G-related Parkinson's disease. Neurobiol Aging. 2014;35(11):2656.e17–23.
11. Funayama M, Hasegawa K, Ohta E, Kawashima N, Komiyama M, Kowa H, Tsuji S, Obata F. An LRRK2 mutation as a cause for the parkinsonism in the original PARK8 family. Ann Neurol. 2005;57:918–21.
12. Aasly JO, Vilarino-Guell C, Dachsel JC, et al. Novel pathogenic LRRK2 p.Asn1437His substitution in familial Parkinson's disease. Mov Disord. 2010;25:2156–63.
13. Puschmann A, Englund E, Ross OA, et al. First neuropathological description of a patient with Parkinson's disease and LRRK2 p.N1437H mutation. Parkinsonism Relat Disord. 2012;18(4):332–8.
14. Tan EK. The role of common genetic risk variants in Parkinson disease. Clin Genet. 2007;72:387–93.
15. Simon-Sanchez J, Schulte C, Bras JM, et al. Genome-wide association study reveals genetic risk underlying Parkinson's disease. Nat Genet. 2009;41:1308–12.
16. Satake W, Nakabayashi Y, Mizuta I, et al. Genome-wide association study identifies common variants at four loci as genetic risk factors for Parkinson's disease. Nat Genet. 2009;41:1303–7.
17. Goldwurm S, Zini M, Mariani L, et al. Evaluation of LRRK2 G2019S penetrance: relevance for genetic counseling in Parkinson disease. Neurology. 2007;68:1141–3.
18. Healy DG, Falchi M, O'Sullivan SS, et al. Phenotype, genotype, and worldwide genetic penetrance of LRRK2-associated Parkinson's disease: a case-control study. Lancet Neurol. 2008;7:583–90.
19. Latourelle JC, Sun M, Lew MF, et al. The Gly2019Ser mutation in LRRK2 is not fully penetrant in familial Parkinson's disease: the GenePD study. BMC Med. 2008;6:32.
20. Lesage S, Janin S, Lohmann E, et al. LRRK2 exon 41 mutations in sporadic Parkinson disease in Europeans. Arch Neurol. 2007;64:425–30.
21. Lesage S, Leclere L, Lohmann E, et al. Frequency of the LRRK2 G2019S mutation in siblings with Parkinson's disease. Neurodegener Dis. 2007;4:195–8.
22. Kay DM, Kramer P, Higgins D, Zabetian CP, Payami H. Escaping Parkinson's disease: a neurologically healthy octogenarian with the LRRK2 G2019S mutation. Mov Disord. 2005;20:1077–8.
23. Ishihara L, Warren L, Gibson R, et al. Clinical features of Parkinson disease patients with homozygous leucine-rich repeat kinase 2 G2019S mutations. Arch Neurol. 2006;63:1250–4.
24. Wszolek ZK, Vieregge P, Uitti RJ, et al. German-Canadian family (family A) with parkinsonism, amyotrophy, and dementia – Longitudinal observations. Parkinsonism Relat Disord. 1997;3:125–39.
25. Ross OA, Toft M, Whittle AJ, et al. Lrrk2 and Lewy body disease. Ann Neurol. 2006;59:388–93.
26. Chen-Plotkin AS, Yuan W, Anderson C, et al. Corticobasal syndrome and primary progressive aphasia as manifestations of LRRK2 gene mutations. Neurology. 2008;70:521–7.
27. Lesage S, Belarbi S, Troiano A, et al. Is the common LRRK2 G2019S mutation related to dyskinesias in North African Parkinson disease? Neurology. 2008;71:1550–2.
28. Wszolek ZK, Pfeiffer RF, Tsuboi Y, et al. Autosomal dominant parkinsonism associated with variable synuclein and tau pathology. Neurology. 2004;62:1619–22.
29. Gilks WP, Abou-Sleiman PM, Gandhi S, et al. A common LRRK2 mutation in idiopathic Parkinson's disease. Lancet. 2005;365:415–6.
30. Giasson BI, Covy JP, Bonini NM, Hurtig HI, Farrer MJ, Trojanowski JQ, Van Deerlin VM. Biochemical and pathological characterization of Lrrk2. Ann Neurol. 2006;59:315–22.
31. Gaig C, Marti MJ, Ezquerra M, Rey MJ, Cardozo A, Tolosa E. G2019S LRRK2 mutation causing Parkinson's disease without Lewy bodies. J Neurol Neurosurg Psychiatry. 2007;78:626–8.
32. Cookson MR. The role of leucine-rich repeat kinase 2 (LRRK2) in Parkinson's disease. Nat Rev Neurosci. 2010;11:791–7.

33. Deng X, Choi HG, Buhrlage SJ, Gray NS. Leucine-rich repeat kinase 2 inhibitors: a patent review (2006–2011). Expert Opin Ther Pat. 2012;22:1415–26.
34. Russo I, Bubacco L, Greggio E. LRRK2 and neuroinflammation: partners in crime in Parkinson's disease? J Neuroinflammation. 2014;11:52.
35. Chartier-Harlin MC, Kachergus J, Roumier C, et al. Alpha-synuclein locus duplication as a cause of familial Parkinson's disease. Lancet. 2004;364:1167–9.
36. Ibanez P, Bonnet AM, Debarges B, et al. Causal relation between alpha-synuclein gene duplication and familial Parkinson's disease. Lancet. 2004;364:1169–71.
37. Singleton AB, Farrer M, Johnson J, et al. alpha-Synuclein locus triplication causes Parkinson's disease. Science. 2003;302:841.
38. Polymeropoulos MH, Lavedan C, Leroy E, et al. Mutation in the alpha-synuclein gene identified in families with Parkinson's disease. Science. 1997;276:2045–7.
39. Athanassiadou A, Voutsinas G, Psiouri L, et al. Genetic analysis of families with Parkinson disease that carry the Ala53Thr mutation in the gene encoding alpha-synuclein. Am J Hum Genet. 1999;65:555–8.
40. Michell AW, Barker RA, Raha SK, Raha-Chowdhury R. A case of late onset sporadic Parkinson's disease with an A53T mutation in alpha-synuclein. J Neurol Neurosurg Psychiatry. 2005;76:596–7.
41. Ki CS, Stavrou EF, Davanos N, Lee WY, Chung EJ, Kim JY, Athanassiadou A. The Ala53Thr mutation in the alpha-synuclein gene in a Korean family with Parkinson disease. Clin Genet. 2007;71:471–3.
42. Choi JM, Woo MS, Ma HI, Kang SY, Sung YH, Yong SW, Chung SJ, Kim JS, Shin HW, Lyoo CH, Lee PH, Baik JS, Kim SJ, Park MY, Sohn YH, Kim JH, Kim JW, Lee MS, Lee MC, Kim DH, Kim YJ. Analysis of PARK genes in a Korean cohort of early-onset Parkinson disease. Neurogenetics. 2008;9:263–9.
43. Puschmann A, Ross OA, Vilarino-Guell C, et al. A Swedish family with de novo alpha-synuclein A53T mutation: evidence for early cortical dysfunction. Parkinsonism Relat Disord. 2009;15:627–32.
44. Kruger R, Kuhn W, Muller T, et al. Ala30Pro mutation in the gene encoding alpha-synuclein in Parkinson's disease. Nat Genet. 1998;18:106–8.
45. Zarranz JJ, Alegre J, Gomez-Esteban JC, et al. The new mutation, E46K, of alpha-synuclein causes Parkinson and Lewy body dementia. Ann Neurol. 2004;55:164–73.
46. Proukakis C, Dudzik CG, Brier T, et al. A novel alpha-synuclein missense mutation in Parkinson disease. Neurology. 2013;80:1062–4.
47. Appel-Cresswell S, Vilarino-Guell C, Encarnacion M, et al. Alpha-synuclein p.H50Q, a novel pathogenic mutation for Parkinson's disease. Mov Disord. 2013;28:811–3.
48. Kiely AP, Asi YT, Kara E, et al. alpha-Synucleinopathy associated with G51D SNCA mutation: a link between Parkinson's disease and multiple system atrophy? Acta Neuropathol. 2013;125:753–69.
49. Lesage S, Anheim M, Letournel F, et al. G51D alpha-synuclein mutation causes a novel parkinsonian-pyramidal syndrome. Ann Neurol. 2013;73:459–71.
50. Tokutake T, Ishikawa A, Yoshimura N, et al. Clinical and neuroimaging features of patient with early-onset Parkinson's disease with dementia carrying SNCA p.G51D mutation. Parkinsonism Relat Disord. 2014;20:262–4.
51. Pasanen P, Myllykangas L, Siitonen M, et al. A novel alpha-synuclein mutation A53E associated with atypical multiple system atrophy and Parkinson's disease-type pathology. Neurobiol Aging. 2014;35:2180.e1–5.
52. Hoffman-Zacharska D, Koziorowski D, Ross OA, et al. Novel A18T and pA29S substitutions in alpha-synuclein may be associated with sporadic Parkinson's disease. Parkinsonism Relat Disord. 2013;19:1057–60.
53. Markopoulou K, Dickson DW, McComb RD, et al. Clinical, neuropathological and genotypic variability in SNCA A53T familial Parkinson's disease. Variability in familial Parkinson's disease. Acta Neuropathol. 2008;116:25–35.
54. Maraganore DM, de Andrade M, Elbaz A, et al. Collaborative analysis of alpha-synuclein gene promoter variability and Parkinson disease. JAMA. 2006;296:661–70.

55. Fuchs J, Tichopad A, Golub Y, et al. Genetic variability in the SNCA gene influences alpha-synuclein levels in the blood and brain. FASEB J. 2008;22:1327–34.
56. Edwards TL, Scott WK, Almonte C, et al. Genome-wide association study confirms SNPs in SNCA and the MAPT region as common risk factors for Parkinson disease. Ann Hum Genet. 2010;74:97–109.
57. Hamza TH, Zabetian CP, Tenesa A, et al. Common genetic variation in the HLA region is associated with late-onset sporadic Parkinson's disease. Nat Genet. 2010;42:781–5.
58. Saad M, Lesage S, Saint-Pierre A, et al. Genome-wide association study confirms BST1 and suggests a locus on 12q24 as the risk loci for Parkinson's disease in the European population. Hum Mol Genet. 2011;20:615–27.
59. Spencer CC, Plagnol V, Strange A, et al. Dissection of the genetics of Parkinson's disease identifies an additional association 5' of SNCA and multiple associated haplotypes at 17q21. Hum Mol Genet. 2011;20:345–53.
60. Nalls MA, Plagnol V, Hernandez DG, et al. Imputation of sequence variants for identification of genetic risks for Parkinson's disease: a meta-analysis of genome-wide association studies. Lancet. 2011;377:641–9.
61. Cookson MR. The biochemistry of Parkinson's disease. Annu Rev Biochem. 2005;74: 29–52.
62. Conway KA, Lee SJ, Rochet JC, Ding TT, Williamson RE, Lansbury Jr PT. Acceleration of oligomerization, not fibrillization, is a shared property of both alpha-synuclein mutations linked to early-onset Parkinson's disease: implications for pathogenesis and therapy. Proc Natl Acad Sci U S A. 2000;97:571–6.
63. Vilarino-Guell C, Wider C, Ross OA, et al. VPS35 mutations in Parkinson disease. Am J Hum Genet. 2011;89:162–7.
64. Zimprich A, Benet-Pages A, Struhal W, et al. A mutation in VPS35, encoding a subunit of the retromer complex, causes late-onset Parkinson disease. Am J Hum Genet. 2011;89:168–75.
65. Lesage S, Condroyer C, Klebe S, et al. Identification of VPS35 mutations replicated in French families with Parkinson disease. Neurology. 2012;78:1449–50.
66. Sharma M, Ioannidis JP, Aasly JO, et al. A multi-centre clinico-genetic analysis of the VPS35 gene in Parkinson disease indicates reduced penetrance for disease-associated variants. J Med Genet. 2012;49:721–6.
67. Deng H, Gao K, Jankovic J. The VPS35 gene and Parkinson's disease. Mov Disord. 2013;28: 569–75.
68. Ando M, Funayama M, Li Y, et al. VPS35 mutation in Japanese patients with typical Parkinson's disease. Mov Disord. 2012;27:1413–7.
69. Verstraeten A, Wauters E, Crosiers D, et al. Contribution of VPS35 genetic variability to LBD in the Flanders-Belgian population. Neurobiol Aging. 1844;2012(33):e11–3.
70. Vilarino-Guell C, Rajput A, Milnerwood AJ, Shah B, Szu-Tu C, Trinh J, et al. DNAJC13 mutations in Parkinson disease. Hum Mol Genet. 2014;23:1794–801.
71. Chartier-Harlin MC, Dachsel JC, Vilarino-Guell C, et al. Translation initiator EIF4G1 mutations in familial Parkinson disease. Am J Hum Genet. 2011;89:398–406.
72. Schulte EC, Mollenhauer B, Zimprich A, et al. Variants in eukaryotic translation initiation factor 4G1 in sporadic Parkinson's disease. Neurogenetics. 2012;13:281–5.
73. Tucci A, Charlesworth G, Sheerin UM, Plagnol V, Wood NW, Hardy J. Study of the genetic variability in a Parkinson's Disease gene: EIF4G1. Neurosci Lett. 2012;518:19–22.
74. Gwinn-Hardy K, Chen JY, Liu HC, et al. Spinocerebellar ataxia type 2 with parkinsonism in ethnic Chinese. Neurology. 2000;55:800–5.
75. Charles P, Camuzat A, Benammar N, et al. Are interrupted SCA2 CAG repeat expansions responsible for parkinsonism? Neurology. 2007;69:1970–5.
76. Modoni A, Contarino MF, Bentivoglio AR, et al. Prevalence of spinocerebellar ataxia type 2 mutation among Italian Parkinsonian patients. Mov Disord. 2007;22:324–7.
77. Wang JL, Xiao B, Cui XX, et al. Analysis of SCA2 and SCA3/MJD repeats in Parkinson's disease in mainland China: genetic, clinical, and positron emission tomography findings. Mov Disord. 2009;24:2007–11.

78. Kim JM, Hong S, Kim GP, et al. Importance of low-range CAG expansion and CAA interruption in SCA2 Parkinsonism. Arch Neurol. 2007;64:1510–8.
79. Socal MP, Emmel VE, Rieder CR, Hilbig A, Saraiva-Pereira ML, Jardim LB. Intrafamilial variability of Parkinson phenotype in SCAs: novel cases due to SCA2 and SCA3 expansions. Parkinsonism Relat Disord. 2009;15:374–8.
80. Lwin A, Orvisky E, Goker-Alpan O, LaMarca ME, Sidransky E. Glucocerebrosidase mutations in subjects with parkinsonism. Mol Genet Metab. 2004;81:70–3.
81. Lesage S, Anheim M, Condroyer C, et al. Large-scale screening of the Gaucher's disease-related glucocerebrosidase gene in Europeans with Parkinson's disease. Hum Mol Genet. 2011;20:202–10.
82. Sidransky E, Nalls MA, Aasly JO, et al. Multicenter analysis of glucocerebrosidase mutations in Parkinson's disease. N Engl J Med. 2009;361:1651–61.
83. Neumann J, Bras J, Deas E, et al. Glucocerebrosidase mutations in clinical and pathologically proven Parkinson's disease. Brain. 2009;132:1783–94.
84. Winder-Rhodes SE, Evans JR, Ban M, et al. Glucocerebrosidase mutations influence the natural history of Parkinson's disease in a community-based incident cohort. Brain. 2013;136:392–9.
85. Anheim M, Elbaz A, Lesage S, et al. Penetrance of Parkinson disease in glucocerebrosidase gene mutation carriers. Neurology. 2012;78:417–20.
86. DePaolo J, Goker-Alpan O, Samaddar T, Lopez G, Sidransky E. The association between mutations in the lysosomal protein glucocerebrosidase and parkinsonism. Mov Disord. 2009;24:1571–8.
87. Clot F, Grabli D, Cazeneuve C, et al. Exhaustive analysis of BH4 and dopamine biosynthesis genes in patients with Dopa-responsive dystonia. Brain. 2009;132:1753–63.
88. Nygaard TG, Trugman JM, de Yebenes JG, Fahn S. Dopa-responsive dystonia: the spectrum of clinical manifestations in a large North American family. Neurology. 1990;40:66–9.
89. Mencacci NE, Isaias IU, Reich MM, et al. Parkinson's disease in GTP cyclohydrolase 1 mutation carriers. Brain. 2014;137(9):2480–92.
90. DeJesus-Hernandez M, Mackenzie IR, Boeve BF, et al. Expanded GGGGCC hexanucleotide repeat in noncoding region of C9ORF72 causes chromosome 9p-linked FTD and ALS. Neuron. 2011;72:245–56.
91. Renton AE, Majounie E, Waite A, et al. A hexanucleotide repeat expansion in C9ORF72 is the cause of chromosome 9p21-linked ALS-FTD. Neuron. 2011;72:257–68.
92. Lesage S, Le Ber I, Condroyer C, et al. C9orf72 repeat expansions are a rare genetic cause of parkinsonism. Brain. 2013;136:385–91.
93. Kitada T, Asakawa S, Hattori N, et al. Mutations in the parkin gene cause autosomal recessive juvenile parkinsonism. Nature. 1998;392:605–8.
94. Lohmann E, Periquet M, Bonifati V, et al. How much phenotypic variation can be attributed to parkin genotype? Ann Neurol. 2003;54:176–85.
95. Shimura H, Hattori N, Kubo S, et al. Familial Parkinson disease gene product, parkin, is a ubiquitin-protein ligase. Nat Genet. 2000;25:302–5.
96. Valente EM, Abou-Sleiman PM, Caputo V, et al. Hereditary early-onset Parkinson's disease caused by mutations in PINK1. Science. 2004;304:1158–60.
97. Valente EM, Salvi S, Ialongo T, et al. PINK1 mutations are associated with sporadic early-onset parkinsonism. Ann Neurol. 2004;56:336–41.
98. Kilarski LL, Pearson JP, Newsway V, et al. Systematic review and UK-based study of PARK2 (parkin), PINK1, PARK7 (DJ-1) and LRRK2 in early-onset Parkinson's disease. Mov Disord. 2012;27:1522–9.
99. Samaranch L, Lorenzo-Betancor O, Arbelo JM, et al. PINK1-linked parkinsonism is associated with Lewy body pathology. Brain. 2010;133:1128–42.
100. van Duijn CM, Dekker MC, Bonifati V, et al. Park7, a novel locus for autosomal recessive early-onset parkinsonism, on chromosome 1p36. Am J Hum Genet. 2001;69:629–34.
101. Bonifati V, Rizzu P, van Baren MJ, et al. Mutations in the DJ-1 gene associated with autosomal recessive early-onset parkinsonism. Science. 2003;299:256–9.

102. Ramirez A, Heimbach A, Grundemann J, et al. Hereditary parkinsonism with dementia is caused by mutations in ATP13A2, encoding a lysosomal type 5 P-type ATPase. Nat Genet. 2006;38:1184–91.
103. Khateeb S, Flusser H, Ofir R, et al. PLA2G6 mutation underlies infantile neuroaxonal dystrophy. Am J Hum Genet. 2006;79:942–8.
104. Morgan NV, Westaway SK, Morton JE, et al. PLA2G6, encoding a phospholipase A2, is mutated in neurodegenerative disorders with high brain iron. Nat Genet. 2006;38:752–4.
105. Paisan-Ruiz C, Bhatia KP, Li A, et al. Characterization of PLA2G6 as a locus for dystonia-parkinsonism. Ann Neurol. 2009;65:19–23.
106. Shojaee S, Sina F, Banihosseini SS, et al. Genome-wide linkage analysis of a Parkinsonian-pyramidal syndrome pedigree by 500 K SNP arrays. Am J Hum Genet. 2008;82:1375–84.
107. Sun GY, Shelat PB, Jensen MB, He Y, Sun AY, Simonyi A. Phospholipases A2 and inflammatory responses in the central nervous system. Neuromolecular Med. 2010;12:133–48.
108. Edvardson S, Cinnamon Y, Ta-Shma A, et al. A deleterious mutation in DNAJC6 encoding the neuronal-specific clathrin-uncoating co-chaperone auxilin, is associated with juvenile parkinsonism. PLoS One. 2012;7:e36458.
109. Koroglu C, Baysal L, Cetinkaya M, Karasoy H, Tolun A. DNAJC6 is responsible for juvenile parkinsonism with phenotypic variability. Parkinsonism Relat Disord. 2013;19:320–4.
110. Quadri M, Fang M, Picillo M, et al. Mutation in the SYNJ1 gene associated with autosomal recessive, early-onset Parkinsonism. Hum Mutat. 2013;34:1208–15.
111. Krebs CE, Karkheiran S, Powell JC, et al. The Sac1 domain of SYNJ1 identified mutated in a family with early-onset progressive Parkinsonism with generalized seizures. Hum Mutat. 2013;34:1200–7.
112. Olgiati S, De Rosa A, Quadri M, et al. PARK20 caused by SYNJ1 homozygous Arg258Gln mutation in a new Italian family. Neurogenetics. 2014;15:183–8.
113. Yang Y, Gehrke S, Imai Y, et al. Mitochondrial pathology and muscle and dopaminergic neuron degeneration caused by inactivation of Drosophila Pink1 is rescued by Parkin. Proc Natl Acad Sci U S A. 2006;103:10793–8.
114. Vives-Bauza C, Zhou C, Huang Y, et al. PINK1-dependent recruitment of Parkin to mitochondria in mitophagy. Proc Natl Acad Sci U S A. 2010;107:378–83.
115. Ziviani E, Tao RN, Whitworth AJ. Drosophila parkin requires PINK1 for mitochondrial translocation and ubiquitinates mitofusin. Proc Natl Acad Sci U S A. 2010;107:5018–23.
116. Canet-Aviles RM, Wilson MA, Miller DW, et al. The Parkinson's disease protein DJ-1 is neuroprotective due to cysteine-sulfinic acid-driven mitochondrial localization. Proc Natl Acad Sci U S A. 2004;101:9103–8.
117. Holmans P, Moskvina V, Jones L, et al. A pathway-based analysis provides additional support for an immune-related genetic susceptibility to Parkinson's disease. Hum Mol Genet. 2013;22:1039–49.
118. Nalls MA, Pankratz N, Lill CM, et al. Large-scale meta-analysis of genome-wide association data identifies six new risk loci for Parkinson's disease. Nat Genet. 2014;46(9):989–93.

Chapter 2
Genetics of Parkinson's Disease

Dena G. Hernandez and Andrew B. Singleton

Abstract Tremendous progress has been made over the last 10 years in the identification of genetic risk factors for Parkinson's disease (PD). This work began with candidate gene-based assessments, where variability in the genes encoding alpha-synuclein, glucocerebrosidase, and leucine-rich repeat kinase 2 was assessed and shown to be linked to risk for disease. This work has been considerably extended upon using genome-wide association studies, which have thus far identified a large number of risk loci. Here we discuss these advances, the current picture of genetic risk factors in PD, and the path forward.

Keywords Genetic risk loci • Candidate gene association • Genome-wide association • Risk profiling • Complex genetics

Introduction

Our understanding of the entity that is Parkinson's disease (PD) has evolved a tremendous amount over the last 20 years. Genetics has been particularly influential in guiding this evolution, and in this regard, the identification of rare mutations that cause disease has been the primary driving force. The discovery of mutations in the gene that encodes alpha-synuclein marked the first of these discoveries and perhaps still the most influential, but the identification of mutations in genes such as *PARK2*, *PINK1*, *PARK7*, and perhaps most notably *LRRK2* also changed the fields perspective on PD [4, 27, 40, 44, 53, 65, 71]. Most immediately these discoveries showed that there were genetic causes of rare familial forms of disease and that these findings lead to insight that was more generalizable to the general PD population – the

D.G. Hernandez, PhD
Laboratory of Neurogenetics, Genomic Technologies Group, National Institute on Aging, National Institutes of Health, Bethesda, MD 20892, USA

A.B. Singleton, PhD (✉)
Laboratory of Neurogenetics, National Institute on Aging, National Institutes of Health, Bethesda, MD 20892, USA
e-mail: singleta@mail.nih.gov

S.A. Schneider, J.M.T. Brás (eds.), *Movement Disorder Genetics*,
DOI 10.1007/978-3-319-17223-1_2

discovery of alpha-synuclein as a major protein component of Lewy bodies was driven by the discovery of mutations in this gene [56], and the discovery of *LRRK2* mutations revealed the genetic cause of disease in a very large number of apparently sporadic typical PD patients [7, 16, 39].

A primary aim of this type of genetic work was, and remains, the use of these findings to understand the disease process and to identify viable points of therapeutic intervention based on etiology not symptomatology. The beginnings of this longer term aim are just now beginning to manifest, with a greater understanding of the molecular processes that represent disease using genetic models. Our progress thus far in understanding the disease process has been highly reliant on these genetic discoveries made in rare families, and we have developed methods and tools specifically to investigate the mechanisms linked to these mutations.

We believe that the research driven by our identification of the causes of monogenic forms of disease will continue to be exceedingly valuable in the effort to understand and treat PD; however, we also believe that the identification of genetic risk factors will both stimulate new areas of research and take previous etiologic investigations in a new exciting direction. Over this chapter, we will discuss the progress that has been made in identifying risk loci in PD and describe our current understanding of the genetic architecture of this disease. We will also discuss the next steps in identifying additional risk genes for this disease and how best to move forward.

Early Attempts at Finding Risk Loci

In the broad research community, a great deal of time was spent searching for genetic risk factors for apparently sporadic diseases from the mid-1990s on. A very high percentage of this work was unfruitful, and there are two primary reasons for this lack of success. First, our ability to identify the correct gene to test, and the correct variants within that gene, based purely on a perceived understanding of the disease process, was rather poor. For many of the early studies, only one or two variants were assessed, and given that there are millions of known single-nucleotide variants and that most do not measurably affect disease, the odds of choosing the correct variant were vanishingly small. Second, the vast majority of studies were performed in rather small sample sizes and thus were only powered to detect major risk effects; we know that such risk alleles, particularly in the context of common variation, are the exception not the rule. The result of these two limitations, and the relative ease with which these studies could be executed and published, was a large body of literature that reported positive genetic association findings that failed to stand the test of time. During this period, however, there were some rare but notable successes, coming from the assessment of genes already known to be linked to PD (through disease causing mutations) or as a result of keen clinical observation.

Shortly after the identification of rare alpha-synuclein mutations as the first known genetic cause of PD, Kruger and colleagues examined common variability at this gene to determine whether this may be linked to risk for typical idiopathic PD [28, 44]. This initial report suggested an interaction between *APOE* genotype and the genotype of a variable dinucleotide repeat, called REP1, ~10 kb 5′ to the transcription start site of *SNCA* in modulating risk for PD. While the interaction between *APOE* and *SNCA* genotypes seems to have been spurious, the association of genetic variability at the *SNCA* locus with risk for PD is now unequivocal. The first truly compelling evidence of this arose from a meta-analysis of existing REP1 genotype data, which showed a consistent association across diseases, with an odds ratio of ~1.4 ($p < 0.001$) [34]. Association at this locus was eventually shown to be overwhelmingly positive in genome-wide association studies, and these have revealed more about the architecture of genetic risk at this locus (this will be discussed later).

Following the identification of *LRRK2* mutations as a cause of PD [40, 71], this gene was sequenced extensively across many populations. In one of these studies, the p.G2385R variant was identified as a possible cause of PD in a parent child pair of patients from Taiwan [36]. Subsequent analyses of this variant showed that this was too common in the general population to be causative of disease; however, they supported a role for this variant in increasing risk for PD within Asian populations [8]. Di Fonzo and colleagues efforts suggested that carrying this variant, normally present in about 5 % of the general population, doubled an individual's risk of PD. This finding has been extensively replicated in varied Asian populations including those from Singapore, Taiwan, Hong Kong (Chinese), Korea, Japan, and mainland China (Han) and is considered a robust association [5, 6, 11–13, 26, 30, 57–59, 66, 70]. Also in Asian populations, the variant p.R1628P in *LRRK2* has been associated with increased risk for PD. This variant, originally described in 2008, appears to also increase risk for PD ~2 fold, being present in ~6 % of PD cases and ~3 % of controls [47]. This finding has also been replicated, although not as widely as p.G2385R, in various Asian populations including Thai, Taiwanese, and Chinese [12, 45, 67, 68]. Notably, meta-analysis of all existing studies as of 2012 revealed a consistent risk effect of ~2.5 in typical PD [67]. In addition, several other exonic variants have been assessed for association with risk for disease, including p.A419V, p.P755L, p.M1646T, and a three-SNP haplotype (p.N551K-p.R1398H-p.K1423K) [46, 67]. These each have varying levels of support, and to date none have been unequivocally linked to risk of PD.

While common variability at *SNCA* and at *LRRK2* was initially implicated in risk for PD because of the known link between rare mutations in these genes and familial forms of PD, another gene was associated with risk for PD because of astute clinical observation. Mutations in the gene encoding glucocerebrosidase (*GBA*) have long been linked to the autosomal recessive lysosomal storage disorder Gaucher's disease [63]. Phenotypic characterization of Gaucher's patients revealed that some would manifest with parkinsonism [60], and it appeared that this feature was more common than one would expect by chance. This led to the early hypothesis that glucocerebrosidase deficiency may lead to a vulnerability to parkinsonism [61]. In the following year, Aharon-Peretz and colleagues provided compelling evidence that extended this idea and showed that carrying a single *GBA* mutation increased the risk for PD [2]. This work was initially viewed with some skepticism, as the effect size was surprisingly high, and the clinical and pathologic link between PD and Gaucher's disease was not immediately obvious. This association however has been borne out. Again, the application of meta-analysis of existing data has provided the most compelling results thus far, with an analysis of *GBA* mutations in ~6,000 PD patients and ~5,000 controls [51]. This work showed that in Ashkenazi Jewish populations, the frequency of the common p.L444P and p.N370S mutations was 15 % in PD patients and 3 % in controls, and in non-Ashkenazi Jewish populations, the frequency of these variants was 3 % in cases and <1 % in controls. Collectively, these data suggest that carrying a single *GBA* mutation, while insufficient to cause Gaucher's disease, increases the risk for PD ~5 fold. It is notable that the same risk variants have also been linked to risk for dementia with Lewy bodies and PD with dementia [37].

Genome-Wide Association

If the criticism of candidate-based association analyses was that they were not broad enough, then a viable solution to finding risk should, at least in part, be the application of genome-wide association (GWA) studies. GWA studies leverage a massively parallel genotyping technology that allows the accurate and efficient typing of hundreds of thousands to millions of variants in a large series of subjects. The understanding of population genetic structure, garnered from such studies as the International Haplotype Map Project, and 1,000 genomes, allows this data to be taken even further, as it facilitates the prediction of genotypes in an individual at untyped variants based on the genotype at neighboring SNPs [1, 62]. This method, broadly called imputation, allows investigators to predict an individual's genotype at tens of millions of positions using actual genotypes at only a few hundred thousand variants. While this method has been responsible for a fundamental shift in our understanding of many diseases and traits, including PD, there are some inherent limitations to GWA that bear consideration. First and foremost, this method aims to identify common variability associated with disease; typically, variants with an allele frequency less than ~2 % are prone to imputation and genotype errors, and are excluded. Thus a traditional GWA design will not detect rare mutations or risk variants. Second, the coverage of GWA studies is not complete; there are variants/regions that are difficult to type and/or impute, and thus not all common variants can be assessed effectively. While difficult to type variants may include SNPs, this also extends to copy number variants and repeats. Despite these limitations, GWA continues to be a valuable tool and has certainly been successfully employed in PD genetics.

One of the first, albeit small, genome-wide association studies performed for any disease or trait was done in PD, but in the context of identifying replicable risk, this was unsuccessful [35]. A second study, performed less than a year later, and still of small size, also failed to identify risk variants at the genome-wide level of significance [14]; however, the deposition of these data into the public domain formed the basis of many GWA studies to come in PD.

Since this time, there have been a number of well-powered GWA in PD, and these have iteratively improved our resolution of the genetic architecture of this complex disease. In 2009 Pankratz and colleagues published a GWA study that showed suggestive evidence for association between alleles at 3 loci, *GAK*, *SNCA*, and *MAPT*, and risk for disease in a series of 850 familial PD cases and a similar number of controls [42]. Shortly after this, two collaborative studies published back-to-back reported several genome-wide significant association results [49, 52]. Satake and colleagues identified significant associations at *SNCA* and *LRRK2*, at the time both linked to risk for PD, and at two novel loci, *BST1* and *PARK16*, in a Japanese population [49]. The work by Simon-Sanchez, which examined Caucasian patients and controls, also showed significant association at *SNCA* and *PARK16*, supportive evidence for the association of common variants at *LRRK2*, and identified a strong association between risk for disease and variants at the *MAPT* locus [52]. Notably, while there was much in common between these studies, there was, and appears to remain, a complete lack of association between PD and *MAPT* variants in Asian populations, illustrating genetic heterogeneity of common risk between disparate populations.

In the following year, Hamza and colleagues used GWA in a series of 2,000 PD patients and a similar number of controls. This effort replicated the previous associations in *GAK*, *SNCA*, and *MAPT* but perhaps surprisingly also implicated variability at the *HLA* locus in risk for PD, genetically implicating the immune system in the pathogenesis of PD [18].

Over the next 4 years, several GWA studies were performed, many of which replicated previous loci and implicated additional risk loci [9, 10, 20, 22, 23, 31, 32, 41, 43, 48, 50, 64], Much of this work incorporated a meta-analysis of existing public data, and it has certainly been of great benefit to the field that PD investigators have deposited their data in public repositories such as the database of Genotypes and Phenotypes (www.ncbi.nlm.nih.gov/gap).

Most recently much of these GWA data have been combined in a large international meta-analysis [38]. This work combined genome-wide SNP data on more than 13,000 PD cases and 80,000 controls. Approximately eight million variants were tested for association across these series, and those SNPs that reached genome-wide significant association were tested for association in an independent series of ~7,000 cases and ~7,000 controls. The net result of this work was the identification of 28 independent risk loci for PD (Table 2.1). The nature of GWA is that these identify loci, not genes, and therefore, while each locus is usually given a gene name as an identifier, these are often just the most proximal gene or nominated based on known function or expression profile. In some instances, one can be relatively sure of the gene that is being affected by the risk variants, for example, the loci proximal to *SNCA* and *LRRK2* are most likely mediating their effect through these genes; for others, there is far less certainty. Likewise, it is worth noting that the identity of the actual variant that mediates the biological risk is usually not immediately apparent. GWA signals are haplotype-tagging signals and therefore delimit a region of association within which the biologically relevant risk allele resides. This raises the question of how to identify the effector variant and the gene it modulates

Table 2.1 Loci identified by a large international collaborative study

SNP ID	Locus name	Chromosome (bp)	Odds ratio
rs35749011	GBA/SYT11	1 (155,135,036)	1.824
rs114138760[a]	GBA/SYT12	1 (154,898,185)	1.519
rs823118	RAB7L1/NUCKS1	1 (205,723,572)	1.122
rs10797576	SIPA1L2	1 (232,664,611)	1.131
rs6430538	ACMSD/TMEM163	2 (135,539,967)	0.875
rs1474055	STK39	2 (169,110,394)	1.214
rs12637471	MCCC1	3 (182,762,437)	0.842
rs34311866	TMEM175/GAK/DGKQ	4 (951,947)	0.786
rs34884217[a]	TMEM175/GAK/DGKQ	4 (944,210)	1.232
rs11724635	BST1	4 (15,737,101)	1.126
rs6812193	FAM47E/SCARB2	4 (77,198,986)	0.907
rs356182	SNCA	4 (90,626,111)	0.760
rs7681154[a]	SNCA	4 (90,763,703)	0.854
rs9275326	HLA-DQB1	6 (32,666,660)	0.826
rs13201101[a]	HLA-DQB1	6 (32,343,604)	1.185
rs199347	GPNMB	7 (23,293,746)	1.110
rs591323	FGF20	8 (16,697,091)	0.916
rs117896735	INPP5F	10 (121,536,327)	1.624
rs329648	MIR4697	11 (133,765,367)	1.105
rs76904798	LRRK2	12 (40,614,434)	1.155
rs11060180	CCDC62	12 (123,303,586)	1.105
rs11158026	GCH1	14 (55,348,869)	0.904
rs2414739	VPS13C	15 (61,994,134)	1.113
rs14235	BCKDK/ STX1B	16 (31,121,793)	1.103
rs11868035	SREBF/RAI1	17 (17,715,101)	0.939
rs17649553	MAPT	17 (43,994,648)	0.769
rs12456492	RIT2	18 (40,673,380)	0.904
rs8118008[a]	DDRGK1	20 (3,168,166)	1.111

[a]Denotes a second risk allele at a described locus

at these loci and how to use these results to understand disease; we will discuss this later.

As with most GWA, the effect sizes identified in this recent GWA are in the range of an odds ratio of ~1.3 per allele (the odds ratio at a locus may change considerably once the effect allele is determined). A common question that is levied is "what is the use of identifying low-risk alleles." There are two aspects of this criticism, and these are both worth consideration: what is the value of these alleles in the context of understanding risk for disease, and what can these loci tell us about the etiology of disease? As noted above, the individual risk conferred by these alleles is relatively modest; however, on a population level, because the alleles are so common, they contribute far more to the risk of PD than, for example, synuclein, parkin, pink1, and dj1 mutations combined. Also, the risk attributed to these alleles is cumulative; thus, they can be combined, and for any individual, it is possible to generate a risk score based on their possession of multiple risk alleles. When this type of risk profile is performed, we can then rank individuals in a population based on the amount of total known genetic risk they possess. If we then look at those individuals with the highest 20 % of genetic risk, and compare them to the group with the lowest 20 % of risk, the former group are about 4 times as likely to get PD. This, by any measure, is a substantive amount of risk. The second aspect of this criticism, that low risk signifies low etiologic importance, is a logical fallacy. The odds ratio tells us about the risk conferred by an allele, and when we have confidence in this signal, we can be sure that this allele is altering the regulation of a gene and that this gene is involved in the disease process. The effect size tells us nothing about the importance of this gene in the disease process. Again, we will provide an illustrative example of this point later, in the description of work that represents a major step forward in PD research and which leveraged GWA results.

So in the context of GWA, is there an appetite for further studies? It is likely that a substantive increase in sample size will continue to identify additional risk loci, and this is certainly an approach that has been successfully applied to diseases such as type II diabetes and schizophrenia, where risk loci number in the hundreds. There are two primary challenges to taking such a route in PD; first significant advances are likely to require substantive increases in sample size, certainly more than double the size of current studies. Collecting these samples, both for discovery and replication stages, represents a significant challenge. Unlike (e.g., type II diabetes), hundreds of thousands of DNA samples from PD patients are not currently available. Second, because the sample size increase will need to be so large, the financial cost associated with sample collection and genotyping is extremely large. It is unlikely that any single funding body will support such an endeavor outside of a large philanthropic donation.

Outside of expanding current genotyping, there are several approaches that may be used to garner more information from the current datasets. In perhaps the most simple, the current GWA data can be mined more deeply, taking forward alleles that did not meet the stringent level of genome-wide significance but that were suggestive in nature. Additional typing of these in replication series is warranted and is certainly ongoing. This represents a fairly cost-efficient approach to wringing more from the current data; however, this approach alone will not identify all of the common risk alleles associated with disease.

Beyond Simple Association for Common Variants

There are many things outside of simple association that can be accomplished with dense genotype data of the type produced by GWA studies. One approach that has become increasingly popular over the last 2 or 3 years is the use of GWA data to estimate the heritable component of disease [29, 69]. The method GCTA (genome-wide complex trait analysis) estimates the proportion of phenotypic variance explained by common SNPs for complex traits, including disease. This is essentially achieved by estimating the degree of genetic relationship between individuals at a very fine genetic scale and comparing this metric between cases and controls, effectively determining how much more cases are related to each other than controls. This method has been applied to PD and the results are revealing. First, this work establishes an autosome-wide heritable component of PD of 0.3 [25]. While this is a substantial number, it is worth noting that this is likely an underestimate of the total heritable component of PD and certainly an underestimate of the total genetic component of this disease. The underestimate of the heritable component is because this method does not effectively capture the impact of very rare variants; a large number of individually rare mutations could account for a substantive proportion of the heritability of PD, but would not be reflected by this method. The genetic component of this disease would also not be completely reflected by this method, as it fails to capture the contribution of *de novo* mutations to disease. Thus the true heritable component is likely to be higher than 0.3 and the genetic component certainly so. Another notable aspect of this GCTA work in PD was a calculation of the proportion of the identified heritable component where the gene or locus is already known. The authors showed that when they repeated the analysis including only the genetic regions already associated with disease, including those identified by GWA and those identified by linkage and positional cloning, the heritable component was ~0.03 [25]. This data suggests that although a large number of loci and genes have been identified, only ~10 % of the heritable component of the disease has thus far been explained; there is much more to find.

In addition to a straightforward approach of association testing, there have been a number of other attempts to garner more etiologic understanding from GWA data. A fairly popular approach centers on pathway-based analysis. In this general scheme, investigators take significant SNPs (and here, significance may be defined quite loosely) and look for a pattern in the associated genes. This can be performed using data from existing pathway-based databases, for example, the Kyoto Encyclopedia of Genes and Genomes (KEGG; http://www.genome.jp/kegg/), and looking for an enrichment of genes associated with the GWA signals in a particular functional group of genes. Broadly, this is the type of approach that was used by Holmans and colleagues, which suggested an enrichment of immune-related genes within the PD identified loci [21]. While this type of pathway-based approach is not ideally suited to identifying individual risk alleles/genes with confidence, it does have the benefit of implicating functional networks/pathways in the disease process and thus may broadly indicate therapeutic opportunities.

As discussed above, the net effect of risk allele burden for each individual can be calculated using genetic risk profiling to give an estimate of an individuals cumulative known genetic risk. It is unlikely that this genetic risk profile alone will be sufficient to predict disease likelihood, onset, or course. It is, however, likely that this risk profile will be a critical component of a multifactorial disease prediction model that may include other easily accessible phenotypic and biological markers. Thus, the development of programs such as the Parkinson's Progression Markers Initiative (http://www.ppmi-info.org) and the Parkinson's Disease

Biomarkers Project (https://pdbp.ninds.nih.gov) has included a substantive genetic component. It is also worth considering that, as we move from risk loci, to identifying the actual biologically relevant risk allele, the effect size at these loci will increase, in some instances substantially; this advance will have a significant impact on risk prediction models.

Next Approaches

A much-lauded tool in our efforts to understand the genetic risk underlying complex disease is second-generation sequencing (also called next-generation sequencing or massively parallel sequencing). This method allows the production of extremely large-scale nucleotide sequence data, of sufficient size to sequence whole genomes or whole exomes. Whole-exome sequencing is a method that centers on taking a genomic DNA sample and enriching that sample for the protein-coding regions of the genome, which represent about 1 % of the total genome or ~30 million base pairs of sequence. This exon-enriched "exome" sample can then be readily sequenced revealing both common and rare variants within an individual's genetic makeup. Thus, this method has been suggested as an answer to find the missing heritability of complex disorders, which is believed in part to exist in the space of rare protein-coding variants. One would expect that, given the variants are individually rare, sample sizes for simple association would need to be extremely large, likely in the tens of thousands. This high bar can perhaps be lowered somewhat by assessing the gene as the unit of association, rather than the variant, for example, by assessing the cumulative number of rare variants in a gene in cases compared to controls. There are several proposed approaches for this type of gene burden test, but no consensus as to the best approach has been established to date. While large unbiased "exome-wide" sequencing efforts have not yet borne fruit in the search for rare risk variants in PD, some success has been had in Alzheimer's disease, for example, with the identification of *TREM2* mutations as moderate-risk alleles [17, 24].

Exome sequence offers speed, reduced cost per individual, and to a certain extent reduced data storage and analytical burden, when compared to whole-genome sequencing. It is inevitable that the field will turn toward whole-genome sequencing as the discovery engine for genetics in complex disease and traits. In many ways, the sample preparation is more simple, and of course more can be gleaned from the data, not only because the whole-genome sequence is generated rather than just the protein-coding exons but also because it is less challenging to analyze structural genomic variants in whole-genome data. While the current cost remains high, at ~ $1,200 for a mid-coverage genome sequence, this is a somewhat accessible price point, and it is to be expected that for many diseases and cohorts, population level genome sequence data will be produced. There are currently no public genome sequencing projects of a large scale in PD at the time of writing, but this will likely change over the next few years.

The Challenge of Understanding Risk

As outlined above, GWA has been very successful in identifying risk loci, with 28 independent risk loci identified to date for PD [38]. It is important to note though that GWA identifies loci, not genes. There are two immediate challenges that follow from the identification of a risk locus: determining the variant at that locus that is mediating the biological effect and establishing which gene is being altered by that locus and how it is being influenced. As with most disease, this effort in PD is still in fairly early days. There are some loci where the likely gene is immediately apparent, for example, it is highly likely (though not 100 % proven) that the risk variants at the *SNCA* and *LRRK2* loci exert their effects through *SNCA* and *LRRK2* rather than some other proximal gene. For the majority of loci such a candidate is not immediately apparent. A common approach to identify the likely effector gene is the use of expression quantitative trait locus mapping (eQTL) [19]. For the most part, GWA signals are not linked to protein-coding variants, and thus it is clear that these risk alleles must be exerting their effect through transcript expression (here expression is defined quite broadly to include transcript splicing, half-life of the transcript, basal amount of the transcript, or induced transcript levels). Several reference sets have been devised that compile genetic data and gene expression data and correlate individual variants with levels of proximally encoded transcripts. Within our own laboratory, we have generated such a set in human brain tissue, and this resource allows us to interrogate risk variants from PD GWA for their association with gene expression levels [15, 19]. Within PD GWA loci, several expression QTLs have been identified, and some of these make biologic sense, for example, the demonstration that PD risk alleles at *SNCA* appear to increase *SNCA* expression fits entirely with our notion of increasing *SNCA* and increasing risk [52, 53]. For the majority of loci, however, an eQTL is not apparent, and even for those where an eQTL exists, association does not imply causation; the transcript could be correlated with genotype by chance, or it could be biologically related to the genotype but irrelevant to the disease process. Clearly, careful functional characterization of proteins encoded by genes within GWA loci is an essential next step in our understanding of the disease process.

One such study was recently performed which sheds some light on the pathologically relevant proteins at two GWA loci. Beilina and colleagues performed a screen that looked for protein interactors of Lrrk2 [3]. The initial screening phase of this effort identified a large number of potential protein interactors with Lrrk2 from a screened pool of ~10,000. The large number of positive hits was too great to take forward through the essential steps of reductionist validation; however, a comparison of these interactor data with GWA data from PD revealed that two of the key proteins were under GWA peaks. This group went on to show that the proteins Rab7L1 and Gak form a complex with Lrrk2, the former of which had been independently shown previously [33]. We predict that the application of unbiased high-content screening methods integrated with the results from broad-scale genetics efforts such as GWA will be the initial key to the identification of proteins critical to the pathogenesis of PD; this work, in our opinion, should be a priority for the field.

Identifying the biologically relevant variants within GWA is challenging. Because genomic regions are inherited in chunks even within a population, extensive linkage disequilibrium exists in the human genome. Thus, it is extremely difficult to separate the true disease-related variant from those variants that are benign and coinherited with the causal variant because they are physically close. Again, we believe that success in this regard will rely on a combination of dense genetic data and functional efforts. One key observation that has been made within PD is that of the pleomorphic risk locus (PRL); this posits that for some genes, many types of disease-related genetic variants will exist, including mutations that cause disease, common noncoding variants that impart risk for disease, and coding variants that impart risk for disease [54]. Within PD thus far the phenomenon of PRL seems to be true for *SNCA*, *LRRK2*, and perhaps also *GBA*. It is reasonable to suggest therefore that some of the GWA-identified loci will contain genes that not only harbor common risk variants but that will also contain rare disease causing mutations or rare risk variants. In this regard resequencing of GWA-identified loci in many thousands of samples would be predicted to provide data for fine mapping of the risk signal and may also identify rare causal mutations, which in effect would both nominate the disease-related gene within the locus and expand the known risk architecture. While this approach is likely being pursued by many laboratories, no systematic investigation of GWA loci through extensive resequencing has been published to date.

Another important step in understanding the causal variant and its effect involves overlaying functional mapping data. The EnCODE project (Encyclopedia Of DNA Elements) is a decade long effort that aims to identify all functional elements in the human genome sequence (http://www.genome.gov/encode/). These functional elements are mapped using a variety of approaches including the mapping of histone modifications, transcription start points, and transcription factor binding sites, each performed in a variety of cell types (for more information, see http://www.genome.gov/26524238). Thus, the data identifying key functional elements can be overlaid on risk SNPs with GWA loci in an attempt to identifying the key DNA element and the critical nucleotide. This approach has been used successfully to both identify the critical variant and the gene effected, although not yet in PD [55]. Again, we believe using this type of data, and indeed creating a catalog of functional elements in PD-related cell types, is a critical need for the field.

Conclusion

The past 10 years has been an incredible period of discovery for Parkinson's disease genetics, particularly in the context of understanding the architecture of genetic risk in this complex disease. Many challenges remain, the most apparent of which is the application of methods to identify the remaining risk loci and determining the effector allele responsible for mediating this risk. The successful translation of this knowledge into an understanding of the etiology and pathogenesis of PD presents new challenges to both our paradigm of disease etiology and to the traditional framework of disease gene investigation. With these challenges lie substantial opportunity however, and this opportunity lies not only in understanding etiology but also in the investigation of genetics in other areas such as prognosis, onset, subtyping, and response to treatment. We predict that genetics will continue to serve as the foundation of our investigation into PD but that progress will rely on extensive collaboration and the integration of disparate data types.

References

1. 1000 Genomes Project Consortium, Abecasis GR, Altshuler D, Auton A, Brooks LD, Durbin RM, Gibbs RA, Hurles ME, McVean GA. A map of human genome variation from population-scale sequencing. Nature. 2010;467(7319):1061–73. doi:10.1038/nature09534.
2. Aharon-Peretz J, Rosenbaum H, Gershoni-Baruch R. Mutations in the glucocerebrosidase gene and Parkinson's disease in Ashkenazi Jews. N Engl J Med. 2004;351(19):1972–7. doi:10.1056/NEJMoa033277.
3. Beilina A, Rudenko IN, Kaganovich A, Civiero L, Chau H, Kalia SK, Kalia LV, et al. Unbiased screen for interactors of leucine-rich repeat kinase 2 supports a common pathway for sporadic and familial Parkinson disease. Proc Natl Acad Sci U S A. 2014;111(7):2626–31. doi:10.1073/pnas.1318306111.
4. Bonifati V, Rizzu P, van Baren MJ, Schaap O, Breedveld GJ, Krieger E, Dekker MCJ, et al. Mutations in the DJ-1 gene associated with autosomal recessive early-onset parkinsonism. Science. 2003;299(5604):256–9. doi:10.1126/science.1077209.
5. Chan DKY, Ng PW, Mok V, Yeung J, Fang ZM, Clarke R, Leung E, Wong L. LRRK2 Gly2385Arg mutation and clinical features in a Chinese population with early-onset Parkinson's disease compared to late-onset patients. J Neural Transm. 2008;115(9):1275–7. doi:10.1007/s00702-008-0065-0.
6. Choi JM, Woo MS, Hyeo M, Kang SY, Sung Y-H, Yong SW, Chung SJ, et al. Analysis of PARK genes in a Korean cohort of early-onset Parkinson disease. Neurogenetics. 2008;9(4):263–9. doi:10.1007/s10048-008-0138-0.
7. Di Fonzo A, Rohé CF, Ferreira J, Chien HF, Vacca L, Stocchi F, Guedes L, et al. A frequent LRRK2 gene mutation associated with autosomal dominant Parkinson's disease. Lancet. 2005;365(9457):412–5. doi:10.1016/S0140-6736(05)17829-5.
8. Di Fonzo A, Wu-Chou Y-H, Lu C-S, van Doeselaar M, Simons EJ, Rohé CF, Chang H-C, et al. A common missense variant in the LRRK2 gene, Gly2385Arg, associated with Parkinson's disease risk in Taiwan. Neurogenetics. 2006;7(3):133–8. doi:10.1007/s10048-006-0041-5.
9. Do CB, Tung JY, Dorfman E, Kiefer AK, Drabant EM, Francke U, Mountain JL, et al. Web-based genome-wide association study identifies two novel loci and a substantial genetic component for Parkinson's disease. PLoS Genet. 2011;7(6):e1002141. doi:10.1371/journal.pgen.1002141, PGENETICS-D-11-00444 [pii].
10. Edwards TL, Scott WK, Almonte C, Burt A, Powell EH, Beecham GW, Wang L, et al. Genome-wide association study confirms SNPs in SNCA and the MAPT region as common risk factors for Parkinson disease. Ann Hum Genet. 2010;74(2):97–109. doi:10.1111/j.1469-1809.2009.00560.x.
11. Farrer MJ, Stone JT, Lin C-H, Dächsel JC, Hulihan MM, Haugarvoll K, Ross OA, Ruey-Meei W. Lrrk2 G2385R is an ancestral risk factor for Parkinson's disease in Asia. Parkinsonism Relat Disord. 2007;13(2):89–92. doi:10.1016/j.parkreldis.2006.12.001.
12. Fu X, Zheng Y, Hong H, He Y, Zhou S, Guo C, Liu Y, et al. LRRK2 G2385R and LRRK2 R1628P increase risk of Parkinson's disease in a Han Chinese population from southern mainland china. Parkinsonism Relat Disord. 2012. doi:10.1016/j.parkreldis.2012.08.007.

13. Funayama M, Li Y, Tomiyama H, Yoshino H, Imamichi Y, Yamamoto M, Murata M, Toda T, Mizuno Y, Hattori N. Leucine-rich repeat kinase 2 G2385R variant is a risk factor for Parkinson disease in Asian population. Neuroreport. 2007;18(3):273–5. doi:10.1097/WNR.0b013e32801254b6.
14. Fung H-C, Scholz S, Matarin M, Simón-Sánchez J, Hernandez D, Angela B, Gibbs JR, et al. Genome-wide genotyping in Parkinson's disease and neurologically normal controls: first stage analysis and public release of data. Lancet Neurol. 2006;5(11):911–6. doi:10.1016/S1474-4422(06)70578-6.
15. Gibbs JR, van der Brug MP, Hernandez DG, Traynor BJ, Nalls MA, Lai S-L, Arepalli S, et al. Abundant quantitative trait loci exist for DNA methylation and gene expression in human brain. PLoS Genet. 2010;6(5):e1000952. doi:10.1371/journal.pgen.1000952.
16. Gilks WP, Abou-Sleiman PM, Gandhi S, Jain S, Singleton A, Lees AJ, Shaw K, et al. A common LRRK2 mutation in idiopathic Parkinson's disease. Lancet. 2005;365(9457):415–6. doi:10.1016/S0140-6736(05)17830-1.
17. Guerreiro R, Wojtas A, Bras J, Carrasquillo M, Rogaeva E, Majounie E, Cruchaga C, et al. TREM2 variants in Alzheimer's disease. N Engl J Med. 2012. doi:10.1056/NEJMoa1211851.
18. Hamza TH, Zabetian CP, Albert T, Laederach A, Montimurro J, Yearout D, Kay DM, et al. Common genetic variation in the HLA region is associated with late-onset sporadic Parkinson's disease. Nat Genet. 2010;42(9):781–5. doi:10.1038/ng.642.
19. Hernandez DG, Nalls MA, Moore M, Chong S, Dillman A, Trabzuni D, Gibbs JR, et al. Integration of GWAS SNPs and tissue specific expression profiling reveal discrete eQTLs for human traits in blood and brain. Neurobiol Dis. 2012;47(1):20–8. doi:10.1016/j.nbd.2012.03.020.
20. Hernandez DG, Nalls MA, Ylikotila P, Keller M, Hardy JA, Majamaa K, Singleton AB. Genome wide assessment of young onset Parkinson's disease from Finland. PLoS One. 2012;7(7):e41859. doi:10.1371/journal.pone.0041859.
21. Holmans P, Moskvina V, Jones L, Sharma M, Vedernikov A, Buchel F, Sadd M, et al. A pathway-based analysis provides additional support for an immune-related genetic susceptibility to Parkinson's disease. Hum Mol Genet. 2012. doi:10.1093/hmg/dds492.
22. International Parkinson Disease Genomics Consortium, Nalls MA, Plagnol V, Hernandez DG, Sharma M, Sheerin UM, Saad M et al. Imputation of sequence variants for identification of genetic risks for Parkinson's disease: a meta-analysis of genome-wide association studies. Lancet. 2011;377(9766):641–49. doi:S0140-6736(10)62345-8 [pii] 10.1016/S0140-6736(10)62345-8.
23. International Parkinson's Disease Genomics Consortium (IPDGC), and Wellcome Trust Case Control Consortium 2 (WTCCC2). A two-stage meta-analysis identifies several new loci for Parkinson's disease. PLoS Genet. 2011;7(6):e1002142. doi:10.1371/journal.pgen.1002142.
24. Jonsson T, Stefansson H, Steinberg S, Jonsdottir I, Jonsson PV, Snaedal J, Bjornsson S, et al. Variant of TREM2 associated with the risk of Alzheimer's disease. N Engl J Med. 2013;368(2):107–16. doi:10.1056/NEJMoa1211103.
25. Keller MF, Saad M, Bras J, Bettella F, Nicolaou N, Simón-Sánchez J, Mittag F, et al. Using genome-wide complex trait analysis to quantify 'missing heritability' in Parkinson's disease. Hum Mol Genet. 2012;21(22):4996–5009. doi:10.1093/hmg/dds335.
26. Kim J-M, Lee J-Y, Kim HJ, Kim JS, Shin E-S, Cho J-H, Park SS, Jeon BS. The LRRK2 G2385R variant is a risk factor for sporadic Parkinson's disease in the Korean population. Parkinsonism Relat Disord. 2010;16(2):85–8. doi:10.1016/j.parkreldis.2009.10.004.
27. Kitada T, Asakawa S, Hattori N, Matsumine H, Yamamura Y, Minoshima S, Yokochi M, Mizuno Y, Shimizu N. Mutations in the parkin gene cause autosomal recessive juvenile parkinsonism. Nature. 1998;392(6676):605–8. doi:10.1038/33416.
28. Krüger R, Vieira-Saecker AM, Kuhn W, Berg D, Müller T, Kühnl N, Fuchs GA, et al. Increased susceptibility to sporadic Parkinson's disease by a certain combined alpha-synuclein/apolipoprotein E genotype. Ann Neurol. 1999;45(5):611–7.
29. Lee SH, Wray NR, Goddard ME, Visscher PM. Estimating missing heritability for disease from genome-wide association studies. Am J Hum Genet. 2011;88(3):294–305. doi:10.1016/j.ajhg.2011.02.002.

30. Li C, Ting Z, Qin X, Ying W, Li B, Guo Qiang L, Fang Jian M, Jing Z, Jian Qing D, Sheng Di C. The prevalence of LRRK2 Gly2385Arg variant in Chinese Han population with Parkinson's disease. Mov Disord. 2007;22(16):2439–43. doi:10.1002/mds.21763.
31. Lill CM, Roehr JT, McQueen MB, Kavvoura FK, Bagade S, Schjeide B-M, Schjeide LM, et al. Comprehensive research synopsis and systematic meta-analyses in Parkinson's disease genetics: the PDGene database. PLoS Genet. 2012;8(3):e1002548. doi:10.1371/journal.pgen.1002548.
32. Liu X, Cheng R, Verbitsky M, Kisselev S, Browne A, Mejia-Sanatana H, Louis ED, et al. Genome-wide association study identifies candidate genes for Parkinson's disease in an Ashkenazi Jewish population. BMC Med Genet. 2011;12:104. doi:10.1186/1471-2350-12-104.
33. Macleod DA, Rhinn H, Kuwahara T, Zolin A, Di Paolo G, Maccabe BD, Marder KS, et al. RAB7L1 interacts with LRRK2 to modify intraneuronal protein sorting and Parkinson's disease risk. Neuron. 2013;77(3):425–39. doi:10.1016/j.neuron.2012.11.033.
34. Maraganore DM, de Andrade M, Elbaz A, Farrer MJ, Ioannidis JP, Krüger R, Rocca WA, et al. Collaborative analysis of alpha-synuclein gene promoter variability and Parkinson disease. JAMA. 2006;296(6):661–70. doi:10.1001/jama.296.6.661.
35. Maraganore DM, de Andrade M, Lesnick TG, Strain KJ, Farrer MJ, Rocca WA, Pant PVK, Frazer KA, Cox DR, Ballinger DG. High-resolution whole-genome association study of Parkinson disease. Am J Hum Genet. 2005;77(5):685–93. doi:10.1086/496902.
36. Mata IF, Kachergus JM, Taylor JP, Lincoln S, Aasly J, Lynch T, Hulihan MM, et al. Lrrk2 pathogenic substitutions in Parkinson's disease. Neurogenetics. 2005;6(4):171–7. doi:10.1007/s10048-005-0005-1.
37. Nalls MA, Duran R, Lopez G, Kurzawa-Akanbi M, McKeith IG, Chinnery PF, Morris CM, et al. A multicenter study of glucocerebrosidase mutations in dementia with Lewy bodies. JAMA Neurol. 2013;70(6):727–35. doi:10.1001/jamaneurol.2013.1925.
38. Nalls MA, Pankratz N, Lill CM, Do CB, Hernandez DG, Saad M, DeStefano AL, et al. Large-scale meta-analysis of genome-wide association data identifies six new risk loci for Parkinson's disease. Nat Genet. 2014;46(9):989–93. doi:10.1038/ng.3043.
39. Nichols WC, Pankratz N, Hernandez D, Paisán-Ruíz C, Jain S, Halter CA, Michaels VE, et al. Genetic screening for a single common LRRK2 mutation in familial Parkinson's disease. Lancet. 2005;365(9457):410–2. doi:10.1016/S0140-6736(05)17828-3.
40. Paisan-Ruiz C, Jain S, Evans EW, Gilks WP, Simon J, van der Brug M, Lopez de Munain A, et al. Cloning of the gene containing mutations that cause PARK8-linked Parkinson's disease. Neuron. 2004;44(4):595–600. doi:10.1016/j.neuron.2004.10.023.
41. Pankratz N, Beecham GW, Destefano AL, Dawson TM, Doheny KF, Factor SA, Hamza TH, et al. Meta-analysis of Parkinson's disease: identification of a novel locus, RIT2. Ann Neurol. 2012;71(3):370–84. doi:10.1002/ana.22687.
42. Pankratz N, Wilk JB, Latourelle JC, DeStefano AL, Halter C, Pugh EW, Doheny KF, et al. Genomewide association study for susceptibility genes contributing to familial Parkinson disease. Hum Genet. 2009;124(6):593–605. doi:10.1007/s00439-008-0582-9.
43. Pihlstrøm L, Axelsson G, Bjørnarå KA, Dizdar N, Fardell C, Forsgren L, Holmberg B, et al. Supportive evidence for 11 loci from genome-wide association studies in Parkinson's disease. Neurobiol Aging. 2013;34(6):1708.e7–13. doi:10.1016/j.neurobiolaging.2012.10.019.
44. Polymeropoulos MH, Lavedan C, Leroy E, Ide SE, Dehejia A, Dutra A, Pike B, et al. Mutation in the alpha-synuclein gene identified in families with Parkinson's disease. Science. 1997;276(5321):2045–7.
45. Pulkes T, Papsing C, Mahasirimongkol S, Busabaratana M, Kulkantrakorn K, Tiamkao S. Frequencies of LRRK2 variants in Thai patients with Parkinson's disease: evidence for an R1628P founder. J Neurol Neurosurg Psychiatry. 2011;82(10):1179–80. doi:10.1136/jnnp.2009.194597.
46. Ross OA, Soto-Ortolaza AI, Heckman MG, Aasly JO, Abahuni N, Annesi G, Bacon JA, et al. Association of LRRK2 exonic variants with susceptibility to Parkinson's disease: a case-control study. Lancet Neurol. 2011. doi:10.1016/S1474-4422(11)70175-2.
47. Ross OA, Wu Y-R, Lee M-C, Funayama M, Chen M-L, Soto AI, Mata IF, et al. Analysis of Lrrk2 R1628P as a risk factor for Parkinson's disease. Ann Neurol. 2008;64(1):88–92. doi:10.1002/ana.21405.

48. Saad M, Lesage S, Saint-Pierre A, Corvol J-C, Zelenika D, Lambert J-C, Vidailhet M, et al. Genome-wide association study confirms BST1 and suggests a locus on 12q24 as the risk loci for Parkinson's disease in the European population. Hum Mol Genet. 2011;20(3):615–27. doi:10.1093/hmg/ddq497.
49. Satake W, Nakabayashi Y, Mizuta I, Hirota Y, Ito C, Kubo M, Kawaguchi T, et al. Genome-wide association study identifies common variants at four loci as genetic risk factors for Parkinson's disease. Nat Genet. 2009;41(12):1303–7. doi:10.1038/ng.485.
50. Sharma M, Ioannidis JPA, Aasly JO, Annesi G, Brice A, Van Broeckhoven C, Bertram L, et al. Large-scale replication and heterogeneity in Parkinson disease genetic loci. Neurology. 2012;79(7):659–67. doi:10.1212/WNL.0b013e318264e353.
51. Sidransky E, Nalls MA, Aasly JO, Aharon-Peretz J, Annesi G, Barbosa ER, Bar-Shira A, et al. Multicenter analysis of glucocerebrosidase mutations in Parkinson's disease. N Engl J Med. 2009;361(17):1651–61. doi:10.1056/NEJMoa0901281.
52. Simon-Sanchez J, Schulte C, Bras JM, Sharma M, Gibbs JR, Berg D, Paisan-Ruiz C, et al. Genome-wide association study reveals genetic risk underlying Parkinson's disease. Nat Genet. 2009;41(12):1308–12. doi:10.1038/ng.487, ng.487 [pii].
53. Singleton AB, Farrer M, Johnson J, Singleton A, Hague S, Kachergus J, Hulihan M, et al. Alpha-synuclein locus triplication causes Parkinson's disease. Science. 2003;302(5646):841. doi:10.1126/science.1090278.
54. Singleton A, Hardy J. A generalizable hypothesis for the genetic architecture of disease: pleomorphic risk loci. Hum Mol Genet. 2011;20(R2):R158–62. doi:10.1093/hmg/ddr358.
55. Smemo S, Tena JJ, Kim K-H, Gamazon ER, Sakabe NJ, Gómez-Marín C, Aneas I, et al. Obesity-associated variants within FTO form long-range functional connections with IRX3. Nature. 2014;507(7492):371–5. doi:10.1038/nature13138.
56. Spillantini MG, Schmidt ML, Lee VM, Trojanowski JQ, Jakes R, Goedert M. Alpha-synuclein in Lewy bodies. Nature. 1997;388(6645):839–40. doi:10.1038/42166.
57. Tan EK, Peng R, Wu YR, Wu RM, Wu-Chou YH, Tan LC, An XK, Chen CM, Fook-Chong S, Lu CS. LRRK2 G2385R modulates age at onset in Parkinson's disease: a multi-center pooled analysis. Am J Med Genet B Neuropsychiatr Genet. 2009;150B(7):1022–3. doi:10.1002/ajmg.b.30923.
58. Tan EK, Zhao Y, Skipper L, Tan MG, Di Fonzo A, Sun L, Fook-Chong S, et al. The LRRK2 Gly2385Arg variant is associated with Parkinson's disease: genetic and functional evidence. Hum Genet. 2007;120(6):857–63. doi:10.1007/s00439-006-0268-0.
59. Tan E-K, Zhao Y, Tan L, Lim H-Q, Lee J, Yuen Y, Pavanni R, Wong M-C, Fook-Chong S, Liu J-J. Analysis of LRRK2 Gly2385Arg genetic variant in Non-Chinese Asians. Mov Disord. 2007;22(12):1816–8. doi:10.1002/mds.21658.
60. Tayebi N, Callahan M, Madike V, Stubblefield BK, Orvisky E, Krasnewich D, Fillano JJ, Sidransky E. Gaucher disease and parkinsonism: a phenotypic and genotypic characterization. Mol Genet Metab. 2001;73(4):313–21. doi:10.1006/mgme.2001.3201.
61. Tayebi N, Walker J, Stubblefield B, Orvisky E, LaMarca ME, Wong K, Rosenbaum H, Schiffmann R, Bembi B, Sidransky E. Gaucher disease with Parkinsonian manifestations: does glucocerebrosidase deficiency contribute to a vulnerability to parkinsonism? Mol Genet Metab. 2003;79(2):104–9.
62. The International HapMap Consortium. A haplotype map of the human genome. Nature. 2005;437(7063):1299–320. doi:10.1038/nature04226.
63. Tsuji S, Choudary PV, Martin BM, Stubblefield BK, Mayor JA, Barranger JA, Ginns EI. A mutation in the human glucocerebrosidase gene in neuronopathic Gaucher's disease. N Engl J Med. 1987;316(10):570–5. doi:10.1056/NEJM198703053161002.
64. UK Parkinson's Disease Consortium, Wellcome Trust Case Control Consortium 2, Spencer CCA, Plagnol V, Strange A, Gardner M, Paisan-Ruiz C, et al. Dissection of the genetics of Parkinson's disease identifies an additional association 5' of SNCA and multiple associated haplotypes at 17q21. Hum Mol Genet. 2011;20(2):345–53. doi:10.1093/hmg/ddq469.
65. Valente EM, Abou-Sleiman PM, Caputo V, Muqit MMK, Harvey K, Gispert S, Ali Z, et al. Hereditary early-onset Parkinson's disease caused by mutations in PINK1. Science. 2004;304(5674):1158–60. doi:10.1126/science.1096284.

66. Wang C, Cai Y, Zheng Z, Tang B-S, Yanming X, Wang T, Ma J, et al. Penetrance of LRRK2 G2385R and R1628P is modified by common PD-associated genetic variants. Parkinsonism Relat Disord. 2012;18(8):958–63. doi:10.1016/j.parkreldis.2012.05.003.
67. Wu X, Tang K-F, Li Y, Xiong Y-Y, Shen L, Wei Z-Y, Zhou K-J, et al. Quantitative assessment of the effect of LRRK2 exonic variants on the risk of Parkinson's disease: a meta-analysis. Parkinsonism Relat Disord. 2012;18(6):722–30. doi:10.1016/j.parkreldis.2012.04.013.
68. Wu-Chou Y-H, Chen Y-T, Yeh T-H, Chang H-C, Weng Y-H, Lai S-C, Huang C-L, et al. Genetic variants of SNCA and LRRK2 genes are associated with sporadic PD susceptibility: a replication study in a Taiwanese cohort. Parkinsonism Relat Disord. 2012. doi:10.1016/j.parkreldis.2012.10.019.
69. Yang J, Lee SH, Goddard ME, Visscher PM. GCTA: a tool for genome-wide complex trait analysis. Am J Hum Genet. 2011;88(1):76–82. doi:10.1016/j.ajhg.2010.11.011.
70. Zabetian CP, Yamamoto M, Lopez NA, Ujike H, Mata IF, Izumi Y, Kaji R, et al. LRRK2 mutations and risk variants in Japanese patients with Parkinson's disease. Mov Disord. 2009;24(7):1034–41. doi:10.1002/mds.22514.
71. Zimprich A, Biskup S, Leitner P, Lichtner P, Farrer M, Lincoln S, Kachergus J, et al. Mutations in LRRK2 cause autosomal-dominant parkinsonism with pleomorphic pathology. Neuron. 2004;44(4):601–7. doi:10.1016/j.neuron.2004.11.005.

Chapter 3
Genetics of Atypical Parkinsonism

Maria Stamelou and Kailash P. Bhatia

Abstract In this chapter, we discuss the genetics of sporadic atypical parkinsonism, namely, progressive supranuclear palsy (PSP), corticobasal degeneration (CBD), and multiple system atrophy (MSA). Major new knowledge include new susceptibility loci apart from the H1 haplotype in microtubuli-associated protein tau (*MAPT*) gene for PSP, as well as the discovery of mutations in *COQ2* gene causing familial MSA. Furthermore, we discuss atypical features of new and known PARK-related genes, such as *DNAJC6* and *SYNJ1*. Lastly, we discuss the features of atypical parkinsonism in genetic conditions presenting predominantly with other phenotypes such as dementia (*MAPT, PGRN, C9ORF72, DCTN1*), ataxia (SCAs, FXTAS), dystonia (DRD, DYT12, dopamine transporter deficiency syndrome), and others such as mitochondrial and metabolic disorders.

Keywords Progressive supranuclear palsy • Corticobasal degeneration • Multiple system atrophy • Atypical parkinsonism • PARK • Dystonia–parkinsonism • Dementia • Ataxia • Spasticity

Introduction

Atypical parkinsonian syndromes (APs) are defined as syndromes that present with parkinsonism and features atypical for Parkinson's disease. Classically, the term is used to describe sporadic neurodegenerative conditions of unknown etiology that

M. Stamelou, MD, PhD (✉)
Department of Neurology, Philipps-University Marburg, Marburg, Germany

Second Department of Neurology, National and Kapodistrian
University of Athens, Attiko Hospital, Athens 12462, Greece
e-mail: mariastamelou@gmail.com

K.P. Bhatia, MD, DM, FRCP
Sobell Department, University College London/Institute of Neurology,
London WC1N 3BG, UK

S.A. Schneider, J.M.T. Brás (eds.), *Movement Disorder Genetics*,
DOI 10.1007/978-3-319-17223-1_3

constitute the major differential diagnoses from sporadic Parkinson's disease, namely, progressive supranuclear palsy (PSP), corticobasal degeneration (CBD), and multiple system atrophy (MSA), which are pathological entities distinct from PD.

However, also a number of genetic conditions may cause parkinsonism with clinical features atypical for PD and diverse or yet unknown pathologies, and the term atypical parkinsonism has been used for these disorders as well. Of those, some are identified as causing predominantly parkinsonism and some as causing predominantly other phenotypes that may also include parkinsonism and in rare cases only parkinsonism. Here, we will discuss firstly the genetics of sporadic APs, secondly genes that cause predominantly APs, and thirdly genes that are linked predominantly to other phenotypes that may include atypical parkinsonism.

Genetics of Sporadic Atypical Parkinsonism: PSP, CBD, and MSA

The most common sporadic atypical parkinsonian conditions include progressive supranuclear palsy (PSP), corticobasal degeneration (CBD), and multiple system atrophy (MSA). These are distinct pathological entities.

Genetics of PSP

PSP is a neurodegenerative disease characterized by symmetric parkinsonism, supranuclear palsy of vertical gaze, early postural instability with falls backwards, and subcortical dementia [111]. This typical PSP phenotype is termed Richardson's syndrome (RS), while further phenotypes have been described [161]. The prevalence of PSP is approximately 5 per 100,000, average age at onset is 63, and mean time from symptom onset to death is 7–9 years. PSP is a 4-repeat tauopathy characterized by degeneration of several subcortical structures including the substantia nigra, the subthalamic nucleus, and the midbrain. Neurofibrillary tangles are present in these areas. Tufted astrocytes (Gallyas positive) are the hallmark feature of PSP that differentiates it in pathology from other 4R tauopathies such as CBD [46]. No effective treatments are available [77, 187, 202].

PSP is almost always sporadic. A genome-wide association study has confirmed that the most common risk allele for PSP is the H1 haplotype of the microtubuli-associated tau (*MAPT*) gene, and further risk loci have been identified [78]. The H1 haplotype of the *MAPT* gene (encoding for tau) is found in over 90 % of the patients. It is suggested that the presence of the H1 *MAPT* haplotype affects alternative splicing of exon 10 of the *MAPT* gene, which may result in an increased ratio of the 4R isoform of the tau protein (4R-tau) compared with the 3R isoform (3R-tau). However, the H1 *MAPT* haplotype did not correlate with age of onset, disease severity, or survival in a study on 63 PSP patients, implying the presence of other modifying factors [110]. Interestingly, Li et al. using genome-wide methylation analysis showed that differential methylation at 17q21.31 correlates with the H1 haplotype in a dose-dependent manner in patients with frontotemporal dementia (FTD) and PSP, pointing for the first time to an epigenetic mediator of neurodegeneration that increases risk for PSP [105].

Apart from confirming two independent variants in *MAPT* affecting risk for PSP, this study identified three significant novel signals associated with PSP risk, which may give some insight in the pathophysiology of the disease: EIF2AK3 (eukaryotic translation initiation factor 2-α kinase 3; rs7571971, OR of major allele = 0.75, $p = 3.2 \times 10^{-13}$), STX6 (syntaxin 6; rs1411478, odds ratio [OR] of major allele = 0.79, $p = 2.3 \times 10^{-10}$), and MOBP (myelin-associated oligodendrocyte basic protein; rs1768208, OR of major allele = 0.72, $p = 1.0 \times 10^{-16}$) [78]. EIF2AK3 is a gene that encodes PERK, a component of the endoplasmic reticulum (ER) unfolded protein response (UPR). When excess unfolded proteins accumulate in the ER, PERK is activated and protein synthesis is inhibited allowing the ER to clear mis-folded proteins. However, tau, which is the primary mis-folded protein in PSP, is not expected to traffic through the ER. The second PSP susceptibility gene STX6 encodes syntaxin 6 (Stx6), and genetic variation at STX6 could influence movement of mis-folded proteins from the ER to lysosomes via the endosomal system. Lastly, MOBP encodes a protein (MOBP) that is produced by oligodendrocytes and is present in the major dense line of CNS myelin. MOBP is highly expressed in the white matter of the medulla, pons, cerebellum, and midbrain, regions affected in PSP, suggesting that myelin dysfunction oligodendrocyte misfunction contributes to PSP pathogenesis [78]. Ferrari et al. subsequently identified point mutations in each of these genes in a subset of the PSP cases used in the original GWAS [57]. Although implication of EIF2AK3 and MOBP could not be fully assessed, they showed that the single nucleotide polymorphism rs1411478 (STX6) is a strong expression quantitative trait locus with significantly lower expression of STX6 in white matter in carriers of the risk allele [57]. Further research is needed to identify the functional links between these risk loci and disease pathophysiology.

Genetics of CBD

Corticobasal degeneration (CBD) is a rare neurodegenerative disorder typically characterized by progressive asymmetric levodopa-resistant parkinsonism, dystonia, myoclonus, and further cortical signs (e.g., apraxia, alien limb phenomena, cortical sensory loss) [10, 186]. This typical CBD phenotype is now called corticobasal syndrome (CBS), while further phenotypes have been described [94]. CBD is a 4R tauopathy characterized by widespread deposition of hyperphosphorylated tau protein (specifically 4-repeat tau) in the brain. There is marked neuronal degeneration in the substantia nigra and the frontoparietal cortex. The hallmark feature of

CBD pathology is the characteristic astrocytic plaques that differentiate CBD from other 4R tauopathies such as PSP (tufted astrocytes) [109].

Since CBD is also a tauopathy, several studies have investigated the possible role of *MAPT* variants in the pathogenesis of the disorder. Indeed, the H1 haplotype was also found to be associated with the development of CBD [78, 79]. In a recent study, a systematic sequence analysis of *MAPT* coding and 3′ untranslated region (3′UTR) in a large cohort of autopsy-confirmed CBD patients ($N=109$) was performed. This identified a novel *MAPT* mutation in exon 13 (p.N410H) in a case that was neuropathologically indistinguishable from sporadic CBD and represents the first case meeting neuropathologic diagnostic criteria for CBD harboring a *MAPT* mutation. On immunoblot, the p.N410H mutation carrier had the same insoluble tau profile as seen in CBD. Sequence analysis of the complete *MAPT* 3′UTR in autopsy-confirmed CBD cases further identified two rare variants with nominally significant association with CBD. An ATC nucleotide insertion ("MAPTv8") was found in 4.6 % of CBD patients compared to 1.2 % of controls ($p=0.031$, OR=3.71) and rs186977284 in 4.6 % CBD patients, but only 0.9 % of controls ($p=0.04$, OR=3.58). Rs186977284 was also present in 2.7 % of a large cohort of autopsy-confirmed PSP patients ($N=566$) and only 0.9 % of an additional control series ($p=0.034$, OR=3.08), extending the association to PSP [93].

Genetics of MSA

Multiple system atrophy (MSA) is a neurodegenerative disorder characterized by autonomic failure and parkinsonism and/or cerebellar signs. MSA-parkinsonism (MSA-P) is characterized predominantly by parkinsonism and autonomic failure at presentation, whereas in MSA-cerebellar type (MSA-C), cerebellar signs occur with autonomic failure [13, 213]. The prevalence is about 4 per 100,000, typical age at onset is 53–55 [214], and mean survival time is 9 years [214]. MSA is an a-synucleinopathy characterized by abnormal a-synuclein-positive cytoplasmic inclusions in oligodendrocytes, termed glial cytoplasmic inclusions, mainly found in the basal ganglia, cerebellar structures, and motor cortex. Neuropathological examination often reveals gross abnormalities of the striatonigral and/or olivopontocerebellar systems, which upon microscopic examination are associated with severe neuronal loss, gliosis, myelin pallor, and axonal degeneration [4, 47].

SNCA (α-synuclein) gene is encoding for the a-synuclein protein. *SNCA* variants have been studied as risk factors to develop MSA. 10 single nucleotide variants of *SNCA* most associated with risk of developing PD were tested in 413 MSA cases, and 2/10 *SNCA* variants were significantly associated with a risk of developing MSA [176]. These results were confirmed in an independent cohort of 108 MSA patients (rs11931074, OR=6.2, $p=5.5\times10^{-12}$; rs3857059, OR=5.9, $p=2\times10^{-10}$) [5, 176]. Al-Chalabi et al. examined 32 *SNCA* variants in 239 MSA cases and found that two of the variants were associated specifically with the MSA-C subtype (rs3822086; rs3775444) [5]. A GWAS in MSA is not available as of now, but is under way.

Recently, a combination of linkage analysis and next-generation genome sequencing identified homozygous and compound heterozygous variants of the gene *COQ2* (coenzyme Q2 4-hydroxybenzoate polyprenyltransferase) as a cause of MSA in familial cases from Japan and as a risk factor to develop sporadic MSA [127]. *COQ2* is important for the biosynthesis of coenzyme Q10, which in turn is an important factor for mitochondrial respiratory chain function. The most common of these mutations, p.V343A, was suggested to increase the risk of MSA through functional impairment of coenzyme Q10, which leads to increased oligodendrocyte apoptosis due to oxidative stress [127, 138].

A heterozygous deletion in *SHC2* (src homology 2 domain containing-transforming protein 2) in monozygotic twins discordant for MSA has also been reported [173]. The authors further observed copy number variation in *SHC2* in 32 % (10 of 31 patients) of MSA patients and in no controls of Japanese descent. However, a more recent study did not find copy number variation of the *SHC2* gene to be a significant genetic factor for non-Japanese MSA patients implying that this may only play a role in MSA pathogenesis in Japanese cohorts [56].

Atypical Parkinsonism in PARK-Related Genes

Mutations in the recessive *ATP13A2*/PARK9 gene that encodes a predominantly neuronal lysosomal type 5 P-type ATPase have been detected in patients with the recessively inherited Kufor–Rakeb syndrome. Kufor–Rakeb syndrome is typically characterized by juvenile-onset (12–29 years), levodopa-responsive parkinsonism (with fluctuations and dyskinesias), vertical supranuclear gaze palsy, cognitive dysfunction (dementia and visual hallucinations), and pyramidal signs [128, 218]. Further characteristic features include oculogyric dystonic spasms and facial–faucial–finger mini-myoclonus [15, 48, 115, 160]. T2*-weighted MRI imaging may show evidence of brain iron accumulation in some patients, which can be a helpful clue to suspect this disorder [139, 140, 160, 174]. There is no pathology from a patient with Kufor–Rakeb syndrome reported, but recently exome sequencing in a family with pathologically confirmed neuronal ceroid-lipofuscinosis has identified *ATP13A2* mutations that segregated with the affected family members [29].

Mutations in *PLA2G6*/PARK14 are identified as one cause of adult-onset parkinsonism with additional dystonia and complicated by pyramidal involvement. *PLA2G6* gene mutations were previously known to cause infantile neuroaxonal dystrophy and are also one cause of neurodegeneration with brain iron accumulation. In adult-onset cases, parkinsonism is characterized by the presence of tremor including a pill-rolling rest component, rigidity, and severe bradykinesia with a good response to levodopa. However, there was early development of dyskinesias [139, 184].

Mutations in the F-box only protein 7 gene (*FBXO7*) cause PARK15, a recessive form of juvenile parkinsonism with pyramidal signs. It was identified in one Iranian kindred with predominant pyramidal signs and later demonstrated by different mutations found in further ethnicities with prominent juvenile parkinsonism with varying degrees of levodopa response [106, 114, 139, 184, 222]. The brain pathology in patients with PARK15 remains unknown. However, FBXO7 immunoreactivity in the Lewy bodies of typical PD, and in glial cytoplasmic inclusions of multiple system atrophy, is reported, suggesting an involvement of this protein in the pathogenesis of the common forms of synucleinopathies [86, 223].

DNAJC6 and *SYNJ1* (PARK20) have been recently identified as the cause of autosomal recessive, juvenile parkinsonism, using exome sequencing combined with genome-wide homozygosity mapping [39, 53, 82, 92, 97, 136, 147, 153, 172, 194, 211]. The phenotype of *DNAJC6* mutations ranges from juvenile parkinsonism without further signs or with mental retardation, pyramidal signs, and epilepsy, while a case with obesity, epilepsy, and mental retardation but no signs of parkinsonism has been reported [53, 82, 92]. *DNAJC6* encodes the neuronal co-chaperone auxilin. In the case of *SYNJ1*, the same homozygous mutation, p.Arg258Gln, was identified independently in two consanguineous families of Iranian and Italian origins, with parkinsonism, dystonia, and cognitive deterioration. Response to levodopa was poor and limited by side effects [97, 153]. Neuroimaging revealed brain atrophy, nigrostriatal dopaminergic defects, and cerebral hypometabolism [97, 153]. *SYNJ1* encodes synaptojanin 1, which plays a role in the post-endocytic recycling of synaptic vesicles (Table 3.1).

Atypical Parkinsonism in Genetic Disorders Predominantly Presenting with Other Neurologic Features

Traditionally a gene is tied to the recognition of a characteristic phenotype, but once the genetic defect is identified, the phenotypic characterization broadens. Indeed, genes identified in cohorts of patients presenting with diverse predominant features such as dementia, ataxia, chorea, or dystonia are now well recognized to also cause atypical parkinsonism, and in fact, in some cases atypical parkinsonism may be the predominant phenotype. In some cases, the atypical parkinsonism may resemble the classical PSP, CBD, or MSA phenotypes, leading to diagnostic confusion [190]. These genetic conditions are described below and are given in Table 3.1.

Atypical parkinsonism in Genes Predominantly Causing Dementia

Microtubule-associated protein tau (*MAPT*) and progranulin (*PGRN*) gene mutations both inherited in a dominant pattern and mainly causing frontotemporal dementias (FTDs) (with 3R/4R and TDP-43 pathology, respectively) can present with atypical parkinsonism and PSP as well as CBS phenotypes [31, 32, 34–36, 64, 125, 142, 149, 164, 165, 167, 168, 192, 208]. Clues to test for *MAPT* mutations would be the earlier age at onset (between the third to fifth decade) [6, 142, 149, 166, 168, 192], a positive family history of parkinsonism or dementia [64, 125, 165], and early and prominent behavioral problems that usually precede the classical PSP or CBS signs.

Table 3.1 An incomplete list of genetic conditions that may cause atypical parkinsonism, along with their respective genes, mode of inheritance, mean age of onset, MRI, and DaTSCAN findings

	Gene	Transmission	Age of onset (years)	Major features in MRI brain	DaTSCAN
PARK-related parkinsonism					
PARK8	*LRRK2*	AD	~Mean 60–65	From normal to generalized atrophy	Abnormal
PARK9 (Kufor–Rakeb)	*ATP13A2*	AR	Juvenile	Diffuse moderate cerebral and cerebellar atrophy and in some putaminal and caudate iron accumulation	Abnormal
PARK14	*PLA2G6*	AR	Juvenile	Cortical and cerebellar atrophy, may show iron in Gpi, may show white matter changes	Abnormal
PARK15	*FBXO7*	AR	Juvenile	Brain atrophy or maybe normal	
PARK20	*SYNJ1*	AR	Juvenile to adulthood	Brain atrophy	Abnormal
Genes predominantly causing dementia					
Frontotemporal lobar degeneration	*MAPT*	AD	~Mean 40	Symmetric frontotemporal atrophy	Abnormal
	PGRN	AD	~Mean 60	Asymmetric fronto-temporo-parietal atrophy	Abnormal
	C9ORF72	AD	~Mean 52	Bilateral frontal atrophy with variable degrees of parietal +/−temporal atrophy; usually no striking asymmetry	Abnormal
Alzheimer's dementia	*PSEN1*	AD	~Mean 45	Medial temporal atrophy	May be abnormal
Perry syndrome	*DCTN1*	AD	~Mean 45–50	May show midbrain atrophy	Abnormal

(continued)

Table 3.1 (continued)

	Gene	Transmission	Age of onset (years)	Major features in MRI brain	DaTSCAN
Genes predominantly causing ataxia					
Spinocerebellar ataxias	*ATXN2*	AD	~Mean 32	Pontocerebellar atrophy 25 % have hot cross bun sign	Abnormal
	ATXN3	AD	Range 5–75	Pontocerebellar atrophy	Abnormal
Fragile X tremor-ataxia syndrome	*FMR1*	X-linked dominant	~Mean 60	Increased signal in MCP and CCS in T2-weighted images	~47 % Abnormal
Genes predominantly causing dystonia					
DYT3	*TAF1*	X-linked dominant	~Main 30	Severe atrophy of the caudate and putamen; hyperintensity with an outer rim in the putamen	Abnormal
DYT5a	*GTPCH1*	AD	~6–10	Usually normal	Normal
DTDS	*SLC6A3*	AR	Infantile to adulthood	Maybe normal, in some white matter changes	Abnormal
DYT12	*ATP1A3*	AR	4–58 years	Usually normal	Abnormal
Wilson's disease	*ATP7B*	AR	First decade (but up to adulthood)	Can show the "face of the giant panda" midbrain May show hyperintensities in basal ganglia, midbrain, thalami, and pons	Abnormal
Inborn error of manganese metabolism	*SLC30A10*	AR	First decade (but up to adulthood)	Hyperintensities in basal ganglia and cerebellum in T1-weighted images	
NBIAs	Diverse		First decade (but up to adulthood)	Eye of the tiger in PKAN, further see genetics of NBIAs	Maybe normal or abnormal
Genes causing predominantly spasticity					
HSPs	*SPG11*	AR	First decade (but up to adulthood)	Atrophy of the corpus callosum	Maybe normal or abnormal

Genes causing predominantly chorea					
Huntington's disease	*huntingtin*	AD	Wide range from early childhood to late adulthood	Caudate atrophy	Maybe normal or abnormal
Neuroacanthocytosis	*VPS13A*	AR	Wide range from early childhood to late adulthood	May show striatal atrophy in particular the head of the caudate	Maybe normal or abnormal
Others					
Cerebrotendinous xanthomatosis	*CYP27A1*	AR	~Mean 40	Cerebellar atrophy Hyperintensities in dentate in T2-weighted images	Abnormal
Gaucher's disease	*GBA*	AR	From 3rd to 7th decade	Normal	Abnormal
Niemann–Pick C	*NPC*	AR	Second to third decade	May show frontal atrophy and hyperintensities in parietal-occipital periventricular white matter	Unknown
Mitochondrial	Various	AR, AD	From juvenile to adulthood	Variable changes	Abnormal
Genetic PRION	*PRNP*	AD	Wide range from juvenile to seventh decade	Hyperintensities in putamen and caudate in T2, FLAIR, and DWI sequences	Abnormal
Leukoencephalopathy with axonal spheroids	*CSF1R*	AD	Wide range	Leukoencephalopathy	Abnormal

Abbreviations: MCP middle cerebellar peduncles, *CCS* corpus callosum splenium, *MRI* magnetic resonance imaging, *DaTSCAN* dopamine transporter imaging, *MAPT* microtubule-associated tau, *PGRN* progranulin, *C9ORF72* chromosome 9 open reading frame 72, *PSEN1* presenilin 1, *DCTN1* dynactin, *LRRK2* leucine-rich repeat kinase 2, *ATXN* ataxin, *FMR1* fragile X mental retardation 1, *GBA* glucocerebrosidase, *NPC* Niemann–Pick C, *PRNP* prion protein, *CSF1R* colony-stimulating factor 1, *SPG11* spastic paraplegia 11, *DTDS* dopamine transporter deficiency syndrome

In contrast, the mean age at onset in *PGRN* mutation carriers is 60 years (range: 35–83 years) [14, 64, 177, 221], and the penetrance reaches that of 90 % at age 70 [26], so a positive family history is not always present. Clinical clues to suspect *PGRN* in a patient with RS or CBS would be a long preceding history of frontal dysfunction [203, 221]; signs of parietal lobe involvement (e.g., dyscalculia, limb apraxia, etc.), which are unusual for sporadic PSP (but usual in CBD); and hallucinations that rarely occur in sporadic PSP and CBD. Different studies report CBS as one of the three most common phenotypes seen in *PGRN* mutation carriers (the other two being bvFTD and PNFA) [14, 17, 18, 24, 35, 36, 49, 66, 87, 141, 157, 164, 185, 209]. A careful language evaluation may help to predict *PGRN* mutations in these patients; PNFA is occasionally the initial manifestation, before the CBS phenotype emerges. MRI imaging shows asymmetric fronto-temporo-parietal atrophy [6], rarely the case in PSP, but similar to findings in CBD [91, 188]. Sequential testing for *MAPT* and *PRGN* in patients with a positive family history is recommended and available [64]. Measurement of progranulin plasma levels may also be helpful if genetic testing is not available [58].

Hexanucleotide expansions in the newly described gene, chromosome 9 open reading frame 72 (*C9ORF72*) (TDP-43 pathology), cause FTD–amyotrophic lateral sclerosis (ALS) overlap syndromes [117, 118, 156], and in 35 % of these patients, atypical parkinsonism may be present [25, 37, 38, 76, 108, 117, 118, 134, 156]. A positive family history, signs of upper or lower motor neuron disease, and the presence of hallucinations are important clues to suspect these mutations [25, 37, 38, 108, 134, 156].

Lastly, Perry syndrome, a rare autosomal dominant disorder due to mutations in the dynactin *(DCTN1)* gene (TDP-43 pathology) may present with atypical parkinsonism and an RS, CBS, as well as MSA phenotype [212, 215]. Clinical clues to suspect these mutations include central hypoventilation, weight loss, and psychiatric symptoms (e.g., apathy, hallucinations) [100, 129, 135, 145, 146, 151, 204]. Response to levodopa varies from no response to significant improvement and development of motor fluctuations and dyskinesias [22, 55, 129, 135, 145, 146, 151, 204, 212, 215, 216].

CBS has been described commonly with Alzheimer's disease (AD) pathology in sporadic AD patients [7, 23, 50, 61, 73, 83, 104], and earlier age at onset and myoclonus are thought to be more suggestive of AD rather than CBD pathology [50, 83, 99]. Increased saccadic latency has been described in AD and CBD, and thus this feature may not be helpful in the differential diagnosis [27]. Some mutations in presenilin 1 (*PSEN1*) have been described to cause parkinsonism with myoclonus, dystonia, apraxia, and frontal dementia mimicking CBD, although there is usually no striking asymmetry and there may be seizures, which rarely occur in CBD [99]. Mutations in *APP* and *PSEN2* may also present with parkinsonism but mostly mimicking dementia with Lewy bodies (DLB) [155].

Atypical parkinsonism in Genes Predominantly Causing Ataxia

Spinocerebellar ataxias (SCA) represent a clinically and genetically heterogeneous group of neurodegenerative disorders in which progressive degeneration of the cerebellum and spinocerebellar tracts of the spinal cord are associated with a variable combination of signs of central and peripheral nervous system involvement (see also Chap. 11). Extrapyramidal features, including parkinsonism, have been described in several of these such as SCA2 and SCA3.

SCA2 (due to expansion of a glutamine tract in the ataxin-2 gene) typically presents with ataxia, slowed horizontal saccades, and peripheral neuropathy; however, phenotypes with a parkinsonism-predominant profile or purely parkinsonism, early postural instability, and vertical supranuclear gaze palsy (SGP) have been described [59, 69, 144, 167, 180, 181, 198], mostly in patients of Asian origin, with later age at onset and shorter repeat expansion [59, 69, 112, 144, 198]. SCA3 (Machado–Joseph disease) is the most frequent cause of autosomal dominantly inherited cerebellar ataxia in Europe, Japan, and the United States and is caused by an expanded polyglutamine CAG repeat size of >44 [162]. Age at onset varies from 5 to 75 years and inversely correlates with CAG repeat length. The parkinsonian variant of SCA3 is associated with lower range repeat expansions and a later age at onset, similar to SCA2 [42, 162, 175]. Cerebellar ataxia, parkinsonism, and only mild cognitive dysfunction [89, 107, 207] in addition to cardiovascular and sympathetic sweating dysautonomia (in up to 45 %) can clinically be mistaken for MSA, particularly when family history is negative [96, 197]. Further SCAs, such as SCA8, SCA17, and SCA6, more rarely present with parkinsonism [2].

Fragile X tremor-ataxia syndrome (FXTAS) is a late-onset (>50 years) neurodegenerative disorder, occurring in carriers of a premutation CGG repeat expansion (55–200 repeats) in the fragile X mental retardation 1 (*FMR1*) gene. The penetrance of FXTAS in male carriers over 50 years is ~40 %, and recently it has been postulated that female carriers develop FXTAS more often than previously suggested [199]. Autopsy reveals intranuclear inclusions in neurons and astrocytes and dystrophic white matter [12, 19, 65, 199]. The typical phenotype consists of the combination of intention tremor and ataxia, but parkinsonism, autonomic dysfunction, cognitive decline, psychiatric features, and neuropathy have been described, and tremor is not always present [12]. A family history of mental retardation or premature ovarian failure provides important clues [19]. However, in a recent series 43 % of the FXTAS patients had no family history of fragile X syndrome [9]. Additional features include autonomic dysfunction presenting, as in MSA, with impotence, orthostatic hypotension, urinary frequency, and urinary incontinence [9, 70]. However, MSA is rarely misdiagnosed as FXTAS – among 426 clinically diagnosed MSA cases, only four were found to have FXTAS in a study [84]. Dopamine transporter imaging (DaTSCAN) in few cases may be normal, and in which case, it is helpful in the differential diagnosis with MSA [116].

Atypical parkinsonism in Genes Predominantly Causing Dystonia or Dystonia–Parkinsonism

X-Linked Recessive Dystonia–Parkinsonism (DYT3; XDP; "Lubag")

DYT3 dystonia, which clusters in Filipinos, is an X-linked recessive disorder. Although this disorder typically affects males, rarely, females may also be affected, possibly due to severe X-inactivation or based on homozygosity for the mutation [103]. DYT3 reaches complete penetrance by the end of the fifth decade in males and later in females (up to 75 years) and is associated with specific sequence changes in the TAF1 gene [126, 183]. Usually symptoms start in adulthood as focal dystonia, tend to progress, and generalize. Parkinsonism is often present (up to 36 %) and in some cases may precede the onset of dystonia or can be the predominant or sole feature throughout the disease course [54, 75, 103]. Parkinsonism may improve with levodopa in the early stages but becomes less responsive or unresponsive over the course of the disease. Investigations in XPD patients show an abnormal DaTSCAN and a clearly abnormal IBZM SPECT, implying decreased dopamine D2 receptor expression. On positron emission tomography (PET), striatal glucose metabolism is selectively reduced. Fluorodopa uptake is normal, suggesting that the origin of the extrapyramidal symptoms is localized rather postsynaptically to the nigrostriatal pathway (see also Chap. 7) [196].

Dopa-Responsive Dystonias (DYT5; Segawa's Disease)

DYT5 was initially described by Segawa et al. in 1976 [178] and later by Nygaard and colleagues as dopa-responsive dystonia (DRD) because of the dramatic and sustained response to low dose of levodopa [132]. The disease is inherited as an autosomal dominant trait with reduced penetrance that appears to be gender dependent with females more frequently expressing symptoms. It is caused by mutations in the *GTPCH1* (GTP cyclohydrolase 1) gene [80]. *GTPCH1* is the rate-limiting enzyme in the synthesis of tetrahydrobiopterin, an essential cofactor for tyrosine hydroxylase (TH) which in turn is needed to synthesize dopamine, explaining the remarkable therapeutic effect of levodopa substitution. The typical phenotype includes childhood (average 6 years) limb-onset dystonia with diurnal variation (e.g., worsening of the symptoms as the day progresses), improvement after sleep, and dramatic response to levodopa [60, 193]. Later in the course of the disease, parkinsonian features occur frequently, and patients may also show typical, late-onset isolated parkinsonism, which responds well to levodopa therapy, but, unlike in idiopathic PD, patients usually do not develop motor fluctuations and dyskinesias [133], although this is not exclusive [41, 102]. Early-onset parkinsonism due to mutations in one of the recessive PARK genes (mostly Parkin) has to be considered in the differential diagnosis of a young patient presenting with prominent leg dystonia that is responsive to levodopa therapy. Early-onset DRD patients show normal DaTSCAN in contrast to patients with young-onset Parkinson's disease [28]. The latter concept has been recently challenged, by demonstrating that later-onset DRD cases presenting with PD may have abnormal DaTSCANs; thus, *GTPCH1* mutations may be risk factors to develop classic PD (see also Chap. 7) [123].

In a minority of cases, DRDs can also be inherited as an autosomal recessive disorder with mutations in the genes coding for other enzymes involved in dopamine synthesis including tyrosine hydroxylase (TH) [60, 113], sepiapterin reductase (SR), and aromatic L-amino acid decarboxylase (AADC) deficiency [3]. The clinical manifestations are often more severe and can include mental retardation, oculogyria, hypotonia, severe bradykinesia, drooling, ptosis, and seizures [189]. Recently it has been shown that TH patients may develop dyskinesias [148].

Hereditary Dopamine Transporter Deficiency Syndrome (DTDS)

Hereditary dopamine transporter deficiency syndrome (DTDS) is the first biogenic amine "transportopathy" to be described. It is an autosomal recessive condition leading to infantile parkinsonism– dystonia caused by pathogenic mutations in the *SLC6A3* gene encoding the dopamine transporter (DAT) [98], which mediates the active reuptake of dopamine and regulates the amplitude and duration of dopamine neurotransmission [98]. All children present with irritability, axial hypotonia, and feeding difficulties in infancy, with a hyperkinetic movement disorder that evolves into hypokinetic parkinsonism–dystonia. Ocular abnormalities included eye flutter, saccade initiation failure, slow saccadic eye movements, eyelid myoclonus, and oculogyric crises [98, 130, 131]. However, the phenotypic spectrum of this condition is expanding, with the first adults diagnosed with DTDS now recognized, and the condition is now considered as a differential for juvenile and early-onset parkinsonism [131]. Diagnosis can be based on CSF studies that show a raised ratio of HVA:5-HIAA >5 (normal range 1.3–4.0), a key finding in DTDS diagnosis [98]. The majority of patients are unresponsive to nearly all available therapeutic agents, including levodopa, anticholinergics, benzodiazepines, and deep brain stimulation [98, 120, 130].

Rapid-Onset Dystonia–Parkinsonism (DYT12)

Rapid-onset dystonia–parkinsonism is inherited as an autosomal dominant trait with reduced penetrance. Six heterozygous missense mutations have been identified in the Na^+, K^+-ATPase *ATP1A3* (alpha 3 subunit) gene, and all are shown to impair cell viability in cell culture experiments [30, 40, 101]. The disease phenotype designated rapid-onset dystonia–parkinsonism because of key clinical features including abrupt onset, within hours to weeks, of dystonia with signs of parkinsonism usually triggered by physical or emotional stress (fever, childbirth, running, alcohol binging). The age of onset varies from 4 to 58 years but typically presents in the teens or early twenties, and the distribution follows a rostrocaudal (face > arm > leg) gradient with prominent bulbar involvement. A presentation that could be more easily confused with PD has been recently described in a genetically proven patient with gradual onset at age 38 years of unilateral bradykinesia and rigidity, however, without improvement on levodopa therapy. This was followed by overnight onset of oromandibular dystonia 3.5 years after his first clinical presentation with parkinsonism (see also Chap. 7) [85].

Wilson's Disease

Wilson's disease (WD) is an autosomal recessive disorder with reduced biliary excretion of copper and impaired formation of ceruloplasmin, leading to copper accumulation in the liver, brain, kidney, and cornea. WD is caused by mutations in the *ATP7B* gene and usually manifests in the first decade of life, although late presentations have also been described [72, 74, 119]. Clinical manifestations include liver damage, psychiatric symptoms, and neurologic features. Juvenile and adult-onset parkinsonism are common features, which do not respond to levodopa, but respond well to specific WD treatment [33]. Evaluation should include serum and 24-h urine copper, serum ceruloplasmin, slit lamp examination looking for Kayser-Fleischer rings, free copper estimation, and if necessary, a liver biopsy [119]. Mutational analysis is labor intensive and is thus not used for screening purposes but confirms the exact mutation in patients with suspected Wilson's disease (see also Chap. 14).

Inborn Error of Manganese Metabolism

A recessive inborn error of manganese metabolism [205] due to mutations in the *SLC30A10* (solute carrier family 30, member 10) gene, encoding a manganese transporter, results in manganese accumulation mainly in the basal ganglia and cerebellum, and the liver, and causes a syndrome of early-onset generalized dystonia, cirrhosis, polycythemia, and hypermanganesemia [152, 205, 206]. Patients with parkinsonism–dystonia have also been described [44, 45, 152]. The metabolic signature of this disorder is the extreme hypermanganesemia with polycythemia and depleted iron stores (e.g., low ferritin, increased total iron-binding capacity), while laboratory findings reflecting hepatic dysfunction vary even between members of the same family [152, 205]. Manganese induces erythropoietin gene expression, and this could be the mechanism leading to polycythemia [52]. T1-weighted MRI images show hyperintensities in the basal ganglia and cerebellum [152, 191, 205]. As in Wilson's disease, manganese chelation treatment is helpful for both neurologic and systemic features (see also Chap. 14) [191].

Neurodegeneration with Brain Iron Accumulation (NBIA) Disorders

NBIA disorders cause complex dystonia–parkinsonism phenotypes and are discussed further in Chap. 13.

Atypical parkinsonism in Genes Predominantly Causing Chorea

Huntington's Disease

Huntington's disease (HD), an autosomal dominant disorder due to a trinucleotide CAG repeat expansion in the huntingtin gene (normal: 15–30 repeats; disease associated: >40 repeats), usually begins in adulthood and is characterized by cognitive decline and psychiatric, oculomotor, and motor abnormalities, usually with chorea as the most prominent feature [51, 88, 154]. The Westphal variant of HD is a distinct presentation characterized by a rigid-hypokinetic syndrome and is usually associated with young-onset age (<20 years) and accounts for 5–10 % of all HD cases. Juvenile HD is predominantly paternally inherited and associated with larger trinucleotide expansions in the range of 60–100 repeats, but may be as long as 250 trinucleotides [51, 170]. Clinically, juvenile HD often presents as an akinetic rigid disorder and may occur without concomitant choreic movements, and there may be supranuclear gaze palsy. Caudate volume loss on neuroimaging can be seen in both adult-onset and juvenile HD [154].

Neuroacanthocytosis

Neuroacanthocytosis may also present with parkinsonism (Table 3.1) (see also Chap. 8).

Other Genetic Disorders Causing Atypical Parkinsonism

Mitochondrial Disorders

Mitochondrial disorders may present with atypical parkinsonism and can be associated with specific point mutations, microdeletions, and also multiple mtDNA deletions due to, for example, polymerase gamma (*POLG*) mutations, which can be inherited in dominant or recessive mode [137]. PSP-like patients who presented in their sixties with parkinsonism, vertical SGP, and early cognitive dysfunction have been reported [68, 71]; associated features in these patients were deafness, ataxia, and lower motor neuron signs, which are absent in PSP [68, 71]. Of note, *POLG-related* parkinsonism can show an excellent response to levodopa, in contrast to sporadic PSP (see also Chap. 20) [137, 217].

Neurometabolic Disorders

In particular the adult-onset Niemann–Pick C (NPC1 and NPC2 gene mutations), an autosomal recessive lysosomal lipid storage disorder [81, 179], presents with vertical SGP, cerebellar ataxia, dysarthria, dysphagia, cognitive dysfunction, and psychiatric symptoms and should be thought in the differential of patients with a PSP-like phenotype [179]. Biochemical diagnosis of Niemann–Pick C is made by filipin staining of cultured skin fibroblasts, with subsequent confirmation of the diagnosis made by mutation analysis of the *NPC1* (the majority) and *NPC2* genes [1, 219]. Miglustat is the only approved treatment for the neurologic manifestations of the disease, and patients who begin treatment early respond better, highlighting the need for early diagnosis [1, 143, 219, 220].

In the adult-onset form of Gaucher's disease, patients usually have slow *horizontal* saccades and increased latency launching horizontal saccades [16], which is usual in CBD [162], but not in PSP [11], in which the saccadic latency is normal and vertical saccades are more and earlier affected than horizontal, particularly downwards. However, some Gaucher's disease patients with prominent slowness of vertical saccades and cognitive dysfunction, mimicking PSP, have been reported [62, 63, 122, 200, 201, 210]. Other neurologic features such as head thrusting (55 %), ataxia (20 %), seizures (16 %), and spasticity (15 %), which are not seen in PSP, provide important clues [8, 43, 67, 200, 201, 210]. Systemic associated features such as splenomegaly, hepatomegaly, bone crisis, bone pain, anemia, and thrombocytopenia are helpful diagnostic clues [200, 201, 210].

Prion Disease

Genetic Creutzfeldt–Jakob disease (gCJD) has been linked to a variety of mutations within the prion protein gene (*PRNP*). Patients with disease onset between their fifth and seventh decade, vertical SGP, "worried facial appearance," postural instability, axial rigidity, and frontal dementia mimicking PSP have been described in gCJD, mostly with the E200K but rarely also with further mutations and in sporadic CJD [20, 21, 95, 121, 171, 182]. These patients often have cerebellar and pyramidal signs as well as myoclonus, and the rapidity of evolution is helpful to suspect the disorder.

Atypical Parkinsonism with White Matter Changes

The combination of parkinsonism with leukoencephalopathy should prompt to test for colony-stimulating factor 1 (*CSF1R*) mutations, causing leukoencephalopathy with axonal spheroids [90, 124, 150, 158, 195]. Also in CADASIL due to *NOTCH3* mutations, atypical parkinsonism has been described [159]. Mitochondrial disorders may also present with white matter changes in MRI.

Conclusion

The advent in genetics has changed the field of atypical parkinsonism. With regard to the sporadic conditions, PSP, CBD, and MSA, genetic susceptibility loci and rare mutations in relevant genes causing familial forms may provide important clues for the pathophysiology of these disorders. On the other hand, the list of genetic disorders causing young-onset atypical parkinsonism with various features is growing, and syndromic associations are important to suspect these. In some cases, this is quite important due to treatment implications.

References

1. Abel LA, Walterfang M, Fietz M, Bowman EA, Velakoulis D. Saccades in adult Niemann-Pick disease type C reflect frontal, brainstem, and biochemical deficits. Neurology. 2009;72: 1083–6.
2. Abele M, Burk K, Schols L, Schwartz S, Besenthal I, Dichgans J, Zuhlke C, Riess O, Klockgether T. The aetiology of sporadic adult-onset ataxia. Brain. 2002;125:961–8.
3. Abeling NG, Duran M, Bakker HD, Stroomer L, Thony B, Blau N, Booij J, Poll-The BT. Sepiapterin reductase deficiency an autosomal recessive DOPA-responsive dystonia. Mol Genet Metab. 2006;89:116–20.
4. Ahmed Z, Asi YT, Sailer A, Lees AJ, Houlden H, Revesz T, Holton JL. The neuropathology, pathophysiology and genetics of multiple system atrophy. Neuropathol Appl Neurobiol. 2012;38:4–24.
5. Al-Chalabi A, Durr A, Wood NW, Parkinson MH, Camuzat A, Hulot JS, Morrison KE, Renton A, Sussmuth SD, Landwehrmeyer BG, Ludolph A, Agid Y, Brice A, Leigh PN, Bensimon G. Genetic variants of the alpha-synuclein gene SNCA are associated with multiple system atrophy. PLoS One. 2009;4:e7114.
6. Alberici A, Cosseddu M, Padovani A, Borroni B. Chromosome 17 in FTLD: from MAPT tau to progranulin and back. Curr Alzheimer Res. 2011;8:229–36.
7. Alladi S, Xuereb J, Bak T, Nestor P, Knibb J, Patterson K, Hodges JR. Focal cortical presentations of Alzheimer's disease. Brain. 2007;130:2636–45.
8. Alonso-Canovas A, Katschnig P, Tucci A, Carecchio M, Wood NW, Edwards M, Martinez Castrillo JC, Burke D, Heales S, Bhatia KP. Atypical parkinsonism with apraxia and supranuclear gaze abnormalities in type 1 Gaucher disease. Expanding the spectrum: case report and literature review. Mov Disord. 2010;25:1506–9.
9. Apartis E, Blancher A, Meissner WG, Guyant-Marechal L, Maltete D, De Broucker T, Legrand AP, Bouzenada H, Thanh HT, Sallansonnet-Froment M, Wang A, Tison F, Roue-Jagot C, Sedel F, Charles P, Whalen S, Heron D, Thobois S, Poisson A, Lesca G, Ouvrard-Hernandez AM, Fraix V, Palfi S, Habert MO, Gaymard B, Dussaule JC, Pollak P, Vidailhet M, Durr A, Barbot JC, Gourlet V, Brice A, Anheim M. FXTAS: new insights and the need for revised diagnostic criteria. Neurology. 2012;79:1898–907.
10. Armstrong MJ, Litvan I, Lang AE, Bak TH, Bhatia KP, Borroni B, Boxer AL, Dickson DW, Grossman M, Hallett M, Josephs KA, Kertesz A, Lee SE, Miller BL, Reich SG, Riley DE, Tolosa E, Troster AI, Vidailhet M, Weiner WJ. Criteria for the diagnosis of corticobasal degeneration. Neurology. 2013;80:496–503.
11. Armstrong RA. Visual signs and symptoms of progressive supranuclear palsy. Clin Exp Optom. 2011;94:150–60.
12. Baba Y, Uitti RJ. Fragile X-associated tremor/ataxia syndrome and movements disorders. Curr Opin Neurol. 2005;18:393–8.
13. Batla A, Stamelou M, Mensikova K, Kaiserova M, Tuckova L, Kanovsky P, Quinn N, Bhatia KP. Markedly asymmetric presentation in multiple system atrophy. Parkinsonism Relat Disord. 2013;19:901–5.
14. Beck J, Rohrer JD, Campbell T, Isaacs A, Morrison KE, Goodall EF, Warrington EK, Stevens J, Revesz T, Holton J, Al-Sarraj S, King A, Scahill R, Warren JD, Fox NC, Rossor MN, Collinge J, Mead S. A distinct clinical, neuropsychological and radiological phenotype is associated with progranulin gene mutations in a large UK series. Brain. 2008;131:706–20.
15. Behrens MI, Bruggemann N, Chana P, Venegas P, Kagi M, Parrao T, Orellana P, Garrido C, Rojas CV, Hauke J, Hahnen E, Gonzalez R, Seleme N, Fernandez V, Schmidt A, Binkofski F, Kompf D, Kubisch C, Hagenah J, Klein C, Ramirez A. Clinical spectrum of Kufor-Rakeb syndrome in the Chilean kindred with ATP13A2 mutations. Mov Disord. 2010;25:1929–37.

16. Benko W, Ries M, Wiggs EA, Brady RO, Schiffmann R, Fitzgibbon EJ. The saccadic and neurological deficits in type 3 Gaucher disease. PLoS One. 2011;6:e22410.
17. Benussi L, Binetti G, Sina E, Gigola L, Bettecken T, Meitinger T, Ghidoni R. A novel deletion in progranulin gene is associated with FTDP-17 and CBS. Neurobiol Aging. 2008;29: 427–35.
18. Benussi L, Ghidoni R, Pegoiani E, Moretti DV, Zanetti O, Binetti G. Progranulin Leu271LeufsX10 is one of the most common FTLD and CBS associated mutations worldwide. Neurobiol Dis. 2009;33:379–85.
19. Berry-Kravis E, Abrams L, Coffey SM, Hall DA, Greco C, Gane LW, Grigsby J, Bourgeois JA, Finucane B, Jacquemont S, Brunberg JA, Zhang L, Lin J, Tassone F, Hagerman PJ, Hagerman RJ, Leehey MA. Fragile X-associated tremor/ataxia syndrome: clinical features, genetics, and testing guidelines. Mov Disord. 2007;22:2018–30, quiz 2140.
20. Bertoni JM, Brown P, Goldfarb LG, Rubenstein R, Gajdusek DC. Familial Creutzfeldt-Jakob disease (codon 200 mutation) with supranuclear palsy. JAMA. 1992;268:2413–5.
21. Bertoni JM, Label LS, Sackelleres JC, Hicks SP. Supranuclear gaze palsy in familial Creutzfeldt-Jakob disease. Arch Neurol. 1983;40:618–22.
22. Bhatia KP, Daniel SE, Marsden CD. Familial parkinsonism with depression: a clinicopathological study. Ann Neurol. 1993;34:842–7.
23. Boeve BF. Links between frontotemporal lobar degeneration, corticobasal degeneration, progressive supranuclear palsy, and amyotrophic lateral sclerosis. Alzheimer Dis Assoc Disord. 2007;21:S31–8.
24. Boeve BF, Baker M, Dickson DW, Parisi JE, Giannini C, Josephs KA, Hutton M, Pickering-Brown SM, Rademakers R, Tang-Wai D, Jack Jr CR, Kantarci K, Shiung MM, Golde T, Smith GE, Geda YE, Knopman DS, Petersen RC. Frontotemporal dementia and parkinsonism associated with the IVS1+1G->A mutation in progranulin: a clinicopathologic study. Brain. 2006;129:3103–14.
25. Boeve BF, Boylan KB, Graff-Radford NR, Dejesus-Hernandez M, Knopman DS, Pedraza O, Vemuri P, Jones D, Lowe V, Murray ME, Dickson DW, Josephs KA, Rush BK, Machulda MM, Fields JA, Ferman TJ, Baker M, Rutherford NJ, Adamson J, Wszolek ZK, Adeli A, Savica R, Boot B, Kuntz KM, Gavrilova R, Reeves A, Whitwell J, Kantarci K, Jack Jr CR, Parisi JE, Lucas JA, Petersen RC, Rademakers R. Characterization of frontotemporal dementia and/or amyotrophic lateral sclerosis associated with the GGGGCC repeat expansion in C9ORF72. Brain. 2012;135:765–83.
26. Boeve BF, Hutton M. Refining frontotemporal dementia with parkinsonism linked to chromosome 17: introducing FTDP-17 (MAPT) and FTDP-17 (PGRN). Arch Neurol. 2008;65:460–4.
27. Boxer AL, Garbutt S, Seeley WW, Jafari A, Heuer HW, Mirsky J, Hellmuth J, Trojanowski JQ, Huang E, DeArmond S, Neuhaus J, Miller BL. Saccade abnormalities in autopsy-confirmed frontotemporal lobar degeneration and Alzheimer disease. Arch Neurol. 2012;69: 509–17.
28. Brajkovic LD, Svetel MV, Kostic VS, Sobic-Saranovic DP, Pavlovic SV, Artiko VM, Obradovic VB. Dopamine transporter imaging (123)I-FP-CIT (DaTSCAN) SPET in differential diagnosis of dopa-responsive dystonia and young-onset Parkinson's disease. Hell J Nucl Med. 2012;15:134–8.
29. Bras J, Verloes A, Schneider SA, Mole SE, Guerreiro RJ. Mutation of the parkinsonism gene ATP13A2 causes neuronal ceroid-lipofuscinosis. Hum Mol Genet. 2012;21:2646–50.
30. Brashear A, Dobyns WB, de Carvalho Aguiar P, Borg M, Frijns CJ, Gollamudi S, Green A, Guimaraes J, Haake BC, Klein C, Linazasoro G, Munchau A, Raymond D, Riley D, Saunders-Pullman R, Tijssen MA, Webb D, Zaremba J, Bressman SB, Ozelius LJ. The phenotypic spectrum of rapid-onset dystonia-parkinsonism (RDP) and mutations in the ATP1A3 gene. Brain. 2007;130:828–35.
31. Bugiani O, Murrell JR, Giaccone G, Hasegawa M, Ghigo G, Tabaton M, Morbin M, Primavera A, Carella F, Solaro C, Grisoli M, Savoiardo M, Spillantini MG, Tagliavini F, Goedert M, Ghetti B. Frontotemporal dementia and corticobasal degeneration in a family with a P301S mutation in tau. J Neuropathol Exp Neurol. 1999;58:667–77.

32. Casseron W, Azulay JP, Guedj E, Gastaut JL, Pouget J. Familial autosomal dominant corticobasal degeneration with the P301S mutation in the tau gene: an example of phenotype variability. J Neurol. 2005;252:1546–8.
33. Chan KH, Cheung RT, Au-Yeung KM, Mak W, Cheng TS, Ho SL. Wilson's disease with depression and parkinsonism. J Clin Neurosci. 2005;12:303–5.
34. Chen-Plotkin AS, Lee VM, Trojanowski JQ. TAR DNA-binding protein 43 in neurodegenerative disease. Nat Rev Neurol. 2010;6:211–20.
35. Chen-Plotkin AS, Martinez-Lage M, Sleiman PM, Hu W, Greene R, Wood EM, Bing S, Grossman M, Schellenberg GD, Hatanpaa KJ, Weiner MF, White 3rd CL, Brooks WS, Halliday GM, Kril JJ, Gearing M, Beach TG, Graff-Radford NR, Dickson DW, Rademakers R, Boeve BF, Pickering-Brown SM, Snowden J, van Swieten JC, Heutink P, Seelaar H, Murrell JR, Ghetti B, Spina S, Grafman J, Kaye JA, Woltjer RL, Mesulam M, Bigio E, Llado A, Miller BL, Alzualde A, Moreno F, Rohrer JD, Mackenzie IR, Feldman HH, Hamilton RL, Cruts M, Engelborghs S, De Deyn PP, Van Broeckhoven C, Bird TD, Cairns NJ, Goate A, Frosch MP, Riederer PF, Bogdanovic N, Lee VM, Trojanowski JQ, Van Deerlin VM. Genetic and clinical features of progranulin-associated frontotemporal lobar degeneration. Arch Neurol. 2011;68:488–97.
36. Chen-Plotkin AS, Xiao J, Geser F, Martinez-Lage M, Grossman M, Unger T, Wood EM, Van Deerlin VM, Trojanowski JQ, Lee VM. Brain progranulin expression in GRN-associated frontotemporal lobar degeneration. Acta Neuropathol. 2010;119:111–22.
37. Chio A, Borghero G, Restagno G, Mora G, Drepper C, Traynor BJ, Sendtner M, Brunetti M, Ossola I, Calvo A, Pugliatti M, Sotgiu MA, Murru MR, Marrosu MG, Marrosu F, Marinou K, Mandrioli J, Sola P, Caponnetto C, Mancardi G, Mandich P, La Bella V, Spataro R, Conte A, Monsurro MR, Tedeschi G, Pisano F, Bartolomei I, Salvi F, Lauria Pinter G, Simone I, Logroscino G, Gambardella A, Quattrone A, Lunetta C, Volanti P, Zollino M, Penco S, Battistini S, Renton AE, Majounie E, Abramzon Y, Conforti FL, Giannini F, Corbo M, Sabatelli M. Clinical characteristics of patients with familial amyotrophic lateral sclerosis carrying the pathogenic GGGGCC hexanucleotide repeat expansion of C9ORF72. Brain. 2012;135:784–93.
38. Cooper-Knock J, Hewitt C, Highley JR, Brockington A, Milano A, Man S, Martindale J, Hartley J, Walsh T, Gelsthorpe C, Baxter L, Forster G, Fox M, Bury J, Mok K, McDermott CJ, Traynor BJ, Kirby J, Wharton SB, Ince PG, Hardy J, Shaw PJ. Clinico-pathological features in amyotrophic lateral sclerosis with expansions in C9ORF72. Brain. 2012;135:751–64.
39. Cremona O, Nimmakayalu M, Haffner C, Bray-Ward P, Ward DC, De Camilli P. Assignment of SYNJ1 to human chromosome 21q22.2 and Synj12 to the murine homologous region on chromosome 16C3-4 by in situ hybridization. Cytogenet Cell Genet. 2000;88:89–90.
40. de Carvalho Aguiar P, Sweadner KJ, Penniston JT, Zaremba J, Liu L, Caton M, Linazasoro G, Borg M, Tijssen MA, Bressman SB, Dobyns WB, Brashear A, Ozelius LJ. Mutations in the Na+/K+ –ATPase alpha3 gene ATP1A3 are associated with rapid-onset dystonia parkinsonism. Neuron. 2004;43:169–75.
41. de la Fuente-Fernandez R. Drug-induced motor complications in dopa-responsive dystonia: implications for the pathogenesis of dyskinesias and motor fluctuations. Clin Neuropharmacol. 1999;22:216–9.
42. Degardin A, Dobbelaere D, Vuillaume I, Defoort-Dhellemmes S, Hurtevent JF, Sablonniere B, Destee A, Defebvre L, Devos D. Spinocerebellar ataxia: a rational approach to aetiological diagnosis. Cerebellum. 2012;11:289–99.
43. DePaolo J, Goker-Alpan O, Samaddar T, Lopez G, Sidransky E. The association between mutations in the lysosomal protein glucocerebrosidase and parkinsonism. Mov Disord. 2009;24:1571–8.
44. DeWitt MR, Chen P, Aschner M. Manganese efflux in Parkinsonism: insights from newly characterized SLC30A10 mutations. Biochem Biophys Res Commun. 2013;432:1–4.
45. Di Toro Mammarella L, Mignarri A, Battisti C, Monti L, Bonifati V, Rasi F, Federico A. Two-year follow-up after chelating therapy in a patient with adult-onset parkinsonism and hypermanganesaemia due to SLC30A10 mutations. J Neurol. 2014;261:227–8.

46. Dickson DW, Ahmed Z, Algom AA, Tsuboi Y, Josephs KA. Neuropathology of variants of progressive supranuclear palsy. Curr Opin Neurol. 2010;23:394–400.
47. Dickson DW, Lin W, Liu WK, Yen SH. Multiple system atrophy: a sporadic synucleinopathy. Brain Pathol. 1999;9:721–32.
48. Djarmati A, Hagenah J, Reetz K, Winkler S, Behrens MI, Pawlack H, Lohmann K, Ramirez A, Tadic V, Bruggemann N, Berg D, Siebner HR, Lang AE, Pramstaller PP, Binkofski F, Kostic VS, Volkmann J, Gasser T, Klein C. ATP13A2 variants in early-onset Parkinson's disease patients and controls. Mov Disord. 2009;24:2104–11.
49. Dopper EG, Seelaar H, Chiu WZ, de Koning I, van Minkelen R, Baker MC, Rozemuller AJ, Rademakers R, van Swieten JC. Symmetrical corticobasal syndrome caused by a novel C.314dup progranulin mutation. J Mol Neurosci. 2011;45:354–8.
50. Doran M, du Plessis DG, Enevoldson TP, Fletcher NA, Ghadiali E, Larner AJ. Pathological heterogeneity of clinically diagnosed corticobasal degeneration. J Neurol Sci. 2003;216:127–34.
51. Douglas I, Evans S, Rawlins MD, Smeeth L, Tabrizi SJ, Wexler NS. Juvenile Huntington's disease: a population-based study using the General Practice Research Database. BMJ Open. 2013;3.
52. Ebert BL, Bunn HF. Regulation of the erythropoietin gene. Blood. 1999;94:1864–77.
53. Edvardson S, Cinnamon Y, Ta-Shma A, Shaag A, Yim YI, Zenvirt S, Jalas C, Lesage S, Brice A, Taraboulos A, Kaestner KH, Greene LE, Elpeleg O. A deleterious mutation in DNAJC6 encoding the neuronal-specific clathrin-uncoating co-chaperone auxilin, is associated with juvenile parkinsonism. PLoS One. 2012;7:e36458.
54. Evidente VG, Nolte D, Niemann S, Advincula J, Mayo MC, Natividad FF, Muller U. Phenotypic and molecular analyses of X-linked dystonia-parkinsonism ("lubag") in women. Arch Neurol. 2004;61:1956–9.
55. Farrer MJ, Hulihan MM, Kachergus JM, Dachsel JC, Stoessl AJ, Grantier LL, Calne S, Calne DB, Lechevalier B, Chapon F, Tsuboi Y, Yamada T, Gutmann L, Elibol B, Bhatia KP, Wider C, Vilarino-Guell C, Ross OA, Brown LA, Castanedes-Casey M, Dickson DW, Wszolek ZK. DCTN1 mutations in Perry syndrome. Nat Genet. 2009;41:163–5.
56. Ferguson MC, Garland EM, Hedges L, Womack-Nunley B, Hamid R, Phillips 3rd JA, Shibao CA, Raj SR, Biaggioni I, Robertson D. SHC2 gene copy number in multiple system atrophy (MSA). Clin Auton Res. 2014;24:25–30.
57. Ferrari R, Ryten M, Simone R, Trabzuni D, Nicolaou N, Hondhamuni G, Ramasamy A, Vandrovcova J, Weale ME, Lees AJ, Momeni P, Hardy J, de Silva R. Assessment of common variability and expression quantitative trait loci for genome-wide associations for progressive supranuclear palsy. Neurobiol Aging. 2014;35(1514):e1511–2.
58. Finch N, Baker M, Crook R, Swanson K, Kuntz K, Surtees R, Bisceglio G, Rovelet-Lecrux A, Boeve B, Petersen RC, Dickson DW, Younkin SG, Deramecourt V, Crook J, Graff-Radford NR, Rademakers R. Plasma progranulin levels predict progranulin mutation status in frontotemporal dementia patients and asymptomatic family members. Brain. 2009;132:583–91.
59. Furtado S, Payami H, Lockhart PJ, Hanson M, Nutt JG, Singleton AA, Singleton A, Bower J, Utti RJ, Bird TD, de la Fuente-Fernandez R, Tsuboi Y, Klimek ML, Suchowersky O, Hardy J, Calne DB, Wszolek ZK, Farrer M, Gwinn-Hardy K, Stoessl AJ. Profile of families with parkinsonism-predominant spinocerebellar ataxia type 2 (SCA2). Mov Disord. 2004;19: 622–9.
60. Furukawa Y, Graf WD, Wong H, Shimadzu M, Kish SJ. Dopa-responsive dystonia simulating spastic paraplegia due to tyrosine hydroxylase (TH) gene mutations. Neurology. 2001;56:260–3.
61. Gallo M, Marcello N, Curcio SA, Colao R, Geracitano S, Bernardi L, Anfossi M, Puccio G, Frangipane F, Clodomiro A, Mirabelli M, Vasso F, Smirne N, Muraca G, Di Lorenzo R, Maletta R, Ghidoni E, Bugiani O, Tagliavini F, Giaccone G, Bruni AC. A novel pathogenic PSEN1 mutation in a family with Alzheimer's disease: phenotypical and neuropathological features. J Alzheimers Dis. 2011;25:425–31.
62. Goker-Alpan O, Lopez G, Vithayathil J, Davis J, Hallett M, Sidransky E. The spectrum of parkinsonian manifestations associated with glucocerebrosidase mutations. Arch Neurol. 2008;65:1353–7.

63. Goker-Alpan O, Schiffmann R, LaMarca ME, Nussbaum RL, McInerney-Leo A, Sidransky E. Parkinsonism among Gaucher disease carriers. J Med Genet. 2004;41:937–40.
64. Goldman JS, Rademakers R, Huey ED, Boxer AL, Mayeux R, Miller BL, Boeve BF. An algorithm for genetic testing of frontotemporal lobar degeneration. Neurology. 2011;76:475–83.
65. Greco CM, Berman RF, Martin RM, Tassone F, Schwartz PH, Chang A, Trapp BD, Iwahashi C, Brunberg J, Grigsby J, Hessl D, Becker EJ, Papazian J, Leehey MA, Hagerman RJ, Hagerman PJ. Neuropathology of fragile X-associated tremor/ataxia syndrome (FXTAS). Brain. 2006;129:243–55.
66. Guerreiro RJ, Santana I, Bras JM, Revesz T, Rebelo O, Ribeiro MH, Santiago B, Oliveira CR, Singleton A, Hardy J. Novel progranulin mutation: screening for PGRN mutations in a Portuguese series of FTD/CBS cases. Mov Disord. 2008;23:1269–73.
67. Guimaraes J, Amaral O, Sa Miranda MC. Adult-onset neuronopathic form of Gaucher's disease: a case report. Parkinsonism Relat Disord. 2003;9:261–4.
68. Gupta SR, Brigell M, Gujrati M, Lee JM. Supranuclear eye movement dysfunction in mitochondrial myopathy with tRNA(LEU) mutation. J Neuroophthalmol. 1995;15:20–5.
69. Gwinn-Hardy K, Chen JY, Liu HC, Liu TY, Boss M, Seltzer W, Adam A, Singleton A, Koroshetz W, Waters C, Hardy J, Farrer M. Spinocerebellar ataxia type 2 with parkinsonism in ethnic Chinese. Neurology. 2000;55:800–5.
70. Hagerman RJ, Hall DA, Coffey S, Leehey M, Bourgeois J, Gould J, Zhang L, Seritan A, Berry-Kravis E, Olichney J, Miller JW, Fong AL, Carpenter R, Bodine C, Gane LW, Rainin E, Hagerman H, Hagerman PJ. Treatment of fragile X-associated tremor ataxia syndrome (FXTAS) and related neurological problems. Clin Interv Aging. 2008;3:251–62.
71. Hara K, Yamamoto M, Anegawa T, Sakuta R, Nakamura M. Mitochondrial encephalomyopathy associated with parkinsonism and a point mutation in the mitochondrial tRNA(Leu)(UUR)) gene. Rinsho Shinkeigaku. 1994;34:361–5.
72. Hassan A, Masood F. Wilson's disease: a review. JPMA J Pak Med Assoc. 2004;54:479–84.
73. Hassan A, Whitwell JL, Josephs KA. The corticobasal syndrome-Alzheimer's disease conundrum. Expert Rev Neurother. 2011;11:1569–78.
74. Heller GL. Wilson's disease (hepato-lenticular degeneration): a brief review. Psychiatry Dig. 1965;26:33–9.
75. Herzfeld T, Nolte D, Grznarova M, Hofmann A, Schultze JL, Muller U. X-linked dystonia parkinsonism syndrome (XDP, lubag): disease-specific sequence change DSC3 in TAF1/DYT3 affects genes in vesicular transport and dopamine metabolism. Hum Mol Genet. 2013;22:941–51.
76. Hodges J. Familial frontotemporal dementia and amyotrophic lateral sclerosis associated with the C9ORF72 hexanucleotide repeat. Brain. 2012;135:652–5.
77. Hoglinger GU, Huppertz HJ, Wagenpfeil S, Andres MV, Belloch V, Leon T, Del Ser T. Tideglusib reduces progression of brain atrophy in progressive supranuclear palsy in a randomized trial. Mov Disord. 2014;29:479–87.
78. Hoglinger GU, Melhem NM, Dickson DW, Sleiman PM, Wang LS, Klei L, Rademakers R, de Silva R, Litvan I, Riley DE, van Swieten JC, Heutink P, Wszolek ZK, Uitti RJ, Vandrovcova J, Hurtig HI, Gross RG, Maetzler W, Goldwurm S, Tolosa E, Borroni B, Pastor P, Cantwell LB, Han MR, Dillman A, van der Brug MP, Gibbs JR, Cookson MR, Hernandez DG, Singleton AB, Farrer MJ, Yu CE, Golbe LI, Revesz T, Hardy J, Lees AJ, Devlin B, Hakonarson H, Muller U, Schellenberg GD. Identification of common variants influencing risk of the tauopathy progressive supranuclear palsy. Nat Genet. 2011;43:699–705.
79. Houlden H, Baker M, Morris HR, MacDonald N, Pickering-Brown S, Adamson J, Lees AJ, Rossor MN, Quinn NP, Kertesz A, Khan MN, Hardy J, Lantos PL, St George-Hyslop P, Munoz DG, Mann D, Lang AE, Bergeron C, Bigio EH, Litvan I, Bhatia KP, Dickson D, Wood NW, Hutton M. Corticobasal degeneration and progressive supranuclear palsy share a common tau haplotype. Neurology. 2001;56:1702–6.
80. Ichinose H, Ohye T, Takahashi E, Seki N, Hori T, Segawa M, Nomura Y, Endo K, Tanaka H, Tsuji S, et al. Hereditary progressive dystonia with marked diurnal fluctuation caused by mutations in the GTP cyclohydrolase I gene. Nat Genet. 1994;8:236–42.

81. Imrie J, Dasgupta S, Besley GT, Harris C, Heptinstall L, Knight S, Vanier MT, Fensom AH, Ward C, Jacklin E, Whitehouse C, Wraith JE. The natural history of Niemann-Pick disease type C in the UK. J Inherit Metab Dis. 2007;30:51–9.
82. Jesus S, Gomez-Garre P, Carrillo F, Caceres-Redondo MT, Huertas-Fernandez I, Bernal-Bernal I, Bonilla-Toribio M, Vargas-Gonzalez L, Carballo M, Mir P. Analysis of c.801-2A>G mutation in the DNAJC6 gene in Parkinson's disease in southern Spain. Parkinsonism Relat Disord. 2014;20:248–9.
83. Josephs KA, Whitwell JL, Boeve BF, Knopman DS, Petersen RC, Hu WT, Parisi JE, Dickson DW, Jack Jr CR. Anatomical differences between CBS-corticobasal degeneration and CBS-Alzheimer's disease. Mov Disord. 2010;25:1246–52.
84. Kamm C, Healy DG, Quinn NP, Wullner U, Moller JC, Schols L, Geser F, Burk K, Borglum AD, Pellecchia MT, Tolosa E, del Sorbo F, Nilsson C, Bandmann O, Sharma M, Mayer P, Gasteiger M, Haworth A, Ozawa T, Lees AJ, Short J, Giunti P, Holinski-Feder E, Illig T, Wichmann HE, Wenning GK, Wood NW, Gasser T, European Multiple System Atrophy Study Group. The fragile X tremor ataxia syndrome in the differential diagnosis of multiple system atrophy: data from the EMSA Study Group. Brain. 2005;128:1855–60.
85. Kamphuis DJ, Koelman H, Lees AJ, Tijssen MA. Sporadic rapid-onset dystonia-parkinsonism presenting as Parkinson's disease. Mov Disord. 2006;21:118–9.
86. Kang J, Chung KC. The F-box protein FBXO7 positively regulates bone morphogenetic protein-mediated signaling through Lys-63-specific ubiquitination of neurotrophin receptor-interacting MAGE (NRAGE). Cell Mol Life Sci. 2015;72(1):181–95.
87. Kelley BJ, Haidar W, Boeve BF, Baker M, Graff-Radford NR, Krefft T, Frank AR, Jack Jr CR, Shiung M, Knopman DS, Josephs KA, Parashos SA, Rademakers R, Hutton M, Pickering-Brown S, Adamson J, Kuntz KM, Dickson DW, Parisi JE, Smith GE, Ivnik RJ, Petersen RC. Prominent phenotypic variability associated with mutations in Progranulin. Neurobiol Aging. 2009;30:739–51.
88. Kiferle L, Mazzucchi S, Unti E, Pesaresi I, Fabbri S, Nicoletti V, Volterrani D, Cosottini M, Bonuccelli U, Ceravolo R. Nigral involvement and nigrostriatal dysfunction in Huntington's disease: evidences from an MRI and SPECT study. Parkinsonism Relat Disord. 2013;19:800–5.
89. Kim JY, Kim SY, Kim JM, Kim YK, Yoon KY, Lee BC, Kim JS, Paek SH, Park SS, Kim SE, Jeon BS. Spinocerebellar ataxia type 17 mutation as a causative and susceptibility gene in parkinsonism. Neurology. 2009;72:1385–9.
90. Kinoshita M, Yoshida K, Oyanagi K, Hashimoto T, Ikeda S. Hereditary diffuse leukoencephalopathy with axonal spheroids caused by R782H mutation in CSF1R: case report. J Neurol Sci. 2012;318:115–8.
91. Knake S, Belke M, Menzler K, Pilatus U, Eggert KM, Oertel WH, Stamelou M, Hoglinger GU. In vivo demonstration of microstructural brain pathology in progressive supranuclear palsy: a DTI study using TBSS. Mov Disord. 2010;25:1232–8.
92. Koroglu C, Baysal L, Cetinkaya M, Karasoy H, Tolun A. DNAJC6 is responsible for juvenile parkinsonism with phenotypic variability. Parkinsonism Relat Disord. 2013;19:320–4.
93. Kouri N, Carlomagno Y, Baker M, Liesinger AM, Caselli RJ, Wszolek ZK, Petrucelli L, Boeve BF, Parisi JE, Josephs KA, Uitti RJ, Ross OA, Graff-Radford NR, DeTure MA, Dickson DW, Rademakers R. Novel mutation in MAPT exon 13 (p.N410H) causes corticobasal degeneration. Acta Neuropathol. 2014;127:271–82.
94. Kouri N, Murray ME, Hassan A, Rademakers R, Uitti RJ, Boeve BF, Graff-Radford NR, Wszolek ZK, Litvan I, Josephs KA, Dickson DW. Neuropathological features of corticobasal degeneration presenting as corticobasal syndrome or Richardson syndrome. Brain. 2011; 134:3264–75.
95. Kovacs GG, Seguin J, Quadrio I, Hoftberger R, Kapas I, Streichenberger N, Biacabe AG, Meyronet D, Sciot R, Vandenberghe R, Majtenyi K, Laszlo L, Strobel T, Budka H, Perret-Liaudet A. Genetic Creutzfeldt-Jakob disease associated with the E200K mutation: characterization of a complex proteinopathy. Acta Neuropathol. 2011;121:39–57.
96. Koyama Y, Asahina M, Honma K, Arai K, Hattori T. Altered heart rate control in response to postural change in patients with Machado-Joseph disease (SCA3). Cerebellum. 2009;8:130–6.

97. Krebs CE, Karkheiran S, Powell JC, Cao M, Makarov V, Darvish H, Di Paolo G, Walker RH, Shahidi GA, Buxbaum JD, De Camilli P, Yue Z, Paisan-Ruiz C. The Sac1 domain of SYNJ1 identified mutated in a family with early-onset progressive Parkinsonism with generalized seizures. Hum Mutat. 2013;34:1200–7.
98. Kurian MA, Li Y, Zhen J, Meyer E, Hai N, Christen HJ, Hoffmann GF, Jardine P, von Moers A, Mordekar SR, O'Callaghan F, Wassmer E, Wraige E, Dietrich C, Lewis T, Hyland K, Heales Jr S, Sanger T, Gissen P, Assmann BE, Reith ME, Maher ER. Clinical and molecular characterisation of hereditary dopamine transporter deficiency syndrome: an observational cohort and experimental study. Lancet Neurol. 2011;10:54–62.
99. Larner AJ, Doran M. Clinical phenotypic heterogeneity of Alzheimer's disease associated with mutations of the presenilin-1 gene. J Neurol. 2006;253:139–58.
100. Lechevalier B, Schupp C, Fallet-Bianco C, Viader F, Eustache F, Chapon F, Morin P. Familial parkinsonian syndrome with athymhormia and hypoventilation. Rev Neurol. 1992;148:39–46.
101. Lee JY, Gollamudi S, Ozelius LJ, Kim JY, Jeon BS. ATP1A3 mutation in the first Asian case of rapid-onset dystonia-parkinsonism. Mov Disord. 2007;22:1808–9.
102. Lee JY, Yang HJ, Kim JM, Jeon BS. Novel GCH-1 mutations and unusual long-lasting dyskinesias in Korean families with dopa-responsive dystonia. Parkinsonism Relat Disord. 2013;19:1156–9.
103. Lee LV, Rivera C, Teleg RA, Dantes MB, Pasco PM, Jamora RD, Arancillo J, Villareal-Jordan RF, Rosales RL, Demaisip C, Maranon E, Peralta O, Borres R, Tolentino C, Monding MJ, Sarcia S. The unique phenomenology of sex-linked dystonia parkinsonism (XDP, DYT3, "Lubag"). Int J Neurosci. 2011;121 Suppl 1:3–11.
104. Lee SE, Rabinovici GD, Mayo MC, Wilson SM, Seeley WW, DeArmond SJ, Huang EJ, Trojanowski JQ, Growdon ME, Jang JY, Sidhu M, See TM, Karydas AM, Gorno-Tempini ML, Boxer AL, Weiner MW, Geschwind MD, Rankin KP, Miller BL. Clinicopathological correlations in corticobasal degeneration. Ann Neurol. 2011;70:327–40.
105. Li Y, Chen JA, Sears RL, Gao F, Klein ED, Karydas A, Geschwind MD, Rosen HJ, Boxer AL, Guo W, Pellegrini M, Horvath S, Miller BL, Geschwind DH, Coppola G. An epigenetic signature in peripheral blood associated with the haplotype on 17q21.31, a risk factor for neurodegenerative tauopathy. PLoS Genet. 2014;10:e1004211.
106. Lin CH, Chen ML, Lai TT, Tai CH, Wu RM. Mutational analysis of FBXO7 gene in Parkinson's disease in a Taiwanese population. Neurobiol Aging. 2013;34(1713):e1711–4.
107. Lin IS, Wu RM, Lee-Chen GJ, Shan DE, Gwinn-Hardy K. The SCA17 phenotype can include features of MSA-C, PSP and cognitive impairment. Parkinsonism Relat Disord. 2007;13:246–9.
108. Lindquist S, Duno M, Batbayli M, Puschmann A, Braendgaard H, Mardosiene S, Svenstrup K, Pinborg L, Vestergaard K, Hjermind L, Stokholm J, Andersen B, Johannsen P, Nielsen J. Corticobasal and ataxia syndromes widen the spectrum of C9ORF72 hexanucleotide expansion disease. Clin Genet. 2013;83(3):279–83.
109. Ling H, O'Sullivan SS, Holton JL, Revesz T, Massey LA, Williams DR, Paviour DC, Lees AJ. Does corticobasal degeneration exist? A clinicopathological re-evaluation. Brain. 2010;133: 2045–57.
110. Litvan I, Baker M, Hutton M. Tau genotype: no effect on onset, symptom severity, or survival in progressive supranuclear palsy. Neurology. 2001;57:138–40.
111. Litvan I, Mangone CA, McKee A, Verny M, Parsa A, Jellinger K, D'Olhaberriague L, Chaudhuri KR, Pearce RK. Natural history of progressive supranuclear palsy (Steele-Richardson-Olszewski syndrome) and clinical predictors of survival: a clinicopathological study. J Neurol Neurosurg Psychiatry. 1996;60:615–20.
112. Lu CS, Wu Chou YH, Yen TC, Tsai CH, Chen RS, Chang HC. Dopa-responsive parkinsonism phenotype of spinocerebellar ataxia type 2. Mov Disord. 2002;17:1046–51.
113. Ludecke B, Dworniczak B, Bartholome K. A point mutation in the tyrosine hydroxylase gene associated with Segawa's syndrome. Hum Genet. 1995;95:123–5.
114. Luo LZ, Xu Q, Guo JF, Wang L, Shi CH, Wei JH, Long ZG, Pan Q, Tang BS, Xia K, Yan XX. FBXO7 gene mutations may be rare in Chinese early-onset Parkinsonism patients. Neurosci Lett. 2010;482:86–9.

115. Machner B, Sprenger A, Behrens MI, Ramirez A, Bruggemann N, Klein C, Helmchen C. Eye movement disorders in ATP13A2 mutation carriers (PARK9). Mov Disord. 2010;25:2687–9.
116. Madeo G, Alemseged F, Di Pietro B, Schillaci O, Pisani A. Early abnormalities in 123I-ioflupane (DaTSCAN) imaging in the fragile X-associated tremor ataxia syndrome (FXTAS): a case report. Neurol Sci. 2013;34(8):1475–7.
117. Mahoney CJ, Beck J, Rohrer JD, Lashley T, Mok K, Shakespeare T, Yeatman T, Warrington EK, Schott JM, Fox NC, Rossor MN, Hardy J, Collinge J, Revesz T, Mead S, Warren JD. Frontotemporal dementia with the C9ORF72 hexanucleotide repeat expansion: clinical, neuroanatomical and neuropathological features. Brain. 2012;135:736–50.
118. Majounie E, Renton AE, Mok K, Dopper EG, Waite A, Rollinson S, Chio A, Restagno G, Nicolaou N, Simon-Sanchez J, van Swieten JC, Abramzon Y, Johnson JO, Sendtner M, Pamphlett R, Orrell RW, Mead S, Sidle KC, Houlden H, Rohrer JD, Morrison KE, Pall H, Talbot K, Ansorge O, Hernandez DG, Arepalli S, Sabatelli M, Mora G, Corbo M, Giannini F, Calvo A, Englund E, Borghero G, Floris GL, Remes AM, Laaksovirta H, McCluskey L, Trojanowski JQ, Van Deerlin VM, Schellenberg GD, Nalls MA, Drory VE, Lu CS, Yeh TH, Ishiura H, Takahashi Y, Tsuji S, Le Ber I, Brice A, Drepper C, Williams N, Kirby J, Shaw P, Hardy J, Tienari PJ, Heutink P, Morris HR, Pickering-Brown S, Traynor BJ. Frequency of the C9orf72 hexanucleotide repeat expansion in patients with amyotrophic lateral sclerosis and frontotemporal dementia: a cross-sectional study. Lancet Neurol. 2012;11:323–30.
119. Mak CM, Lam CW. Diagnosis of Wilson's disease: a comprehensive review. Crit Rev Clin Lab Sci. 2008;45:263–90.
120. Marecos C, Ng J, Kurian MA. What is new for monoamine neurotransmitter disorders? J Inherit Metab Dis. 2014;37:619–26.
121. Matej R, Kovacs GG, Johanidesova S, Keller J, Matejckova M, Novakova J, Sigut V, Keller O, Rusina R. Genetic Creutzfeldt-Jakob disease with R208H mutation presenting as progressive supranuclear palsy. Mov Disord. 2012;27:476–9.
122. McNeill A, Duran R, Proukakis C, Bras J, Hughes D, Mehta A, Hardy J, Wood NW, Schapira AH. Hyposmia and cognitive impairment in Gaucher disease patients and carriers. Mov Disord. 2012;27(4):526–32.
123. Mencacci NE, Isaias IU, Reich MM, Ganos C, Plagnol V, Polke JM, Bras J, Hersheson J, Stamelou M, Pittman AM, Noyce AJ, Mok KY, Opladen T, Kunstmann E, Hodecker S, Munchau A, Volkmann J, Samnick S, Sidle K, Nanji T, Sweeney MG, Houlden H, Batla A, Zecchinelli AL, Pezzoli G, Marotta G, Lees A, Alegria P, Krack P, Cormier-Dequaire F, Lesage S, Brice A, Heutink P, Gasser T, Lubbe SJ, Morris HR, Taba P, Koks S, Majounie E, Raphael Gibbs J, Singleton A, Hardy J, Klebe S, Bhatia KP, Wood NW. Parkinson's disease in GTP cyclohydrolase 1 mutation carriers. Brain. 2014;137(Pt 9):2480–92.
124. Mitsui J, Matsukawa T, Ishiura H, Higasa K, Yoshimura J, Saito TL, Ahsan B, Takahashi Y, Goto J, Iwata A, Niimi Y, Riku Y, Goto Y, Mano K, Yoshida M, Morishita S, Tsuji S. CSF1R mutations identified in three families with autosomal dominantly inherited leukoencephalopathy. Am J Med Genet B Neuropsychiatr Genet. 2012;159B:951–7.
125. Morris HR, Osaki Y, Holton J, Lees AJ, Wood NW, Revesz T, Quinn N. Tau exon 10 +16 mutation FTDP-17 presenting clinically as sporadic young onset PSP. Neurology. 2003;61:102–4.
126. Muller U, Herzfeld T, Nolte D. The TAF1/DYT3 multiple transcript system in X-linked dystonia-parkinsonism. Am J Hum Genet. 2007;81:415–7; author reply 417–8.
127. Multiple-System Atrophy Research Collaboration. Mutations in COQ2 in familial and sporadic multiple-system atrophy. N Engl J Med. 2013;369:233–44.
128. Najim al-Din AS, Wriekat A, Mubaidin A, Dasouki M, Hiari M. Pallido-pyramidal degeneration, supranuclear upgaze paresis and dementia: Kufor-Rakeb syndrome. Acta Neurol Scand. 1994;89:347–52.
129. Newsway V, Fish M, Rohrer JD, Majounie E, Williams N, Hack M, Warren JD, Morris HR. Perry syndrome due to the DCTN1 G71R mutation: a distinctive levodopa responsive disorder with behavioral syndrome, vertical gaze palsy, and respiratory failure. Mov Disord. 2010;25:767–70.

130. Ng J, Heales SJ, Kurian MA. Clinical features and pharmacotherapy of childhood monoamine neurotransmitter disorders. Paediatr Drugs. 2014;16:275–91.
131. Ng J, Zhen J, Meyer E, Erreger K, Li Y, Kakar N, Ahmad J, Thiele H, Kubisch C, Rider NL, Morton DH, Strauss KA, Puffenberger EG, D'Agnano D, Anikster Y, Carducci C, Hyland K, Rotstein M, Leuzzi V, Borck G, Reith ME, Kurian MA. Dopamine transporter deficiency syndrome: phenotypic spectrum from infancy to adulthood. Brain. 2014;137:1107–19.
132. Nygaard TG, Marsden CD, Duvoisin RC. Dopa-responsive dystonia. Adv Neurol. 1988;50:377–84.
133. Nygaard TG, Marsden CD, Fahn S. Dopa-responsive dystonia: long-term treatment response and prognosis. Neurology. 1991;41:174–81.
134. O'Dowd S, Curtin D, Waite AJ, Roberts K, Pender N, Reid V, O'Connell M, Williams NM, Morris HR, Traynor BJ, Lynch T. C9ORF72 expansion in amyotrophic lateral sclerosis/frontotemporal dementia also causes parkinsonism. Mov Disord. 2012;27:1072–4.
135. Ohshima S, Tsuboi Y, Yamamoto A, Kawakami M, Farrer MJ, Kira J, Shii H. Autonomic failures in Perry syndrome with DCTN1 mutation. Parkinsonism Relat Disord. 2010;16:612–4.
136. Olgiati S, De Rosa A, Quadri M, Criscuolo C, Breedveld GJ, Picillo M, Pappata S, Quarantelli M, Barone P, De Michele G, Bonifati V. PARK20 caused by SYNJ1 homozygous Arg258Gln mutation in a new Italian family. Neurogenetics. 2014;15:183–8.
137. Orsucci D, Caldarazzo Ienco E, Mancuso M, Siciliano G. POLG1-related and other "mitochondrial Parkinsonisms": an overview. J Mol Neurosci. 2011;44:17–24.
138. Ozawa T. The COQ2 mutations in Japanese multiple system atrophy: impact on the pathogenesis and phenotypic variation. Mov Disord. 2014;29:184.
139. Paisan-Ruiz C, Guevara R, Federoff M, Hanagasi H, Sina F, Elahi E, Schneider SA, Schwingenschuh P, Bajaj N, Emre M, Singleton AB, Hardy J, Bhatia KP, Brandner S, Lees AJ, Houlden H. Early-onset L-dopa-responsive parkinsonism with pyramidal signs due to ATP13A2, PLA2G6, FBXO7 and spatacsin mutations. Mov Disord. 2010;25:1791–800.
140. Park JS, Mehta P, Cooper AA, Veivers D, Heimbach A, Stiller B, Kubisch C, Fung VS, Krainc D, Mackay-Sim A, Sue CM. Pathogenic effects of novel mutations in the P-type ATPase ATP13A2 (PARK9) causing Kufor-Rakeb syndrome, a form of early-onset parkinsonism. Hum Mutat. 2011;32:956–64.
141. Passov V, Gavrilova RH, Strand E, Cerhan JH, Josephs KA. Sporadic corticobasal syndrome with progranulin mutation presenting as progressive apraxic agraphia. Arch Neurol. 2011;68:376–80.
142. Pastor P, Pastor E, Carnero C, Vela R, Garcia T, Amer G, Tolosa E, Oliva R. Familial atypical progressive supranuclear palsy associated with homozygosity for the delN296 mutation in the tau gene. Ann Neurol. 2001;49:263–7.
143. Patterson MC, Hendriksz CJ, Walterfang M, Sedel F, Vanier MT, Wijburg F. Recommendations for the diagnosis and management of Niemann-Pick disease type C: An update. Mol Genet Metab. 2012;106:330–44.
144. Payami H, Nutt J, Gancher S, Bird T, McNeal MG, Seltzer WK, Hussey J, Lockhart P, Gwinn-Hardy K, Singleton AA, Singleton AB, Hardy J, Farrer M. SCA2 may present as levodopa-responsive parkinsonism. Mov Disord. 2003;18:425–9.
145. Perry TL, Bratty PJ, Hansen S, Kennedy J, Urquhart N, Dolman CL. Hereditary mental depression and Parkinsonism with taurine deficiency. Arch Neurol. 1975;32:108–13.
146. Perry TL, Wright JM, Berry K, Hansen S, Perry Jr TL. Dominantly inherited apathy, central hypoventilation, and Parkinson's syndrome: clinical, biochemical, and neuropathologic studies of 2 new cases. Neurology. 1990;40:1882–7.
147. Picillo M, Ranieri A, Orefice G, Bonifati V, Barone P. Clinical progression of SYNJ1-related early onset atypical parkinsonism: 3-year follow up of the original Italian family. J Neurol. 2014;261:823–4.
148. Pons R, Syrengelas D, Youroukos S, Orfanou I, Dinopoulos A, Cormand B, Ormazabal A, Garzia-Cazorla A, Serrano M, Artuch R. Levodopa-induced dyskinesias in tyrosine hydroxylase deficiency. Mov Disord. 2013;28:1058–63.

149. Poorkaj P, Muma NA, Zhukareva V, Cochran EJ, Shannon KM, Hurtig H, Koller WC, Bird TD, Trojanowski JQ, Lee VM, Schellenberg GD. An R5L tau mutation in a subject with a progressive supranuclear palsy phenotype. Ann Neurol. 2002;52:511–6.
150. Pridans C, Sauter KA, Baer K, Kissel H, Hume DA. CSF1R mutations in hereditary diffuse leukoencephalopathy with spheroids are loss of function. Sci Rep. 2013;3:3013.
151. Purdy A, Hahn A, Barnett HJ, Bratty P, Ahmad D, Lloyd KG, McGeer EG, Perry TL. Familial fatal Parkinsonism with alveolar hypoventilation and mental depression. Ann Neurol. 1979;6:523–31.
152. Quadri M, Federico A, Zhao T, Breedveld GJ, Battisti C, Delnooz C, Severijnen LA, Di Toro Mammarella L, Mignarri A, Monti L, Sanna A, Lu P, Punzo F, Cossu G, Willemsen R, Rasi F, Oostra BA, van de Warrenburg BP, Bonifati V. Mutations in SLC30A10 cause parkinsonism and dystonia with hypermanganesemia, polycythemia, and chronic liver disease. Am J Hum Genet. 2012;90:467–77.
153. Quadri M, Fang M, Picillo M, Olgiati S, Breedveld GJ, Graafland J, Wu B, Xu F, Erro R, Amboni M, Pappata S, Quarantelli M, Annesi G, Quattrone A, Chien HF, Barbosa ER, International Parkinsonism Genetics Network, Oostra BA, Barone P, Wang J, Bonifati V. Mutation in the SYNJ1 gene associated with autosomal recessive, early-onset Parkinsonism. Hum Mutat. 2013;34:1208–121.
154. Racette BA, Perlmutter JS. Levodopa responsive parkinsonism in an adult with Huntington's disease. J Neurol Neurosurg Psychiatry. 1998;65:577–9.
155. Raciti L, Nicoletti A, Le Pira F, Andreoli V, Contrafatto D, Lanzafame S, Maci T, Gambardella A, Quattrone A, Zappia M. Presenilin-2 gene mutation presenting as Lewy body dementia? Neurol Sci. 2011;32:533–4.
156. Rademakers R. C9orf72 repeat expansions in patients with ALS and FTD. Lancet Neurol. 2012;11:297–8.
157. Rademakers R, Baker M, Gass J, Adamson J, Huey ED, Momeni P, Spina S, Coppola G, Karydas AM, Stewart H, Johnson N, Hsiung GY, Kelley B, Kuntz K, Steinbart E, Wood EM, Yu CE, Josephs K, Sorenson E, Womack KB, Weintraub S, Pickering-Brown SM, Schofield PR, Brooks WS, Van Deerlin VM, Snowden J, Clark CM, Kertesz A, Boylan K, Ghetti B, Neary D, Schellenberg GD, Beach TG, Mesulam M, Mann D, Grafman J, Mackenzie IR, Feldman H, Bird T, Petersen R, Knopman D, Boeve B, Geschwind DH, Miller B, Wszolek Z, Lippa C, Bigio EH, Dickson D, Graff-Radford N, Hutton M. Phenotypic variability associated with progranulin haploinsufficiency in patients with the common 1477C-->T (Arg493X) mutation: an international initiative. Lancet Neurol. 2007;6:857–68.
158. Rademakers R, Baker M, Nicholson AM, Rutherford NJ, Finch N, Soto-Ortolaza A, Lash J, Wider C, Wojtas A, DeJesus-Hernandez M, Adamson J, Kouri N, Sundal C, Shuster EA, Aasly J, MacKenzie J, Roeber S, Kretzschmar HA, Boeve BF, Knopman DS, Petersen RC, Cairns NJ, Ghetti B, Spina S, Garbern J, Tselis AC, Uitti R, Das P, Van Gerpen JA, Meschia JF, Levy S, Broderick DF, Graff-Radford N, Ross OA, Miller BB, Swerdlow RH, Dickson DW, Wszolek ZK. Mutations in the colony stimulating factor 1 receptor (CSF1R) gene cause hereditary diffuse leukoencephalopathy with spheroids. Nat Genet. 2012; 44:200–5.
159. Ragno M, Berbellini A, Cacchio G, Manca A, Di Marzio F, Pianese L, De Rosa A, Silvestri S, Scarcella M, De Michele G. Parkinsonism is a late, not rare, feature of CADASIL: a study on Italian patients carrying the R1006C mutation. Stroke. 2013;44:1147–9.
160. Ramirez A, Heimbach A, Grundemann J, Stiller B, Hampshire D, Cid LP, Goebel I, Mubaidin AF, Wriekat AL, Roeper J, Al-Din A, Hillmer AM, Karsak M, Liss B, Woods CG, Behrens MI, Kubisch C. Hereditary parkinsonism with dementia is caused by mutations in ATP13A2, encoding a lysosomal type 5 P-type ATPase. Nat Genet. 2006;38:1184–91.
161. Respondek G, Stamelou M, Kurz C, Ferguson LW, Rajput A, Chiu WZ, van Swieten JC, Troakes C, Al Sarraj S, Gelpi E, Gaig C, Tolosa E, Oertel WH, Giese A, Roeber S, Arzberger T, Wagenpfeil S, Höglinger GU. Movement Disorder Society-endorsed PSP Study Group. The phenotypic spectrum of progressive supranuclear palsy: a retrospective multicenter study of 100 definite cases. Mov Disord. 2014;29(14):1758–66.

162. Riess O, Rub U, Pastore A, Bauer P, Schols L. SCA3: neurological features, pathogenesis and animal models. Cerebellum. 2008;7:125–37.
163. Rivaud-Pechoux S, Vidailhet M, Gallouedec G, Litvan I, Gaymard B, Pierrot-Deseilligny C. Longitudinal ocular motor study in corticobasal degeneration and progressive supranuclear palsy. Neurology. 2000;54:1029–32.
164. Rohrer JD, Beck J, Warren JD, King A, Al Sarraj S, Holton J, Revesz T, Collinge J, Mead S. Corticobasal syndrome associated with a novel 1048_1049insG progranulin mutation. J Neurol Neurosurg Psychiatry. 2009;80:1297–8.
165. Rohrer JD, Warren JD. Phenotypic signatures of genetic frontotemporal dementia. Curr Opin Neurol. 2011;24:542–9.
166. Ros R, Thobois S, Streichenberger N, Kopp N, Sanchez MP, Perez M, Hoenicka J, Avila J, Honnorat J, de Yebenes JG. A new mutation of the tau gene, G303V, in early-onset familial progressive supranuclear palsy. Arch Neurol. 2005;62:1444–50.
167. Ross OA, Rutherford NJ, Baker M, Soto-Ortolaza AI, Carrasquillo MM, DeJesus-Hernandez M, Adamson J, Li M, Volkening K, Finger E, Seeley WW, Hatanpaa KJ, Lomen-Hoerth C, Kertesz A, Bigio EH, Lippa C, Woodruff BK, Knopman DS, White 3rd CL, Van Gerpen JA, Meschia JF, Mackenzie IR, Boylan K, Boeve BF, Miller BL, Strong MJ, Uitti RJ, Younkin SG, Graff-Radford NR, Petersen RC, Wszolek ZK, Dickson DW, Rademakers R. Ataxin-2 repeat-length variation and neurodegeneration. Hum Mol Genet. 2011;20:3207–12.
168. Rossi G, Gasparoli E, Pasquali C, Di Fede G, Testa D, Albanese A, Bracco F, Tagliavini F. Progressive supranuclear palsy and Parkinson's disease in a family with a new mutation in the tau gene. Ann Neurol. 2004;55:448.
169. Rossi G, Marelli C, Farina L, Laura M, Maria Basile A, Ciano C, Tagliavini F, Pareyson D. The G389R mutation in the MAPT gene presenting as sporadic corticobasal syndrome. Mov Disord. 2008;23:892–5.
170. Rossi Sebastiano D, Soliveri P, Panzica F, Moroni I, Gellera C, Gilioli I, Nardocci N, Ciano C, Albanese A, Franceschetti S, Canafoglia L. Cortical myoclonus in childhood and juvenile onset Huntington's disease. Parkinsonism Relat Disord. 2012;18:794–7.
171. Rowe DB, Lewis V, Needham M, Rodriguez M, Boyd A, McLean C, Roberts H, Masters CL, Collins SJ. Novel prion protein gene mutation presenting with subacute PSP-like syndrome. Neurology. 2007;68:868–70.
172. Saito T, Guan F, Papolos DF, Lau S, Klein M, Fann CS, Lachman HM. Mutation analysis of SYNJ1: a possible candidate gene for chromosome 21q22-linked bipolar disorder. Mol Psychiatry. 2001;6:387–95.
173. Sasaki H, Emi M, Iijima H, Ito N, Sato H, Yabe I, Kato T, Utsumi J, Matsubara K. Copy number loss of (src homology 2 domain containing)-transforming protein 2 (SHC2) gene: discordant loss in monozygotic twins and frequent loss in patients with multiple system atrophy. Mol Brain. 2011;4:24.
174. Schneider SA, Paisan-Ruiz C, Quinn NP, Lees AJ, Houlden H, Hardy J, Bhatia KP. ATP13A2 mutations (PARK9) cause neurodegeneration with brain iron accumulation. Mov Disord. 2010;25:979–84.
175. Schols L, Peters S, Szymanski S, Kruger R, Lange S, Hardt C, Riess O, Przuntek H. Extrapyramidal motor signs in degenerative ataxias. Arch Neurol. 2000;57:1495–500.
176. Scholz SW, Houlden H, Schulte C, Sharma M, Li A, Berg D, Melchers A, Paudel R, Gibbs JR, Simon-Sanchez J, Paisan-Ruiz C, Bras J, Ding J, Chen H, Traynor BJ, Arepalli S, Zonozi RR, Revesz T, Holton J, Wood N, Lees A, Oertel W, Wullner U, Goldwurm S, Pellecchia MT, Illig T, Riess O, Fernandez HH, Rodriguez RL, Okun MS, Poewe W, Wenning GK, Hardy JA, Singleton AB, Del Sorbo F, Schneider S, Bhatia KP, Gasser T. SNCA variants are associated with increased risk for multiple system atrophy. Ann Neurol. 2009;65:610–4.
177. Seelaar H, Rohrer JD, Pijnenburg YA, Fox NC, van Swieten JC. Clinical, genetic and pathological heterogeneity of frontotemporal dementia: a review. J Neurol Neurosurg Psychiatry. 2011;82:476–86.
178. Segawa M, Hosaka A, Miyagawa F, Nomura Y, Imai H. Hereditary progressive dystonia with marked diurnal fluctuation. Adv Neurol. 1976;14:215–33.

179. Sevin M, Lesca G, Baumann N, Millat G, Lyon-Caen O, Vanier MT, Sedel F. The adult form of Niemann-Pick disease type C. Brain. 2007;130:120–33.
180. Shan DE, Liu RS, Sun CM, Lee SJ, Liao KK, Soong BW. Presence of spinocerebellar ataxia type 2 gene mutation in a patient with apparently sporadic Parkinson's disease: clinical implications. Mov Disord. 2004;19:1357–60.
181. Shan DE, Soong BW, Sun CM, Lee SJ, Liao KK, Liu RS. Spinocerebellar ataxia type 2 presenting as familial levodopa-responsive parkinsonism. Ann Neurol. 2001;50:812–5.
182. Shimamura M, Uyama E, Hirano T, Murakami T, Mita S, Kitamoto T, Uchino M. A unique case of sporadic Creutzfeldt-Jacob disease presenting as progressive supranuclear palsy. Intern Med. 2003;42:195–8.
183. Singleton A, Hague S, Hernandez D. X-linked recessive dystonia parkinsonism (XDP; Lubag; DYT3). Adv Neurol. 2004;94:139–42.
184. Singleton AB, Farrer MJ, Bonifati V. The genetics of Parkinson's disease: progress and therapeutic implications. Mov Disord. 2013;28:14–23.
185. Spina S, Murrell JR, Huey ED, Wassermann EM, Pietrini P, Grafman J, Ghetti B. Corticobasal syndrome associated with the A9D Progranulin mutation. J Neuropathol Exp Neurol. 2007;66:892–900.
186. Stamelou M, Alonso-Canovas A, Bhatia KP. Dystonia in corticobasal degeneration: a review of the literature on 404 pathologically proven cases. Mov Disord. 2012;27:696–702.
187. Stamelou M, de Silva R, Arias-Carrion O, Boura E, Hollerhage M, Oertel WH, Muller U, Hoglinger GU. Rational therapeutic approaches to progressive supranuclear palsy. Brain. 2010;133:1578–90.
188. Stamelou M, Knake S, Oertel WH, Hoglinger GU. Magnetic resonance imaging in progressive supranuclear palsy. J Neurol. 2011;258:549–58.
189. Stamelou M, Mencacci NE, Cordivari C, Batla A, Wood NW, Houlden H, Hardy J, Bhatia KP. Myoclonus-dystonia syndrome due to tyrosine hydroxylase deficiency. Neurology. 2012;79:435–41.
190. Stamelou M, Quinn N, Bhatia K. 'Atypical' atypical parkinsonism: new genetic disorders presenting with features of PSP, MSA or CBD. Mov Disord. 2013;28(9):1184–99.
191. Stamelou M, Tuschl K, Chong WK, Burroughs AK, Mills PB, Bhatia KP, Clayton PT. Dystonia with brain manganese accumulation resulting from SLC30A10 mutations: a new treatable disorder. Mov Disord. 2012;27:1317–22.
192. Stanford PM, Halliday GM, Brooks WS, Kwok JB, Storey CE, Creasey H, Morris JG, Fulham MJ, Schofield PR. Progressive supranuclear palsy pathology caused by a novel silent mutation in exon 10 of the tau gene: expansion of the disease phenotype caused by tau gene mutations. Brain. 2000;123(Pt 5):880–93.
193. Steinberger D, Weber Y, Korinthenberg R, Deuschl G, Benecke R, Martinius J, Muller U. High penetrance and pronounced variation in expressivity of GCH1 mutations in five families with dopa-responsive dystonia. Ann Neurol. 1998;43:634–9.
194. Stopkova P, Vevera J, Paclt I, Zukov I, Lachman HM. Analysis of SYNJ1, a candidate gene for 21q22 linked bipolar disorder: a replication study. Psychiatry Res. 2004;127:157–61.
195. Sundal C, Fujioka S, Van Gerpen JA, Wider C, Nicholson AM, Baker M, Shuster EA, Aasly J, Spina S, Ghetti B, Roeber S, Garbern J, Tselis A, Swerdlow RH, Miller BB, Borjesson-Hanson A, Uitti RJ, Ross OA, Stoessl AJ, Rademakers R, Josephs KA, Dickson DW, Broderick D, Wszolek ZK. Parkinsonian features in hereditary diffuse leukoencephalopathy with spheroids (HDLS) and CSF1R mutations. Parkinsonism Relat Disord. 2013;19: 869–77.
196. Tackenberg B, Metz A, Unger M, Schimke N, Passow S, Hoeffken H, Hoffmann GF, Muller U, Nolte D, Oertel WH, Eggert K, Moller JC. Nigrostriatal dysfunction in X-linked dystonia-parkinsonism (DYT3). Mov Disord. 2007;22:900–2.
197. Takazaki KA, D'Abreu A, Nucci A, Lopes-Cendes I, Franca Jr MC. Dysautonomia is frequent in Machado-Joseph disease: clinical and neurophysiological evaluation. Cerebellum. 2013;12(4):513–9.

198. Tan EK, Tong J, Pavanni R, Wong MC, Zhao Y. Genetic analysis of SCA 2 and 3 repeat expansions in essential tremor and atypical Parkinsonism. Mov Disord. 2007;22:1971–4.
199. Tassone F, Greco CM, Hunsaker MR, Seritan AL, Berman RF, Gane LW, Jacquemont S, Basuta K, Jin LW, Hagerman PJ, Hagerman RJ. Neuropathological, clinical and molecular pathology in female fragile X premutation carriers with and without FXTAS. Genes Brain Behav. 2012;11:577–85.
200. Tayebi N, Callahan M, Madike V, Stubblefield BK, Orvisky E, Krasnewich D, Fillano JJ, Sidransky E. Gaucher disease and parkinsonism: a phenotypic and genotypic characterization. Mol Genet Metab. 2001;73:313–21.
201. Tayebi N, Walker J, Stubblefield B, Orvisky E, LaMarca ME, Wong K, Rosenbaum H, Schiffmann R, Bembi B, Sidransky E. Gaucher disease with parkinsonian manifestations: does glucocerebrosidase deficiency contribute to a vulnerability to parkinsonism? Mol Genet Metab. 2003;79:104–9.
202. Tolosa E, Litvan I, Hoglinger GU, Burn D, Lees A, Andres MV, Gomez-Carrillo B, Leon T, Del Ser T. A phase 2 trial of the GSK-3 inhibitor tideglusib in progressive supranuclear palsy. Mov Disord. 2014;29:470–8.
203. Tremolizzo L, Bertola F, Casati G, Piperno A, Ferrarese C, Appollonio I. Progressive supranuclear palsy-like phenotype caused by progranulin p.Thr272fs mutation. Mov Disord. 2011;26:1964–6.
204. Tsuboi Y, Dickson DW, Nabeshima K, Schmeichel AM, Wszolek ZK, Yamada T, Benarroch EE. Neurodegeneration involving putative respiratory neurons in Perry syndrome. Acta Neuropathol. 2008;115:263–8.
205. Tuschl K, Clayton PT, Gospe Jr SM, Gulab S, Ibrahim S, Singh P, Aulakh R, Ribeiro R, Barsottini O, Zaki M, Del Rosario ML, Dydak S, Price V, Rideout A, Gordon K, Wevers RA, Chong K, Mills PB. Syndrome of hepatic cirrhosis, dystonia, polycythemia and hypermanganesemia- caused by mutation in *SLC30A10*, a manganese transporter in man. Am J Hum Genet. 2012;90:457–66.
206. Tuschl K, Mills PB, Parsons H, Malone M, Fowler D, Bitner-Glindzicz M, Clayton PT. Hepatic cirrhosis, dystonia, polycythaemia and hypermanganesaemia-A new metabolic disorder. J Inherit Metab Dis. 2008;31:151–63.
207. van Gaalen J, Giunti P, van de Warrenburg BP. Movement disorders in spinocerebellar ataxias. Mov Disord. 2011;26:792–800.
208. van Swieten J, Spillantini MG. Hereditary frontotemporal dementia caused by Tau gene mutations. Brain Pathol. 2007;17:63–73.
209. van Swieten JC, Heutink P. Mutations in progranulin (GRN) within the spectrum of clinical and pathological phenotypes of frontotemporal dementia. Lancet Neurol. 2008;7:965–74.
210. Varkonyi J, Rosenbaum H, Baumann N, MacKenzie JJ, Simon Z, Aharon-Peretz J, Walker JM, Tayebi N, Sidransky E. Gaucher disease associated with parkinsonism: four further case reports. Am J Med Genet A. 2003;116A:348–51.
211. Vauthier V, Jaillard S, Journel H, Dubourg C, Jockers R, Dam J. Homozygous deletion of an 80 kb region comprising part of DNAJC6 and LEPR genes on chromosome 1P31.3 is associated with early onset obesity, mental retardation and epilepsy. Mol Genet Metab. 2012;106:345–50.
212. Vilarino-Guell C, Wider C, Soto-Ortolaza AI, Cobb SA, Kachergus JM, Keeling BH, Dachsel JC, Hulihan MM, Dickson DW, Wszolek ZK, Uitti RJ, Graff-Radford NR, Boeve BF, Josephs KA, Miller B, Boylan KB, Gwinn K, Adler CH, Aasly JO, Hentati F, Destee A, Krygowska-Wajs A, Chartier-Harlin MC, Ross OA, Rademakers R, Farrer MJ. Characterization of DCTN1 genetic variability in neurodegeneration. Neurology. 2009;72:2024–8.
213. Wenning GK, Ben Shlomo Y, Magalhaes M, Daniel SE, Quinn NP. Clinical features and natural history of multiple system atrophy. An analysis of 100 cases. Brain. 1994;117(Pt 4): 835–45.
214. Wenning GK, Geser F, Krismer F, Seppi K, Duerr S, Boesch S, Kollensperger M, Goebel G, Pfeiffer KP, Barone P, Pellecchia MT, Quinn NP, Koukouni V, Fowler CJ, Schrag A, Mathias CJ, Giladi N, Gurevich T, Dupont E, Ostergaard K, Nilsson CF, Widner H, Oertel W, Eggert KM, Albanese A, Del Sorbo F, Tolosa E, Cardozo A, Deuschl G, Hellriegel H,

Klockgether T, Dodel R, Sampaio C, Coelho M, Djaldetti R, Melamed E, Gasser T, Kamm C, Meco G, Colosimo C, Rascol O, Meissner WG, Tison F, Poewe W, European Multiple System Atrophy Study Group. The natural history of multiple system atrophy: a prospective European cohort study. Lancet Neurol. 2013;12:264–74.

215. Wider C, Dachsel JC, Farrer MJ, Dickson DW, Tsuboi Y, Wszolek ZK. Elucidating the genetics and pathology of Perry syndrome. J Neurol Sci. 2010;289:149–54.
216. Wider C, Wszolek ZK. Rapidly progressive familial parkinsonism with central hypoventilation, depression and weight loss (Perry syndrome)–a literature review. Parkinsonism Relat Disord. 2008;14:1–7.
217. Wilcox RA, Churchyard A, Dahl HH, Hutchison WM, Kirby DM, Thyagarajan D. Levodopa response in Parkinsonism with multiple mitochondrial DNA deletions. Mov Disord. 2007;22:1020–3.
218. Williams DR, Hadeed A, al-Din AS, Wreikat AL, Lees AJ. Kufor Rakeb disease: autosomal recessive, levodopa-responsive parkinsonism with pyramidal degeneration, supranuclear gaze palsy, and dementia. Mov Disord. 2005;20:1264–71.
219. Wraith JE, Baumgartner MR, Bembi B, Covanis A, Levade T, Mengel E, Pineda M, Sedel F, Topcu M, Vanier MT, Widner H, Wijburg FA, Patterson MC. Recommendations on the diagnosis and management of Niemann-Pick disease type C. Mol Genet Metab. 2009;98: 152–65.
220. Wraith JE, Vecchio D, Jacklin E, Abel L, Chadha-Boreham H, Luzy C, Giorgino R, Patterson MC. Miglustat in adult and juvenile patients with Niemann-Pick disease type C: long-term data from a clinical trial. Mol Genet Metab. 2010;99:351–7.
221. Yu CE, Bird TD, Bekris LM, Montine TJ, Leverenz JB, Steinbart E, Galloway NM, Feldman H, Woltjer R, Miller CA, Wood EM, Grossman M, McCluskey L, Clark CM, Neumann M, Danek A, Galasko DR, Arnold SE, Chen-Plotkin A, Karydas A, Miller BL, Trojanowski JQ, Lee VM, Schellenberg GD, Van Deerlin VM. The spectrum of mutations in progranulin: a collaborative study screening 545 cases of neurodegeneration. Arch Neurol. 2010;67: 161–70.
222. Zhao T, De Graaff E, Breedveld GJ, Loda A, Severijnen LA, Wouters CH, Verheijen FW, Dekker MC, Montagna P, Willemsen R, Oostra BA, Bonifati V. Loss of nuclear activity of the FBXO7 protein in patients with parkinsonian-pyramidal syndrome (PARK15). PLoS One. 2011;6:e16983.
223. Zhao T, Severijnen LA, van der Weiden M, Zheng PP, Oostra BA, Hukema RK, Willemsen R, Kros JM, Bonifati V. FBXO7 immunoreactivity in alpha-synuclein-containing inclusions in Parkinson disease and multiple system atrophy. J Neuropathol Exp Neurol. 2013;72: 482–8.

Chapter 4
Genetics of Dementia with Lewy Bodies

José M. Tomás Brás

Abstract Dementia with Lewy bodies (DLB) is one of the most underserved common diseases. From clinical to pathological aspects, DLB is often a difficult disease to diagnose. This and other factors that I will discuss in this chapter have added to the complexity in determining the full genetic landscape of DLB.

Over the last few years, advances in technology have allowed us to test the genome in an unprecedented manner. These novel technologies have been applied to many diseases with great success but are only now starting to be used in large enough cohorts of DLB cases. Here, I will discuss and review the most recent data arising from this field that are, slowly, starting to allow us to have a better picture of the genetic architecture of this disorder. Lastly, I discuss what the next few years should bring in terms of molecular studies in DLB.

Keywords Dementia with Lewy bodies • Genetic risk factor • Genetic mutation • Genetic architecture of disease • Association study • Lysosomal function

Lewy Bodies and Alpha-Synuclein

Lewy bodies (LBs) are commonly known as the neuropathological hallmark of Parkinson's disease (PD). They are protein inclusions, formed of insoluble polymers of alpha-synuclein that are present in the neuronal body, forming round lamellated eosinophilic cytoplasmic inclusions [1]. In addition to LBs, alpha-synuclein can also be deposited in neuronal processes (Lewy neurites) and in astrocytes and oligodendroglial cells. It is thought that LBs cause neuronal degeneration and eventually lead to cell death [2].

Using standard histological methods, "classic" or "brainstem" LBs are seen as spherical, intraneuronal, cytoplasmic, eosinophilic inclusions in the neuromelanin-containing dopaminergic neurons of the substantia nigra and in the locus coeruleus.

J.M. Tomás Brás, PhD
Department of Molecular Neuroscience, Institute of Neurology,
University College London, London WC1N 3AR, England, UK
e-mail: j.bras@ucl.ac.uk

S.A. Schneider, J.M.T. Brás (eds.), *Movement Disorder Genetics*,
DOI 10.1007/978-3-319-17223-1_4

These structures are characterized by a hyaline core and a pale halo. Compared with these "classical" LBs, cortical LBs are less well defined and may occur in the limbic and neocortical regions. Because of their small size, they are not always easy to identify with classical histological stainings and frequently require the use of immunohistochemical techniques for their identification, namely, with anti-alpha-synuclein and anti-ubiquitin antibodies [3]. However, some LBs are immunoreactive for alpha-synuclein but not for ubiquitin, so alpha-synuclein positivity may outnumber that of ubiquitin. As a consequence, alpha-synuclein immunohistochemistry is currently the most sensitive and specific technique for detecting and quantifying LBs [4].

The exact function of alpha-synuclein is not known, but it is assumed to help in the regulation of synaptic-vesicle release and to provide a stabilizing effect on complexes of SNARE family proteins [5]. Genetic mutation of alpha-synuclein typically leads to autosomal dominant PD, and copy number changes of the wild-type gene have been associated with aggressive forms of Parkinson's disease with dementia [6, 7]. The latter suggests that the simple increase in normal protein quantity may be sufficient to induce the phenotype, which is remarkable for diseases of protein accumulation. Although, whether total alpha-synuclein concentrations are increased in the brains of patients with PD remains unclear.

Alpha-synuclein is degraded by the lysosome [8], hinting at a role for lysosomal waste-clearing mechanism in diseases of alpha-synuclein accumulation. However, lysosomal function also seems to be affected by alpha-synuclein in a way that leads to neurotoxic effects. The PD-associated Ala53Thr and Ala30Pro mutations inhibit chaperone-mediated autophagy and, therefore, prevent the degradation not only of alpha-synuclein but of related substrates as well [9].

LBs are the pathological common denominator for a number of neurodegenerative diseases. Although the exact mechanism through which they are formed is not entirely clear, they are present in cases where the only known pathogenic defect is an increased amount of normal alpha-synuclein [6, 10]. This suggests that the mechanism through which alpha-synuclein should be removed from the cell is impaired, further suggesting an important role for the lysosome in the pathobiological processes of these diseases.

General Aspects in the Diagnosis of Dementia with Lewy Bodies (DLB)

Despite the fact that LBs within the cerebral cortex of demented patients were recognized as early as 1961, it was only by the mid-1990s that dementia with Lewy bodies (DLB) was recognized as a relatively common form of dementia [11]. This, of course, means that over the years there was much less research efforts devoted to DLB than, for example, PD or AD (Fig. 4.1). Ultimately this leads to the fact that DLB is probably one of the most underserved common diseases.

The most recent consensus for diagnosis was devised in 2005 and was divided in clinical and neuropathological criteria [12]. There is currently no molecular diagnosis for DLB.

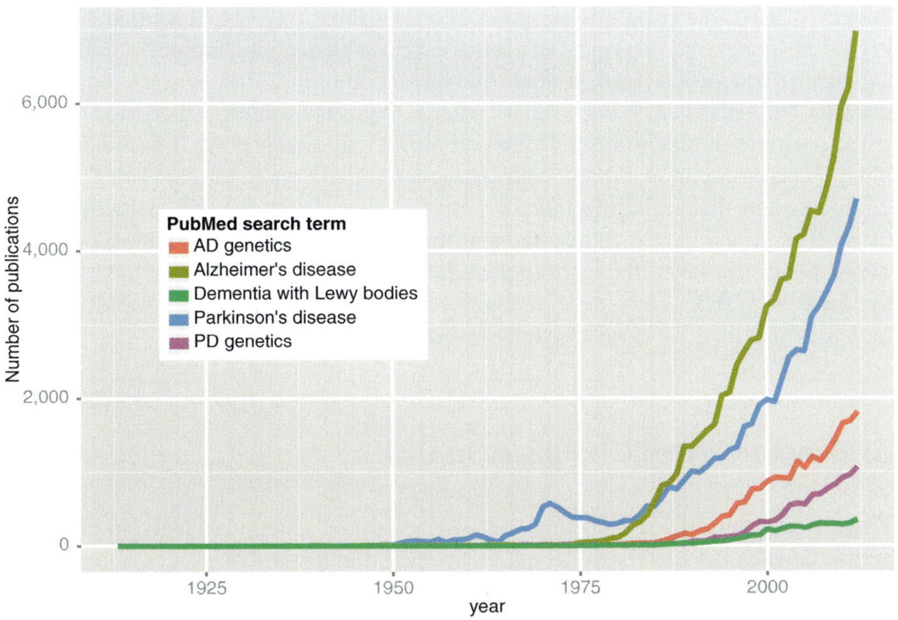

Fig. 4.1 To exemplify how much underserved DLB has been, this figure shows the number of publications in PubMed with each of the search terms in their title. Even in recent years, it is clear that there has not been as much research devoted to DLB when compared with Parkinson's or Alzheimer's disease

From a clinical perspective the consensus recognizes central, core, suggestive, and supportive features for the diagnosis of dementia with Lewy bodies. Additionally, other confounding clinical conditions and the temporal sequence of appearance of cognitive and motor symptoms are also taken into account.

The central clinical feature of DLB is dementia; although unlike in AD, dementia does not need to be a very prominent early feature and can instead occur with disease progression.

There are three core features for diagnosis: fluctuating cognition with pronounced variation in attention and alertness, recurrent visual hallucinations, and spontaneous features of parkinsonism. Two of these features should be present for a diagnosis of probable DLB, while one core feature should be present for a diagnosis of possible DLB.

There are also three suggestive features for diagnosis: REM sleep behavior disorder, severe neuroleptic sensitivity, and low dopamine transporter uptake in the basal ganglia demonstrated by SPECT or PET imaging. In the presence of one core feature, the additional finding of a suggestive feature justifies a diagnosis of probable DLB. In the absence of any core features, the presence of a suggestive feature justifies a diagnosis of possible DLB [12].

The clinical distinction between DLB and PD with dementia is made solely on the basis of the temporal sequence of onset of cognitive and motor symptoms [13].

From a pathological perspective, the diagnosis of DLB is made by determining the frequency of LBs in several brain regions. Taking the tissue distribution and the frequency of LBs, the patient is assigned to one of three types of Lewy body disease: brainstem-predominant (typical of classic Parkinson's disease), limbic or transitional, and diffuse neocortical. Concomitant Alzheimer pathology is a common feature in LB disease. This data is taken into account when making a postmortem diagnosis of DLB: in the presence of little or no AD-type pathology, a diagnosis of DLB becomes "more likely," decreasing in likelihood with an increase in AD-type changes [14].

Because of the similarities and overlaps between DLB and PD/AD, a diagnosis of DLB is generally a difficult one and thus misdiagnosis rate is almost certainly high (this is true even for pathological diagnosis) [15]. Despite this fact, the vast majority of publications have focused on clinically diagnosed samples, which increases the chances of misdiagnosis even more.

Evidence of Genetic Influence in DLB

There is still very limited information with regard to genetic influence in DLB. As with other neurodegenerative diseases, the fact that disease onset generally occurs late in life means that, in many cases, there are no longer living relatives from previous generations, which can lead to cases being potentially mislabeled as sporadic. Additionally, there are also reports of discordant twin pairs for DLB, in this case neuropathologically confirmed cases [16]. However, the same was true for PD [17, 18] before causative genes were found, and today we have more than 30 genes that we know play a role in some form of that disease.

The fact that both AD and PD have multiple disease-causing genes strongly suggests that the same also occurs in DLB. This is particularly true when so much of clinical and pathological characteristics are shared between these diseases.

However, the unequivocal identification of disease-causing genes in families generally requires large and informative pedigrees, and there have not been many of these identified for DLB. To date, there has been a single genome-wide linkage study for DLB. Looking at an autosomal dominant family with autopsy-confirmed DLB, the authors identified a region on chromosome two that segregated with the disease [19]. Despite very promising, these data did not yield the expected results. After detailed genetic screening of all genes in the linkage region, the authors failed to identify any genetic variant (sequence or copy number variant) that could account for the phenotype in that family [20]. These results suggest one of two possibilities: either the original linkage data was incorrect or the causal defect is a more complex one than what we commonly see in Mendelian forms of disease. A good example of such a case is the *C9ORF72* gene in ALS and FTD [21]. Here, the causal mutation is an intronic hexanucleotide repeat, which, to this day, is difficult to identify and characterize.

Mutation of the alpha-synuclein gene (*SNCA*) is a rare cause of familial PD. However, many patients carrying *SNCA* missense mutations or gene multiplications show neurological features beyond typical idiopathic PD, such as cognitive decline, dementia, hallucinations, or autonomic dysfunction. For example, *SNCA* triplications and the missense mutations p.E46K and p.A53T are associated with clinical and pathological phenotypes ranging from PD to PD with dementia to DLB [22].

In addition to *SNCA*, previously reported pathogenic mutations in other PD and AD genes have been shown to occur in probable and definite DLB cases [23]. This is not entirely surprising given the overlap in characteristics between these diseases; however, it should be noted that in all cases reported by Meeus and colleagues, segregation of the mutation was not possible to ascertain.

The fact that no bona fide pathogenic gene defects have been identified does not mean however that there are no genetic factors at play in DLB.

Over the last years, two genes have been shown to be a factor in DLB: the apolipoprotein E gene (*APOE*) and β-glucocerebrosidase (*GBA*).

The epsilon-4 allele of *APOE* is the strongest genetic risk factor for AD, although the exact mechanism of how this allele causes such a dramatic effect remains to be fully determined.

The first report suggesting the involvement of *APOE* in LB disease dates from 1994 [24]. Here, the authors showed that the frequency of the APOE epsilon-4 haplotype has an intermediate frequency in DLB when compared with PD and AD. This result has been widely replicated [25–27] and recently it was shown that it is true even when looking at pure DLB cases (those without neuropathological changes typical of AD) [28].

This data suggests that, in some cases, APOE might contribute to neurodegeneration through mechanisms unrelated to amyloid processing. It is possible that this occurs in cases somehow predisposed to LB disease instead of amyloid disease.

The second gene shown to be involved is the gene encoding the glucocerebrosidase protein. *GBA* is a lysosomal enzyme responsible for breaking down the chemical glucocerebroside, an intermediate in glycolipid metabolism. When homozygous mutations occur in *GBA*, these lead to a recessive lysosomal storage disorder called Gaucher disease. GBA was also linked with Parkinson's disease, where it was shown that the same mutations, but when heterozygous, increase an individual's risk for PD by about fivefold [29]. Subsequently it was shown to also be involved in DLB, with a similar effect [30]. Although the function of GBA is much better understood than that of APOE, it is still not clear how heterozygous mutations increase risk for LB disease. A clear hypothesis is that a single variant impairs lysosome function to a point that leads to alpha-synuclein accumulation, but not sufficiently as to cause overt lysosomal storage disease, though this has not been conclusively shown. Interestingly, it has been shown that GBA-linked PD patients are more prone to develop dementia [31], a result that clearly fits with an association of DLB with GBA.

Taken together, the data from *GBA*, *APOE,* and the few families where DLB segregates clearly point towards a role for genetics in the etiology of this disease.

Genetic Susceptibility Factors for DLB

Over the last decade we have started to be able to test genes for association with phenotypes in a truly unbiased manner. This has proven to be immensely successful for a variety of diseases, where novel genetic risk factors have been identified.

The two aforementioned genes (*APOE* and *GBA*) were identified as risk genes for DLB using candidate gene association studies. There are few examples of successful candidate gene association studies in the literature, mainly because selecting candidate genes requires some prior knowledge of the disease pathobiology. Otherwise, the prior odds of selecting the correct gene to test from a pool of ~20,000 genes in the human genome were very small. In the case of DLB, however, what was used was prior genetic knowledge from related diseases.

The first study to look at a large number of genetic variants in DLB cases was published in 2014 [32]. Here, the authors selected all of the known genetic risk factors for both PD and AD from previously published genome-wide association studies (GWAS) and genotyped them in a large cohort of DLB cases and controls. This study tested approximately 700 DLB cases and 2,600 controls for 6,078 loci. A majority of the cases were neuropathologically diagnosed, reducing the potential misdiagnosis rate.

The most significantly associated region was found on chromosome 19 overlapping the *APOE* locus. Although this can be seen as a replication of previous studies, the association of *APOE* had never been shown in such a large cohort of neuropathologically proven DLB cases. Also, despite the fact that the authors did not test the epsilon4 haplotype specifically, the most associated marker is known to be in very high linkage disequilibrium with that allele and thus the association is, in all likelihood, identical to that seen in AD.

Only two other genomic regions showed levels of association in that study. The first was at the alpha-synuclein locus and the second was at the *SCARB2* locus. Both of these regions were previously associated with PD.

The association at *SNCA* is not entirely surprising given the protein's involvement in LBs, although unlike *APOE*, there are no previous reports in the literature associating *SNCA* genetic variants with DLB.

The association at the *SCARB2* locus is entirely novel. *SCARB2* encodes a lysosomal protein, and homozygous or compound heterozygous mutations in this gene are reported to cause an autosomal recessive progressive myoclonic epilepsy-4 (EPM4) [33–35]. However, its precise function has, thus far, not been described.

One interesting result from this report is the fact that, although the associations are at the same loci previously described in PD, the profile of the association is actually quite different. For example, the association at *SNCA* in PD occurs 3′ to the gene and in DLB it occurs just 5′. One possible explanation is that the different association profiles are related to differential gene expression regulation in each disease, which could potentially lead to differential tissue localization of the pathological features.

In summary, of the known risk genes for DLB, one is likely amyloid-related and is a known dementia risk factor (*APOE*), one is the gene encoding the major component of LBs (*SNCA*), and two are known to have lysosomal functions (*SCARB2* and *GBA*). These data strongly support a role for the lysosomal pathway in the etiology of DLB, similarly to what we now know occurs in PD.

Lessons from Other Diseases

Over the last decade our understanding of the molecular basis of several neurodegenerative diseases has been greatly improved. At the basis of these improvements was the development of methods that allow us to study the genome in an unbiased manner. This meant that we would not have to rely on prior knowledge to create study hypotheses; in fact study hypotheses started to not really be applicable, since we could simply test the entire genome of large numbers of individuals. This apparently simplistic approach has been tremendously successful and has led to the identification of over 30 genes involved in the most common neurodegenerative diseases [36–39].

Unfortunately, we have not yet seen these approaches applied to DLB; so far, molecular studies in DLB have focused on relatively small families or cohorts of patients, tested for a small number of genetic markers.

Another lesson from other diseases is sample size. Clearly, for common diseases, large sample sizes are a requirement for any genetic study. More often than not, this means that properly powered studies can only be accomplished when groups enter into collaboration and share samples or data. As an example, the latest GWAS in PD included 15,000 cases and about 95,000 control subjects [37], numbers that are only possible with collaborative approaches. Estimates point to a need for over 25,000 cases when designing a study that aims at identifying variants that are not very common in the general population [40]. For a disease like DLB, where diagnosis is not always an easy task, these numbers may need to be even higher to account for a proportion of misdiagnosed cases.

One interesting result from the field of AD relates to the finding of the gene *TREM2* as a strong risk factor for that disease. *TREM2* had been described as the causal gene for a rare neurological condition with bone involvement named Nasu-Hakola disease [41, 42]. The finding that the same gene and perhaps even the same variants, when heterozygous, confer risk for the most common form of Alzheimer's disease was far from expected [43, 44]. There are several examples of this type of unpredicted results in recent literature (for a review see [45]). In the case of AD, *TREM2* brought to center stage the role of inflammation in the disease pathobiology, something that had for long been alluded to, but for which molecular evidence was still lacking. These unexpected results are sometimes the easiest to interpret and it is expected that in DLB we will come to see some of them in the future.

Future Perspectives on the Research of DLB

DLB has been a tremendously underserved disease. There are several factors contributing to this, such as the difficulty in diagnosis, the availability of a small number of cases to study, or even the fact that DLB was only recently recognized as a disease entity.

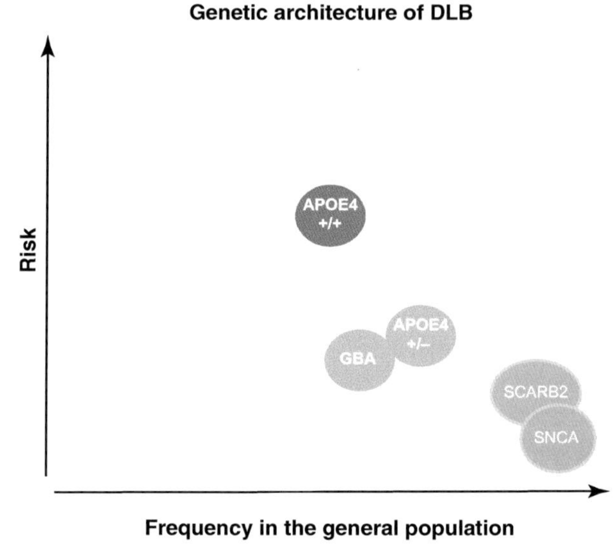

Fig. 4.2 The paradigm proposed by Manolio and co-workers [46] detailed the feasibility of finding genetic variants according to their frequency in the general population and their effect size on the phenotype. Variants that are common tend to have small effect sizes and are identified by GWAS, while variants that are rare tend to have high effect sizes and are only found by sequencing approaches. In DLB we can see that there is much missing from the plot with only four genes identified to play a role in this disease

Current data strongly implies that DLB has a genetic component that, in many aspects, is not very different from the ones we know are involved in other common neurological diseases. Familial aggregation suggests Mendelian forms of disease, while positive association studies suggest the contribution of genetic risk factors.

In 2009 Manolio and colleagues published a manuscript that aimed at identifying the reasons why we had not yet found all of the missing heritability for many diseases [46]. As part of that article, they proposed a paradigm that looked at the feasibility of identifying disease-associated genetic variants by their frequency in the general population. Figure 4.2 shows the application of the same paradigm to DLB, where it is clear how much is left to do. Currently, no Mendelian genes have been identified and only four genes are known to modulate the risk for disease.

The next stage in DLB's genetic research clearly needs to bring it up to speed with other diseases. Large-scale genetic studies need to be performed to identify genes involved in modulating risk; sequencing studies are needed to identify rare disease-specific variants; multinational teams need to come together to share and/or meta-analyze their data. All of these approaches are currently starting and it is hoped that results from them will greatly improve our understanding of DLB's etiology, eventually leading to the creation of effective therapeutic approaches.

References

1. George S et al. Alpha-synuclein: the long distance runner. Brain Pathol. 2013;23(3):350–7.
2. Spillantini MG et al. Alpha-synuclein in filamentous inclusions of Lewy bodies from Parkinson's disease and dementia with lewy bodies. Proc Natl Acad Sci USA. 1998;95(11): 6469–73.

3. Burn DJ. Cortical Lewy body disease. J Neurol Neurosurg Psychiatry. 2004;75(2):175–8.
4. Kovari E, Horvath J, Bouras C. Neuropathology of Lewy body disorders. Brain Res Bull. 2009;80(4–5):203–10.
5. Vekrellis K et al. Pathological roles of alpha-synuclein in neurological disorders. Lancet Neurol. 2011;10(11):1015–25.
6. Singleton AB et al. Alpha-synuclein locus triplication causes Parkinson's disease. Science. 2003;302(5646):841.
7. Devine MJ et al. Parkinson's disease and alpha-synuclein expression. Mov Disord. 2011; 26(12):2160–8.
8. Mak SK et al. Lysosomal degradation of alpha-synuclein in vivo. J Biol Chem. 2010;285(18): 13621–9.
9. Cuervo AM et al. Impaired degradation of mutant alpha-synuclein by chaperone-mediated autophagy. Science. 2004;305(5688):1292–5.
10. Chartier-Harlin MC et al. Alpha-synuclein locus duplication as a cause of familial Parkinson's disease. Lancet. 2004;364(9440):1167–9.
11. McKeith IG et al. Consensus guidelines for the clinical and pathologic diagnosis of dementia with Lewy bodies (DLB): report of the consortium on DLB international workshop. Neurology. 1996;47(5):1113–24.
12. McKeith IG et al. Diagnosis and management of dementia with Lewy bodies: third report of the DLB Consortium. Neurology. 2005;65(12):1863–72.
13. Lippa CF et al. DLB and PDD boundary issues: diagnosis, treatment, molecular pathology, and biomarkers. Neurology. 2007;68(11):812–9.
14. Mrak RE, Griffin WS. Dementia with Lewy bodies: Definition, diagnosis, and pathogenic relationship to Alzheimer's disease. Neuropsychiatr Dis Treat. 2007;3(5):619–25.
15. Hohl U et al. Diagnostic accuracy of dementia with Lewy bodies. Arch Neurol. 2000;57(3):347–51.
16. Wang CS et al. Twin pairs discordant for neuropathologically confirmed Lewy body dementia. J Neurol Neurosurg Psychiatry. 2009;80(5):562–5.
17. Duvoisin RC et al. Twin study of Parkinson disease. Neurology. 1981;31(1):77–80.
18. Pembrey ME. Discordant identical twins. II. Parkinsonism. Practitioner. 1972;209(250): 240–3.
19. Bogaerts V et al. A novel locus for dementia with Lewy bodies: a clinically and genetically heterogeneous disorder. Brain. 2007;130(Pt 9):2277–91.
20. Meeus B et al. Comprehensive genetic and mutation analysis of familial dementia with Lewy bodies linked to 2q35–q36. J Alzheimers Dis. 2010;20(1):197–205.
21. Renton AE et al. A hexanucleotide repeat expansion in C9ORF72 is the cause of chromosome 9p21-linked ALS-FTD. Neuron. 2011;72(2):257–68.
22. Meeus B, Theuns J, Van Broeckhoven C. The genetics of dementia with Lewy bodies: what are we missing? Arch Neurol. 2012;69(9):1113–8.
23. Meeus B et al. DLB and PDD: a role for mutations in dementia and Parkinson disease genes? Neurobiol Aging. 2012;33(3):629 e5–18.
24. Hardy J et al. Senile dementia of the Lewy body type has an apolipoprotein E epsilon 4 allele frequency intermediate between controls and Alzheimer's disease. Neurosci Lett. 1994;182(1):1–2.
25. Engelborghs S et al. Dose dependent effect of APOE epsilon4 on behavioral symptoms in frontal lobe dementia. Neurobiol Aging. 2006;27(2):285–92.
26. Pickering-Brown SM et al. Apolipoprotein E4 and Alzheimer's disease pathology in Lewy body disease and in other beta-amyloid-forming diseases. Lancet. 1994;343(8906):1155.
27. Singleton AB et al. Clinical and neuropathological correlates of apolipoprotein E genotype in dementia with Lewy bodies. Dement Geriatr Cogn Disord. 2002;14(4):167–75.
28. Tsuang D et al. APOE epsilon4 increases risk for dementia in pure synucleinopathies. JAMA Neurol. 2013;70(2):223–8.
29. Sidransky E et al. Multicenter analysis of glucocerebrosidase mutations in Parkinson's disease. N Engl J Med. 2009;361(17):1651–61.

30. Nalls MA et al. A multicenter study of glucocerebrosidase mutations in dementia with Lewy bodies. JAMA Neurol. 2013;70(6):727–35.
31. Alcalay RN et al. Cognitive performance of GBA mutation carriers with early-onset PD: the CORE-PD study. Neurology. 2012;78(18):1434–40.
32. Bras J, et al. Genetic analysis implicates APOE, SNCA and suggests lysosomal dysfunction in the etiology of dementia with Lewy bodies. Hum Mol Genet. 2014;23(23):6139–46.
33. Balreira A et al. A nonsense mutation in the LIMP-2 gene associated with progressive myoclonic epilepsy and nephrotic syndrome. Hum Mol Genet. 2008;17(14):2238–43.
34. Berkovic SF et al. Array-based gene discovery with three unrelated subjects shows SCARB2/LIMP-2 deficiency causes myoclonus epilepsy and glomerulosclerosis. Am J Hum Genet. 2008;82(3):673–84.
35. Dibbens LM et al. Mutation of SCARB2 in a patient with progressive myoclonus epilepsy and demyelinating peripheral neuropathy. Arch Neurol. 2011;68(6):812–3.
36. Lambert JC et al. Meta-analysis of 74,046 individuals identifies 11 new susceptibility loci for Alzheimer's disease. Nat Genet. 2013;45(12):1452–8.
37. Nalls MA et al. Large-scale meta-analysis of genome-wide association data identifies six new risk loci for Parkinson's disease. Nat Genet. 2014;46:989–93.
38. Vilarino-Guell C et al. VPS35 mutations in Parkinson disease. Am J Hum Genet. 2011;89(1):162–7.
39. Zimprich A et al. A mutation in VPS35, encoding a subunit of the retromer complex, causes late-onset Parkinson disease. Am J Hum Genet. 2011;89(1):168–75.
40. Zuk O et al. Searching for missing heritability: designing rare variant association studies. Proc Natl Acad Sci USA. 2014;111(4):E455–64.
41. Hakola HP, Iivanainen M. A new hereditary disease with progressive dementia and polycystic osteodysplasia: neuroradiological analysis of seven cases. Neuroradiology. 1973;6(3):162–8.
42. Klunemann HH et al. The genetic causes of basal ganglia calcification, dementia, and bone cysts: DAP12 and TREM2. Neurology. 2005;64(9):1502–7.
43. Guerreiro R et al. TREM2 variants in Alzheimer's disease. N Eng J Med. 2013;368(2):117–27.
44. Jonsson T et al. Variant of TREM2 associated with the risk of Alzheimer's disease. N Eng J Med. 2013;368(2):107–16.
45. Guerreiro R et al. Next generation sequencing techniques in neurological diseases: redefining clinical and molecular associations. Hum Mol Genet. 2014;23:R47–53.
46. Manolio TA et al. Finding the missing heritability of complex diseases. Nature. 2009;461(7265):747–53.

Chapter 5
Genetics of Frontotemporal Dementia

Sasja Heetveld, Patrizia Rizzu, and Peter Heutink

Abstract Frontotemporal dementia (FTD) is a progressive brain disease characterized by atrophy of the frontal and anterior temporal lobes. The prevalence has been estimated between 10 and 30 per 100,000, and patients have severe changes in personality and behavior. The disease has a strong genetic component, and in up to 40 % of cases, a positive family history has been observed. To date, seven disease genes have been identified, of which *MAPT*, *GRN*, and *C9orf72* are most frequently mutated. In contrast to familial FTD, far less is known about sporadic FTD. GWAS reported *TMEM106B* as an important risk factor for FTD, and recently, new loci have been associated with the disease. In this chapter, we summarize the current insights into the genetics of FTD based on neuropathological and functional data.

Keywords *C9orf72* • Frontotemporal dementia • Frontotemporal lobar degeneration • *GRN* • *MAPT* • Neurodegeneration

Abbreviations

aFTLD-U	Atypical frontotemporal lobar degeneration with ubiquitinated inclusions
AGD	Argyrophilic grain disease
BIBD	Basophilic inclusion body disease
C9orf72	Chromosome 9 open reading frame 72
CBD	Corticobasal degeneration
CHMP2B	Charged multivesicular body protein 2B
FTD-3	Frontotemporal dementia linked to chromosome 3

S. Heetveld, MSc • P. Heutink, MSc, PhD (✉)
Genome Biology of Neurodegenerative Diseases, Tübingen 72076, Germany

Eberhard Karls University, Tübingen, Germany
e-mail: peter.heutink@dzne.de

P. Rizzu, PhD
Applied Genomics of Neurodegenerative Diseases, Tübingen 72076, Germany

S.A. Schneider, J.M.T. Brás (eds.), *Movement Disorder Genetics*,
DOI 10.1007/978-3-319-17223-1_5

FTLD	Frontotemporal lobar degeneration
FUS	Fused in sarcoma
GRN	Granulin
MAPT	Microtubule-associated protein tau
MSTD	Multiple system tauopathy with dementia
NFT-dementia	Neurofibrillary tangle predominant dementia
ni	No inclusions
NIFID	Neuronal intermediate filament inclusion disease
PiD	Pick's disease
PSP	Progressive supranuclear palsy
TARDBP	TAR DNA-binding protein
TDP	TDP-43
UPS	Ubiquitin proteasome system
VCP	Valosin-containing protein
WMT-GGI	White matter tauopathy with globular glial inclusions

Introduction

Frontotemporal dementia (FTD) is a devastating presenile dementia characterized by atrophy of the frontal and anterior temporal lobes, and the prevalence, in the age group between 45 and 65 years, has been estimated between 10 and 30 per 100,000 [1]. It is a heterogeneous group of disorders and associated with genes that typically cause a clinical picture of amyotrophic lateral sclerosis (ALS), the most common type of motor neuron disease (MND) [2].

Clinically, there is progressive deterioration of either behavior or language, which translates into two FTD subtypes: the behavioral variant of frontotemporal dementia (bvFTD) and primary progressive aphasia (PPA). In bvFTD, patients have severe changes in behavior and personality, as indicated by early disinhibition, apathy, loss of sympathy, perseverative and stereotypic behavior, and hyperorality [3]. PPA can be further subdivided into semantic variant PPA (svPPA) and nonfluent variant PPA (nfvPPA), based on specific speech and language features. A third recognized subtype for patients not fitting either category is logopenic variant primary progressive aphasia (lvPPA) [4, 5]. The bvFTD accounts for more than 50 % of the FTD patients, and PNFA is the second most prevalent presentation of FTD, accounting for 25 %. The svPPA presents in 20–25 % of the FTD patients, and lvPPA is not considered part of the FTD group of disorders [6, 7]. Other conditions closely related to FTD are MND, progressive supranuclear palsy (PSP) syndromes, corticobasal syndrome (CBS), FTD with parkinsonism (FTDP), and argyrophilic grain disease (AGD) [8].

At the neuropathological level, the different subtypes of FTD present with diverse patterns of frontal and anterior temporal lobe atrophy. The term "frontotemporal lobar degeneration" (FTLD) is often used for these pathological conditions that present with FTD. FTLD is a proteinopathy characterized by abnormal, ubiquitinated protein inclusions in the cytoplasm or nuclei of neuronal and glial cells. Neuronal loss and astrocytosis are seen in cortices of atrophied frontal and temporal lobes, and neuropathological subcategories are based on the major constituent of inclusions [9]. Initially, two pathological categories were described: FTLD-tau including Pick's disease, in which neurons and glial cells contained inclusions of hyperphosphorylated tau protein, and FTLD-Ubiquitin or FTLD-U with unknown inclusions. In 80–95 % of the FTLD-U group, inclusions were later found to be mainly composed of TDP-43 (FTLD-TDP), and a considerable number of TDP-43-negative FTLD-U cases had inclusion of FUS (FTLD-FUS) [10, 11]. In a small number of FTLD-U patients, the inclusion protein remains unknown (FTLD-UPS) [12].

In up to 40 % of FTD cases, a positive family history is observed and inheritance varies among the different clinical subtypes [13–15]. Family history is most prominent in bvFTD, especially when MND is present. Research on these families has led to the discovery of multiple disease-causing genes. Mutations in microtubule-associated protein tau (*MAPT*) [16–18], granulin (*GRN*) [19, 20], and chromosome 9 open reading frame 72 (*C9orf72*) [21, 22] together explain the majority of familial FTD cases [1, 23]. Mutations in valosin-containing protein (*VCP*) and charged multivesicular body protein 2B (*CHMP2B*) are rare, each explaining less than 1 % of the familial FTD [1]. Mutations in common ALS genes TAR DNA-binding protein (*TARDBP*) and fused in sarcoma (*FUS*) are a very rare cause of familial FTD [24–27]. Association between affected gene and associated neuropathology is observed, and the association between disease gene and clinical phenotype is limited (Table 5.1) [1]. In contrast to familial forms of FTD, far less is known about the genetics of sporadic forms of the disease. To date, two genome-wide association studies (GWAS) have been published in which *TMEM106B* at chromosome 7p21

Table 5.1 Molecular classification of FTLD with pathological subtypes and associated genes [9, 12]

Molecular class	Major pathological subtypes	Associated genes
FTLD-tau	PiD CBD PSP AGD MSTD NFT-dementia WMT-GGI Unclassifiable	*MAPT*
FTLD-TDP	Types 1–4 Unclassifiable	*GRN* *VCP* *C9orf72* (*TARDBP*)
FTLD-FUS	aFTLD-U NIFID BIBD	(*FUS*)
FTLD-UPS	FTD-3	*CHMP2B*
FTLD-ni		

has been reported as a risk factor for FTLD-TDP [28] and novel genetic risk loci and pathways have been associated with FTD [29].

MAPT

In the late 1990s, linkage at chromosome 17q21 was found for multiple families in FTD and parkinsonism linked to chromosome 17 (FTDP-17). Three research groups found mutations in and around *MAPT* exon 10 and proved that dysfunction of the protein tau is sufficient to cause neurodegeneration and dementia [16–18]. Accumulation of tau occurs primarily as insoluble fibrils in neuronal cell bodies (neurofibrillary tangles (NFTs)) and processes (neuropil threads or dystrophic neurites), but can also accumulate in astrocytes and microglia. Tau deposits are characteristic for a large number of neurodegenerative diseases known as the "tauopathies," which include Alzheimer's disease (AD), Pick's disease (PiD), PSP, corticobasal degeneration (CBD), and AGD [30]. In AD, all six brain isoforms of tau are found in inclusions [31], and in FTDP-17, inclusions are heterogeneous, with different mutations associated with a different isoform composition. For PSP, CBD, and AGD, inclusions consist mainly of 4-repeat tau [32–34], and PiD has predominantly 3-repeat tau deposits [35]. In populations of European descent, *MAPT* is characterized by two haplotypes, H1 and H2, which result from a 900-kb inversion polymorphism. Inheritance of the H1 haplotype is a risk factor for PSP, CBD, and idiopathic Parkinson's disease. The H2 haplotype is associated with increased expression of exon 3, suggesting that inclusion of this exon might be protective [36–39].

Tau proteins are microtubule-associated proteins that are abundant in the central nervous system (CNS) and mainly concentrated in axons [40]. The *MAPT* gene is located on chromosome 17q21 and consists of 16 exons, as depicted in Fig. 5.1. In adult human brain, alternative mRNA splicing of exons 2, 3, and 10 produces six tau isoforms ranging from 352 to 441 amino acids. Three of these isoforms contain 4 microtubule-binding repeats (4R), whereas the other three contain only 3 microtubule-binding repeats (3R). The extra repeat domain is encoded by exon 10. The presence or absence of a 29 amino acid (exon 2) or a 58 amino acid (exons 2 and 3) insert in the N-terminal half of the protein divides the isoforms further in 0N, 1N, and 2N (Fig. 5.1). The ratio of 4R and 3R tau isoforms in the cerebral cortex of healthy adults is equal, while in fetal brain, only 3R0N is expressed. Most adult rodents express isoforms with four repeats [41]. Tau is enriched in neurons and has an important function in promoting microtubule assembly and stability [42–44]. The C-terminal repeat domains bind microtubules directly, and 4R tau promotes microtubule assembly 3-fold stronger than 3R tau [45, 46]. The N-terminal inserts are part of the projection domain, establishing the interaction of tau and microtubules with the plasma membrane [47, 48]. In addition to its role in microtubule assembly, tau mediates transport of vesicles and organelles along the microtubules by regulating attachment and detachment of motor proteins [49, 50]. The motility of motor proteins dynein and kinesin is differentially regulated and dependent on tau

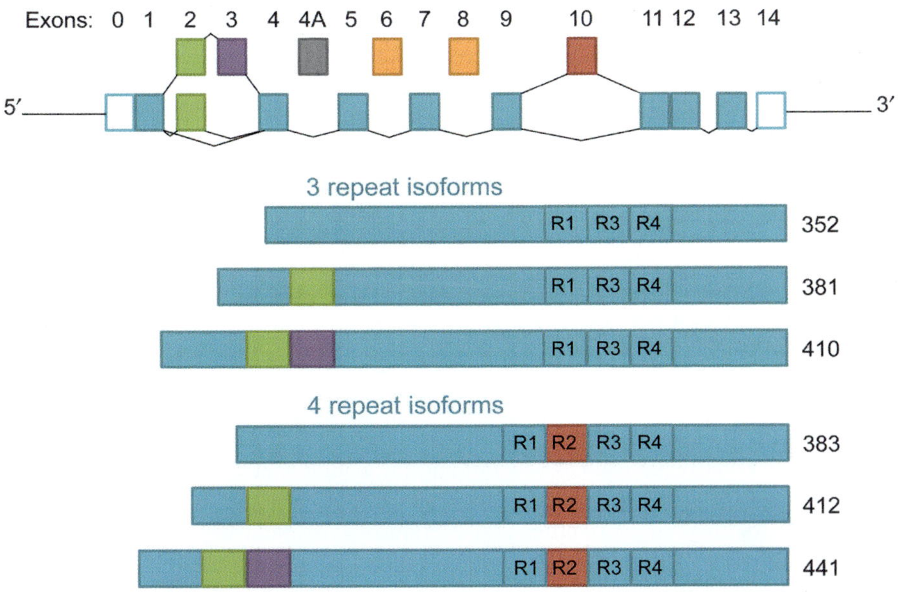

Fig. 5.1 Human brain MAPT isoforms. MAPT and the six isoforms found in adult human brain. Exons 1, 4, 5, 7, 9, and 11–13 are constitutively spliced (*blue*), and exons 0, which is part of the promoter, and 14 are noncoding (*white*). Exons 6 and 8 are not transcribed in human brain (*orange*), and the unusually long exon 4a (*gray*) is expressed only in the peripheral nervous system in higher-molecular-weight proteins termed "big tau." Alternative splicing of exons 2 (*green*), 3 (*purple*), and 10 (*red*) gives rise to the six isoforms (352–441 amino acids), and the repeats of tau (R1–R4) are indicated

concentration and isoform, pointing to a balanced spatiotemporal regulation of axonal transport [51]. Literature also suggests a physiological role for tau in dendrites, which might be an important function mediating synaptic impairment early in the disease process [52, 53].

Phosphorylation is the major posttranslational modification of tau protein, and in diseased brain, tau is abnormally hyperphosphorylated, generating paired helical filaments (PHFs) and neurofibrillary tangles [54–56]. The degree of tau phosphorylation influences its interaction with microtubules. Abnormal hyperphosphorylated tau sequesters normal tau, leading to misfolding, co-aggregation, and inhibition of microtubule assembly [57]. Microtubule-associated proteins 1 and 2 are also sequestered from pre-assembled microtubules, leading to their disruption [58–61]. There are 80 serine/threonine and 5 tyrosine potential phosphorylation sites, and normal brain tau contains 2–3 mol of phosphate per mole of tau protein. Mass spectrometry and antibody staining have identified more than 40 serine/threonine hyperphosphorylation sites of tau in AD [62, 63]. The phosphorylation of tau itself is developmentally regulated, and fetal tau is more phosphorylated than adult brain tau [64]. Several protein kinases are known to phosphorylate tau, and hyperphosphorylation probably involves coordinated action of several of them [65, 66]. When tau hyperphosphorylation induces dissociation from microtubules, it is redistributed from axonal to somatodendritic compartments. The increased pool of hyperphosphorylated tau is thought to promote assembly into fibrillar aggregates. In addition to phosphorylation, tau undergoes other posttranslation modifications, such as acetylation, glycation, glycosylation with O-linked N-acetylglucosamine, nitration, ubiquitination, sumoylation, prolyl isomerization, and truncation, all of which affect tau phosphorylation and/or aggregation [30].

Pathological MAPT *Mutations*

Up to 44 different clinical *MAPT* mutations in 134 FTD families have been reported in exons 1, 9, 10, 11, 12, and 13, intron 9, and the first 19 nucleotides of intron 10 (detailed information on each *MAPT* mutation is available at www.molgen.ua.ac.be/ftdmutations) [67, 68]. Except for mutations P301L in exon 10 and E10+16 in intron 10, identified in 32 families and 27 families, respectively, *MAPT* mutations are rare and seen in single families. Mutations are mainly clustered in exons 9–12, encoding the four microtubule-binding domains of tau, and can be divided into two functional groups. The first group has a primary effect at the protein level and includes missense and deletion mutations in the coding region of the gene. These mutations reduce the ability of tau to interact with microtubules, and some mutations promote filament assembly [68, 69]. The second group affects alternative splicing of tau pre-mRNA. This includes intronic and exonic mutations that alter alternative mRNA splicing of *MAPT* exon 10. The intronic mutations are clustered at the exon 10/intron 10 junction that is predicted to form a stem-loop structure protecting the 5′-splice site [70, 71]. Most of these mutations increase exon 10 inclusion and raise the normal 4R/3R isoform ratio from 1 to 2–3 [16]. However, a few mutations such as Δ(delta)K280 enhance exon 10 exclusion and result in increased expression of 3R tau [72]. In FTDP-17, the early clinical symptoms vary with the type of mutation found, and there is considerable phenotypic variability [73].

Tau Animal Models

After the identification of pathogenic mutations in *MAPT* in FTDP-17, several groups reported on the formation of NFTs and neuronal death in mouse models expressing human mutant tau, reviewed by Götz et al. [74]. To study the link between NFTs and brain dysfunction, transgenic mice were created expressing human P301L mutant tau that could be suppressed by doxycycline. This model (rTg4510) develops progressive age-related NFTs, neuronal loss, and behavioral impairment [75]. After switching off transgenic tau expression, memory function recovers and the number of neurons stabilizes, while NFTs continue to accumulate. Additional studies in rTg4510 showed that neuron loss can occur independently of NFT pathology and not all regions with NFT pathology undergo neuron loss, together implying that NFTs alone are not sufficient to cause cognitive decline or neuronal death [76, 77]. In vivo imaging shows that tangle-bearing neurons are long-lived and soluble tau species may be the critical components underlying neurodegeneration [78]. In transgenic mice expressing mutant repeat domains of human tau, similar observations were made [79]. After turning off expression of pro-aggregant Δ(delta)K280 mutant repeat domains of tau, memory and long-term potentiation recovers, while neuronal loss and aggregates persist. When anti-aggregant mutations were added, neuronal death was prevented, but tau aggregates are still formed [80].

There is accumulating evidence for intercellular transfer of tau aggregates [81–83]. In one of the first studies, brain homogenates from mice expressing human mutant P301S tau protein (with silver-positive tau inclusions) were injected into mice expressing human wild-type tau. This induced filament formation of wild-type human tau and spreading of pathology over time to anatomically connected brain regions [81]. Additional work showed that synthetic tau fibrils assembled from human mutant tau protein promoted the formation of tau inclusions in presymptomatic mice transgenic for human mutant P301S tau protein. In these mice, spreading of tau pathology was also initiated [84]. This has been further supported by experiments in a mouse model expressing human tau P301L restricted to layer II of the entorhinal cortex, recreating an early stage of NFT pathology [85]. Recently, similar results were obtained after injection of brain homogenates from cases of human tauopathies (including AD, PiD, AGD, PSP, and CBD) [86]. One other study demonstrated the induction and propagation of pathology when tau oligomers from AD brain were injected into wild-type mice, suggesting that they might play a critical role in initiation and spreading of tau pathology [87]. In vitro studies also showed induction and propagation of tau misfolding, and involvement of the endocytic pathway has been suggested [83, 88–91]. These studies show that tau fibrils spread from cell to cell by converting soluble tau into aggregates, and this mechanism might be responsible for disease propagation.

Besides the mouse, other organisms have been used to study FTD, such as the fruit fly *Drosophila melanogaster*, the nematode *Caenorhabditis elegans*, and the zebrafish *Danio rerio*. When wild-type and FTDP-17 mutant forms of human tau (R406W) were expressed in *Drosophila*, flies exhibited adult-onset progressive neurodegeneration, early death, enhanced toxicity of mutant tau, and abnormal tau accumulation without NFT formation [92]. Expression of wild-type and mutant human tau (P301L and V337M) in the *C. elegans* led to progressive uncoordinated locomotion, accumulation of insoluble tau species, neurodegeneration, and loss of neurons [93]. Expression of mutant tau caused an earlier and more severe phenotype compared to wild-type tau. Stable expression of human tau with the P301L mutation in the zebrafish also recapitulates key pathological features of tauopathies, including tau hyperphosphorylation, tangle formation, behavioral disturbances, and neuronal cell death [94].

GRN

In a large number of families linked to chromosome 17q21, mutations in *MAPT* could not be identified. In 2006, systematic analyses of the 17q21 region led to the discovery of mutations in *GRN* as a cause of FTLD-U [19, 20]. All *GRN*-associated FTLD patients present with TDP-43-positive inclusions in the affected cortical regions and basal ganglia (FTLD-TDP), often accompanied by irregular and short dystrophic neurites [95, 96]. The inclusions are found in neurons and glial cells and can be cytoplasmic as well as intranuclear. NFTs, neuritic plaques, and Lewy bodies have occasionally been observed in *GRN* brains [97–100].

In humans, the *GRN* gene is located upstream to the *MAPT* gene and comprises 12 coding exons (Fig. 5.2) [101]. The gene encodes progranulin, a 593-amino-acid-long protein containing a secretory signal sequence and seven and a half repeats of a unique 10–12 cysteine-containing motif. This motif is highly conserved in evolution and a reminiscent of the epithelial growth factor [102–105]. Progranulin is expressed in several tissues of the periphery as well as in neurons and microglia in the central nervous system, and little or no expression has been detected in adult astrocytes and oligodendrocytes [102, 106–108]. A GWAS implicated sortilin (*SORT1*) as an important regulator of GRN levels in human plasma, and cellular studies showed that SORT1 is a major neuronal receptor for GRN [109, 110]. SORT1 facilitates extracellular GRN clearance via endocytosis and delivery to the

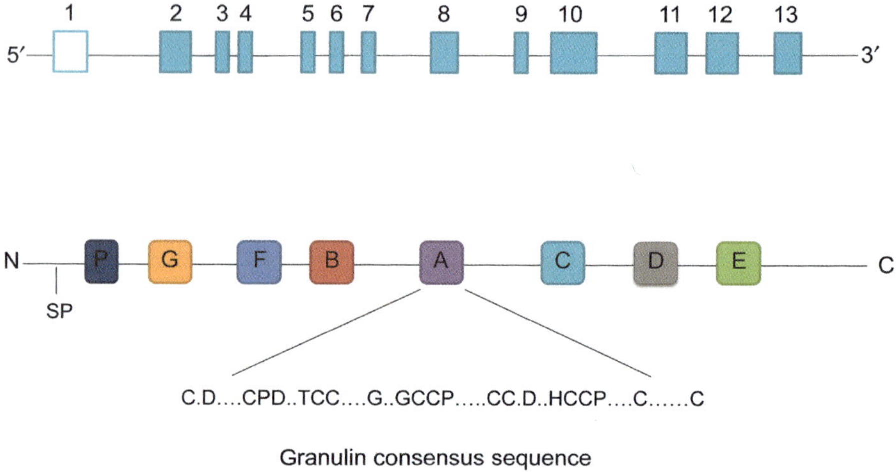

Fig. 5.2 GRN gene and protein structure. Schematic representation of human GRN gene structure (*top*) and progranulin protein structure (*bottom*). The GRN gene spans approximately 8 kb genomic sequence on chromosome 17q21. The gene structure indicates noncoding exon 1 (*white*) and the coding exons 2–13 (*blue*). The full-length progranulin protein presents a signal peptide (*SP*) and seven and a half tandem repeats of a conserved 10–12 cysteine-containing motif (granulins A to G and paragranulin P). Once the signal peptide is cleaved off, the mature protein gets secreted; it can be further processed by cleavage in the linker regions between the granulin domains. The lettered boxes in progranulin refer to individual granulin domains (~6 kDa)

lysosomes. When GRN interaction with SORT1 is impaired, it is possible to restore extracellular GRN levels in FTD patient-derived lymphocytes and induced pluripotent stem cells (iPSC) differentiated to neurons [111].

GRN plays a key role in several biological processes including cell growth, wound repair, inflammation, and neuron development [112]. Studies in different cellular models show that GRN expression enhances neuronal survival and promotes neurite outgrowth and branching, while siRNA-mediated *GRN* knockdown results in reduced neurite arborization and dendritic protrusions [113–117]. The exact mechanism through which GRN exerts its neurotrophic function is not completely understood; however, compelling evidence suggests the involvement of the phosphatidylinositol 3-kinase/Akt signaling pathway and glycogen synthase kinase-3 beta regulation [118–120]. *GRN*-deficient cells show increased caspase activation, decrease in cellular survival, and vulnerability to a number of cellular stressors, including oxygen and glucose deprivation, oxidative stress, and sublethal doses of N-methyl-D-aspartic acid, kinase inhibitors, and proteasomal inhibitors [118, 121–123].

It has been hypothesized that GRN performs a neuroprotective role in the CNS by stimulating production of anti-inflammatory Th2 cytokines and supporting neuroprotective inflammation by binding to TNF receptors [124, 125]. The anti-inflammatory effects of GRN are evident in *Grn−/−* mice that show an exacerbated inflammatory reaction [123]. Moreover, increased GRN expression has been observed in microglia following a variety of acute and chronic insults in several neurodegenerative disorders including Creutzfeldt-Jakob disease [126], ALS [127, 128] and FTLD [99]. It also attracts and activates microglia, enhancing endocytosis of extracellular peptides such as amyloid β (beta) 1–42 [129]. Interestingly, microglia of patients with *GRN* mutations are able to upregulate GRN despite reduced levels in blood, cerebrospinal fluid, and neurons in unaffected brain regions [99] suggesting GRN plays a central role in the inflammatory response.

Pathological *GRN* Mutations

Confirmed pathogenic mutations in *GRN* cases have been so far identified only in FTLD-TDP, and *GRN* mutation screening in patients with ALS [130, 131], Parkinson's disease [132], and non-FTD cases with TDP-43 pathology [133] yields no positive results. To date, 69 pathogenic mutations have been observed in patients with FTLD-TDP, mostly being loss-of-function mutations suggesting that *GRN* haploinsufficiency is the major pathogenic mechanism (detailed information on each *GRN* mutation is available at www.molgen.ua.ac.be/ftdmutations) [67]. *GRN* deficiency occurs through frame-shift, splice site, and nonsense mutations, introducing a premature termination codon with activation of nonsense-mediated mRNA decay and reduction of progranulin protein levels [19, 20, 134]. Loss of mRNA translation and consequent protein haploinsufficiency is also observed when mutations are present in the Kozak sequence of the *GRN* gene preventing translation [19, 20, 135, 136] or result in genomic deletion of one copy of the gene [137, 138].

The *GRN* R493X and T272fs mutations are among the most frequent mutations found in *GRN* patients [139, 140]. Patients carrying these mutations do not show significant phenotypic differences with other *GRN* mutation carriers. Interestingly, the occurrence of a founder effect has been suggested for both mutations [139, 141]. In addition, missense and silent mutations have been observed scattered along the *GRN* gene. For a large number of them, it is still debated if they play an active role in the disease pathogenesis. Some mutations are predicted to affect protein function in silico, they have been found in patients only, or experimental studies demonstrated a potential pathogenic effect causing reduced protein expression by cellular mechanisms other than *GRN* mRNA reduction [142, 143]. Mutations A9D, P248L, and R432C have been reported to affect protein secretion and stability thereby reducing the amount of available GRN. The A9D mutation [144] occurs within the hydrophobic core of the signal peptide sequence of *GRN* impairing its secretion. The mutated protein fails to undergo N-glycosylation, suggesting its missorting into the cytosol [135, 143]. The P248L and R432C mutations might contribute to disease phenotype by adversely affecting the neurotrophic properties of GRN [114].

GRN mutations pathologically confirmed in FTD with TDP-43 pathology are so far all heterozygote. The only exception is a single report of two siblings clinically diagnosed with adult-onset neuronal ceroid lipofuscinosis (NCL), a lysosomal storage disorder with severe accumulation of lipofuscin, and progressive neurodegeneration [145]. Interestingly, *Grn–/–* mice also show an increase of the aging pigment lipofuscin accompanied by tissue vacuolization in the hippocampus. Although we are still awaiting for the neuropathological assessment, the inclusion of *GRN* as genetic cause of NCL [146] has important consequences for the role of *GRN* in lysosome biology.

GRN Animal Models

To date, five independent *Grn–/–* mouse models have been established and extensively characterized (reviewed in [112, 147]). Although in humans *GRN* loss alone is sufficient to cause neurodegeneration, none of the mouse models fully recapitulate the human disease. Their most consistent behavioral phenotype is reduction in social interactions already observed at young age. Neuropathologically, *Grn–/–* mice all display pronounced progressive microgliosis and astrocytosis as well as ubiquitin accumulation in the cortex, hippocampus, thalamus, and brain stem. Accumulation of ubiquitinated proteins suggests disturbance of the proteasomal and/or autophagy-lysosomal pathways, which is supported by accumulation of the autophagy-related receptor p62 and increased expression of lysosomal protease cathepsin D [148]. Neuronal loss is in general not remarkable, and it is present only in selected areas; however, *Grn–/–* mice show impaired neuronal function with reduced synaptic connectivity and impaired synaptic plasticity. These findings support in part the results from *GRN* knockdown or knockout studies in primary hippocampal neuronal and slice cultures [149, 150]. Interestingly, altered synaptic vesicle numbers are also found in FTD patients carrying *GRN* mutations [149]. *Grn–/–* mice do not show TDP-43 fragmentation, cytoplasmic mislocalization, abnormal phosphorylation, and accumulation in aggregates typical of FTLD-TDP associated with *GRN* mutations [148, 151]. In the insoluble fraction of *Grn–/–* mice brain lysates, only full-length TDP-43 has been detected with a significant increase from 12 months forward. One study did show the appearance of phosphorylated TDP-43 in the cytosol of neurons in the hippocampal and thalamic areas [123, 152], and studies in mouse cortical neurons and *GRN* patient iPSC differentiated to neurons demonstrated increased translocation of TDP-43 from the nucleus to the cytoplasm [118, 121].

C9orf72

In 2011, two independent consortia identified the pathological expansion of a non-coding GGGGCC hexanucleotide repeat in *C9orf72* as a cause of familial FTD and ALS, explaining several linkages and GWAS performed since 2006 linking chromosome 9p to these disorders [21, 22, 153, 154]. The findings where confirmed by other studies in a wide series of populations [155, 156], and repeat expansions for *C9orf72* have since then also been confirmed in families affected with AD, CBS, and ataxia syndromes [157, 158].

The *C9orf72* gene is transcribed in three major transcripts and located on the short arm of chromosome 9. The location of the repeat is between noncoding exons 1a and 1b, which is the first intron following noncoding exon 1 of transcript variants 1 and 3 and the upstream regulatory region of transcript variant 2 (Fig. 5.3). In the general population, the median length of the hexanucleotide repeat sequence is two repeats (range 0 to ±20). The *C9orf72* transcript variants 1 and 3 encode for a 481 amino acid protein, whereas transcript variant 2 encodes for a shorter 222 amino acid protein. These protein isoforms share the first 221 N-terminal amino acids but differ in their C-terminal region. *C9orf72* is detected throughout the CNS, with the highest expression level observed within the cerebellum [21, 22, 154, 159, 160]. Currently, there are no specific antibodies for C9orf72, and therefore, the exact subcellular localization is not very well established. In neuronal cell lines transfected with C9orf72, the protein is detected both in the nucleus and cytoplasm and in the medium [161], and additional studies have suggested C9orf72 is also present in the membrane fraction of cells after subcellular fractionation experiments [162, 163]. Further experiments are needed to conclusively determine where the protein is localized.

C9orf72 is highly conserved in evolution, and bioinformatics approaches showed that the protein is a novel homologue of differentially expressed in normal and neoplastic (DENN) proteins [164, 165]. DENN proteins are guanine exchange factors (GEF) that activate Rab GTPases, and these findings suggest a role for C9orf72 in Rab GTPase-dependent membrane trafficking. Support comes from a study in which several Rab proteins involved in endocytosis and autophagy were found to

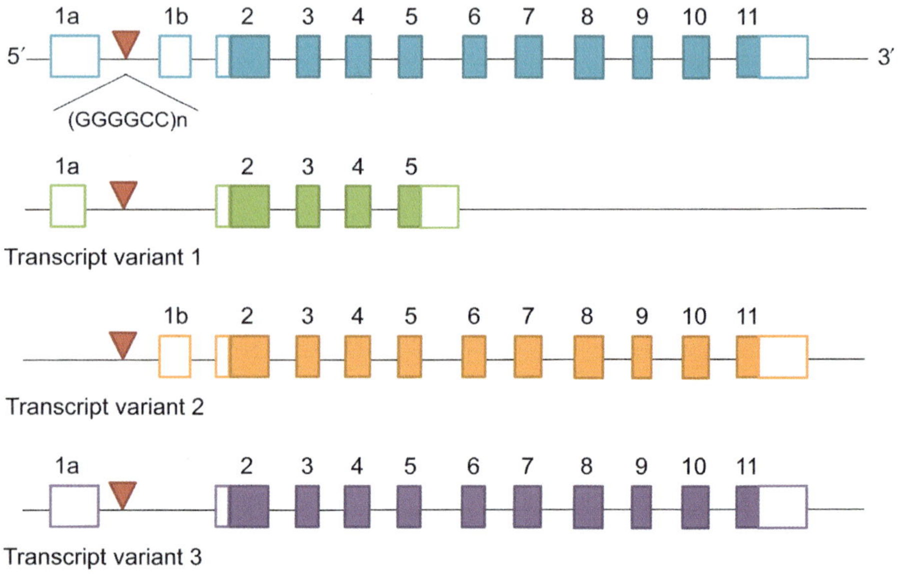

Fig. 5.3 Human C9orf72 gene structure. The structure of the C9orf72 gene and its major transcripts. Transcript variant 1 (NM_145005.5) in *green*, transcript variant 2 (NM_018325.3) in *orange*, and transcript variant 3 (NM_001256054.1) in *purple* according to the NCBI RefSeq Database. The *arrow* (*red*) marks the hexanucleotide repeat location. (GGGGCC)n indicates repetition of this sequence n times, with a median length of two repeats in the general population (range 0 to ±20). *Colored blocks* indicate coding exons and *white blocks* indicate noncoding exons

co-localize or co-immunoprecipitate with C9orf72 [161]. Knockdown of *C9orf72* in neuronal cell lines also led to defects in autophagic processing as well as endocytosis. Furthermore, human neurons differentiated from iPSC with the *C9orf72* repeat expansion were more sensitive to autophagy-inhibiting drugs [166]. Functional studies are required in order to conclusively demonstrate that *C9orf72* encodes a GEF and Rab proteins might be activated.

Effect of the Pathogenic *C9orf72* Mutation

The frequency of C9orf72 repeat expansions ranges from 12 to 25 % in familial and 6–7 % in sporadic FTD patients and 10–50 % in familial and 5–7 % in sporadic ALS cases. This makes *C9orf72* repeat expansions the most common cause of the FTD/ALS complex of diseases [155, 167, 168]. The causal effect of the *C9orf72* mutation is not yet completely understood, and currently, three mechanisms have been implicated for the disease.

There is accumulating evidence that the expanded repeat is associated with reduced expression of *C9orf72* transcripts, and studies in human postmortem brain tissue, patient-derived iPSC, and lymphoblasts suggest that a loss of function might be relevant for the disease pathogenesis [21, 154, 159, 160, 162, 166, 169, 170].

Epigenetic changes could be responsible for the decrease in C9orf72 expression levels observed in patients, and this mechanism has been described previously for Friedreich's ataxia and fragile X syndrome [171, 172]. This hypothesis is supported by two studies describing hypermethylation of CpG islands and abnormal histone binding associated with the repeat expansion [159, 173].

A second mechanism associated with repeat expansion diseases is RNA toxicity, caused by sequestration of normal transcripts and RNA-binding proteins by RNA molecules including the expanded repeat [174]. The presence of the expanded repeat in pre-mRNA transcripts could prevent normal splicing toward a mature mRNA, and the resulting repeat-containing RNA species could then aggregate into RNA foci and have a toxic effect. In support of this hypothesis, repeat-containing RNA aggregates have been reported in brains of patients and in patient-derived iPSC [21, 162, 163, 175, 176]. In vitro experiments using GGGGCC-repeat RNA oligonucleotides showed that they fold into stable RNA G-quadruplex structures, which suggests that the inclusion of the expanded repeat into the *C9orf72* transcripts in vivo could interfere with the normal processing of the pre-mRNA for transcripts 1 and 3 [177, 178]. This is supported by in vitro transcription assays that show the presence of abortive transcripts caused by G-quadruplex assembly, and these findings were confirmed in patient-derived B lymphocytes [179]. There is also evidence for the sequestration of RNA-binding proteins (RBPs) by RNA molecules including the transcribed repeat expansion, which could cause a depletion of RBPs available for normal RNA metabolism. RNA-binding assays, using $r(GGGGCC)_{10}$ repeat sequences, identified Pur α as a repeat binding protein. Loss of Pur α reduced cell viability of Neuro-2a cells and overexpression of Pur α in *Drosophila*, and Neuro-2a cells mitigated the repeat-mediated neurotoxicity [180]. The interaction of Pur α is supported by co-localization studies, and also binding of several heterogeneous nuclear ribonucleoprotein (hnRNP) family members to the hexanucleotide repeat has been reported [163, 181].

A third hypothesis is that repeat-associated non-ATG-initiated (RAN) translation takes place within the expanded repeat sequence, resulting in the production and aggregation of dipeptide repeat proteins. In support of this hypothesis, aggregates positively stained with antibodies raised against putative hexanucleotide repeat RAN-translated peptides have been detected in human postmortem brain and cultured patient-derived iPSC [162, 170, 182]. The presence of stable RNA G-quadruplex structures could induce RAN translation similar to what has been reported for expanded CAG repeats in spinocerebellar ataxia 8 and myotonic dystrophy type 1 [183]. Sequencing results of DNAse 1-treated pre-mRNA from postmortem tissue matched the *C9orf72* genomic sequence and therefore support this hypothesis [182]. Interestingly, a *C9orf72* antisense transcript containing intron 1 sequences including repeat sequences was detected raising the possibility that the dipeptide repeat proteins might be translated from this transcript [184]. Foci containing this antisense RNA transcript are observed in the same brain regions as sense foci, but they are present in fewer cells and the average number of foci per cell appears higher [175]. Recently, a study in U2OS cancer cells and human astrocytes showed that synthetic dipeptides containing 20 repeats of sense glycine-proline (GR) or antisense proline-arginine (PR) associate with nucleoli and affect cell morphology and viability.

Exposure of cultured cells to these GR and PR translation products also led to altered pre-mRNA splicing and changes in ribosomal RNA biogenesis [185].

Animal Models for *C9orf72*

One of the first animal models created for *C9orf72* was a zebrafish model in which the translation of the z*C9orf72* orthologue was blocked using antisense morpholino oligonucleotides (AMO). This model system provided evidence that a decrease in *C9orf72* expression level could be important for the disease process [169]. The knockdown resulted in disrupted branching and shortening of motor neuron axons when compared to noninjected or mismatch AMO-injected fish; this phenotype could be rescued by injecting the mRNA for the human *C9orf72* long transcript. In addition, knockdown of *C9orf72* in zebrafish resulted in motor deficits associated with axonopathy, such as deficits in touch-evoked escape response and reduced mobility. Partial knockdown of endogenous *C9orf72* to 30–40 % of normal levels in a mouse model by antisense oligonucleotide administration was well tolerated for 18 weeks, which does not support that a loss of function is the main mechanism of the mutation [176]. Studies in patient fibroblasts and motor neurons derived from patient iPSC also did not confirm this hypothesis [163, 176]. A *Drosophila* model expressing the expanded hexanucleotide repeat (rGGGGCC) provides evidence that RNA foci or aberrantly processed pre-mRNAs are toxic. Neuronal toxicity in *Drosophila* and Neuro-2a cells was observed, and the expression of rGGGGCC repeats caused progressive neurodegeneration in *Drosophila* eye and a reduction in locomotor activity [180]. A more recent study differentiated between repeat RNA and DPR protein toxicity and showed that the major toxic species in their *Drosophila* model system are the DPR proteins; however, additional contribution of RNA toxicity is not ruled out [186].

VCP and *CHMP2B*

Mutations in two other genes, *VCP* and *CHMP2B*, lead to FTLD-TDP and account for a minority of familial cases [1]. Mutations in *VCP* were identified in 2004 by linkage analysis studies in families with inclusion body myopathy associated with Paget disease of bone and frontotemporal dementia (IBMPFD) [187]. *VCP* mutations are also a cause of familial ALS [188]. The protein is ubiquitously expressed and a highly conserved member of the AAA(+)-ATPase superfamily. The protein is associated with a wide variety of cellular activities, including cell cycle control and membrane fusion. It is also a multi-ubiquitin chain-targeting factor and is required in the degradation of many ubiquitin-proteasome pathway substrates [189]. IBMPFD mutations cluster in the N-terminal CDC48 domain, mediating substrate recognition and cofactor binding. Studies in patient tissue, transgenic mice, and cell models suggest that *VCP* is a key regulator at the intersection of autophagy and the ubiquitin-proteasome system [190, 191]. Mouse models expressing mutant *VCP* recapitulate aspects of the disease, including age-dependent degeneration in muscle, brain, and bone, and progressive widespread TDP-43 pathology [192, 193].

Mutations in *CHMP2B* were found in 2005 via linkage analysis in a large Danish FTD family [194], and mutations are also a cause of familial ALS [195]. The ubiquitinated neuronal cytoplasmic inclusions do not stain for tau, TDP-43, or FUS, and the classification is FTLD-UPS. CHMP2B is a component of the endosomal sorting complex required for transport III (ESCRT-III) and expressed in neurons of all major brain regions. The ESCRT-III complex is required for function of the multivesicular body (MVB), an endosomal structure that fuses with the lysosome to degrade endocytosed proteins. Mutations affect the C-terminal region of the protein due to aberrant splicing, and mutant *CHMP2B* disrupts the fusion of endosomes with lysosomes in cell culture models [196]. Mice expressing C-terminally truncated and mutant *CHMP2B* develop axonal swellings and have reduced survival. The mice also develop ubiquitinated protein inclusions negative for TDP-43 and FUS, mimicking the inclusions found in patients with *CHMP2B* mutations [197].

TARDBP and *FUS*

Mutations in *TARDBP* and *FUS* are found, although these are very rare in FTD and more common in ALS [24–27]. FTD associated with mutations in *GRN*, *VCP*, or *C9orf72* is consistently characterized by the presence of TDP-43 pathology, and a considerable number of tau-/TDP-negative FTLD cases have inclusion of FUS, suggesting that dysregulation of both proteins might be important in the pathogenesis of FTD [10, 95].

TDP-43 is a 414 amino acid protein with two RNA recognition motifs and a carboxy-terminal glycine-rich domain, encoded by the *TARDBP* gene on chromosome 1. TDP-43 is a member of the hnRNP family of proteins and regulates RNA processing in a variety of ways. It is involved in mRNA transport, stability and turnover, splicing, and translation. The protein is highly conserved, is predominantly nuclear, and can shuttle between the nucleus and the cytoplasm [198–200]. Essentially, all ALS- and FTD-associated mutations are missense changes in the C-terminal glycine-rich region, involved in protein-protein interactions. In FTLD-TDP brains, TDP-43 is redistributed to the cytoplasm, hyperphosphorylated, ubiquitinated, and cleaved into the C-terminal fragments (CTFs) [95]. Experimental studies do not conclusively demonstrate whether TDP-43-mediated neurodegeneration results from a gain or loss of function of the protein. There is evidence for both: gains of functions mediated by aggregation and abnormal cytoplasmic function or loss of functions mediated by nuclear depletion, CTFs, and RNA dysregulation [201, 202].

FUS was first reported in 2009 to be the cause of ~3 % familial ALS cases and subsequently found to be the marker for the pathology of many remaining tau-/TDP-negative FTLD cases [10, 203, 204]. The *FUS* gene encodes a 526 amino acid protein and forms a gene family together with *EWSR1* and *TAF15* (*FET*). Increased insolubility of all FET proteins has been found in FTLD-FUS, but not in ALS-FUS [205]. It is highly conserved, ubiquitously expressed, and mainly localized to the nucleus. The protein has a high degree of functional homology with TDP-43 and is involved in multiple steps of RNA processing [206]. Most mutations are missense mutations affecting the C-terminus, disrupting the binding of FUS to Transportin. This nuclear import receptor shuttles proteins from the cytoplasm to the nucleus leading to an accumulation of mutant FUS in the cytoplasm [207]. Also for FUS, it is still unclear whether the cytosolic deposition causes loss of essential nuclear functions, a gain of toxic functions in the cytosol, or both.

Susceptibility Genes and Risk Loci

Compared to Mendelian FTD genes, little is known about susceptibility genes contributing to the risk of developing the disease. In 2010, Van Deerlin and colleagues identified *TMEM106B* in a genome-wide association study as a risk factor for FTLD-TDP [28]. Three SNPs encompassing the *TMEM106B* gene were found significant in a series of 515 FTLD-TDP patients, and variants specifically increased the risk in *GRN* mutation carriers. The initial GWAS finding has been successfully replicated in several FTD cohorts, strongly supporting a key role for *TMEM106B* in FTLD-TDP pathogenesis [208–210]. *TMEMB106B* is a 274 amino acid transmembrane type 2 protein with a highly glycosylated luminal domain [211]. It is cytoplasmically expressed in neurons, glia, and endothelial cells/pericytes of human brain samples from normal individuals, while in neurons of FTLD-TDP cases, TMEM106B appears to extend beyond the cell body into neuronal processes. In multiple immortalized cell lines and primary cortical neurons, TMEM106B is localized to late endosomes or lysosomes, and increased levels affect endolysosomal and progranulin pathways [212–214]. A recent GWAS points to novel associations, and the immune system processes, lysosomal, and autophagy pathways are potentially involved in FTD. The new loci need to be replicated in future studies to determine their possible association with the disease [29].

In 2011, *UBQLN2* was added to the list of ALS-FTD genes [215]. The gene encodes the ubiquitin-like protein ubiquilin 2, a member of the ubiquitin family, which regulates the degradation of ubiquitinated proteins. In ~20 % of *UBQLN2* mutation carriers, progressive dementia similar to FTD was identified, but all patients eventually developed motor symptoms. P62, encoded for by the *SQSTM1* gene, is another protein at the intersection of ALS and FTD. It was found following the observation of involvement of P62 in ALS and has been subsequently reported in ALS and in FTD [216–218]. Inclusion positive for p62 can be found in *C9orf72* expansion mutation patients, both with and without TDP-43 pathology [219].

Another risk factor for FTLD-TDP comes from a variant located in the 3′UTR of *GRN* in a binding site for the microRNA mir-659 [220]. In a series of pathologically confirmed FTLD-TDP patients without *GRN* mutations, Rademakers and colleagues observed that homozygous T-allele carriers had a 3.2-fold increase risk to develop FTLD-TDP as compared to homozygote C-allele carriers. They hypothesized that this variant reduces GRN protein expression through mir-659-dependent translational inhibition. It is still unclear whether GRN levels play a direct role in general FTLD population as two other studies failed to replicate the original findings [221, 222]. However, the risk allele is overrepresented in cases with hippocampal sclerosis [223, 224] and was found associated with a lower GRN serum level in two independent studies [225, 226], suggesting that decreased *GRN* expression may be a risk factor for FTLD-TDP and other dementias.

Conclusion

In recent years, remarkable progress has been made regarding the understanding of the genetic causes and neuropathological features of FTD. The recent discovery of the *C9orf72* repeat expansions as the most common cause of the FTD/ALS complex of diseases showed that there is still a lot to be discovered. We know, for example, very little about susceptibility genes contributing to the risk of developing FTD and not all proteinopathies are fully characterized. The biological significance of the identified FTD genes has been studied extensively in cellular and animal models, as described in this chapter. However, diagnosis of FTD remains challenging, and no cure is available yet. Interestingly, many of the FTD genes seem to be connected at the molecular level. *TMEM106B* has originally been found as a risk factor for *GRN* mutation carriers, and several studies now describe *TMEM106B* as a genetic modifier for FTD with the *C9orf72* repeat expansions [227, 228]. Patients with mutations in *C9orf72* in combination with mutations in other genes involved in FTD/ALS have also been reported [229, 230]. Furthermore, FTD cases associated with *GRN* and *C9orf72* mutations both present with TDP-43 pathology, and several studies showed that TDP-43 binds the 3′-UTR of *GRN* and regulates its expression [199, 231]. Understanding the full biology and connecting all identified FTD genes and risk factors with clinical phenotypes are of high importance for developing therapeutic approaches and offering reliable genetic advice to patients.

Disclosure Peter Heutink is a co-applicant on a patent application related to *MAPT* (PCT/US1999/009529) and *C9orf72* (PCT/GB2012/052140) and is co-owner of Synaptologics BV.

References

1. Sieben A, Van Langenhove T, Engelborghs S, Martin J-J, Boon P, Cras P, et al. The genetics and neuropathology of frontotemporal lobar degeneration. Acta Neuropathol. 2012;124(3):353–72.
2. Bennion Callister J, Pickering-Brown SM. Pathogenesis/genetics of frontotemporal dementia and how it relates to ALS. Exp Neurol. 2014;262:84–90. PubMed PMID: 24915640.
3. Rascovsky K, Hodges JR, Knopman D, Mendez MF, Kramer JH, Neuhaus J, et al. Sensitivity of revised diagnostic criteria for the behavioural variant of frontotemporal dementia. Brain. 2011;134(Pt 9):2456–77. PubMed PMID: 21810890. PubMed Central PMCID: 3170532.
4. Gorno-Tempini ML, Hillis AE, Weintraub S, Kertesz A, Mendez M, Cappa SF, et al. Classification of primary progressive aphasia and its variants. Neurology. 2011;76(11):1006–14. PubMed PMID: 21325651. PubMed Central PMCID: 3059138.
5. Rascovsky K, Grossman M. Clinical diagnostic criteria and classification controversies in frontotemporal lobar degeneration. Int Rev Psychiatry. 2013;25(2):145–58. PubMed PMID: 23611345. PubMed Central PMCID: 3906583.
6. Johnson JK, Diehl J, Mendez MF, Neuhaus J, Shapira JS, Forman M, et al. Frontotemporal lobar degeneration: demographic characteristics of 353 patients. Arch Neurol. 2005;62(6):925–30. PubMed PMID: 15956163.
7. Josephs KA, Hodges JR, Snowden JS, Mackenzie IR, Neumann M, Mann DM, et al. Neuropathological background of phenotypical variability in frontotemporal dementia. Acta Neuropathol. 2011;122(2):137–53. PubMed PMID: 21614463. PubMed Central PMCID: 3232515.
8. Riedl L, Mackenzie IR, Forstl H, Kurz A, Diehl-Schmid J. Frontotemporal lobar degeneration: current perspectives. Neuropsychiatr Dis Treat. 2014;10:297–310. PubMed PMID: 24600223. PubMed Central PMCID: 3928059.
9. Mackenzie IR, Neumann M, Bigio EH, Cairns NJ, Alafuzoff I, Kril J, et al. Nomenclature for neuropathologic subtypes of frontotemporal lobar degeneration: consensus recommendations. Acta Neuropathol. 2009;117(1):15–8. PubMed PMID: 19015862. Pubmed Central PMCID: 2710877.
10. Neumann M, Rademakers R, Roeber S, Baker M, Kretzschmar HA, Mackenzie IR. A new subtype of frontotemporal lobar degeneration with FUS pathology. Brain. 2009;132(Pt 11):2922–31. PubMed PMID: 19674978. Pubmed Central PMCID: 2768659.
11. Roeber S, Mackenzie IR, Kretzschmar HA, Neumann M. TDP-43-negative FTLD-U is a significant new clinico-pathological subtype of FTLD. Acta Neuropathol. 2008;116(2):147–57. PubMed PMID: 18536926.
12. Mackenzie IR, Neumann M, Bigio EH, Cairns NJ, Alafuzoff I, Kril J, et al. Nomenclature and nosology for neuropathologic subtypes of frontotemporal lobar degeneration: an update. Acta Neuropathol. 2010;119(1):1–4. PubMed PMID: 19924424. Pubmed Central PMCID: 2799633.
13. Goldman JS, Adamson J, Karydas A, Miller BL, Hutton M. New genes, new dilemmas: FTLD genetics and its implications for families. Am J Alzheimers Dis Other Demen. 2007–2008;22(6):507–15. PubMed PMID: 18166610.
14. Rohrer JD, Guerreiro R, Vandrovcova J, Uphill J, Reiman D, Beck J, et al. The heritability and genetics of frontotemporal lobar degeneration. Neurology. 2009;73(18):1451–6. PubMed PMID: 19884572. PubMed Central PMCID: 2779007.
15. Seelaar H, Kamphorst W, Rosso SM, Azmani A, Masdjedi R, de Koning I, et al. Distinct genetic forms of frontotemporal dementia. Neurology. 2008;71(16):1220–6. PubMed PMID: 18703462.
16. Hutton M, Lendon CL, Rizzu P, Baker M, Froelich S, Houlden H, et al. Association of missense and 5′-splice-site mutations in tau with the inherited dementia FTDP-17. Nature. 1998;393(6686):702–5. PubMed PMID: 9641683.

17. Poorkaj P, Bird TD, Wijsman E, Nemens E, Garruto RM, Anderson L, et al. Tau is a candidate gene for chromosome 17 frontotemporal dementia. Ann Neurol. 1998;43(6):815–25. PubMed PMID: 9629852.
18. Spillantini MG, Murrell JR, Goedert M, Farlow MR, Klug A, Ghetti B. Mutation in the tau gene in familial multiple system tauopathy with presenile dementia. Proc Natl Acad Sci U S A. 1998;95(13):7737–41. PubMed PMID: 9636220. PubMed Central PMCID: 22742.
19. Baker M, Mackenzie IR, Pickering-Brown SM, Gass J, Rademakers R, Lindholm C, et al. Mutations in progranulin cause tau-negative frontotemporal dementia linked to chromosome 17. Nature. 2006;442(7105):916–9. PubMed PMID: 16862116.
20. Cruts M, Gijselinck I, van der Zee J, Engelborghs S, Wils H, Pirici D, et al. Null mutations in progranulin cause ubiquitin-positive frontotemporal dementia linked to chromosome 17q21. Nature. 2006;442(7105):920–4. PubMed PMID: 16862115.
21. DeJesus-Hernandez M, Mackenzie IR, Boeve BF, Boxer AL, Baker M, Rutherford NJ, et al. Expanded GGGGCC hexanucleotide repeat in noncoding region of C9ORF72 causes chromosome 9p-linked FTD and ALS. Neuron. 2011;72(2):245–56. PubMed PMID: 21944778. Pubmed Central PMCID: 3202986.
22. Renton AE, Majounie E, Waite A, Simon-Sanchez J, Rollinson S, Gibbs JR, et al. A hexanucleotide repeat expansion in C9ORF72 is the cause of chromosome 9p21-linked ALS-FTD. Neuron. 2011;72(2):257–68. PubMed PMID: 21944779. Pubmed Central PMCID: 3200438.
23. Cohn-Hokke PE, Elting MW, Pijnenburg YA, van Swieten JC. Genetics of dementia: update and guidelines for the clinician. Am J Med Genet B Neuropsychiatr Genet. 2012;159B(6):628–43. PubMed PMID: 22815225.
24. Benajiba L, Le Ber I, Camuzat A, Lacoste M, Thomas-Anterion C, Couratier P, et al. TARDBP mutations in motoneuron disease with frontotemporal lobar degeneration. Ann Neurol. 2009;65(4):470–3. PubMed PMID: 19350673.
25. Borroni B, Archetti S, Del Bo R, Papetti A, Buratti E, Bonvicini C, et al. TARDBP mutations in frontotemporal lobar degeneration: frequency, clinical features, and disease course. Rejuvenation Res. 2010;13(5):509–17. PubMed PMID: 20645878.
26. Huey ED, Ferrari R, Moreno JH, Jensen C, Morris CM, Potocnik F, et al. FUS and TDP43 genetic variability in FTD and CBS. Neurobiol Aging. 2012;33(5):1016 e9–17. PubMed PMID: 21943958.
27. Van Langenhove T, van der Zee J, Sleegers K, Engelborghs S, Vandenberghe R, Gijselinck I, et al. Genetic contribution of FUS to frontotemporal lobar degeneration. Neurology. 2010;74(5):366–71. PubMed PMID: 20124201.
28. Van Deerlin VM, Sleiman PM, Martinez-Lage M, Chen-Plotkin A, Wang LS, Graff-Radford NR, et al. Common variants at 7p21 are associated with frontotemporal lobar degeneration with TDP-43 inclusions. Nat Genet. 2010;42(3):234–9. PubMed PMID: 20154673. Pubmed Central PMCID: 2828525.
29. Ferrari R, Hernandez DG, Nalls MA, Rohrer JD, Ramasamy A, Kwok JB, et al. Frontotemporal dementia and its subtypes: a genome-wide association study. Lancet Neurol. 2014;13(7):686–99. PubMed PMID: 24943344.
30. Spillantini MG, Goedert M. Tau pathology and neurodegeneration. Lancet Neurol. 2013;12(6):609–22. PubMed PMID: 23684085.
31. Goedert M, Spillantini MG, Cairns NJ, Crowther RA. Tau proteins of Alzheimer paired helical filaments: abnormal phosphorylation of all six brain isoforms. Neuron. 1992;8(1):159–68. PubMed PMID: 1530909.
32. Flament S, Delacourte A, Verny M, Hauw JJ, Javoy-Agid F. Abnormal Tau proteins in progressive supranuclear palsy. Similarities and differences with the neurofibrillary degeneration of the Alzheimer type. Acta Neuropathol. 1991;81(6):591–6. PubMed PMID: 1831952.
33. Ksiezak-Reding H, Morgan K, Mattiace LA, Davies P, Liu WK, Yen SH, et al. Ultrastructure and biochemical composition of paired helical filaments in corticobasal degeneration. Am J

Pathol. 1994;145(6):1496–508. PubMed PMID: 7992852. Pubmed Central PMCID: 1887493.
34. Togo T, Sahara N, Yen SH, Cookson N, Ishizawa T, Hutton M, et al. Argyrophilic grain disease is a sporadic 4-repeat tauopathy. J Neuropathol Exp Neurol. 2002;61(6):547–56. PubMed PMID: 12071638.
35. Delacourte A, Robitaille Y, Sergeant N, Buee L, Hof PR, Wattez A, et al. Specific pathological Tau protein variants characterize Pick's disease. J Neuropathol Exp Neurol. 1996;55(2):159–68. PubMed PMID: 8786374.
36. Baker M, Litvan I, Houlden H, Adamson J, Dickson D, Perez-Tur J, et al. Association of an extended haplotype in the tau gene with progressive supranuclear palsy. Hum Mol Genet. 1999;8(4):711–5. PubMed PMID: 10072441.
37. Houlden H, Baker M, Morris HR, MacDonald N, Pickering-Brown S, Adamson J, et al. Corticobasal degeneration and progressive supranuclear palsy share a common tau haplotype. Neurology. 2001;56(12):1702–6. PubMed PMID: 11425937.
38. Pastor P, Ezquerra M, Munoz E, Marti MJ, Blesa R, Tolosa E, et al. Significant association between the tau gene A0/A0 genotype and Parkinson's disease. Ann Neurol. 2000;47(2):242–5. PubMed PMID: 10665497.
39. Stefansson H, Helgason A, Thorleifsson G, Steinthorsdottir V, Masson G, Barnard J, et al. A common inversion under selection in Europeans. Nat Genet. 2005;37(2):129–37. PubMed PMID: 15654335.
40. Binder LI, Frankfurter A, Rebhun LI. The distribution of tau in the mammalian central nervous system. J Cell Biol. 1985;101(4):1371–8. PubMed PMID: 3930508. Pubmed Central PMCID: 2113928.
41. Andreadis A, Brown WM, Kosik KS. Structure and novel exons of the human tau gene. Biochemistry. 1992;31(43):10626–33. PubMed PMID: 1420178.
42. Cleveland DW, Hwo SY, Kirschner MW. Purification of tau, a microtubule-associated protein that induces assembly of microtubules from purified tubulin. J Mol Biol. 1977;116(2):207–25. PubMed PMID: 599557.
43. Hirokawa N. Microtubule organization and dynamics dependent on microtubule-associated proteins. Curr Opin Cell Biol. 1994;6(1):74–81. PubMed PMID: 8167029.
44. Drechsel DN, Hyman AA, Cobb MH, Kirschner MW. Modulation of the dynamic instability of tubulin assembly by the microtubule-associated protein tau. Mol Biol Cell. 1992;3(10):1141–54. PubMed PMID: 1421571. Pubmed Central PMCID: 275678.
45. Goode BL, Chau M, Denis PE, Feinstein SC. Structural and functional differences between 3-repeat and 4-repeat tau isoforms. Implications for normal tau function and the onset of neurodegenerative disease. J Biol Chem. 2000;275(49):38182–9. PubMed PMID: 10984497.
46. Gustke N, Trinczek B, Biernat J, Mandelkow EM, Mandelkow E. Domains of tau protein and interactions with microtubules. Biochemistry. 1994;33(32):9511–22. PubMed PMID: 8068626.
47. Brandt R, Leger J, Lee G. Interaction of tau with the neural plasma membrane mediated by tau's amino-terminal projection domain. J Cell Biol. 1995;131(5):1327–40. PubMed PMID: 8522593. Pubmed Central PMCID: 2120645.
48. Pooler AM, Hanger DP. Functional implications of the association of tau with the plasma membrane. Biochem Soc Trans. 2010;38(4):1012–5. PubMed PMID: 20658995.
49. Ebneth A, Godemann R, Stamer K, Illenberger S, Trinczek B, Mandelkow E. Overexpression of tau protein inhibits kinesin-dependent trafficking of vesicles, mitochondria, and endoplasmic reticulum: implications for Alzheimer's disease. J Cell Biol. 1998;143(3):777–94. PubMed PMID: 9813097. Pubmed Central PMCID: 2148132.
50. Trinczek B, Ebneth A, Mandelkow EM, Mandelkow E. Tau regulates the attachment/detachment but not the speed of motors in microtubule-dependent transport of single vesicles and organelles. J Cell Sci. 1999;112(Pt 14):2355–67. PubMed PMID: 10381391.

51. Dixit R, Ross JL, Goldman YE, Holzbaur EL. Differential regulation of dynein and kinesin motor proteins by tau. Science. 2008;319(5866):1086–9. PubMed PMID: 18202255. Pubmed Central PMCID: 2866193.
52. Ittner LM, Ke YD, Delerue F, Bi M, Gladbach A, van Eersel J, et al. Dendritic function of tau mediates amyloid-beta toxicity in Alzheimer's disease mouse models6. Cell. 2010;142(3):387–97. PubMed PMID: 20655099.
53. Hoover BR, Reed MN, Su J, Penrod RD, Kotilinek LA, Grant MK, et al. Tau mislocalization to dendritic spines mediates synaptic dysfunction independently of neurodegeneration. Neuron. 2010;68(6):1067–81. PubMed PMID: 21172610. PubMed Central PMCID: 3026458.
54. Grundke-Iqbal I, Iqbal K, Quinlan M, Tung YC, Zaidi MS, Wisniewski HM. Microtubule-associated protein tau. A component of Alzheimer paired helical filaments. J Biol Chem. 1986;261(13):6084–9. PubMed PMID: 3084478.
55. Grundke-Iqbal I, Iqbal K, Tung YC, Quinlan M, Wisniewski HM, Binder LI. Abnormal phosphorylation of the microtubule-associated protein tau (tau) in Alzheimer cytoskeletal pathology. Proc Natl Acad Sci U S A. 1986;83(13):4913–7. PubMed PMID: 3088567. Pubmed Central PMCID: 323854.
56. Kidd M. Paired helical filaments in electron microscopy of Alzheimer's disease. Nature. 1963;197:192–3. PubMed PMID: 14032480.
57. Alonso AC, Grundke-Iqbal I, Iqbal K. Alzheimer's disease hyperphosphorylated tau sequesters normal tau into tangles of filaments and disassembles microtubules. Nat Med. 1996;2(7):783–7. PubMed PMID: 8673924.
58. Bramblett GT, Goedert M, Jakes R, Merrick SE, Trojanowski JQ, Lee VM. Abnormal tau phosphorylation at Ser396 in Alzheimer's disease recapitulates development and contributes to reduced microtubule binding. Neuron. 1993;10(6):1089–99. PubMed PMID: 8318230.
59. Iqbal K, Grundke-Iqbal I, Zaidi T, Merz PA, Wen GY, Shaikh SS, et al. Defective brain microtubule assembly in Alzheimer's disease. Lancet. 1986;2(8504):412–6. PubMed PMID: 2874414.
60. Alonso AC, Zaidi T, Grundke-Iqbal I, Iqbal K. Role of abnormally phosphorylated tau in the breakdown of microtubules in Alzheimer disease. Proc Natl Acad Sci U S A. 1994;91(12):5562–6. PubMed PMID: 8202528. PubMed Central PMCID: 44036.
61. Alonso AD, Grundke-Iqbal I, Barra HS, Iqbal K. Abnormal phosphorylation of tau and the mechanism of Alzheimer neurofibrillary degeneration: sequestration of microtubule-associated proteins 1 and 2 and the disassembly of microtubules by the abnormal tau. Proc Natl Acad Sci U S A. 1997;94(1):298–303. PubMed PMID: 8990203. PubMed Central PMCID: 19321.
62. Wang JZ, Xia YY, Grundke-Iqbal I, Iqbal K. Abnormal hyperphosphorylation of tau: sites, regulation, and molecular mechanism of neurofibrillary degeneration. J Alzheimers Dis. 2013;33 Suppl 1:S123–39. PubMed PMID: 22710920.
63. Mercken M, Vandermeeren M, Lubke U, Six J, Boons J, Van de Voorde A, et al. Monoclonal antibodies with selective specificity for Alzheimer Tau are directed against phosphatase-sensitive epitopes. Acta Neuropathol. 1992;84(3):265–72. PubMed PMID: 1384266.
64. Kanemaru K, Takio K, Miura R, Titani K, Ihara Y. Fetal-type phosphorylation of the tau in paired helical filaments. J Neurochem. 1992;58(5):1667–75. PubMed PMID: 1560225.
65. Dolan PJ, Johnson GV. The role of tau kinases in Alzheimer's disease. Curr Opin Drug Discovery Dev. 2010;13(5):595–603. PubMed PMID: 20812151. PubMed Central PMCID: 2941661.
66. Hanger DP, Anderton BH, Noble W. Tau phosphorylation: the therapeutic challenge for neurodegenerative disease. Trends Mol Med. 2009;15(3):112–9. PubMed PMID: 19246243.
67. Cruts M, Theuns J, Van Broeckhoven C. Locus-specific mutation databases for neurodegenerative brain diseases. Hum Mutat. 2012;33(9):1340–4. PubMed PMID: 22581678. PubMed Central PMCID: 3465795.

68. Rademakers R, Cruts M, van Broeckhoven C. The role of tau (MAPT) in frontotemporal dementia and related tauopathies. Hum Mutat. 2004;24(4):277–95. PubMed PMID: 15365985.
69. Hong M, Zhukareva V, Vogelsberg-Ragaglia V, Wszolek Z, Reed L, Miller BI, et al. Mutation-specific functional impairments in distinct tau isoforms of hereditary FTDP-17. Science. 1998;282(5395):1914–7. PubMed PMID: 9836646.
70. D'Souza I, Schellenberg GD. Determinants of 4-repeat tau expression. Coordination between enhancing and inhibitory splicing sequences for exon 10 inclusion. J Biol Chem. 2000;275(23):17700–9. PubMed PMID: 10748133.
71. D'Souza I, Schellenberg GD. tau Exon 10 expression involves a bipartite intron 10 regulatory sequence and weak 5′ and 3′ splice sites. J Biol Chem. 2002;277(29):26587–99. PubMed PMID: 12000767.
72. Rizzu P, Van Swieten JC, Joosse M, Hasegawa M, Stevens M, Tibben A, et al. High prevalence of mutations in the microtubule-associated protein tau in a population study of frontotemporal dementia in the Netherlands. Am J Hum Genet. 1999;64(2):414–21. PubMed PMID: 9973279. PubMed Central PMCID: 1377751.
73. D'Souza I, Schellenberg GD. Regulation of tau isoform expression and dementia. Biochim Biophys Acta. 2005;1739(2–3):104–15. PubMed PMID: 15615630.
74. Gotz J, Deters N, Doldissen A, Bokhari L, Ke Y, Wiesner A, et al. A decade of tau transgenic animal models and beyond. Brain Pathol. 2007;17(1):91–103. PubMed PMID: 17493043.
75. Santacruz K, Lewis J, Spires T, Paulson J, Kotilinek L, Ingelsson M, et al. Tau suppression in a neurodegenerative mouse model improves memory function. Science. 2005;309(5733):476–81. PubMed PMID: 16020737. PubMed Central PMCID: 1574647.
76. Roberson ED. Mouse models of frontotemporal dementia. Ann Neurol. 2012;72(6):837–49. PubMed PMID: 23280835. PubMed Central PMCID: 3539234.
77. Spires TL, Orne JD, SantaCruz K, Pitstick R, Carlson GA, Ashe KH, et al. Region-specific dissociation of neuronal loss and neurofibrillary pathology in a mouse model of tauopathy. Am J Pathol. 2006;168(5):1598–607. PubMed PMID: 16651626. PubMed Central PMCID: 1606598.
78. de Calignon A, Fox LM, Pitstick R, Carlson GA, Bacskai BJ, Spires-Jones TL, et al. Caspase activation precedes and leads to tangles. Nature. 2010;464(7292):1201–4. PubMed PMID: 20357768. PubMed Central PMCID: 3091360.
79. Sydow A, Van der Jeugd A, Zheng F, Ahmed T, Balschun D, Petrova O, et al. Tau-induced defects in synaptic plasticity, learning, and memory are reversible in transgenic mice after switching off the toxic Tau mutant. J Neurosci. 2011;31(7):2511–25. PubMed PMID: 21325519.
80. Mocanu MM, Nissen A, Eckermann K, Khlistunova I, Biernat J, Drexler D, et al. The potential for beta-structure in the repeat domain of tau protein determines aggregation, synaptic decay, neuronal loss, and coassembly with endogenous Tau in inducible mouse models of tauopathy. J Neurosci. 2008;28(3):737–48. PubMed PMID: 18199773.
81. Clavaguera F, Bolmont T, Crowther RA, Abramowski D, Frank S, Probst A, et al. Transmission and spreading of tauopathy in transgenic mouse brain. Nat Cell Biol. 2009;11(7):909–13. PubMed PMID: 19503072. PubMed Central PMCID: 2726961.
82. Clavaguera F, Hench J, Lavenir I, Schweighauser G, Frank S, Goedert M, et al. Peripheral administration of tau aggregates triggers intracerebral tauopathy in transgenic mice. Acta Neuropathol. 2014;127(2):299–301. PubMed PMID: 24362441.
83. Frost B, Jacks RL, Diamond MI. Propagation of tau misfolding from the outside to the inside of a cell. J Biol Chem. 2009;284(19):12845–52. PubMed PMID: 19282288. PubMed Central PMCID: 2676015.
84. Iba M, Guo JL, McBride JD, Zhang B, Trojanowski JQ, Lee VM. Synthetic tau fibrils mediate transmission of neurofibrillary tangles in a transgenic mouse model of Alzheimer's-like tauopathy. J Neurosci. 2013;33(3):1024–37. PubMed PMID: 23325240. PubMed Central PMCID: 3575082.

85. de Calignon A, Polydoro M, Suarez-Calvet M, William C, Adamowicz DH, Kopeikina KJ, et al. Propagation of tau pathology in a model of early Alzheimer's disease. Neuron. 2012;73(4):685–97. PubMed PMID: 22365544. PubMed Central PMCID: 3292759.
86. Clavaguera F, Akatsu H, Fraser G, Crowther RA, Frank S, Hench J, et al. Brain homogenates from human tauopathies induce tau inclusions in mouse brain. Proc Natl Acad Sci U S A. 2013;110(23):9535–40. PubMed PMID: 23690619. PubMed Central PMCID: 3677441.
87. Lasagna-Reeves CA, Castillo-Carranza DL, Sengupta U, Guerrero-Munoz MJ, Kiritoshi T, Neugebauer V, et al. Alzheimer brain-derived tau oligomers propagate pathology from endogenous tau. Sci Rep. 2012;2:700. PubMed PMID: 23050084. PubMed Central PMCID: 3463004.
88. Wu JW, Herman M, Liu L, Simoes S, Acker CM, Figueroa H, et al. Small misfolded Tau species are internalized via bulk endocytosis and anterogradely and retrogradely transported in neurons. J Biol Chem. 2013;288(3):1856–70. PubMed PMID: 23188818. PubMed Central PMCID: 3548495.
89. Guo JL, Lee VM. Seeding of normal Tau by pathological Tau conformers drives pathogenesis of Alzheimer-like tangles. J Biol Chem. 2011;286(17):15317–31. PubMed PMID: 21372138. PubMed Central PMCID: 3083182.
90. Kfoury N, Holmes BB, Jiang H, Holtzman DM, Diamond MI. Trans-cellular propagation of Tau aggregation by fibrillar species. J Biol Chem. 2012;287(23):19440–51. PubMed PMID: 22461630. PubMed Central PMCID: 3365982.
91. Santa-Maria I, Varghese M, Ksiezak-Reding H, Dzhun A, Wang J, Pasinetti GM. Paired helical filaments from Alzheimer disease brain induce intracellular accumulation of Tau protein in aggresomes. J Biol Chem. 2012;287(24):20522–33. PubMed PMID: 22496370. PubMed Central PMCID: 3370237.
92. Wittmann CW, Wszolek MF, Shulman JM, Salvaterra PM, Lewis J, Hutton M, et al. Tauopathy in Drosophila: neurodegeneration without neurofibrillary tangles. Science. 2001;293(5530):711–4. PubMed PMID: 11408621.
93. Kraemer BC, Zhang B, Leverenz JB, Thomas JH, Trojanowski JQ, Schellenberg GD. Neurodegeneration and defective neurotransmission in a Caenorhabditis elegans model of tauopathy. Proc Natl Acad Sci U S A. 2003;100(17):9980–5. PubMed PMID: 12872001. PubMed Central PMCID: 187908.
94. Paquet D, Bhat R, Sydow A, Mandelkow EM, Berg S, Hellberg S, et al. A zebrafish model of tauopathy allows in vivo imaging of neuronal cell death and drug evaluation. J Clin Invest. 2009;119(5):1382–95. PubMed PMID: 19363289. PubMed Central PMCID: 2673864.
95. Neumann M, Sampathu DM, Kwong LK, Truax AC, Micsenyi MC, Chou TT, et al. Ubiquitinated TDP-43 in frontotemporal lobar degeneration and amyotrophic lateral sclerosis. Science. 2006;314(5796):130–3. PubMed PMID: 17023659.
96. Mackenzie IR. The neuropathology and clinical phenotype of FTD with progranulin mutations. Acta Neuropathol. 2007;114(1):49–54. PubMed PMID: 17458552.
97. Behrens MI, Mukherjee O, Tu PH, Liscic RM, Grinberg LT, Carter D, et al. Neuropathologic heterogeneity in HDDD1: a familial frontotemporal lobar degeneration with ubiquitin-positive inclusions and progranulin mutation. Alzheimer Dis Assoc Disord. 2007;21(1):1–7. PubMed PMID: 17334266.
98. Leverenz JB, Yu CE, Montine TJ, Steinbart E, Bekris LM, Zabetian C, et al. A novel progranulin mutation associated with variable clinical presentation and tau, TDP43 and alpha-synuclein pathology. Brain. 2007;130(Pt 5):1360–74. PubMed PMID: 17439980.
99. Mackenzie IR, Baker M, Pickering-Brown S, Hsiung GY, Lindholm C, Dwosh E, et al. The neuropathology of frontotemporal lobar degeneration caused by mutations in the progranulin gene. Brain. 2006;129(Pt 11):3081–90. PubMed PMID: 17071926.
100. Spina S, Murrell JR, Huey ED, Wassermann EM, Pietrini P, Baraibar MA, et al. Clinicopathologic features of frontotemporal dementia with progranulin sequence variation. Neurology. 2007;68(11):820–7. PubMed PMID: 17202431.
101. Bhandari V, Bateman A. Structure and chromosomal location of the human granulin gene. Biochem Biophys Res Commun. 1992;188(1):57–63. PubMed PMID: 1417868.

102. Bateman A, Bennett HP. Granulins: the structure and function of an emerging family of growth factors. J Endocrinol. 1998;158(2):145–51. PubMed PMID: 9771457.
103. Cadieux B, Chitramuthu BP, Baranowski D, Bennett HP. The zebrafish progranulin gene family and antisense transcripts. BMC Genomics. 2005;6:156. PubMed PMID: 16277664. PubMed Central PMCID: 1310530.
104. Kao AW, Eisenhut RJ, Martens LH, Nakamura A, Huang A, Bagley JA, et al. A neurodegenerative disease mutation that accelerates the clearance of apoptotic cells. Proc Natl Acad Sci U S A. 2011;108(11):4441–6. PubMed PMID: 21368173. PubMed Central PMCID: 3060230.
105. Pera EM, Hou S, Strate I, Wessely O, De Robertis EM. Exploration of the extracellular space by a large-scale secretion screen in the early Xenopus embryo. Int J Dev Biol. 2005;49(7):781–96. PubMed PMID: 16172975.
106. Bhandari V, Giaid A, Bateman A. The complementary deoxyribonucleic acid sequence, tissue distribution, and cellular localization of the rat granulin precursor. Endocrinology. 1993;133(6):2682–9. PubMed PMID: 8243292.
107. Daniel R, He Z, Carmichael KP, Halper J, Bateman A. Cellular localization of gene expression for progranulin. J Histochem Cytochem. 2000;48(7):999–1009. PubMed PMID: 10858277.
108. Petkau TL, Neal SJ, Orban PC, MacDonald JL, Hill AM, Lu G, et al. Progranulin expression in the developing and adult murine brain. J Comp Neurol. 2010;518(19):3931–47. PubMed PMID: 20737593.
109. Carrasquillo MM, Nicholson AM, Finch N, Gibbs JR, Baker M, Rutherford NJ, et al. Genome-wide screen identifies rs646776 near sortilin as a regulator of progranulin levels in human plasma. Am J Hum Genet. 2010;87(6):890–7. PubMed PMID: 21087763. PubMed Central PMCID: 2997361.
110. Hu F, Padukkavidana T, Vaegter CB, Brady OA, Zheng Y, Mackenzie IR, et al. Sortilin-mediated endocytosis determines levels of the frontotemporal dementia protein, progranulin. Neuron. 2010;68(4):654–67. PubMed PMID: 21092856. PubMed Central PMCID: 2990962.
111. Lee WC, Almeida S, Prudencio M, Caulfield TR, Zhang YJ, Tay WM, et al. Targeted manipulation of the sortilin-progranulin axis rescues progranulin haploinsufficiency. Hum Mol Genet. 2014;23(6):1467–78. PubMed PMID: 24163244. PubMed Central PMCID: 3929086.
112. Kleinberger G, Capell A, Haass C, Van Broeckhoven C. Mechanisms of granulin deficiency: lessons from cellular and animal models. Mol Neurobiol. 2013;47(1):337–60. PubMed PMID: 23239020. PubMed Central PMCID: 3538123.
113. Chitramuthu BP, Baranowski DC, Kay DG, Bateman A, Bennett HP. Progranulin modulates zebrafish motoneuron development in vivo and rescues truncation defects associated with knockdown of Survival motor neuron 1. Mol Neurodegener. 2010;5:41. PubMed PMID: 20946666. PubMed Central PMCID: 2974670.
114. Gass J, Lee WC, Cook C, Finch N, Stetler C, Jansen-West K, et al. Progranulin regulates neuronal outgrowth independent of sortilin. Mol Neurodegener. 2012;7:33. PubMed PMID: 22781549. PubMed Central PMCID: 3508877.
115. Laird AS, Van Hoecke A, De Muynck L, Timmers M, Van den Bosch L, Van Damme P, et al. Progranulin is neurotrophic in vivo and protects against a mutant TDP-43 induced axonopathy. PLoS One. 2010;5(10):e13368. PubMed PMID: 20967127. PubMed Central PMCID: 2954192.
116. Ryan CL, Baranowski DC, Chitramuthu BP, Malik S, Li Z, Cao M, et al. Progranulin is expressed within motor neurons and promotes neuronal cell survival. BMC Neurosci. 2009;10:130. PubMed PMID: 19860916. PubMed Central PMCID: 2779192.
117. Van Damme P, Van Hoecke A, Lambrechts D, Vanacker P, Bogaert E, van Swieten J, et al. Progranulin functions as a neurotrophic factor to regulate neurite outgrowth and enhance neuronal survival. J Cell Biol. 2008;181(1):37–41. PubMed PMID: 18378771. PubMed Central PMCID: 2287280.
118. Almeida S, Zhang Z, Coppola G, Mao W, Futai K, Karydas A, et al. Induced pluripotent stem cell models of progranulin-deficient frontotemporal dementia uncover specific reversible neuronal defects. Cell Rep. 2012;2(4):789–98. PubMed PMID: 23063362. PubMed Central PMCID: 3532907.

119. Gao X, Joselin AP, Wang L, Kar A, Ray P, Bateman A, et al. Progranulin promotes neurite outgrowth and neuronal differentiation by regulating GSK-3beta. Protein Cell. 2010;1(6):552–62. PubMed PMID: 21204008.
120. Nedachi T, Kawai T, Matsuwaki T, Yamanouchi K, Nishihara M. Progranulin enhances neural progenitor cell proliferation through glycogen synthase kinase 3beta phosphorylation. Neuroscience. 2011;185:106–15. PubMed PMID: 21540081.
121. Guo A, Tapia L, Bamji SX, Cynader MS, Jia W. Progranulin deficiency leads to enhanced cell vulnerability and TDP-43 translocation in primary neuronal cultures. Brain Res. 2010;1366:1–8. PubMed PMID: 20888804.
122. Kleinberger G, Wils H, Ponsaerts P, Joris G, Timmermans J-P, Van Broeckhoven C, et al. Increased caspase activation and decreased TDP-43 solubility in progranulin knockout cortical cultures. J Neurochem. 2010;115(3):735–47.
123. Yin F, Banerjee R, Thomas B, Zhou P, Qian L, Jia T, et al. Exaggerated inflammation, impaired host defense, and neuropathology in progranulin-deficient mice. J Exp Med. 2010;207(1):117–28. PubMed PMID: 20026663. PubMed Central PMCID: 2812536.
124. De Muynck L, Van Damme P. Cellular effects of progranulin in health and disease. J Mol Neurosci. 2011;45(3):549–60. PubMed PMID: 21611805.
125. Tang W, Lu Y, Tian QY, Zhang Y, Guo FJ, Liu GY, et al. The growth factor progranulin binds to TNF receptors and is therapeutic against inflammatory arthritis in mice. Science. 2011;332(6028):478–84. PubMed PMID: 21393509. PubMed Central PMCID: 3104397.
126. Baker CA, Manuelidis L. Unique inflammatory RNA profiles of microglia in Creutzfeldt-Jakob disease. Proc Natl Acad Sci U S A. 2003;100(2):675–9. PubMed PMID: 12525699. PubMed Central PMCID: 141055.
127. Malaspina A, Kaushik N, de Belleroche J. Differential expression of 14 genes in amyotrophic lateral sclerosis spinal cord detected using gridded cDNA arrays. J Neurochem. 2001;77(1):132–45. PubMed PMID: 11279269.
128. Philips T, De Muynck L, Thu HN, Weynants B, Vanacker P, Dhondt J, et al. Microglial upregulation of progranulin as a marker of motor neuron degeneration. J Neuropathol Exp Neurol. 2010;69(12):1191–200. PubMed PMID: 21107132.
129. Pickford F, Marcus J, Camargo LM, Xiao Q, Graham D, Mo JR, et al. Progranulin is a chemoattractant for microglia and stimulates their endocytic activity. Am J Pathol. 2011;178(1):284–95. PubMed PMID: 21224065. PubMed Central PMCID: 3070582.
130. Del Bo R, Corti S, Santoro D, Ghione I, Fenoglio C, Ghezzi S, et al. No major progranulin genetic variability contribution to disease etiopathogenesis in an ALS Italian cohort. Neurobiol Aging. 2011;32(6):1157–8. PubMed PMID: 19632744. PubMed Central PMCID: 3511779.
131. Schymick JC, Yang Y, Andersen PM, Vonsattel JP, Greenway M, Momeni P, et al. Progranulin mutations and amyotrophic lateral sclerosis or amyotrophic lateral sclerosis-frontotemporal dementia phenotypes. J Neurol Neurosurg Psychiatry. 2007;78(7):754–6. PubMed PMID: 17371905. PubMed Central PMCID: 2117704.
132. Nuytemans K, Pals P, Sleegers K, Engelborghs S, Corsmit E, Peeters K, et al. Progranulin variability has no major role in Parkinson disease genetic etiology. Neurology. 2008;71(15):1147–51. PubMed PMID: 18838661.
133. Yu CE, Bird TD, Bekris LM, Montine TJ, Leverenz JB, Steinbart E, et al. The spectrum of mutations in progranulin: a collaborative study screening 545 cases of neurodegeneration. Arch Neurol. 2010;67(2):161–70. PubMed PMID: 20142524. PubMed Central PMCID: 2901991.
134. Behm-Ansmant I, Kashima I, Rehwinkel J, Sauliere J, Wittkopp N, Izaurralde E. mRNA quality control: an ancient machinery recognizes and degrades mRNAs with nonsense codons. FEBS Lett. 2007;581(15):2845–53. PubMed PMID: 17531985.
135. Gass J, Cannon A, Mackenzie IR, Boeve B, Baker M, Adamson J, et al. Mutations in progranulin are a major cause of ubiquitin-positive frontotemporal lobar degeneration. Hum Mol Genet. 2006;15(20):2988–3001. PubMed PMID: 16950801.
136. Le Ber I, Camuzat A, Hannequin D, Pasquier F, Guedj E, Rovelet-Lecrux A, et al. Phenotype variability in progranulin mutation carriers: a clinical, neuropsychological, imaging and genetic study. Brain. 2008;131(Pt 3):732–46. PubMed PMID: 18245784.

137. Gijselinck I, van der Zee J, Engelborghs S, Goossens D, Peeters K, Mattheijssens M, et al. Progranulin locus deletion in frontotemporal dementia. Hum Mutat. 2008;29(1):53–8. PubMed PMID: 18157829.
138. Rovelet-Lecrux A, Deramecourt V, Legallic S, Maurage CA, Le Ber I, Brice A, et al. Deletion of the progranulin gene in patients with frontotemporal lobar degeneration or Parkinson disease. Neurobiol Dis. 2008;31(1):41–5. PubMed PMID: 18479928.
139. Chen-Plotkin AS, Martinez-Lage M, Sleiman PM, Hu W, Greene R, Wood EM, et al. Genetic and clinical features of progranulin-associated frontotemporal lobar degeneration. Arch Neurol. 2011;68(4):488–97. PubMed PMID: 21482928. PubMed Central PMCID: 3160280.
140. Benussi L, Ghidoni R, Pegoiani E, Moretti DV, Zanetti O, Binetti G. Progranulin Leu271LeufsX10 is one of the most common FTLD and CBS associated mutations worldwide. Neurobiol Dis. 2009;33(3):379–85. PubMed PMID: 19101631.
141. Borroni B, Bonvicini C, Galimberti D, Tremolizzo L, Papetti A, Archetti S, et al. Founder effect and estimation of the age of the Progranulin Thr272fs mutation in 14 Italian pedigrees with frontotemporal lobar degeneration. Neurobiol Aging. 2011;32(3):555 e1–8. PubMed PMID: 20947212.
142. Gijselinck I, Van Broeckhoven C, Cruts M. Granulin mutations associated with frontotemporal lobar degeneration and related disorders: an update. Human Mutat. 2008;29(12):1373–86. PubMed PMID: 18543312.
143. Shankaran SS, Capell A, Hruscha AT, Fellerer K, Neumann M, Schmid B, et al. Missense mutations in the progranulin gene linked to frontotemporal lobar degeneration with ubiquitin-immunoreactive inclusions reduce progranulin production and secretion. J Biol Chem. 2008;283(3):1744–53. PubMed PMID: 17984093.
144. Mukherjee O, Pastor P, Cairns NJ, Chakraverty S, Kauwe JS, Shears S, et al. HDDD2 is a familial frontotemporal lobar degeneration with ubiquitin-positive, tau-negative inclusions caused by a missense mutation in the signal peptide of progranulin. Ann Neurol. 2006;60(3):314–22. PubMed PMID: 16983685. PubMed Central PMCID: 2803024.
145. Smith KR, Damiano J, Franceschetti S, Carpenter S, Canafoglia L, Morbin M, et al. Strikingly different clinicopathological phenotypes determined by progranulin-mutation dosage. Am J Hum Genet. 2012;90(6):1102–7. PubMed PMID: 22608501. PubMed Central PMCID: 3370276.
146. Kollmann K, Uusi-Rauva K, Scifo E, Tyynela J, Jalanko A, Braulke T. Cell biology and function of neuronal ceroid lipofuscinosis-related proteins. Biochim Biophys Acta. 2013;1832(11):1866–81. PubMed PMID: 23402926.
147. Petkau TL, Leavitt BR. Progranulin in neurodegenerative disease. Trends Neurosci. 2014;37(7):388–98. PubMed PMID: 24800652.
148. Wils H, Kleinberger G, Pereson S, Janssens J, Capell A, Van Dam D, et al. Cellular ageing, increased mortality and FTLD-TDP-associated neuropathology in progranulin knockout mice. J Pathol. 2012;228(1):67–76. PubMed PMID: 22733568.
149. Tapia L, Milnerwood A, Guo A, Mills F, Yoshida E, Vasuta C, et al. Progranulin deficiency decreases gross neural connectivity but enhances transmission at individual synapses. J Neurosci. 2011;31(31):11126–32. PubMed PMID: 21813674.
150. Petkau TL, Neal SJ, Milnerwood A, Mew A, Hill AM, Orban P, et al. Synaptic dysfunction in progranulin-deficient mice. Neurobiol Dis. 2012;45(2):711–22. PubMed PMID: 22062772.
151. Ahmed Z, Sheng H, Xu YF, Lin WL, Innes AE, Gass J, et al. Accelerated lipofuscinosis and ubiquitination in granulin knockout mice suggest a role for progranulin in successful aging. Am J Pathol. 2010;177(1):311–24. PubMed PMID: 20522652. PubMed Central PMCID: 2893674.
152. Yin F, Dumont M, Banerjee R, Ma Y, Li H, Lin MT, et al. Behavioral deficits and progressive neuropathology in progranulin-deficient mice: a mouse model of frontotemporal dementia. FASEB J. 2010;24(12):4639–47. PubMed PMID: 20667979. PubMed Central PMCID: 2992364.
153. Englund E, Gustafson L, Passant U, Majounie E, Renton AE, Traynor BJ, et al. Familial Lund frontotemporal dementia caused by C9ORF72 hexanucleotide expansion. Neurobiol Aging. 2012;33(8):1850 e13–6. PubMed PMID: 22483864.

154. Gijselinck I, Van Langenhove T, van der Zee J, Sleegers K, Philtjens S, Kleinberger G, et al. A C9orf72 promoter repeat expansion in a Flanders-Belgian cohort with disorders of the frontotemporal lobar degeneration-amyotrophic lateral sclerosis spectrum: a gene identification study. Lancet Neurol. 2012;11(1):54–65. PubMed PMID: 22154785.
155. Cruts M, Gijselinck I, Van Langenhove T, van der Zee J, Van Broeckhoven C. Current insights into the C9orf72 repeat expansion diseases of the FTLD/ALS spectrum. Trends Neurosci. 2013;36(8):450–59. PubMed PMID: 23746459.
156. Heutink P, Jansen IE, Lynes EM. C9orf72; abnormal RNA expression is the key. Exp Neurol. 2014;262:102–10. PubMed PMID: 24873727.
157. Lindquist SG, Duno M, Batbayli M, Puschmann A, Braendgaard H, Mardosiene S, et al. Corticobasal and ataxia syndromes widen the spectrum of C9ORF72 hexanucleotide expansion disease. Clin Genet. 2013;83(3):279–83. PubMed PMID: 22650353.
158. Majounie E, Abramzon Y, Renton AE, Perry R, Bassett SS, Pletnikova O, et al. Repeat expansion in C9ORF72 in Alzheimer's disease. N Eng J Med. 2012;366(3):283–4. PubMed PMID: 22216764. PubMed Central PMCID: 3513272.
159. Belzil VV, Bauer PO, Prudencio M, Gendron TF, Stetler CT, Yan IK, et al. Reduced C9orf72 gene expression in c9FTD/ALS is caused by histone trimethylation, an epigenetic event detectable in blood. Acta Neuropathol. 2013;126(6):895–905. PubMed PMID: 24166615. PubMed Central PMCID: 3830740.
160. Waite AJ, Baumer D, East S, Neal J, Morris HR, Ansorge O, et al. Reduced C9orf72 protein levels in frontal cortex of amyotrophic lateral sclerosis and frontotemporal degeneration brain with the C9ORF72 hexanucleotide repeat expansion. Neurobiol Aging. 2014;35(7):1779.e5–1779.e13. PubMed PMID: 24559645.
161. Farg MA, Sundaramoorthy V, Sultana JM, Yang S, Atkinson RA, Levina V, et al. C9ORF72, implicated in amyotrophic lateral sclerosis and frontotemporal dementia, regulates endosomal trafficking. Hum Mol Genet. 2014;23(13):3579–595. PubMed PMID: 24549040.
162. Donnelly CJ, Zhang PW, Pham JT, Heusler AR, Mistry NA, Vidensky S, et al. RNA toxicity from the ALS/FTD C9ORF72 expansion is mitigated by antisense intervention. Neuron. 2013;80(2):415–28. PubMed PMID: 24139042.
163. Sareen D, O'Rourke JG, Meera P, Muhammad AK, Grant S, Simpkinson M, et al. Targeting RNA foci in iPSC-derived motor neurons from ALS patients with a C9ORF72 repeat expansion. Sci Transl Med. 2013;5(208):208ra149. PubMed PMID: 24154603.
164. Zhang D, Iyer LM, He F, Aravind L. Discovery of novel DENN proteins: implications for the evolution of eukaryotic intracellular membrane structures and human disease. Front Genet. 2012;3:283. PubMed PMID: 23248642. PubMed Central PMCID: 3521125.
165. Levine TP, Daniels RD, Gatta AT, Wong LH, Hayes MJ. The product of C9orf72, a gene strongly implicated in neurodegeneration, is structurally related to DENN Rab-GEFs. Bioinformatics. 2013;29(4):499–503. PubMed PMID: 23329412. PubMed Central PMCID: 3570213.
166. Almeida S, Gascon E, Tran H, Chou HJ, Gendron TF, Degroot S, et al. Modeling key pathological features of frontotemporal dementia with C9ORF72 repeat expansion in iPSC-derived human neurons. Acta Neuropathol. 2013;126(3):385–99. PubMed PMID: 23836290. PubMed Central PMCID: 3753484.
167. Majounie E, Renton AE, Mok K, Dopper EG, Waite A, Rollinson S, et al. Frequency of the C9orf72 hexanucleotide repeat expansion in patients with amyotrophic lateral sclerosis and frontotemporal dementia: a cross-sectional study. Lancet Neurol. 2012;11(4):323–30. PubMed PMID: 22406228. PubMed Central PMCID: 3322422.
168. van der Zee J, Gijselinck I, Dillen L, Van Langenhove T, Theuns J, Engelborghs S, et al. A pan-European study of the C9orf72 repeat associated with FTLD: geographic prevalence, genomic instability, and intermediate repeats. Hum Mutat. 2013;34(2):363–73. PubMed PMID: 23111906. PubMed Central PMCID: 3638346.
169. Ciura S, Lattante S, Le Ber I, Latouche M, Tostivint H, Brice A, et al. Loss of function of C9orf72 causes motor deficits in a zebrafish model of amyotrophic lateral sclerosis. Ann Neurol. 2013;74(2):180–87. PubMed PMID: 23720273.

170. Mori K, Weng SM, Arzberger T, May S, Rentzsch K, Kremmer E, et al. The C9orf72 GGGGCC repeat is translated into aggregating dipeptide-repeat proteins in FTLD/ALS. Science. 2013;339(6125):1335–8. PubMed PMID: 23393093.
171. Greene E, Mahishi L, Entezam A, Kumari D, Usdin K. Repeat-induced epigenetic changes in intron 1 of the frataxin gene and its consequences in Friedreich ataxia. Nucleic Acids Res. 2007;35(10):3383–90. PubMed PMID: 17478498. PubMed Central PMCID: 1904289.
172. Sutcliffe JS, Nelson DL, Zhang F, Pieretti M, Caskey CT, Saxe D, et al. DNA methylation represses FMR-1 transcription in fragile X syndrome. Hum Mol Genet. 1992;1(6):397–400. PubMed PMID: 1301913.
173. Xi Z, Zinman L, Moreno D, Schymick J, Liang Y, Sato C, et al. Hypermethylation of the CpG island near the G4C2 repeat in ALS with a C9orf72 expansion. Am J Hum Genet. 2013;92(6):981–9. PubMed PMID: 23731538. PubMed Central PMCID: 3675239.
174. Wojciechowska M, Krzyzosiak WJ. Cellular toxicity of expanded RNA repeats: focus on RNA foci. Hum Mol Genet. 2011;20(19):3811–21. PubMed PMID: 21729883. PubMed Central PMCID: 3168290.
175. Mizielinska S, Lashley T, Norona FE, Clayton EL, Ridler CE, Fratta P, et al. C9orf72 frontotemporal lobar degeneration is characterised by frequent neuronal sense and antisense RNA foci. Acta Neuropathol. 2013;126(6):845–57. PubMed PMID: 24170096.
176. Lagier-Tourenne C, Baughn M, Rigo F, Sun S, Liu P, Li HR, et al. Targeted degradation of sense and antisense C9orf72 RNA foci as therapy for ALS and frontotemporal degeneration. Proc Natl Acad Sci U S A. 2013;110(47):E4530–9. PubMed PMID: 24170860.
177. Fratta P, Mizielinska S, Nicoll AJ, Zloh M, Fisher EM, Parkinson G, et al. C9orf72 hexanucleotide repeat associated with amyotrophic lateral sclerosis and frontotemporal dementia forms RNA G-quadruplexes. Sci Rep. 2012;2:1016. PubMed PMID: 23264878. PubMed Central PMCID: 3527825.
178. Zamiri B, Reddy K, Macgregor Jr RB, Pearson CE. TMPyP4 porphyrin distorts RNA G-quadruplex structures of the disease-associated r(GGGGCC)n repeat of the C9orf72 gene and blocks interaction of RNA-binding proteins. J Biol Chem. 2014;289(8):4653–9. PubMed PMID: 24371143.
179. Haeusler AR, Donnelly CJ, Periz G, Simko EA, Shaw PG, Kim MS, et al. C9orf72 nucleotide repeat structures initiate molecular cascades of disease. Nature. 2014;507(7491):195–200. PubMed PMID: 24598541.
180. Xu Z, Poidevin M, Li X, Li Y, Shu L, Nelson DL, et al. Expanded GGGGCC repeat RNA associated with amyotrophic lateral sclerosis and frontotemporal dementia causes neurodegeneration. Proc Natl Acad Sci U S A. 2013;110(19):7778–83. PubMed PMID: 23553836. PubMed Central PMCID: 3651485.
181. Mori K, Lammich S, Mackenzie IR, Forne I, Zilow S, Kretzschmar H, et al. hnRNP A3 binds to GGGGCC repeats and is a constituent of p62-positive/TDP43-negative inclusions in the hippocampus of patients with C9orf72 mutations. Acta Neuropathol. 2013;125(3):413–23. PubMed PMID: 23381195.
182. Ash PE, Bieniek KF, Gendron TF, Caulfield T, Lin WL, Dejesus-Hernandez M, et al. Unconventional translation of C9ORF72 GGGGCC expansion generates insoluble polypeptides specific to c9FTD/ALS. Neuron. 2013;77(4):639–46. PubMed PMID: 23415312. Pubmed Central PMCID: 3593233.
183. Zu T, Gibbens B, Doty NS, Gomes-Pereira M, Huguet A, Stone MD, et al. Non-ATG-initiated translation directed by microsatellite expansions. Proc Natl Acad Sci U S A. 2011;108(1):260–5. PubMed PMID: 21173221. PubMed Central PMCID: 3017129.
184. Mori K, Arzberger T, Grasser FA, Gijselinck I, May S, Rentzsch K, et al. Bidirectional transcripts of the expanded C9orf72 hexanucleotide repeat are translated into aggregating dipeptide repeat proteins. Acta Neuropathol. 2013;126(6):881–93. PubMed PMID: 24132570.
185. Kwon I, Xiang S, Kato M, Wu L, Theodoropoulos P, Wang T, et al. Poly-dipeptides encoded by the C9ORF72 repeats bind nucleoli, impede RNA biogenesis, and kill cells. Science. 2014;345(6201):1139–145. PubMed PMID: 25081482.

186. Mizielinska S, Gronke S, Niccoli T, Ridler CE, Clayton EL, Devoy A, et al. C9orf72 repeat expansions cause neurodegeneration in Drosophila through arginine-rich proteins. Science. 2014;345(6201):1192–194. PubMed PMID: 25103406.
187. Watts GD, Wymer J, Kovach MJ, Mehta SG, Mumm S, Darvish D, et al. Inclusion body myopathy associated with Paget disease of bone and frontotemporal dementia is caused by mutant valosin-containing protein. Nat Genet. 2004;36(4):377–81. PubMed PMID: 15034582.
188. Johnson JO, Mandrioli J, Benatar M, Abramzon Y, Van Deerlin VM, Trojanowski JQ, et al. Exome sequencing reveals VCP mutations as a cause of familial ALS. Neuron. 2010;68(5):857–64. PubMed PMID: 21145000. PubMed Central PMCID: 3032425.
189. Dai RM, Li CC. Valosin-containing protein is a multi-ubiquitin chain-targeting factor required in ubiquitin-proteasome degradation. Nat Cell Biol. 2001;3(8):740–4. PubMed PMID: 11483959.
190. Ju JS, Weihl CC. Inclusion body myopathy, Paget's disease of the bone and fronto-temporal dementia: a disorder of autophagy. Hum Mol Genet. 2010;19(R1):R38–45. PubMed PMID: 20410287. PubMed Central PMCID: 2875057.
191. Weihl CC, Pestronk A, Kimonis VE. Valosin-containing protein disease: inclusion body myopathy with Paget's disease of the bone and fronto-temporal dementia. Neuromuscul Disord: NMD. 2009;19(5):308–15. PubMed PMID: 19380227. PubMed Central PMCID: 2859037.
192. Badadani M, Nalbandian A, Watts GD, Vesa J, Kitazawa M, Su H, et al. VCP associated inclusion body myopathy and paget disease of bone knock-in mouse model exhibits tissue pathology typical of human disease. PLoS One. 2010;5(10):pii:e13183.
193. Custer SK, Neumann M, Lu H, Wright AC, Taylor JP. Transgenic mice expressing mutant forms VCP/p97 recapitulate the full spectrum of IBMPFD including degeneration in muscle, brain and bone. Hum Mol Genet. 2010;19(9):1741–55. PubMed PMID: 20147319.
194. Skibinski G, Parkinson NJ, Brown JM, Chakrabarti L, Lloyd SL, Hummerich H, et al. Mutations in the endosomal ESCRTIII-complex subunit CHMP2B in frontotemporal dementia. Nat Genet. 2005;37(8):806–8. PubMed PMID: 16041373.
195. Cox LE, Ferraiuolo L, Goodall EF, Heath PR, Higginbottom A, Mortiboys H, et al. Mutations in CHMP2B in lower motor neuron predominant amyotrophic lateral sclerosis (ALS). PLoS One. 2010;5(3):e9872. PubMed PMID: 20352044. PubMed Central PMCID: 2844426.
196. Urwin H, Authier A, Nielsen JE, Metcalf D, Powell C, Froud K, et al. Disruption of endocytic trafficking in frontotemporal dementia with CHMP2B mutations. Hum Mol Genet. 2010;19(11):2228–38. PubMed PMID: 20223751. PubMed Central PMCID: 2865375.
197. Ghazi-Noori S, Froud KE, Mizielinska S, Powell C, Smidak M, et al. Progressive neuronal inclusion formation and axonal degeneration in CHMP2B mutant transgenic mice. Brain. 2012;135(Pt 3):819–32. PubMed PMID: 22366797.
198. Buratti E, Dork T, Zuccato E, Pagani F, Romano M, Baralle FE. Nuclear factor TDP-43 and SR proteins promote in vitro and in vivo CFTR exon 9 skipping. EMBO J. 2001;20(7):1774–84. PubMed PMID: 11285240. PubMed Central PMCID: 145463.
199. Colombrita C, Onesto E, Megiorni F, Pizzuti A, Baralle F, Buratti E, et al. TDP-43 and FUS RNA-binding proteins bind distinct sets of cytoplasmic messenger RNAs and differently regulate their post-transcriptional fate in motoneuron-like cells. J Biol Chem. 2012;287(19):15635–47.
200. Ou SH, Wu F, Harrich D, Garcia-Martinez LF, Gaynor RB. Cloning and characterization of a novel cellular protein, TDP-43, that binds to human immunodeficiency virus type 1 TAR DNA sequence motifs. J Virol. 1995;69(6):3584–96. PubMed PMID: 7745706. PubMed Central PMCID: 189073.
201. Da Cruz S, Cleveland DW. Understanding the role of TDP-43 and FUS/TLS in ALS and beyond. Curr Opin Neurobiol. 2011;21(6):904–19. PubMed PMID: 21813273. PubMed Central PMCID: 3228892.
202. Lee EB, Lee VM, Trojanowski JQ. Gains or losses: molecular mechanisms of TDP43-mediated neurodegeneration. Nat Rev Neurosci. 2012;13(1):38–50. PubMed PMID: 22127299. PubMed Central PMCID: 3285250.

203. Kwiatkowski Jr TJ, Bosco DA, Leclerc AL, Tamrazian E, Vanderburg CR, Russ C, et al. Mutations in the FUS/TLS gene on chromosome 16 cause familial amyotrophic lateral sclerosis. Science. 2009;323(5918):1205–8. PubMed PMID: 19251627.
204. Vance C, Rogelj B, Hortobagyi T, De Vos KJ, Nishimura AL, Sreedharan J, et al. Mutations in FUS, an RNA processing protein, cause familial amyotrophic lateral sclerosis type 6. Science. 2009;323(5918):1208–11. PubMed PMID: 19251628.
205. Neumann M, Bentmann E, Dormann D, Jawaid A, DeJesus-Hernandez M, Ansorge O, et al. FET proteins TAF15 and EWS are selective markers that distinguish FTLD with FUS pathology from amyotrophic lateral sclerosis with FUS mutations. Brain. 2011;134(Pt 9):2595–609. PubMed PMID: 21856723. PubMed Central PMCID: 3170539.
206. Lagier-Tourenne C, Polymenidou M, Cleveland DW. TDP-43 and FUS/TLS: emerging roles in RNA processing and neurodegeneration. Hum Mol Genet. 2010;19(R1):R46–64. PubMed PMID: 20400460. PubMed Central PMCID: 3167692.
207. Dormann D, Haass C. Fused in sarcoma (FUS): an oncogene goes awry in neurodegeneration. Mol Cell Neurosci. 2013;56:475–86. PubMed PMID: 23557964.
208. van der Zee J, Van Langenhove T, Kleinberger G, Sleegers K, Engelborghs S, Vandenberghe R, et al. TMEM106B is associated with frontotemporal lobar degeneration in a clinically diagnosed patient cohort. Brain. 2011;134(Pt 3):808–15. PubMed PMID: 21354975. PubMed Central PMCID: 3044834.
209. Finch N, Carrasquillo MM, Baker M, Rutherford NJ, Coppola G, Dejesus-Hernandez M, et al. TMEM106B regulates progranulin levels and the penetrance of FTLD in GRN mutation carriers. Neurology. 2011;76(5):467–74. PubMed PMID: 21178100. PubMed Central PMCID: 3034409.
210. Cruchaga C, Graff C, Chiang HH, Wang J, Hinrichs AL, Spiegel N, et al. Association of TMEM106B gene polymorphism with age at onset in granulin mutation carriers and plasma granulin protein levels. Arch Neurol. 2011;68(5):581–6. PubMed PMID: 21220649. PubMed Central PMCID: 3090529.
211. Lang CM, Fellerer K, Schwenk BM, Kuhn PH, Kremmer E, Edbauer D, et al. Membrane orientation and subcellular localization of transmembrane protein 106B (TMEM106B), a major risk factor for frontotemporal lobar degeneration. J Biol Chem. 2012;287(23):19355–65. PubMed PMID: 22511793. PubMed Central PMCID: 3365973.
212. Brady OA, Zheng Y, Murphy K, Huang M, Hu F. The frontotemporal lobar degeneration risk factor, TMEM106B, regulates lysosomal morphology and function. Hum Mol Genet. 2013;22(4):685–95. PubMed PMID: 23136129. PubMed Central PMCID: 3554197.
213. Busch JI, Martinez-Lage M, Ashbridge E, Grossman M, Van Deerlin VM, Hu F, et al. Expression of TMEM106B, the frontotemporal lobar degeneration-associated protein, in normal and diseased human brain. Acta Neuropathol Commun. 2013;1(1):36. PubMed PMID: 24252750. PubMed Central PMCID: 3893524.
214. Chen-Plotkin AS, Unger TL, Gallagher MD, Bill E, Kwong LK, Volpicelli-Daley L, et al. TMEM106B, the risk gene for frontotemporal dementia, is regulated by the microRNA-132/212 cluster and affects progranulin pathways. J Neurosci. 2012;32(33):11213–27. PubMed PMID: 22895706. PubMed Central PMCID: 3446826.
215. Deng HX, Chen W, Hong ST, Boycott KM, Gorrie GH, Siddique N, et al. Mutations in UBQLN2 cause dominant X-linked juvenile and adult-onset alS and ALS/dementia. Nature. 2011;477(7363):211–5. PubMed PMID: 21857683. PubMed Central PMCID: 3169705.
216. Fecto F, Yan J, Vemula SP, Liu E, Yang Y, Chen W, et al. SQSTM1 mutations in familial and sporadic amyotrophic lateral sclerosis. Arch Neurol. 2011;68(11):1440–6. PubMed PMID: 22084127.
217. Le Ber I, Camuzat A, Guerreiro R, Bouya-Ahmed K, Bras J, Nicolas G, et al. SQSTM1 mutations in French patients with frontotemporal dementia or frontotemporal dementia with amyotrophic lateral sclerosis. JAMA Neurol. 2013;70(11):1403–10. PubMed PMID: 24042580.
218. Rubino E, Rainero I, Chio A, Rogaeva E, Galimberti D, Fenoglio P, et al. SQSTM1 mutations in frontotemporal lobar degeneration and amyotrophic lateral sclerosis. Neurology. 2012;79(15):1556–62. PubMed PMID: 22972638. PubMed Central PMCID: 3655323.

219. Liu Y, Yu JT, Sun FR, Ou JR, Qu SB, Tan L. The clinical and pathological phenotypes of frontotemporal dementia with C9ORF72 mutations. J Neurol Sci. 2013;335(1–2):26–35. PubMed PMID: 24090760.
220. Rademakers R, Eriksen JL, Baker M, Robinson T, Ahmed Z, Lincoln SJ, et al. Common variation in the miR-659 binding-site of GRN is a major risk factor for TDP43-positive frontotemporal dementia. Hum Mol Genet. 2008;17(23):3631–42. PubMed PMID: 18723524. PubMed Central PMCID: 2581433.
221. Simon-Sanchez J, Seelaar H, Bochdanovits Z, Deeg DJ, van Swieten JC, Heutink P. Variation at GRN 3′-UTR rs5848 is not associated with a risk of frontotemporal lobar degeneration in Dutch population. PLoS One. 2009;4(10):e7494. PubMed PMID: 19847305. PubMed Central PMCID: 2761542.
222. Rollinson S, Rohrer JD, van der Zee J, Sleegers K, Mead S, Engelborghs S, et al. No association of PGRN 3′UTR rs5848 in frontotemporal lobar degeneration. Neurobiol Aging. 2011;32(4):754–5. PubMed PMID: 19446372.
223. Dickson DW, Baker M, Rademakers R. Common variant in GRN is a genetic risk factor for hippocampal sclerosis in the elderly. Neurodegener Dis. 2010;7(1–3):170–4. PubMed PMID: 20197700. PubMed Central PMCID: 2859236.
224. Pao WC, Dickson DW, Crook JE, Finch NA, Rademakers R, Graff-Radford NR. Hippocampal sclerosis in the elderly: genetic and pathologic findings, some mimicking Alzheimer disease clinically. Alzheimer Dis Assoc Disord. 2011;25(4):364–8. PubMed PMID: 21346515. PubMed Central PMCID: 3107353.
225. Hsiung GY, Fok A, Feldman HH, Rademakers R, Mackenzie IR. rs5848 polymorphism and serum progranulin level. J Neurol Sci. 2011;300(1–2):28–32. PubMed PMID: 21047645. PubMed Central PMCID: 3085023.
226. Kamalainen A, Viswanathan J, Natunen T, Helisalmi S, Kauppinen T, Pikkarainen M, et al. GRN variant rs5848 reduces plasma and brain levels of granulin in Alzheimer's disease patients. J Alzheimers Dis. 2013;33(1):23–7. PubMed PMID: 22890097.
227. van Blitterswijk M, Mullen B, Nicholson AM, Bieniek KF, Heckman MG, Baker MC, et al. TMEM106B protects C9ORF72 expansion carriers against frontotemporal dementia. Acta Neuropathol. 2014;127(3):397–406. PubMed PMID: 24385136.
228. Gallagher MD, Suh E, Grossman M, Elman L, McCluskey L, Van Swieten JC, et al. TMEM106B is a genetic modifier of frontotemporal lobar degeneration with C9orf72 hexanucleotide repeat expansions. Acta Neuropathol. 2014;127(3):407–18. PubMed PMID: 24442578.
229. van Blitterswijk M, Baker MC, DeJesus-Hernandez M, Ghidoni R, Benussi L, Finger E, et al. C9ORF72 repeat expansions in cases with previously identified pathogenic mutations. Neurology. 2013;81(15):1332–41. PubMed PMID: 24027057. PubMed Central PMCID: 3806926.
230. Lashley T, Rohrer JD, Mahoney C, Gordon E, Beck J, Mead S, et al. A pathogenic progranulin mutation and C9orf72 repeat expansion in a family with frontotemporal dementia. Neuropath Appl Neurobiol. 2013;40(4):502–13. PubMed PMID: 24286341.
231. Polymenidou M, Lagier-Tourenne C, Hutt K, Huelga S, Moran J, Liang T, et al. Long pre-mRNA depletion and RNA missplicing contribute to neuronal vulnerability from loss of TDP-43. Nat Neurosci. 2011;14(4):459–68.

Chapter 6
Genetics of Primary Tremor Disorders

Gregor Kuhlenbäumer

Abstract Tremor, defined as rhythmical, involuntary oscillatory movement of a body part, is a symptom of numerous disorders of the central and peripheral nervous system. This chapter will deal with primary tremor disorders with a recognizable genetic component not discussed elsewhere in this book. These are essential tremor (ET), orthostatic tremor (OT), and cortical myoclonic "tremor." ET has a high genetic component and has been the subject of intense genetic investigation. Despite these efforts genes causing monogenic ET or genetic risk factors for genetically complex ET have not been reliably and reproducibly identified to date. OT is mostly a sporadic disease but has been described in sib pairs and identical twins. Cortical myoclonic "tremor" is characterized by irregular, rapid myoclonic jerks mimicking a tremor. Geniospasm (chin tremor) is also briefly discussed. Three loci and two putative candidate genes have been identified. In summary, the genetic investigation of tremor has been difficult and not overly successful up to now.

Keywords Tremor • Genetics • Essential tremor • Cortical tremor • Orthostatic tremor • Myoclonic epilepsy • Chin tremor • Geniospasm • ETM locus • FUS gene • Benign adult familial myoclonic epilepsy (BAFME) • Familial cortical myoclonic tremor with epilepsy (FCMTE) • Familial adult myoclonic epilepsy (FAME)

Introduction

Tremor, defined as rhythmical, involuntary oscillatory movement of a body part, is a symptom of numerous disorders of the central and peripheral nervous system. Tremor may either be the main symptom of a primary tremor disorder or one of the symptoms of other neurological diseases – many of them being movement disorders – defined by different main symptoms. The scope of this chapter will encompass only primary tremor disorders with a recognizable genetic component, i.e.,

G. Kuhlenbäumer, MD, PhD
Department of Neurology, University Hospital Schleswig Holstein,
Kiel, Kiel 24105, Germany
e-mail: g.kuhlenbaeumer@neurologie.uni-kiel.de

S.A. Schneider, J.M.T. Brás (eds.), *Movement Disorder Genetics*,
DOI 10.1007/978-3-319-17223-1_6

Table 6.1 Monogenic neurologic disorders commonly associated with tremor

Ataxia telangiectasia
Dystonia, monogenic forms
Hereditary peripheral neuropathies, monogenic forms
Hereditary spastic paraplegias, monogenic forms
Huntington disease
Neurodegeneration with brain iron accumulation (NBIA), monogenic forms
Parkinson disease, monogenic forms
Paroxysmal dystonic choreoathetosis
Spinal muscular atrophies
Spinobulbar muscular atrophy (Kennedy syndrome)
Spinocerebellar ataxias, monogenic forms
Wilson's disease

essential tremor (ET), orthostatic tremor (OT), cortical myoclonic tremor, and hereditary geniospasm. The genetics of dystonic tremor (in particular DYT1, DYT24, and DYT18 and others; see Chap. 7), the tremor of Parkinson disease (Chaps. 2 and 3), tremor associated with cerebellar ataxias (including fragile x-associated tremor/ataxia syndrome (FXTAS), see Chaps. 11 and 12), and other tremors associated with movement disorders (such as Wilson's disease (Chap. 14), hereditary spastic paraplegias (Chap. 16), mitochondrial disease (Chap. 18), etc.) will be dealt with in the respective chapters of this book. Table 6.1 presents a non-exhaustive list of the most common monogenic disorders associated with tremor.

Essential Tremor

Definition

ET, often referred to as "classic ET," is an idiopathic tremor syndrome, defined by a mainly postural and often also kinetic tremor of the hands, arms, and sometimes the head which is more accurately defined by a set of diagnostic criteria detailed in the section "Clinical phenotype and diagnostic criteria" [1].

Epidemiology

The term "essential tremor" has been coined in 1874 by the Italian physician Pietro Burresi, but the basic clinical phenotype has been described much earlier [2]. ET occurs worldwide. ET is a very common disorder, possibly the second most common movement disorder after restless legs syndrome (RLS), and the prevalence is increasing due to an aging population [3]. Estimates vary considerably, but a prevalence of

~1 % in the general population and ~5 in the population older than 65 years is a reasonable estimate [4]. ET might be slightly more common in men compared to women (~1.1 times) [4]. The age of onset of ET varies widely from childhood to senescence. It is not entirely clear whether the age of onset of ET shows a unimodal distribution with an age-dependent increase of the incidence or a bimodal distribution with a young-onset peak around 20 years of age and another peak centered around 60 years of age [5–7]. The young-onset peak has been attributed to the fact that many studies were done in tertial referral centers [6]. However, our own unpublished data in a sample of 913 ET patients mostly recruited via newspaper articles supports the notion of a young-onset peak mostly attributable to patients with a positive family history. It is unknown whether ET has an impact on life expectancy [8, 9]. One Spanish/US study addressed this issue and found a small but statistically significant reduction of life expectancy in ET patients [9]. However, this study examined an aged population with a mean age at inclusion of 74 years. After stratification for tremor duration in long (>5 years) and short (<5 years), a reduction in life expectancy was observed only in the short tremor duration group. These patients had a senile onset of tremor, and it is currently unknown if this form of tremor is etiologically comparable to ET or represents a separate "senile tremor" entity.

Clinical Phenotype and Diagnostic Criteria

ET is probably best defined looking at a four slightly different but widely overlapping sets of diagnostic criteria proposed in the last 20 years. The first set of criteria was published by a specialist subgroup of the Movement Disorders Society (MDS), the Tremor Investigation Group (TRIG) in 1995 [10]. The core feature is a "bilateral postural tremor with or without kinetic tremor, involving hands and forearms, that is visible and persistent." Exclusion criteria for "definite" and "probable" ET are other causes of tremor and additional neurological signs except "increased resistance to passive movements of a limb about a joint upon voluntary activity of another body part" (Froment's sign). In addition a tremor duration of >5 years for "definite" and >3 years for "probable" ET is required. "Possible" Et allows for a number of other neurologic signs or a concomitant neurologic disorder, e.g., parkinsonism or dystonia. The second set of criteria proposed in 1998 by the MDS discards the duration criterion and differentiates between "classic" ET, encompassing "definite" and "probable" ET according to the TRIG criteria and – unchanged – "possible" ET [1]. The third set of criteria by essentially the same authors proposes "core" and "secondary" criteria [11]. In addition to the tremor of the hands, an isolated tremor of the head is listed among the core criteria, and a cogwheel phenomenon is generally permitted. A fourth set of diagnostic criteria, the Washington Heights-Inwood Genetic Study of Essential Tremor (WHIGET) criteria, were published in 1997 [12]. These criteria are similar to the previously described ones but include tremor amplitude criteria while lacking some of the criteria of the aforementioned diagnostic criteria.

Table 6.2 Summary of diagnostic criteria for ET

Core criteria
1. Bilateral postural and kinetic tremor of the hands and forearms (but not rest tremor) (T, MD, B)
2. Absence of other neurologic signs (T, MD, B), with the exception of the cogwheel phenomenon (T, B)
3. May have isolated head tremor with no signs of dystonia (MD, B)
Duration and level of certainty
1. "Definite ET": duration >5 years + comprehensive exclusion of other causes + no stepwise deterioration (T)
2. "Probable ET": duration >3 years + same criteria as "definite ET" (T)
3. "Possible ET": no duration criterion + type I, some other neurologic symptoms allowed; type II, monosymptomatic or isolated tremors of uncertain relation to essential tremor (T)
Secondary criteria
1. Positive family history (present in 30–60 % of patients) (B)
2. Beneficial alcohol response (present in 50–75 % of patients) (B)

According to TRIG (T, [10]), Movement Disorders Society (MD, [1]) and Bain et al. (B, [11])

Table 6.2 summarizes the key features of the three sets of criteria created by task forces of the MDS.

The tremor amplitude in ET patients usually increases, while the tremor frequency decreases with advancing age. Patients with mild ET rarely show a significant rest tremor, while ~10–15 % of patients with advanced ET show a mild rest tremor. The tremor in ET patients with rest tremor is – in contrast to PD – not suppressed but enhanced upon voluntary movement [13]. While older studies emphasize the preponderance of a postural tremor in ET, more recent studies often report an increase of the tremor upon (goal-directed) movement [14]. The kinetic tremor is a gait disturbance in advanced ET, and kinematic analyses demonstrate cerebellar dysfunction in ET [15]. Ethanol ameliorates the tremor in many ET patients [16]. Up to now ethanol sensitivity has not been sufficiently studied to determine whether it might serve as a useful diagnostic marker. The full differential diagnosis of ET comprises a large number of diseases, but only few of these are commonly encountered. The tremor frequency in ET is mostly in the 4–8 Hertz (Hz) range but might be up to 12 Hz. Physiologic tremor and enhanced physiologic tremor present with a frequency in the 8–12 Hz range and might be difficult to distinguish from mild ET in the upper frequency range [17]. A common condition exacerbating physiologic tremor is hyperthyroidism. The relationship between dystonia and ET is a longstanding matter of debate [18]. While dystonia is an exclusion criterion in the different sets of diagnostic criteria, many clinicians would regard mild, subclinical signs of dystonia, mostly not recognized by the patients who complain of tremor as being compatible with ET. This problem is most pronounced in studies of familial ET because a closer examination of all family members often reveals mild dystonic signs in conjunction with obvious tremor in a subset of family members [19, 20]. It is unclear whether these individuals suffer from dystonic tremor or from ET with a dystonic component. Tremor-dominant PD is in most cases differentiated by a preponderant rest tremor and additional neurologic signs in PD patients. Drug-induced

Table 6.3 Additional clinical features possibly associated with ET

Cognitive deficits (frontal executive and memory)
Dementia
Personality changes
Depression
Mild olfactory dysfunction
Hearing impairment
Increased mortality

tremor should be ruled out by an appropriate drug history. Psychogenic tremor can be difficult to differentiate from ET [21].

A number of additional clinical features have been reported in ET patients (Table 6.3). Most of these features are relatively mild and therefore subclinical. Keeping in mind that ET might be an etiologically heterogeneous group of biologically different diseases, it is not clear whether the reported features affect only certain subgroups or all ET patients. Some of the studies reporting additional features studied only ET with an age of onset >65 years, e.g., [22, 23]. Whether these patients represent a distinct subform of "senile (essential) tremor" is unknown. Therefore, these results might not be completely applicable to young-onset ET patients. Clarifying these issues would require an extremely large and very long-term prospective study. An association between ET and Parkinson disease (PD) has been analyzed by numerous studies which show inconsistent results.

Etiology and Pathogenesis

Genetic and environmental factors play a role in the etiology of ET. Environmental risk factors might be harmane and lead. Both substances have been found in higher concentrations in the serum of ET patients compared to controls [24, 25]. Harmala alkaloids are potent tremor inducers in rodents. Two hypotheses regarding the pathogenesis of ET exist. One hypothesis, mainly based on neurophysiological data states that ET is a neurofunctional disorder caused by abnormal oscillations in the cortico-bulbo-cerebello-thalamo-cortical loop which is also involved in the generation of other tremor forms [26]. The other hypothesis, based on autopsy findings, states that ET is a neurodegenerative disorder, mainly involving the cerebellum [27]. However, in the published autopsy studies, all ET patients were very old at the time of autopsy and the pathological changes were mild compared to other neurodegenerative disorders. In addition, these findings have not been replicated by other groups [28].

Heritability

ET patients can tentatively be separated into at least two subgroups. Predominantly young-onset patients (onset <~40–50 years) with a strongly positive family history suggesting monogenic, mostly autosomal dominant inheritance form one subgroup, while sporadic patients, often with a higher age of onset, form the other subgroup [22, 29, 30]. It is currently not clear whether patients with a very high age at onset (>~65–75 years) form a third subgroup which could be termed "senile tremor" [31, 32]. Heritability of sporadic ET has been assessed using family history and twin studies. A number of studies have shown that family history studies in ET are unreliable and tend to underestimate the genetic component. Twin studies are a better way to estimate heritability [33–35]. Two twin studies of ET have been conducted – one in a US population and the other one employing the Danish twin registry [36, 37]. The US study found a pairwise concordance rate of 0.60 (United States, definite ET), whereas the Danish/German study one of 0.93 (Denmark/Germany, definite and probable ET) for monozygotic twins versus 0.27 (United States) and 0.29 (Denmark/Germany) for dizygotic twins which translate into rough heritability estimates between 45 and 90 %.

Molecular Genetics

Presumably Monogenic ET

Linkage Studies. Three chromosomal loci have been identified for presumably monogenic ET using genome-wide linkage analysis. The results of genome-wide linkage scans are usually expressed as logarithm of odds (LOD) scores. In monogenic disorders an LOD score >3.3 in a single family is regarded as conclusive, while an LOD score >2 is usually regarded as suggestive for a novel locus and as confirmatory for a known locus.

ETM1 was mapped to chromosome 13q13 in 16 small Icelandic families [38]. The maximum LOD score in a single family was 1.42, the maximum LOD score across all families was 3.71. Eight follow-up studies were not able to confirm the locus [39–46]. Co-segregation of the Gly allele of the dopamine receptor 3 gene (*DRD3*) Ser9Gly (rs6280) polymorphism located in the ETM1 locus was observed in 23 out of 30 French families with 1–5 affected individuals and showed a weak association of the same polymorphism with ET in sporadic US ET patients [47]. Three follow-up studies found co-segregation of the Gly allele in 8/46 families of varying size which is not surprising considering an allele frequency of the Gly allele of rs6280 ranging from 0.3 (dpSNP database, Asian) to 0.5 (Exome Sequencing Project database) [44, 48, 49]. Out of six association studies attempting replication between rs6280 and ET, only one yielded a significant *p*-value [44, 48–52]. Therefore, it is questionable whether ETM1 harbors a gene causing monogenic ET. It also seems unlikely that the *DRD3* polymorphism rs6280 is a major risk factor for sporadic ET.

The *ETM2* locus has been convincingly mapped to chromosome 2p24 in a very large Czech/American family with a conclusive LOD score of 5.92 [53]. Eight follow-up analyses of 34 additional families with 3–19 affected individuals did not confirm these results [40, 42–46, 54]. The group that mapped the locus described a genetic variant (Ala265Gly) in the hematopoietic lineage cell-specific protein binding protein 3 (*HS1BP3*) that segregated with ET in two families, one of them containing 10 affected family members [55]. It is not reported if this variant has been analyzed in the original family which allowed mapping of the locus. Out of two association studies, one found association between the *HS1BP3* variant and ET and one did not [56, 57]. The ETM2 locus is based on a convincing linkage result in one large family and could well harbor a gene for monogenic ET, but it is unlikely that the Ala265Gly variant in the *HS1BP3* gene is causative.

The *ETM3* locus has been mapped to chromosome 6p23 in one large American family with a nonconclusive maximum LOD score of 2.93 [20]. The LOD score was obtained in an "affected-only" analysis. The published pedigree shows that – if this locus harbors a gene for monogenic ET – a very low penetrance and extremely high phenocopy rate of ~20 % has to be postulated. In a second family, co-segregation of markers in the ETM3 region was shown but LOD scores were below 2 [20]. Four independent follow-up studies examining 21 additional families with 3–15 affected individuals were not able to demonstrate linkage to this locus in any of the families [39, 40, 43, 44].

Exome sequencing, the DNA sequencing of all protein coding exons in the genome, is a novel method made possible by the rapid advances in DNA sequencing technology, collectively called "next-generation sequencing" (NGS). A Canadian group identified a stop mutation in the fused in sarcoma (*FUS*) gene in a large Franco-Canadian family [58]. The mutation segregated well with the ET phenotype in the family. Follow-up studies identified a number of additional mutations in *FUS* in sporadic and familial ET patients [59–63]. However, it is not clear whether the frequency of these mutations exceeds the mutation frequency of *FUS* in controls. In order to confirm the causative role of *FUS* further, large ET families showing co-segregation of *FUS* mutations with ET are needed.

Genetically Complex ET

Currently the method of choice for the analysis of genetically complex disorders is the genetic association study. Genetic association studies are usually conducted either as candidate gene studies or as genome-wide association studies (GWAS).

Candidate gene association studies in ET were not successful, and none of the associations found in these studies have been consistently replicated [64]. They will therefore not be discussed in detail. Candidate gene selection followed different approaches: (1) assuming a pathogenetic overlap between ET and PD (genes studied: *SNCA*, *LRRK2*, *MAPT*, *GBA*, Parkin); (2) a number of short-tandem-repeat (STR) expansions analyzed because anticipation has been observed in some families with ET (genes/repeats studied: *FMR1*, *PP2APR55beta*, *C9orf72*, *ATX2*, *MJD1* repeat expansions were analyzed and the "repeat-expansion-detection" (RED) method was used for the detection CAG expansions); and (3) genes acting in the gamma-amino-butyric-acid (GABA) neurotransmitter system. GABA is the most important inhibitory neurotransmitter in the central nervous system and most likely

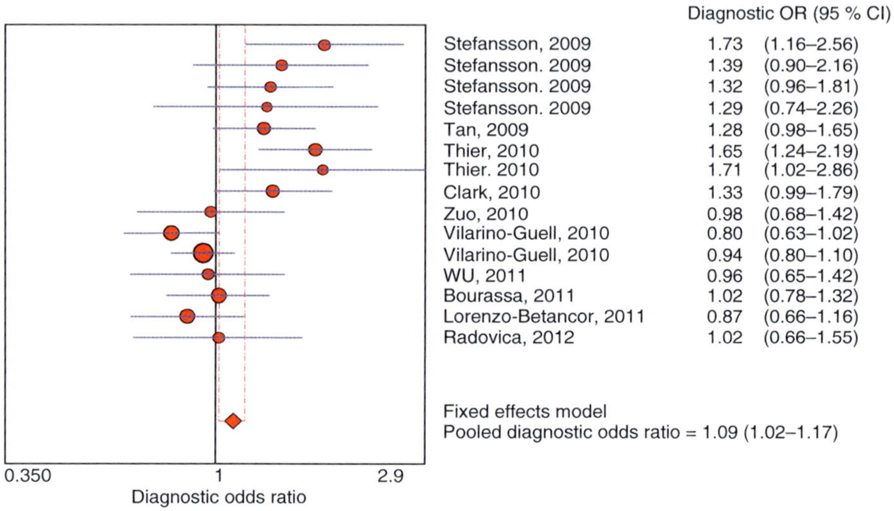

Fig. 6.1 Meta-analysis of the association between LINO1 rs9652490 and ET

involved in the pathogenesis of ET. GABA receptor alpha 1 subunit-deficient mice exhibit a spontaneous tremor; a GABAergic deficit has been demonstrated in ET patients by positron emission tomography (PET), and autopsy findings in ET patients suggest that the GABA receptor density is reduced in the dentate nucleus of the cerebellum [65–67]. Unfortunately, four studies investigating numerous genes in the GABA system were negative, and GWAS studies did not highlight GABA-related genes either [68–70]. It needs to be mentioned that most candidate gene association studies suffered from relatively small sample sizes and were therefore not able to reliably exclude weak to moderate associations.

Genome-wide association studies (*GWAS*) examine a large number of genetic markers which are distributed over the whole genome. GWA studies are usually regarded as conclusive if they fulfill the following requirements: (I) a two-stage design with a discovery stage and a replication stage, (II) achieving "genome-wide significance" in the discovery stage, (III) obtaining p-values in the replication stage which remain significant after Bonferroni correction, and (IV) replication in different patients samples in independent laboratories.

Two GWAS of ET have been performed to date. The first GWAS study by the Icelandic deCODE consortium found an association between ET and a single nucleotide polymorphism in the leucine-rich repeat and Ig domain containing 1 gene (*LINGO1*) which did not reach genome-wide significance in the discovery stage (SNP, rs9652490, $p=3.0\times10^{-7}$) but was significant in the replication stage ($p=0.0010$) [71]. Subsequent independent replication studies showed mixed results. The result of a meta-analysis of all available studies for SNP rs9652490 excluding the discovery cohort is shown in Fig. 6.1 (pooled odds ratio, 95 % confidence interval, 1.09 (1.02–1.17)) [71–81]. One study reported association with the opposite allele of the one found to be associated in the initial Icelandic study, leading to

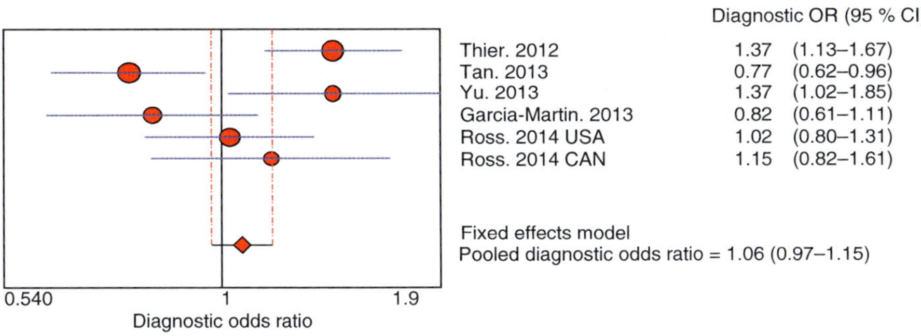

Fig. 6.2 Meta-analysis of the association between SLC1A2 rs3794087 and ET

substantial interstudy heterogeneity [78]. A second SNP in the same gene (rs11856808) found in the Icelandic study did not reach significance in most replication studies [71]. *LINGO1* is a signaling molecule in the NOGO receptor pathway and regulates neuroregeneration and neuronal survival in a negative way [82]. Recently two studies reported increased *LINGO1* expression in the cerebellum of ET patients [83–85].

The second GWAS conducted in a German/Austrian/Danish ET sample identified an SNP (rs3794087) in the solute carrier family 1 member 2 gene (*SLC1A2*) which did not reach genome-wide significance in the discovery stage ($p = 6.95 \times 10^{-5}$) but was significant in the replication stage ($p = 1.25 \times 10^{-3}$) [86]. This study included only patients with "probable" and "definite" ET according to the TRIG criteria. *SLC1A2* encodes the excitatory amino acid transporter 2 (EAAT2), the major transporter limiting the action of the excitatory transmitter glutamate in the brain [87–90]. Up to date, four studies attempting replication with mixed results have been published. A meta-analysis of all studies shown in Fig. 6.2, again without the discovery sample, does not support an association between the rs3794087 and ET (pooled odds ratio, 95 % confidence interval, 1.09 (0.97–1.15)) [86, 91–94].

In summary it has not been possible to identify beyond doubt any genetic cause or risk factor of ET despite a high heritability shown in multiple studies.

Primary Orthostatic Tremor

Primary orthostatic tremor is a very rare disorder of unknown etiology and pathogenesis characterized by a high-frequency (13–18 Hz) tremor of the legs when standing, ameliorated or disappearing when walking and not present when sitting or lying [95]. The condition has also been described in conjunction with Parkinson disease. Although primary orthostatic tremor has been described mainly in sporadic patients, three reports of affected sibs exist, one of them in a brother/sister pair [96], one in male monozygotic twins [97], and one in three brothers [98]. The parents of the patients – except for anecdotal evidence concerning the mother in one study – were not affected by primary orthostatic tremor suggesting either autosomal recessive inheritance or, in the families with male patients only, X-linked inheritance. The molecular genetic basis of primary orthostatic tremor has not been investigated.

Cortical Myoclonic Tremor

Cortical myoclonic tremor designates a group of rare, mostly autosomal dominant, genetically heterogeneous disorders characterized by similar clinical features, comprising an irregular, high-frequency myoclonus of cortical origin mimicking an irregular tremor and in most patients epileptic fits of different semiology and interictual EEG abnormalities [99]. A large number of synonymous acronyms have been coined for these disorders including autosomal dominant cortical myoclonus and epilepsy (ADCME), benign adult familial myoclonic epilepsy (BAFME), familial cortical myoclonic tremor with epilepsy (FCMTE), and familial adult myoclonic epilepsy (FAME). The first symptom of the disease is in most cases an "irregular action tremor" of the upper limbs [99]. Polymyography shows arrhythmic high-frequency burst-like discharges of very short duration (50 ms), typical for cortical myoclonus [100, 101]. The cortical origin of the myoclonus was confirmed with EEG-EMG coherence and EMG functional MRI studies [100, 101]. In addition features of cortical reflex myoclonus, e.g., giant somatosensory-evoked potentials (g-SEP) and abnormalities of the long loop reflexes (LLR) suggesting cortical hyperexcitability, are found [100–102]. A number of additional clinical features suggesting involvement of the cerebellum (e.g., eye movement abnormalities, gait ataxia) and slowly progressive cognitive decline in some families have been described. Neuropathologic data are very scarce. Published autopsy data suggest cerebellar degeneration with Purkinje cell loss [100]. Three loci for cortical myoclonic tremor have been mapped. *FAME/BAFME 1* was mapped to chromosome 8q23.3-q24.11 in Japanese families with conclusive LOD scores [103, 104]. This entity seems to have a later age of onset and milder course than the other loci which were mapped in European families. *FAME/BAFME 2* was mapped with conclusive LOD scores to chromosome 2p11.1-q12.2 in a number of Italian families [102, 105, 106]. *FAME/BAFME 3* was mapped to chromosome 5p15.31-p15.1 in a large French family with a conclusive maximum LOD score of 6.3 [107]. A fourth locus (*FAME/BAFME 4*) has been mapped with a maximum LOD score of 5.4 to chromosome 3q26.32-q28 in a Thai family [108]. Recently a similar phenotype involving myoclonic tremor and epilepsy with autosomal recessive inheritance has been described in a consanguineous Egyptian family [109]. The clinical features showed clear differences compared to the previously described families with autosomal dominant inheritance. All patients experienced focal temporal lobe seizures as manifesting symptom, and the SEP were normal. MRI revealed temporal mesial sclerosis in one patient. The underlying genetic defect was mapped using homozygosity mapping to chromosome 1q31-q32.2 with a conclusive LOD score of 3.6 and three possibly deleterious rare variants in the genes *DDX59* probably encoding an RNA helicase with very low expression in the brain; *TNNI1*, a gene implied in slow-twitch skeletal muscle contraction, and *CNTN2* (*Contactin 2*), a neuronal membrane protein, were found in the homozygous state in all 5 patients and in the heterozygous state in the parents [109], and *CNTN2* was highlighted as the most likely causal gene. Another putatively causal gene was identified in a Spanish family with presumably autosomal dominant cortical myoclonic tremor using whole-exome sequencing [110]. Two possibly deleterious rare variants showing full co-segregation with the disease in the available family members were identified, one in the tumor suppressor gene *MYBBP1A* and the other one in the *ACMSD* gene encoding an enzyme involved in the kynurenine pathway of tryptophan degradation [110]. Based on the fact that the kynurenine pathway has been shown to be involved in the pathogenesis of neurological disorders including epilepsies, the *ACMSD* gene was highlighted as the most likely causal gene. *ACMSD* maps to chromosome 2q21.3 outside the FAME/BAFME 2 locus.

In summary five chromosomal loci (4 AD, 1 AR) for cortical myoclonic tremor have been mapped with conclusive LOD scores in at least one family. Two candidate genes – *CNTN2* and *ACMSD* – have been identified, but none of the gene findings have so far been replicated.

Hereditary Geniospasm

Hereditary geniospasm is a rare, autosomal dominant, early onset, often stress-induced involuntary tremulous movement of the skin overlying the chin ("trembling of the chin") already observed at the end of the nineteenth century [111]. The disease is usually not associated with other neurologic abnormalities and is not progressive. Around 25 families have been described in total. Botulinum toxin is the therapy of choice. Hereditary geniospasm has been mapped to chromosome 9q13-q21 with a conclusive maximum LOD score of 5.24 in a large British family [112]. The underlying genetic defect is unknown. The 9q13-q21 locus was excluded in another family from Canada suggesting genetic heterogeneity of the disease [113].

References

1. Deuschl G, Bain P, Brin M. Consensus statement of the Movement Disorder Society on Tremor. Ad Hoc Scientific Committee. Mov Disord. 1998;13 Suppl 3:2–23. Epub 1998/11/25.
2. Louis ED, Broussolle E, Goetz CG, Krack P, Kaufmann P, Mazzoni P. Historical underpinnings of the term essential tremor in the late 19th century. Neurology. 2008;71(11):856–9. Epub 2008/09/10.
3. Bach JP, Ziegler U, Deuschl G, Dodel R, Doblhammer-Reiter G. Projected numbers of people with movement disorders in the years 2030 and 2050. Mov Disord. 2011;26(12):2286–90. Epub 2011/10/25.

4. Louis ED, Ferreira JJ. How common is the most common adult movement disorder? Update on the worldwide prevalence of essential tremor. Mov Disord. 2010;25(5):534–41. Epub 2010/02/23.
5. Lou JS, Jankovic J. Essential tremor: clinical correlates in 350 patients. Neurology. 1991;41(2(Pt 1)):234–8. Epub 1991/02/01.
6. Louis ED, Dogu O. Does age of onset in essential tremor have a bimodal distribution? Data from a tertiary referral setting and a population-based study. Neuroepidemiology. 2007;29 (3–4):208–12. Epub 2007/11/29.
7. Whaley NR, Putzke JD, Baba Y, Wszolek ZK, Uitti RJ. Essential tremor: phenotypic expression in a clinical cohort. Parkinsonism Relat Disord. 2007;13(6):333–9. Epub 2007/02/13.
8. Jankovic J, Beach J, Schwartz K, Contant C. Tremor and longevity in relatives of patients with Parkinson's disease, essential tremor, and control subjects. Neurology. 1995;45(4): 645–8. Epub 1995/04/01.
9. Louis ED, Benito-Leon J, Ottman R, Bermejo-Pareja F. A population-based study of mortality in essential tremor. Neurology. 2007;69(21):1982–9. Epub 2007/11/21.
10. Deuschl G, Zimmermann R, Genger H, Lücking C. Physiologic classification of essential tremor. In: Findley L, Koller W, editors. Handbook of tremor disorders. New York: Marcel Dekker; 1995. p. 195–208.
11. Bain P, Brin M, Deuschl G, Elble R, Jankovic J, Findley L, et al. Criteria for the diagnosis of essential tremor. Neurology. 2000;54(11 Suppl 4):S7. Epub 2000/06/15.
12. Louis ED, Ford B, Lee H, Andrews H, Cameron G. Diagnostic criteria for essential tremor: a population perspective. Arch Neurol. 1998;55(6):823–8. Epub 1998/06/17.
13. Papengut F, Raethjen J, Binder A, Deuschl G. Rest tremor suppression may separate essential from parkinsonian rest tremor. Parkinsonism Relat Disord. 2013;19(7):693–7. Epub 2013/04/30.
14. Louis ED. The primary type of tremor in essential tremor is kinetic rather than postural: cross-sectional observation of tremor phenomenology in 369 cases. Eur J Neurol. 2013;20(4): 725–7. Epub 2012/08/29.
15. Deuschl G, Wenzelburger R, Loffler K, Raethjen J, Stolze H. Essential tremor and cerebellar dysfunction clinical and kinematic analysis of intention tremor. Brain. 2000;123(Pt 8):1568–80. Epub 2000/07/25.
16. Koller WC, Biary N. Effect of alcohol on tremors: comparison with propranolol. Neurology. 1984;34(2):221–2. Epub 1984/02/01.
17. Elble RJ. What is essential tremor? Curr Neurol Neurosci Rep. 2013;13(6):353. Epub 2013/04/18.
18. Quinn NP, Schneider SA, Schwingenschuh P, Bhatia KP. Tremor–some controversial aspects. Mov Disord. 2011;26(1):18–23. Epub 2011/02/16.
19. Louis ED, Hernandez N, Alcalay RN, Tirri DJ, Ottman R, Clark LN. Prevalence and features of unreported dystonia in a family study of "pure" essential tremor. Parkinsonism Relat Disord. 2013;19(3):359–62. Epub 2012/10/24.
20. Shatunov A, Sambuughin N, Jankovic J, Elble R, Lee HS, Singleton AB, et al. Genomewide scans in North American families reveal genetic linkage of essential tremor to a region on chromosome 6p23. Brain. 2006;129(Pt 9):2318–31. Epub 2006/05/17.
21. Bhatia KP, Schneider SA. Psychogenic tremor and related disorders. J Neurol. 2007;254(5): 569–74. Epub 2007/04/10.
22. Benito-Leon J, Louis ED, Bermejo-Pareja F. Elderly-onset essential tremor is associated with dementia. Neurology. 2006;66(10):1500–5. Epub 2006/05/24.
23. Benito-Leon J, Louis ED, Bermejo-Pareja F. Population-based case–control study of cognitive function in essential tremor. Neurology. 2006;66(1):69–74. Epub 2006/01/13.
24. Louis ED, Applegate L, Graziano JH, Parides M, Slavkovich V, Bhat HK. Interaction between blood lead concentration and delta-amino-levulinic acid dehydratase gene polymorphisms increases the odds of essential tremor. Mov Disord. 2005;20(9):1170–7. Epub 2005/06/15.
25. Louis ED, Zheng W, Applegate L, Shi L, Factor-Litvak P. Blood harmane concentrations and dietary protein consumption in essential tremor. Neurology. 2005;65(3):391–6. Epub 2005/08/10.

26. Muthuraman M, Heute U, Arning K, Anwar AR, Elble R, Deuschl G, et al. Oscillating central motor networks in pathological tremors and voluntary movements. What makes the difference? Neuroimage. 2012;60(2):1331–9. Epub 2012/02/02.
27. Louis ED, Faust PL, Vonsattel JP, Honig LS, Rajput A, Robinson CA, et al. Neuropathological changes in essential tremor: 33 cases compared with 21 controls. Brain. 2007;130(Pt 12): 3297–307. Epub 2007/11/21.
28. Rajput AH, Adler CH, Shill HA, Rajput A. Essential tremor is not a neurodegenerative disease. Neurodegener Dis Manag. 2012;2(3):259–68. Epub 2012/10/30.
29. Louis ED, Ottman R. Study of possible factors associated with age of onset in essential tremor. Mov Disord. 2006;21(11):1980–6. Epub 2006/09/23.
30. Bain PG, Findley LJ, Thompson PD, Gresty MA, Rothwell JC, Harding AE, et al. A study of hereditary essential tremor. Brain. 1994;117(Pt 4):805–24. Epub 1994/08/01.
31. Louis ED, Wendt KJ, Ford B. Senile tremor. What is the prevalence and severity of tremor in older adults? Gerontology. 2000;46(1):12–6. Epub 2000/12/09.
32. Deuschl G, Elble R. Essential tremor–neurodegenerative or nondegenerative disease towards a working definition of ET. Mov Disord. 2009;24(14):2033–41. Epub 2009/09/15.
33. Louis ED, Ford B, Wendt KJ, Ottman R. Validity of family history data on essential tremor. Mov Disord. 1999;14(3):456–61. Epub 1999/05/29.
34. Busenbark K, Barnes P, Lyons K, Ince D, Villagra F, Koller WC. Accuracy of reported family histories of essential tremor. Neurology. 1996;47(1):264–5. Epub 1996/07/01.
35. Louis ED, Ford B, Frucht S, Ottman R. Mild tremor in relatives of patients with essential tremor: what does this tell us about the penetrance of the disease? Arch Neurol. 2001;58(10):1584–9. Epub 2001/10/27.
36. Tanner CM, Goldman SM, Lyons KE, Aston DA, Tetrud JW, Welsh MD, et al. Essential tremor in twins: an assessment of genetic vs environmental determinants of etiology. Neurology. 2001;57(8):1389–91. Epub 2001/10/24.
37. Lorenz D, Frederiksen H, Moises H, Kopper F, Deuschl G, Christensen K. High concordance for essential tremor in monozygotic twins of old age. Neurology. 2004;62(2):208–11. Epub 2004/01/28.
38. Gulcher JR, Jonsson P, Kong A, Kristjansson K, Frigge ML, Karason A, et al. Mapping of a familial essential tremor gene, FET1, to chromosome 3q13. Nat Genet. 1997;17(1):84–7. Epub 1997/09/01.
39. Novelletto A, Gulli R, Ciotti P, Vitale C, Malaspina P, Blasi P, et al. Linkage exclusion in Italian families with hereditary essential tremor. Eur J Neurol. 2011;18(9):e118–20. Epub 2011/08/13.
40. Pasini E, Busolin G, Nobile C, Michelucci R. Autosomal dominant essential tremor: a novel family with anticipation. Neurol Sci. 2013;34(5):761–3. Epub 2012/10/16.
41. Illarioshkin SN, Ivanova-Smolenskaya IA, Rahmonov RA, Markova ED, Stevanin G, Brice A. Clinical and genetic study of familial essential tremor in an isolate of Northern Tajikistan. Mov Disord. 2000;15(5):1020–3. Epub 2000/09/29.
42. Abbruzzese G, Pigullo S, Di Maria E, Martinelli P, Barone P, Marchese R, et al. Clinical and genetic study of essential tremor in the Italian population. Neurol Sci. 2001;22(1):39–40. Epub 2001/08/07.
43. Aridon P, Ragonese P, De Fusco M, Salemi G, Casari G, Savettieri G. Further evidence of genetic heterogeneity in familial essential tremor. Parkinsonism Relat Disord. 2008;14(1): 15–8. Epub 2007/08/21.
44. Lorenz D, Klebe S, Stevanin G, Thier S, Nebel A, Feingold J, et al. Dopamine receptor D3 gene and essential tremor in large series of German, Danish and French patients. Eur J Hum Genet. 2008;17(6):766–73. Epub 2008/12/19.
45. Kovach MJ, Ruiz J, Kimonis K, Mueed S, Sinha S, Higgins C, et al. Genetic heterogeneity in autosomal dominant essential tremor. Genet Med. 2001;3(3):197–9. Epub 2001/06/05.
46. Ma S, Davis TL, Blair MA, Fang JY, Bradford Y, Haines JL, et al. Familial essential tremor with apparent autosomal dominant inheritance: should we also consider other inheritance modes? Mov Disord. 2006;21(9):1368–74. Epub 2006/05/25.

47. Jeanneteau F, Funalot B, Jankovic J, Deng H, Lagarde JP, Lucotte G, et al. A functional variant of the dopamine D3 receptor is associated with risk and age-at-onset of essential tremor. Proc Natl Acad Sci U S A. 2006;103(28):10753–8. Epub 2006/07/01.
48. Blair MA, Ma S, Phibbs F, Fang JY, Cooper MK, Davis TL, et al. Reappraisal of the role of the DRD3 gene in essential tremor. Parkinsonism Relat Disord. 2008;14(6):471–5. Epub 2008/03/05.
49. Tan EK, Prakash KM, Fook-Chong S, Yih Y, Chua E, Lum SY, et al. DRD3 variant and risk of essential tremor. Neurology. 2007;68(10):790–1. Epub 2007/03/07.
50. Inashkina I, Radovica I, Smeltere L, Vitols E, Jankevics E. Case–control study of patients with essential tremor in Latvia. Eur J Neurol. 2008;15(9):988–90. Epub 2008/07/19.
51. Vitale C, Gulli R, Ciotti P, Scaglione C, Bellone E, Avanzino L, et al. DRD3 Ser9Gly variant is not associated with essential tremor in a series of Italian patients. Eur J Neurol. 2008;15(9):985–7. Epub 2008/05/20.
52. Garcia-Martin E, Martinez C, Alonso-Navarro H, Benito-Leon J, Puertas I, Rubio L, et al. Dopamine receptor D3 (DRD3) genotype and allelic variants and risk for essential tremor. Mov Disord. 2009;24(13):1910–5. Epub 2009/08/01.
53. Higgins JJ, Pho LT, Nee LE. A gene (ETM) for essential tremor maps to chromosome 2p22-p25. Mov Disord. 1997;12(6):859–64. Epub 1997/12/17.
54. Higgins JJ, Loveless JM, Jankovic J, Patel PI. Evidence that a gene for essential tremor maps to chromosome 2p in four families. Mov Disord. 1998;13(6):972–7. Epub 1998/11/25.
55. Higgins JJ, Lombardi RQ, Pucilowska J, Jankovic J, Tan EK, Rooney JP. A variant in the HS1-BP3 gene is associated with familial essential tremor. Neurology. 2005;64(3):417–21. Epub 2005/02/09.
56. Deng H, Le WD, Guo Y, Huang MS, Xie WJ, Jankovic J. Extended study of A265G variant of HS1BP3 in essential tremor and Parkinson disease. Neurology. 2005;65(4):651–2. Epub 2005/08/24.
57. Higgins JJ, Lombardi RQ, Pucilowska J, Jankovic J, Golbe LI, Verhagen L. HS1-BP3 gene variant is common in familial essential tremor. Mov Disord. 2006;21(3):306–9. Epub 2005/10/08.
58. Merner ND, Girard SL, Catoire H, Bourassa CV, Belzil VV, Riviere JB, et al. Exome sequencing identifies FUS mutations as a cause of essential tremor. Am J Hum Genet. 2012;91: 313–9. Epub 2012/08/07.
59. Rajput A, Rajput AH, Rajput ML, Encarnacion M, Bernales CQ, Ross JP, et al. Identification of FUS p.R377W in essential tremor. Eur J Neurol. 2014;21(2):361–3. Epub 2013/07/10.
60. Wu YR, Foo JN, Tan LC, Chen CM, Prakash KM, Chen YC, et al. Identification of a novel risk variant in the FUS gene in essential tremor. Neurology. 2013;81(6):541–4. Epub 2013/07/05.
61. Labbe C, Soto-Ortolaza AI, Rayaprolu S, Harriott AM, Strongosky AJ, Uitti RJ, et al. Investigating the role of FUS exonic variants in essential tremor. Parkinsonism Relat Disord. 2013;19(8):755–7. Epub 2013/04/23.
62. Zheng W, Deng X, Liang H, Song Z, Gao K, Yang Y, et al. Genetic analysis of the fused in sarcoma gene in Chinese Han patients with essential tremor. Neurobiol Aging. 2013;34(8):e3–4. Epub 2013/04/16.
63. Parmalee N, Mirzozoda K, Kisselev S, Merner N, Dion P, Rouleau G, et al. Genetic analysis of the FUS/TLS gene in essential tremor. Eur J Neurol. 2012;20(3):534–9. Epub 2012/11/02.
64. Kuhlenbaumer G, Hopfner F, Deuschl G. Genetics of essential tremor: meta-analysis and review. Neurology. 2014;82(11):1000–7. Epub 2014/02/18.
65. Luo C, Rajput AH, Robinson CA, Rajput A. Gamma-aminobutyric acid (GABA)-B receptor 1 in cerebellar cortex of essential tremor. J Clin Neurosci. 2012;19(6):920–1. Epub 2012/02/11.
66. Vicini S, Ferguson C, Prybylowski K, Kralic J, Morrow AL, Homanics GE. GABA(A) receptor alpha1 subunit deletion prevents developmental changes of inhibitory synaptic currents in cerebellar neurons. J Neurosci. 2001;21(9):3009–16. Epub 2001/04/20.
67. Boecker H, Weindl A, Brooks DJ, Ceballos-Baumann AO, Liedtke C, Miederer M, et al. GABAergic dysfunction in essential tremor: an 11C-flumazenil PET study. J Nucl Med. 2010;51(7):1030–5. Epub 2010/06/18.

68. Garcia-Martin E, Martinez C, Alonso-Navarro H, Benito-Leon J, Lorenzo-Betancor O, Pastor P, et al. Gamma-aminobutyric acid (GABA) receptor rho (GABRR) polymorphisms and risk for essential tremor. J Neurol. 2011;258(2):203–11. Epub 2010/09/08.
69. Thier S, Kuhlenbäumer G, Lorenz D, Nothnagel M, Nebel A, Christensen K, et al. $GABA_A$ receptor- and GABA transporter polymorphisms and risk for essential tremor. Eur J Neurol. 2011;18(8):1098–100.
70. Deng H, Xie WJ, Le WD, Huang MS, Jankovic J. Genetic analysis of the GABRA1 gene in patients with essential tremor. Neurosci Lett. 2006;401(1–2):16–9. Epub 2006/03/15.
71. Stefansson H, Steinberg S, Petursson H, Gustafsson O, Gudjonsdottir IH, Jonsdottir GA, et al. Variant in the sequence of the LINGO1 gene confers risk of essential tremor. Nat Genet. 2009;41(3):277–9. Epub 2009/02/03.
72. Tan EK, Teo YY, Prakash KM, Li R, Lim HQ, Angeles D, et al. LINGO1 variant increases risk of familial essential tremor. Neurology. 2009;73(14):1161–2. Epub 2009/10/07.
73. Zuo X, Jiang H, Guo JF, Yu RH, Sun QY, Hu L, et al. Screening for two SNPs of LINGO1 gene in patients with essential tremor or sporadic Parkinson's disease in Chinese population. Neurosci Lett. 2010;481(2):69–72. Epub 2010/07/06.
74. Wu YW, Rong TY, Li HH, Xiao Q, Fei QZ, Tan EK, et al. Analysis of Lingo1 variant in sporadic and familial essential tremor among Asians. Acta Neurol Scand. 2011;124(4):264–8. Epub 2010/12/17.
75. Radovica I, Inashkina I, Smeltere L, Vitols E, Jankevics E. Screening of 10 SNPs of LINGO1 gene in patients with essential tremor in the Latvian population. Parkinsonism Relat Disord. 2012;18(1):93–5. Epub 2011/07/12.
76. Lorenzo-Betancor O, Garcia-Martin E, Cervantes S, Agundez JA, Jimenez-Jimenez FJ, Alonso-Navarro H, et al. Lack of association of LINGO1 rs9652490 and rs11856808 SNPs with familial essential tremor. Eur J Neurol. 2011;18(8):1085–9. Epub 2011/01/12.
77. Bourassa CV, Riviere JB, Dion PA, Bernard G, Diab S, Panisset M, et al. LINGO1 variants in the French-Canadian population. PLoS One. 2011;6(1):e16254. Epub 2011/01/26.
78. Vilarino-Guell C, Ross OA, Wider C, Jasinska-Myga B, Cobb SA, Soto-Ortolaza AI, et al. LINGO1 rs9652490 is associated with essential tremor and Parkinson disease. Parkinsonism Relat Disord. 2010;16(2):109–11. Epub 2009/09/02.
79. Thier S, Lorenz D, Nothnagel M, Stevanin G, Durr A, Nebel A, et al. LINGO1 polymorphisms are associated with essential tremor in Europeans. Mov Disord. 2010;25(6):709–15. Epub 2010/03/24.
80. Vilarino-Guell C, Wider C, Ross OA, Jasinska-Myga B, Kachergus J, Cobb SA, et al. LINGO1 and LINGO2 variants are associated with essential tremor and Parkinson disease. Neurogenetics. 2010;11(4):401–8. Epub 2010/04/07.
81. Clark LN, Park N, Kisselev S, Rios E, Lee JH, Louis ED. Replication of the LINGO1 gene association with essential tremor in a North American population. Eur J Hum Genet. 2010;18(7):838–43. Epub 2010/04/08.
82. Mi S, Lee X, Shao Z, Thill G, Ji B, Relton J, et al. LINGO-1 is a component of the Nogo-66 receptor/p75 signaling complex. Nat Neurosci. 2004;7(3):221–8. Epub 2004/02/18.
83. Delay C, Tremblay C, Brochu E, Paris-Robidas S, Emond V, Rajput AH, et al. Increased LINGO1 in the cerebellum of essential tremor patients. Mov Disord. 2014;29(13):1637–47. Epub 2014/02/18.
84. Zhou ZD, Sathiyamoorthy S, Tan EK. LINGO-1 and neurodegeneration: pathophysiologic clues for essential tremor. Tremor Other Hyperkinet Mov (N Y). 2012;2:1346. Epub 2013/02/27.
85. Kuo SH, Tang G, Louis ED, Ma K, Babji R, Balatbat M, et al. Lingo-1 expression is increased in essential tremor cerebellum and is present in the basket cell pinceau. Acta Neuropathol. 2013;125(6):879–89. Epub 2013/04/02.
86. Thier S, Lorenz D, Nothnagel M, Poremba C, Papengut F, Appenzeller S, et al. Polymorphisms in the glial glutamate transporter SLC1A2 are associated with essential tremor. Neurology. 2012;79(3):243–8. Epub 2012/07/06.
87. Berger UV, Hediger MA. Comparative analysis of glutamate transporter expression in rat brain using differential double in situ hybridization. Anat Embryol (Berl). 1998;198(1):13–30. Epub 1998/07/31.

88. Lauriat TL, McInnes LA. EAAT2 regulation and splicing: relevance to psychiatric and neurological disorders. Mol Psychiatry. 2007;12(12):1065–78. Epub 2007/08/09.
89. Mookherjee P, Green PS, Watson GS, Marques MA, Tanaka K, Meeker KD, et al. GLT-1 loss accelerates cognitive deficit onset in an Alzheimer's disease animal model. J Alzheimers Dis. 2011;26(3):447–55. Epub 2011/06/17.
90. Li Y, Sattler R, Yang EJ, Nunes A, Ayukawa Y, Akhtar S, et al. Harmine, a natural beta-carboline alkaloid, upregulates astroglial glutamate transporter expression. Neuropharmacology. 2011;60(7–8):1168–75. Epub 2010/11/03.
91. Ross JP, Rayaprolu S, Bernales CQ, Soto-Ortolaza AI, van Gerpen J, Uitti RJ, et al. SLC1A2 rs3794087 does not associate with essential tremor. Neurobiol Aging. 2014;35(4):935.e9–10. Epub 2013/10/22.
92. Garcia-Martin E, Martinez C, Alonso-Navarro H, Benito-Leon J, Lorenzo-Betancor O, Pastor P, et al. No association of the SLC1A2 rs3794087 allele with risk for essential tremor in the Spanish population. Pharmacogenet Genomics. 2013;23(11):587–90. Epub 2013/08/21.
93. Yu SW, Chen CM, Chen YC, Chang CW, Chang HS, Lyu RK, et al. SLC1A2 variant is associated with essential tremor in Taiwanese population. PLoS One. 2013;8(8):e71919. Epub 2013/08/21.
94. Tan EK, Foo JN, Tan L, Au WL, Prakash KM, Ng E, et al. SLC1A2 variant associated with essential tremor but not Parkinson disease in Chinese subjects. Neurology. 2013;80(17):1618–9. Epub 2013/04/19.
95. Gerschlager W, Brown P. Orthostatic tremor – a review. Handb Clin Neurol. 2011;100:457–62. Epub 2011/04/19.
96. Virmani T, Louis ED, Waters C, Pullman SL. Familial orthostatic tremor: an additional report in siblings. Neurology. 2012;79(3):288–9. Epub 2012/07/06.
97. Contarino MF, Welter ML, Agid Y, Hartmann A. Orthostatic tremor in monozygotic twins. Neurology. 2006;66(10):1600–1. Epub 2006/05/24.
98. Fischer M, Kress W, Reiners K, Rieckmann P. Orthostatic tremor in three brothers. J Neurol. 2007;254(12):1759–60. Epub 2007/07/28.
99. van Rootselaar AF, van Schaik IN, van den Maagdenberg AM, Koelman JH, Callenbach PM, Tijssen MA. Familial cortical myoclonic tremor with epilepsy: a single syndromic classification for a group of pedigrees bearing common features. Mov Disord. 2005;20(6):665–73. Epub 2005/03/05.
100. Sharifi S, Aronica E, Koelman JH, Tijssen MA, Van Rootselaar AF. Familial cortical myoclonic tremor with epilepsy and cerebellar changes: description of a new pathology case and review of the literature. Tremor Other Hyperkinet Mov (N Y). 2012;2:1–10. Epub 2013/02/27.
101. van Rootselaar AF, Maurits NM, Koelman JH, van der Hoeven JH, Bour LJ, Leenders KL, et al. Coherence analysis differentiates between cortical myoclonic tremor and essential tremor. Mov Disord. 2006;21(2):215–22. Epub 2005/10/04.
102. Striano P, Madia F, Minetti C, Striano S, Zara F. Electroclinical and genetic findings in a family with cortical tremor, myoclonus, and epilepsy. Epilepsia. 2005;46(12):1993–5. Epub 2006/01/06.
103. Plaster NM, Uyama E, Uchino M, Ikeda T, Flanigan KM, Kondo I, et al. Genetic localization of the familial adult myoclonic epilepsy (FAME) gene to chromosome 8q24. Neurology. 1999;53(6):1180–3. Epub 1999/10/16.
104. Mikami M, Yasuda T, Terao A, Nakamura M, Ueno S, Tanabe H, et al. Localization of a gene for benign adult familial myoclonic epilepsy to chromosome 8q23.3-q24.1. Am J Hum Genet. 1999;65(3):745–51. Epub 1999/08/12.
105. Striano P, Chifari R, Striano S, de Fusco M, Elia M, Guerrini R, et al. A new benign adult familial myoclonic epilepsy (BAFME) pedigree suggesting linkage to chromosome 2p11.1-q12.2. Epilepsia. 2004;45(2):190–2. Epub 2004/01/24.
106. Coppola A, Santulli L, Del Gaudio L, Minetti C, Striano S, Zara F, et al. Natural history and long-term evolution in families with autosomal dominant cortical tremor, myoclonus, and epilepsy. Epilepsia. 2011;52(7):1245–50. Epub 2011/03/24.
107. Depienne C, Magnin E, Bouteiller D, Stevanin G, Saint-Martin C, Vidailhet M, et al. Familial cortical myoclonic tremor with epilepsy: the third locus (FCMTE3) maps to 5p. Neurology. 2010;74(24):2000–3. Epub 2010/06/16.

108. Yeetong P, Ausavarat S, Bhidayasiri R, Piravej K, Pasutharnchat N, Desudchit T, et al. A newly identified locus for benign adult familial myoclonic epilepsy on chromosome 3q26.32-3q28. Eur J Hum Genet. 2013;21(2):225–8. Epub 2012/06/21.
109. Stogmann E, Reinthaler E, Eltawil S, El Etribi MA, Hemeda M, El Nahhas N, et al. Autosomal recessive cortical myoclonic tremor and epilepsy: association with a mutation in the potassium channel associated gene CNTN2. Brain. 2013;136(Pt 4):1155–60. Epub 2013/03/23.
110. Marti-Masso JF, Bergareche A, Makarov V, Ruiz-Martinez J, Gorostidi A, de Munain AL, et al. The ACMSD gene, involved in tryptophan metabolism, is mutated in a family with cortical myoclonus, epilepsy, and parkinsonism. J Mol Med (Berl). 2013;91(12):1399–406. Epub 2013/08/21.
111. Danek A, Gams M, Garner C. Erbliches Kinnmuskelzittern ("Geniospasmus"). Akt Neurol. 1991;18:124–7.
112. Jarman PR, Wood NW, Davis MT, Davis PV, Bhatia KP, Marsden CD, et al. Hereditary geniospasm: linkage to chromosome 9q13-q21 and evidence for genetic heterogeneity. Am J Hum Genet. 1997;61(4):928–33. Epub 1997/10/23.
113. Grimes DA, Han F, Bulman D, Nicolson ML, Suchowersky O. Hereditary chin trembling: a new family with exclusion of the chromosome 9q13-q21 Locus. Mov Disord. 2002;17(6):1390–2. Epub 2002/12/05.

Chapter 7
Genetics of Dystonia

Susanne A. Schneider and Kailash P. Bhatia

Abstract Great advances have been made in the field of dystonia in the last decade. This includes the identification of several new genes, and it is likely the number of known genetic causes will continue to grow. Currently 25 DYT loci have been allocated, most of them referring to autosomal dominantly inherited conditions or pure or complex dystonia. In this chapter we discuss genetic causes of dystonia with focus on those variants which have been assigned a DYT locus. We summarize main clinical findings and genetic underpinnings and give a brief discussion of a clinical approach.

Keywords Dystonia • Genetic • DYT locus • Phenotype • THAP1 • TUBB4A • Dopa-responsive dystonia • Myoclonus-dystonia • CIZ1 • GNAL • ATP1A3 • SGCE

Introduction: Definition and the New Classification

Dystonia is a hyperkinetic disorder defined by involuntary twisting and repetitive movements resulting in abnormal postures due to sustained muscle co-contractions of agonist and antagonist muscles [1]. As a first note, the term "dystonia" embraces three different meanings: first, dystonia can be a physical sign, second, dystonia can be a syndrome of sustained muscle contractions, and third, dystonia may refer to a disease such as "idiopathic (or primary) dystonia" [2].

Dystonias can be classified in various ways. Recently, a new classification [3] was proposed, organized along two axes, according to clinical characteristics and to etiology. Briefly, the clinical categorization (axis I) includes classification based on age at onset (i.e., early vs. late), site of onset (i.e., focal, segmental, generalized, etc.),

S.A. Schneider, MD, PhD (✉)
Department of Neurology, University Hospital Kiel,
Arnold-Heller- Str. 3, Kiel 24105, Germany
e-mail: s.schneider@ucl.ac.uk

K.P. Bhatia, MD, DM, FRCP
Sobell Department, University College London/Institute of Neurology,
London WC1N 3BG, UK

S.A. Schneider, J.M.T. Brás (eds.), *Movement Disorder Genetics*,
DOI 10.1007/978-3-319-17223-1_7

Table 7.1 Current definition [3]

Dystonia is a movement disorder characterized by sustained or intermittent muscle contractions causing abnormal, often repetitive, movements, postures, or both. Dystonic movements are typically patterned, twisting, and may be tremulous. Dystonia is often initiated or worsened by voluntary action and associated with overflow muscle activation
Axis I. Clinical characteristics
Age at onset
Body distribution
Temporal pattern
Associated features
Axis II. Etiology
Nervous system pathology
Inherited or acquired
Idiopathic

temporal pattern (i.e., action specific, paroxysmal, presence of diurnal fluctuations, etc.), and presence of associated features (such as myoclonus, etc.). The classification according to axis II (etiology) includes the separation of inherited and acquired forms (see Table 7.1).

Combining the two axes, in general, in patients with a late-onset and a non-progressive focal form of dystonia, a primary cause is most likely. This form usually involves the neck or cranial muscles but spares the lower extremities. This late-onset variant affects more women than men and appears to be sporadic in most cases (for review see [4]), although some 15–30 % of patients do have a positive family history and genetic susceptibility has been proposed (see below).

In contrast, early-onset dystonia typically starts in the lower limbs, tends to generalize, and commonly has a genetic origin. Young-onset cases should thus be investigated further for genetic causes or treatable metabolic diseases. Altogether, the prevalence of primary dystonia has been estimated at 152 per million in a European prevalence study [5].

In recent years, a growing number of genetic causes associated with dystonia have been recognized which are reviewed in this chapter.

Genetic Forms of Dystonia

The monogenic forms of dystonia have been "classified" according to the gene locus. However, this list of differential diagnoses for dystonia is by far complete, as not all genes associated with dystonia have been assigned to a DYT locus (e.g., mutations in *SPR* associated with complicated dopa-responsive dystonia or *SLC6A3* [6] associated with dopamine transporter deficiency syndrome, mutations in *TIMM8A* and other genes associated with dystonia deafness syndromes [7], or mutations in one of the several genes associated with dystonia parkinsonism [8], etc.). These often complicated syndromes where dystonia may be one (prominent) feature are beyond the scope of this chapter.

Currently, 25 DYT loci have been assigned referring to 23 genes (two loci have been abandoned because of redundancy or initial incorrect assignation due to erroneous linkage, e.g., DYT9 or DYT14; see below and Table 7.2 and Fig. 7.1). For most but not all loci, the correlating gene has been identified. With the exception of the five rare forms (DYT2, 3, 5b, 16, and 17), the DYT genes follow an autosomal-dominant pattern of transmission with reduced penetrance. In at least one form (DYT11), maternal imprinting also plays a role [9]. Notably, the designation of some loci has never been replicated and is of questionable significance (e.g., DYT7 or DYT13).

Some have criticized the DYT classification because it is an assortment of clinically and genetically heterogeneous disorders [10]. However, this owes to the historical evolution when loci were assigned chronologically according to appearance in the literature.

Targeted genetic testing for many dystonia genes is commercially available including using gene panels. However, it is important to realize that a negative gene test result does not fully exclude a mutation in the gene tested or an inheritable cause for that matter because introns and promoter regions are usually not sequenced and variations in these areas remain difficult to interpret. Furthermore, routine methods may only involve mutational analysis, while for some genes mutational screening per se may not be sufficient as entire or parts of genes may be deleted or multiplied (whole gene deletion, exon deletion, duplications, etc.), also referred to as gene dosage alterations, e.g., in the context of dystonia in *GTP cyclohydrolase* [11] or *SGCE* [12]. These are only detected if gene dosage analysis is performed.

Genetic testing can confirm the diagnosis in a patient. It can also be used to identify at-risk individuals based on their mutational status. For both symptomatic and non-symptomatic gene mutation carriers, knowledge about the genetic status may have implications for the prognosis and therapeutic management decisions and with respect to family planning. A special role plays prenatal testing which is beyond the focus of this chapter. For DYT1 dystonia testing guidelines have been proposed [13]. For the other forms, genetic testing guidelines are still being formulated.

Autosomal-Dominant Forms of Primary Dystonia with Known Genetic Defect

DYT1 Dystonia (Early-Onset Generalized Dystonia) Associated with TOR1A Gene Mutations

In the 1990s the first gene responsible for some cases of generalized torsion dystonia was identified, termed DYT1 [14]. DYT1 dystonia is the most common cause of monogenic dystonia. The mutation occurs particularly frequent in the Ashkenazi Jewish population (1/9,000), where it is 5–10-fold more common compared to

Table 7.2 Monogenic forms of dystonia (DYT1 – 20)

Designation	Dystonia phenotype	Mode of inheritance	Gene locus	Gene product
DYT1	Early-onset generalized torsion dystonia (TD)	Autosomal dominant	9q34	Deletion in torsinA
DYT2	Autosomal-recessive TD	Autosomal recessive	1p35	HPCA
DYT3	X-linked dystonia parkinsonism, "lubag"	X-chromosomal recessive	Xq	Disease-specific changes 3 in DYT3 region
DYT4	Whispering dysphonia, focal or generalized dystonia, hobby horse gait	Autosomal dominant	19p13	TUBB4A (seems to be a private mutation)
DYT5	Dopa-responsive dystonia, Segawa syndrome	Autosomal dominant	14q22	GCH1
		Autosomal recessive	11p15	TH
DYT6	Adolescent-onset TD of mixed type	Autosomal dominant	8p11	THAP1
DYT7	Adult-onset focal TD	Autosomal dominant	18p	Unknown, locus questionable
DYT8	Paroxysmal nonkinesigenic dyskinesia	Autosomal dominant	2q35	MR1
DYT9	Paroxysmal choreoathetosis with episodic ataxia and spasticity	DYT9 recently omitted and reclassified as DYT18		
DYT10	Paroxysmal kinesigenic choreoathetosis (PKD)	Autosomal dominant	16p11	PRRT2
DYT11	Myoclonus-dystonia	Autosomal dominant	7q21	SGCE
DYT12	Rapid-onset dystonia parkinsonism (allelic to alternating hemiplegia of childhood)	Autosomal dominant[a]	19q13	ATP1A3
DYT13	Multifocal/segmental dystonia	Autosomal dominant	1p36.32-p36.13	Unknown
DYT14	DYT14 was recently omitted and reclassified as DYT5			
DYT15	Myoclonus-dystonia	Autosomal dominant	18p11	Unknown
DYT16	Generalized dystonia parkinsonism	Autosomal recessive	2q31	PRKRA
DYT17	Young-onset generalized dystonia	Autosomal recessive	20p11.2-q13.12	Unknown
DYT18	Paroxysmal exercise-induced dyskinesia	Autosomal dominant	1p35	SLC2A1 (glucose transporter 1)

(continued)

Table 7.2 (continued)

Designation	Dystonia phenotype	Mode of inheritance	Gene locus	Gene product
DYT19	Paroxysmal kinesigenic dyskinesia 2 (episodic kinesigenic dyskinesia 2)	Autosomal dominant	16q13-q22.1	Unknown
DYT20	Paroxysmal non-kinesigenic dyskinesia 2	Autosomal dominant	2q31	Unknown
DYT21	Adult-onset mixed dystonia with generalization in one Swedish family	Autosomal dominant	2q14.3-q21.3	Unknown
DYT22	Reserved, not published	?	?	?
DYT23[b]	Adult-onset (tremulous) craniocervical dystonia +/– upper limb tremor	Autosomal dominant	9q34	CIZ1 (not confirmed by others)
DYT24[b]	(Tremulous) craniocervical dystonia +/– upper limb tremor	Autosomal dominant	11p14	ANO3
DYT25	Segmental, mainly cervical dystonia, often facial involvement	Autosomal dominant	18p11	GNAL

Some gene tests may (only) be available on a research basis. To choose the appropriate gene test, it is helpful clinically and genetically to think of autosomal-recessive syndromes, autosomal-dominant syndromes, and X-linked syndromes. Furthermore, genetic testing in general has implications not only for the diagnosis and therapy but also, of course, for family planning and counseling of family members

ANO3 anoctamin 3, *ATP1A3* Na^+/K^+ ATPase alpha 3, *CIZ1* CDKN1A-interacting zinc finger protein 1, *GCH1* GTP-cyclohydrolase 1, *GNAL* guanidine nucleotide-binding protein, alpha-activating activity polypeptide of the olfactory type, *HPCA* hippocalcin, *MR1* myofibrillogenesis regulator 1, *PRKRA* protein kinase interferon-inducible double-stranded RNA-dependent activator, *PRRT2* proline-rich transmembrane protein 2, *SGCE* epsilon sarcoglycan, *TH* tyrosine hydroxylase, *THAP1* thanatos-associated [THAP] domain containing apoptosis-associated protein 1, *TUBB4A* tubulin beta-4A

[a]Often de novo

[b]Please note that there is some confusion in the literature with regard to assignment of these two loci (see main text for more details)

non-Jewish populations [15]. DYT1 dystonia typically presents as early onset, generalized dystonia, starting in the legs. The clinical course varies, even within the same family (intrafamilial heterogeneity) ranging from severe generalized dystonia to mild focal dystonia (like writer's dystonia) [16, 17]. Unusual phenotypes in gene-proven cases have been described [18, 19]. In addition to solely motor involvement, subclinical changes of the sensory system have been described [20, 21]. Notably, penetrance is markedly reduced: 60–70 % of mutation carriers remain unaffected in that they do not exhibit any dystonia at all. The natural course among the 30–40 % of symptomatic cases is influenced by clinical factors such as age of onset, site of onset, and distribution of symptoms which have prognostic significance, as well as genetic (see below) and extragenetic (such as complications of vaginal delivery)

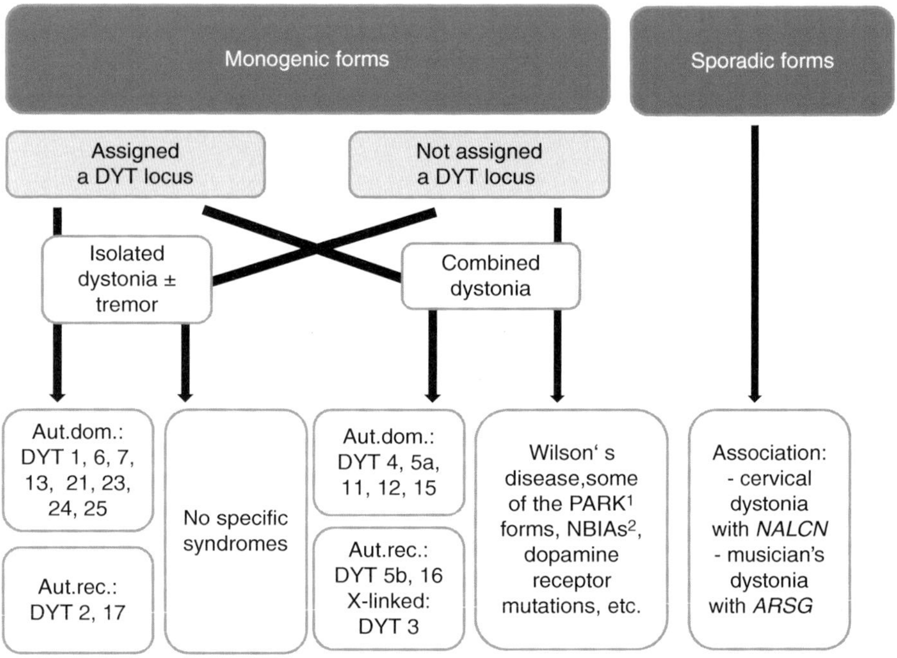

Fig. 7.1 An approach to different genetic forms of dystonia. Paroxysmal dyskinesia is not included in this figure. (1) Parkin-, PINK1-, and DJ-1-associated parkinsonism. (2) Including PANK2- and PLA2G6-associated neurodegeneration, neuroferritinopathy, and others

factors [22]. Clinical experience has shown that mutation carriers usually remain unaffected if symptoms have not developed before 28 years of age. In affected cases there is a tendency for stabilization of the clinical course after the age of 25 years without direct relationship to therapeutic modalities [23]. However, others [21] suggested that earlier treatment may slow disease progression.

Inheritance of DYT1 dystonia is autosomal dominant. It is caused by a mutation (typically a 3 base pair deletion (GAG)) in the *TOR1A* gene located on chromosome 9. Penetrance may be influenced by a "trans" allele. Precisely, the D216H polymorphism in trans (inherited from the non-affected parent) may be protective [24].

The encoded protein, torsinA, is a member of the superfamily of ATPases. Functions include protein processing and degradation, organelle biogenesis, intracellular trafficking, and vesicle recycling [25]. A functional link to DYT6 dystonia has been suggested with repression of DYT1 by the transcription factor THAP1 [26]. Brain pathology is generally normal in DYT1 dystonia except perinuclear inclusion bodies in the midbrain reticular formation and periaqueductal gray [27]. However, this could not be replicated in another case series [28]. The inclusions were located within cholinergic and other neurons in the pedunculopontine nucleus, cuneiform nucleus, and griseum centrale mesencephali and stained positively for ubiquitin, torsinA, and the nuclear envelope protein lamin A/C. Additional tau/ubiquitin-immunoreactive aggregates in pigmented neurons of the substantia nigra pars compacta and locus coeruleus were observed [27].

DYT4 (Whispering Dysphonia) Associated with TUBB4A Gene Mutations

DYT4 dystonia is characterized by whispering dysphonia, craniocervical or, more frequently, generalized dystonia, and a unique ataxic (hobby horse) gait with normal MRI. In 2013 the condition was first described in a large Australian family with more than 30 affected individuals [29]. In 2013, the underlying gene was then identified by two independent research groups [30, 31]. A single missense (p.Arg2Gly) *TUBB4A* mutation in exon 1 located within the autoregulatory methionine–arginine–glutamic acid–isoleucine (MREI) domain was identified as the underlying cause in the original family. So far, no further patients with *TUBB4A* mutations have been identified. It was concluded that the mutation may be private, and the classification as primary dystonia was criticized [32].

Notably, there is allelic association with the distinct syndrome of hypomyelination with atrophy of the basal ganglia and cerebellum (H-ABC). This is a rare sporadic leukodystrophy characterized by developmental delay, a variety of extrapyramidal movement disorders, ataxia, progressive spastic tetraplegia, and seizures with a variable age of onset. Indeed, it has been suggested that H-ABC and DYT4 belong to a continuous phenotypic spectrum associated with *TUBB4A* mutations [33, 34, 35].

The encoded protein, tubulin, beta 4A class IVa of the β-tubulin protein family forms heterodimers with α-tubulins, which ultimately assemble into microtubules, a major cytoskeletal component. TUBB4A is primarily expressed in the nervous system. Functional studies suggested reduced levels (rather than functional changes) of TUBB4 which play a key role in the pathophysiology [31].

DYT5 Dystonia (Dopa-Responsive Dystonia or Segawa Syndrome)

Dopa-responsive dystonia (DRD) is characterized by the triad of childhood-onset dystonia (in the first decade of life) with or without parkinsonism, diurnal fluctuation of symptoms, and a dramatic and sustained response to levodopa [36]. Atypical phenotypes including late-onset parkinsonism have been reported [36]. Some motor features (e.g., writer's cramp, dysphonia, truncal dystonia) may remain levodopa resistant, but overall dopamine treatment is very effective and safe for long-term use including during pregnancy without suggestion that it may cause fetal abnormalities [36].

Cerebrospinal fluid analysis may demonstrate decreased catecholamine metabolites. The most common form of DRD (DYT5a) is dominantly inherited and associated with mutations in the *GTP cyclohydrolase 1* (*GCH1*) gene, a gene which encodes the enzyme GTPCH that catalyzes the first step in the dopamine synthesis. Mutations in *GCH1* can be identified in 40–60 % of clinically typical DRD patients [37]. In addition, exon deletions have been demonstrated [11] that are not detectable by conventional screening methods and may account for at least another 10 % of the "mutation-negative" cases. Notably, heterozygous variants in *GCH1* [38] are associated with an increased risk for Parkinson's disease (even in the absence of a family history for DRD).

Recessive forms of DRD also occur, but their clinical presentation is usually strikingly more complex, characterized by mental retardation, oculogyric crises, and parkinsonism (dopa-responsive dystonia-plus syndromes). Mutations in various genes involved in metabolic pathways of biopterin and dopamine synthesis may be the cause, such as *tyrosine hydroxylase* (*TH*) (DYT5b) but also *6-pyruvoyl-tetrahydropterin synthase* (*6-PTPS*), *sepiapterin reductase* (*SPR*), *dihydropteridine reductase* (*DHPR*), and *aromatic L-amino acid decarboxylase* (*AADC*) (for review see [39]). Notably, mutations in genes involved in distinct (non-dopamine synthesis) metabolic pathways may sometimes also clinically present as DRD phenocopies, e.g., recently, biallelic mutations in the *ATM* gene (traditionally associated with ataxia telangiectasia) were described as one cause of a (recessive) DRD presentation [40].

DYT6 Associated with THAP1 Gene Mutations

Another locus associated with generalized dystonia is DYT6 dystonia, originally described in Mennonite families [41]. The underlying gene, *THAP1*, was identified in 2009 [42, 43]. Since then more than 100 patients have been described in the literature (for review see [44]). Clinically, it presents as focal or generalized dystonia with a mean age at onset of 24 years. Limbs are the most common site at onset (in about 45 % of patients), followed by the cervical region [44]. However, in contrast to DYT1 dystonia, there seems to be a rostrocaudal gradient, and bulbar findings (present in 60 % of patients) may be prominent (which are typically absent in DYT dystonia). Similar to DYT1 dystonia, changes beyond the motor system (i.e., affecting spatial discrimination) have been reported [45].

Inheritance of DYT6 dystonia is autosomal dominant. Notably though, homozygous mutations have also rarely been reported [46]. The penetrance is reduced to about 40 % [10].

THAP1 is a small gene containing 3 exons. Variants mostly affect the THAP1 domain (exon 1 and 2). More than 60 *THAP1* mutations have been reported, mostly missense (>65 %) [44], but small insertions/deletions, nonsense mutations, and splice-site mutations have also been described. No definite obvious genotype–phenotype correlations have yet emerged. However, in a recent review of the literature, Xiromerisiou et al. [44] re-analyzed the pathogenicity of mutations computationally. Interestingly, in the generalized dystonia, 84 % of patients harbored likely damaging mutations versus 4 % that presented with benign variants. On the other hand, in focal dystonia, 65 % harbored benign variants versus 14 % with likely damaging mutations.

The *THAP1*-encoded THAP1 protein belongs to the family of sequence-specific DNA-binding factors. THAP1 regulates endothelial cell proliferation and is a transcription factor [47, 48]. A functional link between THAP1 and torsinA has been suggested: THAP1 binds to the core promoter of TOR1A, and wild-type THAP1 represses the expression of TOR1A [26, 49].

DYT11 (Myoclonus-Dystonia) Associated with SGCE Gene Mutations

As the name suggests, myoclonus-dystonia is characterized by the combination of dystonia and myoclonic jerks, thus rapid, brief lightning-like muscle contractions [50, 51]. Dystonia usually remains focal or segmental as cervical or arm dystonia [50].

Legs are less prominently affected, in contrast to DYT1 dystonia. Myoclonus also most often affects the neck, trunk, and upper limbs. Myoclonus is often dramatically responsive to alcohol, however, with rebound effect.

Again there may also be non-motor features, particularly psychiatric features (including obsessive–compulsive disorder, anxiety, and addiction but also depression, panic attacks, and personality disorders) [52, 53]. In fact, a recent study reported psychiatric symptoms in almost 80 % of cases [53].

Mutations in the underlying *epsilon–sarcoglycan* (*SGCE*) gene [52] are inherited in an autosomal-dominant manner with reduced penetrance due to maternal genomic imprinting [54]. However, family history is positive in more than 80 % of cases with genetically confirmed DYT11 dystonia [12]. Gene function remains unknown. All sorts of mutations have been reported in the *SGCE* gene including nonsense and missense, as well as deletions and insertions leading to frame shifts and splicing errors, but also larger deletions of entire exons and de novo mutations without obvious genotype–phenotype correlations [12, 50, 52, 54]. Notably, such larger deletions may affect areas beyond the *SGCE* gene and involve neighboring genes ("genomic deletions"). This may impinge on the clinical phenotype. For example, if the adjacent *COL1A2* gene is also affected, patients may be affected by additional osteoarthritis, osteoporosis, or delayed skeletal development [12, 55]. Other clinical manifestations associated with neighboring genes include split-hand/split-foot malformations, sensorineural hearing loss, and cavernous cerebral malformations [55]. Such findings emphasize the importance of a careful clinical examination which also includes other (non-motor) features [12].

Finally, there is evidence of genetic heterogeneity after mutations in the *SGCE* gene were excluded in a large Canadian family with a clinical presentation compatible with typical myoclonus-dystonia. This family was linked to chromosome 18p, and this was designated the DYT15 locus, but the gene is yet unknown [56, 57].

DYT12 Dystonia (Rapid-Onset Dystonia Parkinsonism, Allelic to Alternating Hemiplegia of Childhood) Associated with ATP1A3 Gene Mutations

Rapid-onset dystonia parkinsonism is characterized by sudden onset (within hours to weeks) with a rostral–caudal (face > arm > leg) gradient in response to physical or mental stress without evidence of neurodegeneration on brain pathology [58, 59]. The phenotypic spectrum includes dystonic spasms predominantly in the upper limbs, orofacial dystonia, dysarthria, dysphagia, slowness of movement, rigidity and postural instability, and non-responsiveness to levodopa [60]. Notably, intermittent hemidystonia, paroxysmal dystonia, and seizures have been described (see below) [58, 60, 61]. Onset is usually early in life (in adolescence or young adulthood but may be as late as 55 years), and symptoms persist throughout life. Fever, prolonged exercise, childbirth, and even giving oral presentations have been described as triggering factors [58, 59].

Inheritance follows an autosomal-dominant manner with reduced penetrance. The causative gene, *ATP1A3*, located on chromosome 19q13 (23 exons), encodes

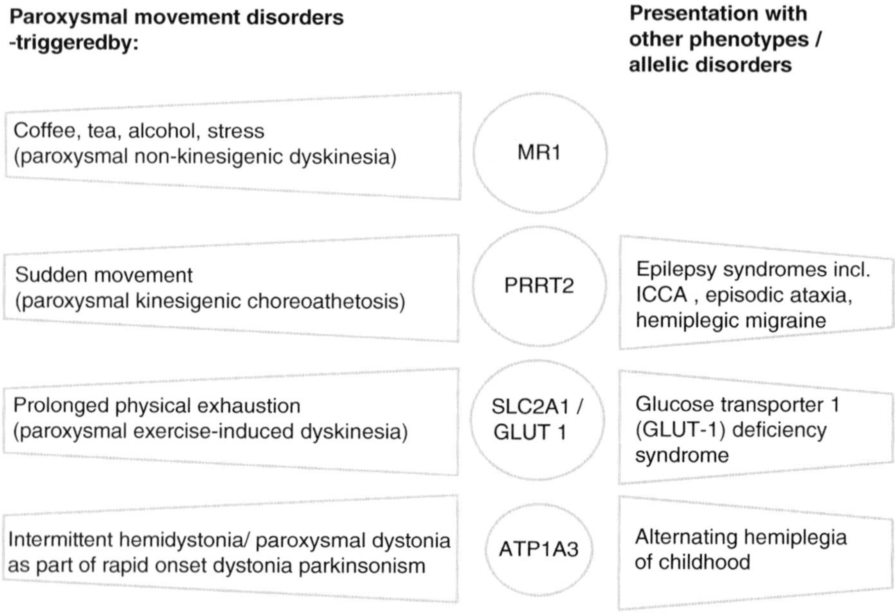

Fig. 7.2 The main phenotypic variability of genes associated with paroxysmal movement disorders

Na^+/K^+ATPase alpha 3 [62], a subunit of a sodium pump responsible for maintenance of ionic gradients across cell membranes. Interestingly, there is phenotypic variability as mutations in this gene are also the major cause of alternating hemiplegia of childhood (AHC) [63–65], a rare, usually sporadic syndrome (due to frequent de novo mutations) with early onset characterized by episodes of hemiplegia on alternating body sides, dystonia or ataxia, seizures, and developmental delay. See also Fig. 7.2 and Chap. 10 for more detailed discussion of this syndrome.

DYT23[1]: Dystonia Associated with Mutations in the CIZ1 Gene

Recently, mutations in *CIZ1* located at the long arm of chromosome 9 were described in several cases of autosomal dominant adult-onset cervical dystonia as identified by exome sequencing [66]. However, this finding has not yet been confirmed by others [67].

[1] Please note that there is some confusion in the literature with regard to the assignment of these two loci. Online Mendelian Inheritance in Man (OMIM) lists *CIZ* as DYT23 (OMIM entry 614860) and *ANO3* as DYT24 (OMIM entry 615034). The HUGO Gene Nomenclature Committee lists *ANO3* as DYT23 but has no entry for DYT24. The latter is in line with a paper entitled "The phenotypic spectrum of DYT24 due to ANO3 mutations" by Stamelou et al. [69].

DYT23[1]/24: Dystonia with Dystonic Tremor (ANO3-Related Dystonia)

Recently, the combination of linkage analysis with whole-exome sequencing led to identification of *ANO3* as a new cause of autosomal-dominant dystonia [68]. The age at onset ranged from early childhood to the forties [69]. The clinical picture consisted of focal dystonia affecting the neck, laryngeal muscles, and upper limbs accompanied by 6-Hz dystonic tremor with or without superimposed myoclonus in some. The duration of the myoclonic bursts was most consistent with a subcortical type. Tremor was the sole initial manifestation in some individuals with *ANO3* mutations, leading to misdiagnosis as essential tremor [69]; however, genetic studies in an independent cohort of essential tremor patients (with a positive autosomal-dominant family history) did not identify further *ANO3* mutations [70].

The *ANO3* gene, located at chromosome 11p14, encodes a protein called anoctamin 3, a predicted $Ca2^{+}$-gated chloride channel with high expression in the striatum. Notably, related genes from the ANO family have also been linked to neurological disease (*ANO5* to several forms of muscular dystrophy and *ANO10* to autosomal-recessive spinocerebellar ataxia) [68].

DYT25: Dystonia Associated with Mutations in the GNAL Gene

Recently, using exome sequencing, mutations in *GNAL* were identified in two families with primary torsion dystonia [71]. A handful of other patients from different ethnic backgrounds were since reported [72–75], while other researchers did not detect any changes in their cohort [76]. The clinical phenotype consists of focal or segmental, mainly cervical dystonia, with a relatively broad range in the age of onset and spreading to other muscles, especially the facial muscles [71].

GNAL has 12 exons and encodes guanine nucleotide-binding protein G(olf), subunit alpha [Gα(olf)]. Gα(olf) plays a role in olfaction, coupling D1 and A2a receptors to adenylyl cyclase, and histone H3 phosphorylation.

The Paroxysmal Dyskinesia (DYT8, DYT9, and DYT10 as well as DYT19 and DYT20)

The group of paroxysmal dyskinesia is defined as abnormal involuntary movements of intermittent or episodic nature. The phenotype varies but tends to be dystonic and/or choreic and may be complex. Episodes are sudden in onset and without change in consciousness. Subtypes include the nonkinesigenic variant (PNKD), the kinesigenic variant (PKD), and the exercise-induced variant (PED) according to the triggering factors (for review see [77, 78]). While secondary causes should be excluded, genetic forms, usually with autosomal-dominant inheritance, are recognized. They are discussed in detail in Chap. 10.

Briefly, of these, PNKD is frequently precipitated by alcohol, caffeine, stress, or fatigue in line with the finding of the underlying gene, *myofibrillogenesis regulator*

1 (*MR1*), which encodes an enzyme in a stress response pathway. PNKD attacks last about minutes to hours and typically improve with benzodiazepine treatment [79]. Genetic heterogeneity has been suggested [80], termed PNKD2 located at chromosome 2q31. The gene underlying PNKD2 remains to be identified.

In contrast, PKD is typically triggered by sudden movements, as the name suggests, and attacks are of very brief duration, lasting only seconds [81]. Onset age is usually in late childhood or early teens. Mutations in the associated gene, *PRRT2*, located at chromosome 16p11.2 may also produce epilepsy syndromes, episodic ataxia, or hemiplegic migraine as well as overlapping phenotypes including (*i*nfantile *c*onvulsions and paroxysmal *c*horeo*a*thetosis, “ICCA”) [82]. PKD attacks usually respond well to carbamazepine.

Finally, PED attacks are triggered by prolonged physical exertion and usually cease in 10–15 min after stopping the exercise. The disorder is due to mutations in the *SLC2A1* gene, which occur often de novo (resulting in PED appearing sporadically) or follows autosomal-dominant transmission [83, 84]. Mutations in the same gene may also cause the much more severe glucose transporter 1 (GLUT-1) deficiency syndrome characterized by infantile-onset drug refractory epilepsy, developmental delay, acquired microcephaly, and complex motor abnormalities [85]. The gene encodes the glucose transporter GLUT1 which impairs transfer of glucose into the brain.

Autosomal-Dominant Forms of Primary Dystonia with Unknown Genetic Defect

DYT7: A Questionable Locus

In 1997, the DYT7 locus was assigned to chromosome 18p based on a single large German family with autosomal-dominant cervical dystonia [86]. However, this finding has not been replicated in other families, and more recent clinical and genetic reanalysis of this family demonstrated that there were no disease-causing mutations or copy-number variants in 18p so the locus was redefined as questionable [87].

DYT13

This locus on chromosome 1p36 was assigned based on a single large Italian family first examined in 1994 [88, 89]. The phenotype consisted of early-onset (age of onset range, 5–43 years) torsion dystonia with the craniocervical region or upper limbs as the typical first affected region. However, even those with generalized dystonia were not severely disabled and progression was mild. Penetrance was incomplete (about 60 %). The gene is unknown, and the locus has not been replicated in other cases.

DYT15 (Also See DYT11)

In 2001, a large Canadian kindred with alcohol-responsive myoclonic dystonia characterized mainly by jerky movements of the upper limbs, hands, and axial muscles was described [90]. Mutations in the SGCE gene (as common cause of myoclonic dystonia/DYT11) were excluded, and subsequently linkage to a 17-cM region on chromosome 18p11 was suggested [56]. The gene is unknown, and the locus has not been replicated in other cases.

DYT21

This locus refers to a single Swedish family reported in 1988 with highly penetrant autosomal-dominant late-onset multifocal or generalized dystonia [91]. The mean age at onset was 25–30 years. Upper body involvement was characteristic affecting the face, neck, and upper limbs or with spasmodic dysphonia. Linkage studies suggested a locus at chromosome 2q14, but the gene remains to be determined [92]. This locus has not been replicated in other cases.

Autosomal-Recessive Forms of Primary Dystonia with Known Genetic Defect

DYT2

Gimenez-Roldan et al. [93, 94] reported autosomal-recessive torsion dystonia in several Spanish gypsy families, some of them with consanguineous background. Mean onset was in the teens. Most recently, using a combination of homozygosity mapping and whole-exome sequencing a homozygous mutations in *hippocalcin* (*HPCA*), a gene encoding a neuronal calcium sensor protein was identified. The protein is almost exclusively expressed in the brain and at particularly high levels in the striatum [95]. The gene plays a role in long-term depression in the hippocampus and neuropsychological testing of one member of the index family showed evidence of cognitive underfunctioning characterized by particular difficulties in encoding verbal and visual information [95]. DYT2-like families have been reported [96, 97], in how far *HPCA* mutations account for these needs to be determined.

DYT5b

This locus refers to mutations in *tyrosine hydroxylase* (TH), one cause of complex dopa-responsive dystonia. See above under DYT5.

DYT16: Dystonia Associated with Mutations in *PRKRA*

In 2008, Camargos et al. reported homozygous missense mutations (c.665C>T;p. P222L in exon 7) in *PRKRA* at chromosome 2q31 identified as the new cause of young-onset generalized dystonia or dystonia parkinsonism by high-density genome-wide SNP genotyping [98]. Dystonia affected the axial muscle and the oromandibular region (sardonic smile). There was intrafamilial phenotypic heterogeneity. Symptoms were refractory to pharmacological therapy [99]. A further case with compound heterozygous mutations (likely to be pathogenic) with imaging abnormalities in the form of T2 hyperintensity and progressive volume loss of the bilateral basal ganglia has more recently been reported [100]. The significance of another case with a heterozygous frameshift mutation in exon 3 remains to be determined [101].

Autosomal-Recessive Forms of Primary Dystonia with Unknown Genetic Defect

DYT17

DYT17 dystonia refers to a single consanguineous Lebanese family with three sisters affected by pure segmental or generalized dystonia and dysphonia/dysarthria beginning in the neck with onset during teenage years. Imaging was normal. Genetic testing revealed a suspicious 20.5-Mb interval on chromosome 20p11-q13.12. The underlying gene remains to be identified [102].

X-Linked Forms of Dystonia

DYT3: Lubag Disease

DYT3 dystonia is associated with specific sequence changes in the *TAF1* gene [103] and inherited in an X-linked recessive fashion with complete penetrance by the end of the fifth decade. Due to a founder effect, a cluster is found on the Philippine Island of Panay (the prevalence rate is highest in the province of Capiz, where 1:4,000 men suffer from the disorder) [104]. Dystonic symptoms usually start in adulthood as focal dystonia [105] and then become generalized. Concurrent parkinsonism is frequent [105, 106] and may also precede the onset of dystonia, including presentation with classical (initially) levodopa-responsive parkinsonism [107, 108].

Reserved, Not-Published DYT Locus: DYT22

One locus, DYT22, has been reserved, but no further details have been published yet.

Further Evidence of Inheritability of Dystonia

In addition to the monogenic forms described above, there is evidence of a strong genetic basis in the late-onset dystonias. While these are often perceived as idiopathic sporadic form, clinical studies found that first-degree relatives of patients with focal dystonia have a 23–36 % risk of developing the same or another form of dystonia [109, 110]. Epidemiological studies suggest that they may be inherited in an autosomal-dominant manner, albeit with a markedly penetrance of 12–15 % [109, 111, 112].

A recent genome-wide association study suggested a possible association of cervical dystonia with the sodium leak channel, *NALCN*. In a genome-wide association study in musician's dystonia, an intronic variant in the *arylsulfatase G* (*ARSG*) gene was observed [113]. However, large-scale genome-wide association studies are needed to confirm this and to further dissect the genetic contribution in these cases. Altogether, the genetic architecture of late-onset dystonia remains largely unknown.

The use of endophenotypes (imaging or neurophysiological testing) may be a helpful approach in order to identify non-penetrant mutation carriers by facilitating segregation and linkage analysis in larger kindreds [114–116].

The Clinical Approach

Certain features may be suggestive of a genetic cause. Besides a positive family history, these include an early age of onset, a specific clinical picture (e.g., diurnal variation of the dystonia with worsening throughout the day suggesting dopa-responsive dystonia or syndromic associations), and certain ethnic backgrounds (e.g., *DYT1* dystonia is more common among Ashkenazi Jews; DYT3 is typically seen in Filipinos [22], DYT6 is more common in Mennonites). However, a genetic etiology should also be considered in those patients with a negative family history, possibly resulting from too small a family size, reduced penetrance, variable expressivity, or de novo mutations. Nonpaternity and adoption may appear as "pseudo"-negative family history.

On practical grounds in young-onset cases, Wilson's disease and DRD (by a trial of levodopa) should be excluded first, as accurate identification of these diseases at an early stage will permit the introduction of potentially life-changing treatments

Table 7.3 Recommended investigations in a patient with dystonia

Investigation	Primary dystonia		In patients with features suggestive of secondary dystonia	Diagnosis to be excluded (incomplete list)
	Early onset	Late onset	Independent of onset age	
CCT, MRT	+	+	+	Vascular disease, malformations, neoplasms, calcifications, iron accumulation
EEG	+		+	
Slit lamp exam	+	+	+	Wilson's disease
Funduscopy			+	NBIA syndromes
Hearing assessment			+	Dystonia deafness syndromes
CSF	+		+	
Muscle biopsy			+	Mitochondrial disease (Leigh's disease)
Gene test (*DYT1*)	+	(+)		*DYT1* dystonia
Blood test				
Full blood count, liver/kidney function test, coagulation parameters	+	+	+	
Ceruloplasmin, copper	+	+	+	Wilson's disease
Serology: syphilis, etc.	+	+	+	Infections (syphilis, Tbc, AIDS, SSPE)
Antinuclear/thyroid antibodies	+		+	Immune disease (SLE)
Immunoelectrophoresis			+	Ataxia telangiectasia
Amino acids			+	Metabolic disease affecting the amino acid metabolism (e.g., homocystinuria)
Lysosomal enzymes, long-chain fatty acids			+	Metabolic disease affecting the fat metabolism (e.g., gangliosidosis, metachromatic leukodystrophy)
Acanthocytes in peripheral blood smear			+	Neuroacanthocytosis and McLeod syndrome
Alpha-fetoprotein			+	Ataxia telangiectasia
Urine				
Copper	+	+	+	Wilson's disease
Amino acids			+	Metabolic disease affecting the amino acid metabolism
Oligosaccharides/ mucopolysaccharides			+	

Reprinted from Schneider and Klein [117]

(see Table 7.3). In practice, an MRI and genetic testing for *TOR1A* and *THAP1* mutations are often also performed. In late-onset patients, genetic testing usually does not reveal the molecular diagnosis; this includes the recently discovered genes *ANO3*, *GNAL*, and *CIZ1* which also appear not to be a common cause of adult-onset cervical dystonia. Of course, the differential diagnosis includes disorders associated with non-DYT genes which are beyond the scope of this chapter.

In summary, great advances have been made in the field of dystonia in the last decade. Several new genes have been identified, and it is likely the number of known genetic causes will continue to grow.

References

1. Fahn S. Concept and classification of dystonia. Adv Neurol. 1988;50:1–8.
2. Quinn N. Parkinsonism and dystonia, pseudo-parkinsonism and pseudodystonia. Adv Neurol. 1993;60:540–3.
3. Albanese A, Bhatia K, Bressman SB, et al. Phenomenology and classification of dystonia: a consensus update. Mov Disord. 2013;28:863–73.
4. Klein C, Breakefield XO, Ozelius LJ. Genetics of primary dystonia. Semin Neurol. 1999;19:271–80.
5. Epidemiological Study of Dystonia in Europe Collaborative G. A prevalence study of primary dystonia in eight European countries. J Neurol. 2000;247:787–92.
6. Ng J, Zhen J, Meyer E, et al. Dopamine transporter deficiency syndrome: phenotypic spectrum from infancy to adulthood. Brain. 2014;137:1107–19.
7. Kojovic M, Parees I, Lampreia T, et al. The syndrome of deafness-dystonia: clinical and genetic heterogeneity. Mov Disord. 2013;28:795–803.
8. Schneider SA, Bhatia KP, Hardy J. Complicated recessive dystonia parkinsonism syndromes. Mov Disord. 2009;24:490–9.
9. Grabowski M, Zimprich A, Lorenz-Depiereux B, et al. The epsilon-sarcoglycan gene (SGCE), mutated in myoclonus-dystonia syndrome, is maternally imprinted. Eur J Hum Genet. 2003;11:138–44.
10. Marras C, Lohmann K, Lang A, Klein C. Fixing the broken system of genetic locus symbols: Parkinson disease and dystonia as examples. Neurology. 2012;78:1016–24.
11. Furukawa Y, Guttman M, Sparagana SP, et al. Dopa-responsive dystonia due to a large deletion in the GTP cyclohydrolase I gene. Ann Neurol. 2000;47:517–20.
12. Grunewald A, Djarmati A, Lohmann-Hedrich K, et al. Myoclonus-dystonia: significance of large SGCE deletions. Hum Mutat. 2008;29:331–2.
13. Bressman SB, Sabatti C, Raymond D, et al. The DYT1 phenotype and guidelines for diagnostic testing. Neurology. 2000;54:1746–52.
14. Ozelius LJ, Hewett JW, Page CE, et al. The early-onset torsion dystonia gene (DYT1) encodes an ATP-binding protein. Nat Genet. 1997;17:40–8.
15. Risch N, de Leon D, Ozelius L, et al. Genetic analysis of idiopathic torsion dystonia in Ashkenazi Jews and their recent descent from a small founder population. Nat Genet. 1995;9:152–9.
16. Opal P, Tintner R, Jankovic J, et al. Intrafamilial phenotypic variability of the DYT1 dystonia: from asymptomatic TOR1A gene carrier status to dystonic storm. Mov Disord. 2002;17:339–45.
17. Kabakci K, Hedrich K, Leung JC, et al. Mutations in DYT1: extension of the phenotypic and mutational spectrum. Neurology. 2004;62:395–400.
18. Edwards M, Wood N, Bhatia K. Unusual phenotypes in DYT1 dystonia: a report of five cases and a review of the literature. Mov Disord. 2003;18:706–11.

19. Yilmaz U, Yuksel D, Atac FB, Yilmaz D, Verdi H, Senbil N. Atypical phenotypes of DYT1 dystonia in three children. Brain Dev. 2013;35:356–9.
20. Tinazzi M, Fiorio M, Fiaschi A, Rothwell JC, Bhatia KP. Sensory functions in dystonia: insights from behavioral studies. Mov Disord. 2009;24(10):1427–36.
21. Fiorio M, Gambarin M, Valente EM, et al. Defective temporal processing of sensory stimuli in DYT1 mutation carriers: a new endophenotype of dystonia? Brain. 2007;130: 134–42.
22. Martino D, Gajos A, Gallo V, et al. Extragenetic factors and clinical penetrance of DYT1 dystonia: an exploratory study. J Neurol. 2013;260:1081–6.
23. Anca MH, Zaccai TF, Badarna S, Lozano AM, Lang AE, Giladi N. Natural history of Oppenheim's dystonia (DYT1) in Israel. J Child Neurol. 2003;18:325–30.
24. Risch NJ, Bressman SB, Senthil G, Ozelius LJ. Intragenic Cis and Trans modification of genetic susceptibility in DYT1 torsion dystonia. Am J Hum Genet. 2007;80:1188–93.
25. Vale RD. AAA proteins. Lords of the ring. J Cell Biol. 2000;150:F13–9.
26. Kaiser FJ, Osmanoric A, Rakovic A, et al. The dystonia gene DYT1 is repressed by the transcription factor THAP1 (DYT6). Ann Neurol. 2010;68:554–9.
27. McNaught KS, Kapustin A, Jackson T, et al. Brainstem pathology in DYT1 primary torsion dystonia. Ann Neurol. 2004;56:540–7.
28. Paudel R, Kiely A, Li A, Lashley T, Bandopadhyay R, Hardy J, et al. Neuropathological features of genetically confirmed DYT1 dystonia: investigating disease-specific inclusions. Acta Neuropathol Commun. 2014;2(1):159. [Epub ahead of print].
29. Parker N. Hereditary whispering dysphonia. J Neurol Neurosurg Psychiatry. 1985;48: 218–24.
30. Hersheson J, Mencacci NE, Davis M, et al. Mutations in the autoregulatory domain of beta-tubulin 4a cause hereditary dystonia. Ann Neurol. 2013;73:546–53.
31. Lohmann K, Wilcox RA, Winkler S, et al. Whispering dysphonia (DYT4 dystonia) is caused by a mutation in the TUBB4 gene. Ann Neurol. 2013;73:537–45.
32. Vemula SR, Xiao J, Bastian RW, Momcilovic D, Blitzer A, LeDoux MS. Pathogenic variants in TUBB4A are not found in primary dystonia. Neurology. 2014;82:1227–30.
33. Hamilton EM, Polder E, Vanderver A, et al. Hypomyelination with atrophy of the basal ganglia and cerebellum: further delineation of the phenotype and genotype-phenotype correlation. Brain. 2014;137:1921–30.
34. Miyatake S, Osaka H, Shiina M, et al. Expanding the phenotypic spectrum of TUBB4A-associated hypomyelinating leukoencephalopathies. Neurology. 2014;82:2230–7.
35. Erro R, Hersheson J, Ganos C, Mencacci NE, Stamelou M, Batla A, et al. H-ABC syndrome and DYT4: Variable expressivity or pleiotropy of TUBB4 mutations? Mov Disord. 2014. [Epub ahead of print].
36. Trender-Gerhard I, Sweeney MG, Schwingenschuh P, et al. Autosomal-dominant GTPCH1-deficient DRD: clinical characteristics and long-term outcome of 34 patients. J Neurol Neurosurg Psychiatry. 2009;80:839–45.
37. Nygaard TG, Wooten GF. Dopa-responsive dystonia: some pieces of the puzzle are still missing. Neurology. 1998;50:853–5.
38. Mencacci NE, Isaias IU, Reich MM, et al. Parkinson's disease in GTP cyclohydrolase 1 mutation carriers. Brain. 2014;137(Pt 9):2480–92.
39. Clot F, Grabli D, Cazeneuve C, et al. Exhaustive analysis of BH4 and dopamine biosynthesis genes in patients with Dopa-responsive dystonia. Brain. 2009;132:1753–63.
40. Charlesworth G, Mohire MD, Schneider SA, Stamelou M, Wood NW, Bhatia KP. Ataxia telangiectasia presenting as dopa-responsive cervical dystonia. Neurology. 2013;81: 1148–51.
41. Almasy L, Bressman SB, Raymond D, Kramer PL, Greene PE, Heiman GA, et al. Idiopathic torsion dystonia linked to chromosome 8 in two Mennonite families. Ann Neurol. 1997;42(4):670–3.
42. Fuchs T, Gavarini S, Saunders-Pullman R, et al. Mutations in the THAP1 gene are responsible for DYT6 primary torsion dystonia. Nat Genet. 2009;41:286–8.

43. Djarmati A, Schneider SA, Lohmann K, et al. Mutations in THAP1 (DYT6) are associated with generalised dystonia with prominent spasmodic dysphonia - a genetic screening study. Lancet Neurol. 2009;8:447–52.
44. Xiromerisiou G, Houlden H, Scarmeas N, et al. THAP1 mutations and dystonia phenotypes: genotype phenotype correlations. Mov Disord. 2012;27:1290–4.
45. Deik AF, O'Riordan S, Luciano MS, et al. Spatial discrimination threshold abnormalities are not detected in a pilot study of DYT6 dystonia mutation carriers. Tremor Other Hyperkinet Mov (N Y) 2012;2. p.ii.
46. Schneider SA, Ramirez A, Shafiee K, et al. Homozygous THAP1 mutations as cause of early-onset generalized dystonia. Mov Disord. 2011;26:858–61.
47. Cayrol C, Lacroix C, Mathe C, et al. The THAP-zinc finger protein THAP1 regulates endothelial cell proliferation through modulation of pRB/E2F cell-cycle target genes. Blood. 2007;109(2):584–94.
48. Roussigne M, Cayrol C, Clouaire T, Amalric F, Girard JP. THAP1 is a nuclear proapoptotic factor that links prostate-apoptosis-response-4 (Par-4) to PML nuclear bodies. Oncogene. 2003;22:2432–42.
49. Gavarini S, Cayrol C, Fuchs T, et al. Direct interaction between causative genes of DYT1 and DYT6 primary dystonia. Ann Neurol. 2010;68:549–53.
50. Asmus F, Zimprich A, Du Tezenas MS, et al. Myoclonus-dystonia syndrome: epsilon-sarcoglycan mutations and phenotype. Ann Neurol. 2002;52:489–92.
51. Quinn NP, Rothwell JC, Thompson PD, Marsden CD. Hereditary myoclonic dystonia, hereditary torsion dystonia and hereditary essential myoclonus: an area of confusion. Adv Neurol. 1988;50:391–401.
52. Zimprich A, Grabowski M, Asmus F, et al. Mutations in the gene encoding epsilon-sarcoglycan cause myoclonus-dystonia syndrome. Nat Genet. 2001;29:66–9.
53. Peall KJ, Smith DJ, Kurian MA, et al. SGCE mutations cause psychiatric disorders: clinical and genetic characterization. Brain. 2013;136:294–303.
54. Hedrich K, Meyer EM, Schule B, et al. Myoclonus-dystonia: detection of novel, recurrent, and de novo SGCE mutations. Neurology. 2004;62:1229–31.
55. Asmus F, Hjermind LE, Dupont E, et al. Genomic deletion size at the epsilon-sarcoglycan locus determines the clinical phenotype. Brain. 2007;130:2736–45.
56. Grimes DA, Han F, Lang AE, George-Hyssop P, Racacho L, Bulman DE. A novel locus for inherited myoclonus-dystonia on 18p11. Neurology. 2002;59:1183–6.
57. Han F, Racacho L, Lang AE, Bulman DE, Grimes DA. Refinement of the DYT15 locus in myoclonus dystonia. Mov Disord. 2007;22:888–92.
58. Pittock SJ, Joyce C, O'Keane V, et al. Rapid-onset dystonia-parkinsonism: a clinical and genetic analysis of a new kindred. Neurology. 2000;55:991–5.
59. Dobyns WB, Ozelius LJ, Kramer PL, et al. Rapid-onset dystonia-parkinsonism. Neurology. 1993;43:2596–602.
60. Brashear A, Dobyns WB, de Carvalho AP, et al. The phenotypic spectrum of rapid-onset dystonia-parkinsonism (RDP) and mutations in the ATP1A3 gene. Brain. 2007;130:828–35.
61. Webb DW, Broderick A, Brashear A, Dobyns WB. Rapid onset dystonia-parkinsonism in a 14-year-old girl. Eur J Paediatr Neurol. 1999;3:171–3.
62. de Carvalho AP, Sweadner KJ, Penniston JT, et al. Mutations in the Na+/K+ – ATPase alpha3 gene ATP1A3 are associated with rapid-onset dystonia parkinsonism. Neuron. 2004;43: 169–75.
63. Heinzen EL, Swoboda KJ, Hitomi Y, et al. De novo mutations in ATP1A3 cause alternating hemiplegia of childhood. Nat Genet. 2012;44:1030–4.
64. Yang X, Gao H, Zhang J, et al. ATP1A3 mutations and genotype-phenotype correlation of alternating hemiplegia of childhood in Chinese patients. PLoS One. 2014;9:e97274.
65. Sasaki M, Ishii A, Saito Y, et al. Genotype-phenotype correlations in alternating hemiplegia of childhood. Neurology. 2014;82:482–90.
66. Xiao J, Uitti RJ, Zhao Y, et al. Mutations in CIZ1 cause adult onset primary cervical dystonia. Ann Neurol. 2012;71:458–69.

67. Ma L, Chen R, Wang L, Yang Y, Wan X. No mutations in CIZ1 in twelve adult-onset primary cervical dystonia families. Mov Disord. 2013;28:1899–901.
68. Charlesworth G, Plagnol V, Holmstrom KM, et al. Mutations in ANO3 cause dominant craniocervical dystonia: ion channel implicated in pathogenesis. Am J Hum Genet. 2012;91: 1041–50.
69. Stamelou M, Charlesworth G, Cordivari C, et al. The phenotypic spectrum of DYT24 due to ANO3 mutations. Mov Disord. 2014;29(7):928–34.
70. Hopfner F, Bungeroth M, Pendziwiat M, et al. Rare variants in ANO3 are not a susceptibility factor in essential tremor. Parkinsonism Relat Disord. 2014;20:134–5.
71. Fuchs T, Saunders-Pullman R, Masuho I, et al. Mutations in GNAL cause primary torsion dystonia. Nat Genet. 2013;45:88–92.
72. Vemula SR, Puschmann A, Xiao J, et al. Role of Galpha(olf) in familial and sporadic adult-onset primary dystonia. Hum Mol Genet. 2013;22:2510–9.
73. Miao J, Wan XH, Sun Y, Feng JC, Cheng FB. Mutation screening of GNAL gene in patients with primary dystonia from Northeast China. Parkinsonism Relat Disord. 2013; 19:910–2.
74. Dufke C, Sturm M, Schroeder C, et al. Screening of mutations in GNAL in sporadic dystonia patients. Mov Disord. 2014;29(9):1193–6.
75. Kumar KR, Lohmann K, Masuho I, et al. Mutations in GNAL: a novel cause of craniocervical dystonia. JAMA Neurol. 2014;71:490–4.
76. Charlesworth G, Bhatia KP, Wood NW. No pathogenic GNAL mutations in 192 sporadic and familial cases of cervical dystonia. Mov Disord. 2014;29:154–5.
77. Schneider SA, Bhatia KP, Jankovic J, Tolosa E. Paroxysmal dyskinesias: an overview. In: Parkinson's disease and movement disorders. Philadelphia: Lippincott Williams & Wilkins; 2007. p. 459–67.
78. Bhatia KP. Paroxysmal dyskinesias. Mov Disord. 2011;26:1157–65.
79. Bruno MK, Lee HY, Auburger GW, et al. Genotype-phenotype correlation of paroxysmal nonkinesigenic dyskinesia. Neurology. 2007;68:1782–9.
80. Spacey SD, Valente EM, Wali GM, et al. Genetic and clinical heterogeneity in paroxysmal kinesigenic dyskinesia: evidence for a third EKD gene. Mov Disord. 2002;17:717–25.
81. Bruno MK, Hallett M, Gwinn-Hardy K, et al. Clinical evaluation of idiopathic paroxysmal kinesigenic dyskinesia: new diagnostic criteria. Neurology. 2004;63:2280–7.
82. Gardiner AR, Bhatia KP, Stamelou M, et al. PRRT2 gene mutations: from paroxysmal dyskinesia to episodic ataxia and hemiplegic migraine. Neurology. 2012;79:2115–21.
83. Weber YG, Storch A, Wuttke TV, et al. GLUT1 mutations are a cause of paroxysmal exertion-induced dyskinesias and induce hemolytic anemia by a cation leak. J Clin Invest. 2008;118:2157–68.
84. Schneider SA, Paisan-Ruiz C, Garcia-Gorostiaga I, et al. GLUT1 gene mutations cause sporadic paroxysmal exercise-induced dyskinesias. Mov Disord. 2009;24(11):1684–8.
85. Pascual JM, Wang D, Lecumberri B, et al. GLUT1 deficiency and other glucose transporter diseases. Eur J Endocrinol. 2004;150:627–33.
86. Leube B, Rudnicki D, Ratzlaff T, Kessler KR, Benecke R, Auburger G. Idiopathic torsion dystonia: assignment of a gene to chromosome 18p in a German family with adult onset, autosomal dominant inheritance and purely focal distribution. Hum Mol Genet. 1996;5:1673–7.
87. Winter P, Kamm C, Biskup S, et al. DYT7 gene locus for cervical dystonia on chromosome 18p is questionable. Mov Disord. 2012;27:1819–21.
88. Valente EM, Bentivoglio AR, Cassetta E, et al. DYT13, a novel primary torsion dystonia locus, maps to chromosome 1p36.13–36.32 in an Italian family with cranial-cervical or upper limb onset. Ann Neurol. 2001;49:362–6.
89. Bentivoglio AR, Ialongo T, Contarino MF, Valente EM, Albanese A. Phenotypic characterization of DYT13 primary torsion dystonia. Mov Disord. 2004;19:200–6.
90. Grimes DA, Bulman D, George-Hyslop PS, Lang AE. Inherited myoclonus-dystonia: evidence supporting genetic heterogeneity. Mov Disord. 2001;16:106–10.

91. Forsgren L, Holmgren G, Almay BG, Drugge U. Autosomal dominant torsion dystonia in a Swedish family. Adv Neurol. 1988;50:83–92.
92. Norgren N, Mattson E, Forsgren L, Holmberg M. A high-penetrance form of late-onset torsion dystonia maps to a novel locus (DYT21) on chromosome 2q14.3-q21.3. Neurogenetics. 2011;12:137–43.
93. Gimenez-Roldan S, Delgado G, Marin M, Villanueva JA, Mateo D. Hereditary torsion dystonia in gypsies. Adv Neurol. 1988;50:73–81.
94. Gimenez-Roldan S, Lopez-Fraile IP, Esteban A. Dystonia in Spain: study of a Gypsy family and general survey. Adv Neurol. 1976;14:125–36.
95. Charlesworth G, Angelova PR, Bartolomé-Robledo F, Ryten M, Trabzuni D, Stamelou M, et al. Mutations in HPCA Cause Autosomal-Recessive Primary Isolated Dystonia. Am J Hum Gen 2015. [Published online].
96. Khan NL, Wood NW, Bhatia KP. Autosomal recessive, DYT2-like primary torsion dystonia: a new family. Neurology. 2003;61:1801–3.
97. Zlotogora J. Autosomal recessive, DYT2-like primary torsion dystonia: a new family. Neurology. 2004;63:1340.
98. Camargos S, Scholz S, Sim¢n-Sánchez J, et al. DYT16, a novel young-onset dystonia-parkinsonism disorder: identification of a segregating mutation in the stress response protein prkra. Lancet Neurol. 2008;7:207–15.
99. Camargos S, Lees AJ, Singleton A, Cardoso F. DYT16: the original cases. J Neurol Neurosurg Psychiatry. 2012;83:1012–4.
100. Lemmon ME, Lavenstein B, Applegate CD, Hamosh A, Tekes A, Singer HS. A novel presentation of DYT 16: acute onset in infancy and association with MRI abnormalities. Mov Disord. 2013;28:1937–8.
101. Seibler P, Djarmati A, Langpap B, et al. A heterozygous frameshift mutation in PRKRA (DYT16) associated with generalised dystonia in a German patient. Lancet Neurol. 2008;7:380–1.
102. Chouery E, Kfoury J, Delague V, et al. A novel locus for autosomal recessive primary torsion dystonia (DYT17) maps to 20p11.22-q13.12. Neurogenetics. 2008;9:287–93.
103. Makino S, Kaji R, Ando S, et al. Reduced neuron-specific expression of the TAF1 gene is associated with X-linked dystonia-parkinsonism. Am J Hum Genet. 2007;80: 393–406.
104. Lee LV, Rivera C, Teleg RA, et al. The unique phenomenology of sex-linked dystonia parkinsonism (XDP, DYT3, "Lubag"). Int J Neurosci. 2011;121 Suppl 1:3–11.
105. Lee LV, Kupke KG, Caballar-Gonzaga F, Hebron-Ortiz M, Muller U. The phenotype of the X-linked dystonia-parkinsonism syndrome. An assessment of 42 cases in the Philippines. Medicine (Baltimore). 1991;70:179–87.
106. Müller U, Steinberger D, Nemeth A. Clinical and molecular genetics of primary dystonias. Neurogenetics. 1998;1:165–77.
107. Evidente VG, Advincula J, Esteban R, et al. Phenomenology of "Lubag" or X-linked dystonia-parkinsonism. Mov Disord. 2002;17:1271–7.
108. Gwinn-Hardy K. Genetics of parkinsonism. Mov Disord. 2002;17:645–56.
109. Waddy HM, Fletcher NA, Harding AE, Marsden CD. A genetic study of idiopathic focal dystonias. Ann Neurol. 1991;29:320–4.
110. Schmidt A, Jabusch HC, Altenmuller E, et al. Etiology of musician's dystonia: familial or environmental? Neurology. 2009;72:1248–54.
111. Stojanovic M, Cvetkovic D, Kostic VS. A genetic study of idiopathic focal dystonias. J Neurol. 1995;242:508–11.
112. Leube B, Kessler KR, Goecke T, Auburger G, Benecke R. Frequency of familial inheritance among 488 index patients with idiopathic focal dystonia and clinical variability in a large family. Mov Disord. 1997;12:1000–6.
113. Lohmann K, Schmidt A, Schillert A, et al. Genome-wide association study in musician's dystonia: a risk variant at the arylsulfatase G locus? Mov Disord. 2014;29: 921–7.

114. Kimmich O, Bradley D, Whelan R, et al. Sporadic adult onset primary torsion dystonia is a genetic disorder by the temporal discrimination test. Brain. 2011;134:2656–63.
115. Defazio G, Berardelli A, Hallett M. Do primary adult-onset focal dystonias share aetiological factors? Brain. 2007;130:1183–93.
116. Hutchinson M, Kimmich O, Molloy A, et al. The endophenotype and the phenotype: temporal discrimination and adult-onset dystonia. Mov Disord. 2013;28:1766–74.
117. Schneider SAK, Klein C. Dystonic syndromes. In: Galvez-Jimenez N, Tuite PJ, editors. Uncommon causes of movement disorders. Cambridge/New York: Cambridge University Press; 2011. p. 121–30.

Chapter 8
Genetic Choreas

Ruth H. Walker, Dobrila D. Rudnicki, and Russell L. Margolis

Abstract The "genetic choreas" consist of a heterogeneous group of disorders, similar in that chorea is typically the most prominent or presenting clinical feature and that degeneration of the striatum is the most characteristic neuropathological feature. Here we discuss the prototypical hereditary choreiform disorder, Huntington's disease (HD), and a series of other familial disorders in which chorea is more or less part of the clinical syndrome and that may resemble HD, including Huntington's disease-like 2 (HDL2), the neuroacanthocytoses, benign hereditary chorea, the iron accumulation diseases, and paroxysmal movement disorders. We conclude by providing comprehensive tables of the dominant and nondominant genetic choreas.

Keywords Chorea • Huntington's disease • Neuroacanthocytosis • Dyskinesia • Basal ganglia • Hereditary

The Prototypic Hereditary Chorea: Huntington's Disease

Since the first description by George Huntington in 1872 [1], HD has held a prominent place as an archetypical neurological and genetic disorder. Here we will review only key details relevant to other forms of chorea; more complete reviews are available elsewhere [2, 3]. As Huntington recognized, it is a tripartite condition of movement, emotion, and cognition, with autosomal dominant inheritance, typically a midlife onset, and inevitable progression to death. Chorea is often the first

R.H. Walker, MB, ChB, PhD
Department of Neurology, James J. Peters Veterans Affairs Medical Center, Bronx, NY 10468, USA

D.D. Rudnicki, PhD
Department of Psychiatry, Johns Hopkins University, Baltimore, MD 21210, USA

R.L. Margolis, MD (✉)
Department of Psychiatry, Johns Hopkins University School of Medicine, Baltimore, MD 21287, USA
e-mail: rmargoli@jhmi.edu

S.A. Schneider, J.M.T. Brás (eds.), *Movement Disorder Genetics*,
DOI 10.1007/978-3-319-17223-1_8

manifestation noted by family members of the affected individual [4] and its prominence is such that the disease was known until recently as Huntington's chorea. HD prevalence, at about 1/10,000 in much of the Western world, makes it the most common of the genetic choreas in these regions [5], with considerably lower prevalence in other regions, including Japan [6–8] and Africa [5]. For this reason, and for multiple historical factors, HD is by far the best studied of the genetic choreas and is often the first consideration in the differential diagnosis of an individual with chorea.

The formal diagnosis of HD is based on motor signs and symptoms in the presence of a family history of HD, although cognitive and psychiatric manifestations may precede motor abnormalities in some individuals. Early chorea may manifest as nonspecific fidgeting, as patients disguise involuntary movements (parakinesias). Chorea typically becomes increasingly prominent, accompanied by other motor symptoms, including ataxia and other disruptions of voluntary movement, dystonia, tics, and myoclonus. Weight loss is common and may stem from direct disruption by the disease mutation of central and peripheral metabolic regulation [9–12]. As disease progresses, affected individuals tend to become more bradykinetic and rigid, with a parkinsonian appearance and further disruption of voluntary motor function, but often a decrease in chorea. In advanced disease, patients are often quite parkinsonian. Young people who develop HD before the age of 20 typically have the "Westphal variant," characterized by parkinsonism and sometimes seizures [13]. Occasionally, adults may present with L-dopa-responsive parkinsonism [14]. Impairment of postural reflexes can be a major cause of falls and morbidity throughout the illness. On eye movement evaluation, square-wave jerks can be seen, with intrusion of involuntary saccades when the patient holds a fixed gaze. Patients may find it necessary to blink or use a head thrust in order to generate a saccadic eye movement.

Imaging data demonstrate that both structural [15, 16] and functional [17] abnormalities are detectable in individuals with the HD mutation more than a decade before clinical diagnosis. Correspondingly, rigorous examination using approaches not routinely employed at the bedside can detect subtle motor and cognitive manifestations of the disease, including abnormalities of fine motor function [18, 19] eye movements [20], cognitive processing [17, 21], and sleep [22].

While motor dysfunction is often considered the defining feature of HD, psychiatric disorders and impaired cognition often cause more difficulty for patients and their families [23]. The most common psychiatric abnormalities include depression, irritability, and apathy. Obsessive-compulsive phenomena are not uncommon [24], while hallucinations and delusions are less frequent [3]. Depression, often mistakenly attributed to the demoralization of suffering from an incurable illness, can have devastating consequences, including suicide. However, this symptom responds reasonably well to antidepressants and, if particularly severe, electroconvulsive therapy. Irritability can often be managed medically with antidepressants, mood stabilizers, or low doses of antipsychotics and psychologically by teaching family members and care providers how to interact with the affected individual. Apathy is much more difficult to treat and often requires family and care providers to lower their expectations of the affected individual. The cognitive changes in HD can be conceptualized, at least at a superficial level, as subcortical. As opposed to cortical dementias, most prominently Alzheimer's disease, language and memory are relatively preserved early in the course of disease, while processing speed and executive function, among other functions, are relatively impaired [25]. The consequence is that individuals may be more functionally disabled than is apparent on superficial interaction, which in turn can lead to frustration on the part of employers or family members. Rosenblatt and others have defined an executive function syndrome, characterized by a combination of apathy, disinhibition, and specific cognitive deficits, which can be particularly troublesome [23, 26]. While the hereditary choreas differ from each other, and from HD, in etiology, pathology, and associated symptoms, the prominence of psychiatric and cognitive dysfunction in HD, at least in part a reflection of disruption of striatal-cortical pathways, clearly points out the need for vigilance about the cognitive and psychiatric manifestations of other diseases characterized by chorea.

HD neuropathology is marked by early prominent striatal atrophy and particularly of loss of striatal neurons that project to the external segment of the globus pallidus (marked by the presence of encephalin) and the substantia nigra (marked by substance P), while striatal neurons projecting to the internal segment of the globus pallidus are relatively spared [27–29]. Loss of cortical neurons is also prominent, including pyramidal neurons that project to the striatum [30], and neuronal loss ultimately becomes widespread as the disease progresses. The spatial and temporal pattern of neuropathology correlates well with the clinical course of the illness: early chorea followed by parkinsonism, with eventual global deterioration of function.

HD is caused by a CAG repeat expansion in exon 1 of the *huntingtin* (*HTT*) gene on chromosome 4p16.3 (Huntington Study Group, 1993). Extensive exploration of HD genetics has substantially contributed to understanding this form of mutation, first described in 1991 for spinal bulbar muscular atrophy (SBMA) [31]. In HD, alleles with <27 consecutive CAG triplets are considered normal. Alleles with 27–35 triplets, termed intermediate alleles, are not typically associated with disease, with a few controversial exceptions [32–34], but can on occasion expand during vertical transmission into the disease-causing range. Alleles with repeats of 36–39 triplets are of variable penetrance [35], while alleles with >39 repeats will cause disease in any individual by about age 65. Somatic mosaicism of repeat expansion can occur, with particularly large expansions found in striatal neurons [36, 37].

Repeat length of normal alleles rarely changes during vertical transmission, but, in the expanded range, as repeat length increases, instability becomes increasingly common. Transmissions from a mother with a repeat expansion in the disease range changes by only a few repeats, with about an equal number of expansions and contractions. Transmissions from an affected father lead, on average, to longer repeats in their offspring, and large increases in repeat length are not uncommon. Contractions from a mutation length allele (>39 triplets) to an allele in the incomplete inheritance range (36–39 triplets) may rarely occur [38]. Anticipation (earlier disease onset in subsequent generations of an affected family) arises from the tendency of allele length to increase, on average, during vertical transmission, combined with the inverse correlation of repeat length and onset age [39].

While an autosomal dominant pattern of inheritance is present in most families with HD, odd patterns of inheritance or de novo cases occasionally come to clinical attention. Possible explanations include (1) lack of sufficient information about family history of HD, (2) adoption or "false" paternity, (3) extreme anticipation (see below) in which a child develops the disease before his or her affected parent (usually a father), (4) expansion of repeat from the intermediate range to disease range in transmission from parent to child [40], and (5) misdiagnosis of either the individual with HD or of family members (e.g., HD misdiagnosed as Parkinson's disease or psychiatric disorder).

Approximately 70 % of the variance of age of onset can be explained by repeat length [41]. The relationship between repeat length and age of onset and to a lesser extent disease progression [40, 42, 43] and older age of onset [44] is of major significance in guiding HD genetic counseling, clinical research, and the search for mechanisms of disease pathogenesis. For instance, formulas have been developed to estimate age of disease onset for individuals with a given repeat length, facilitating investigations into brain changes that develop prior to the onset of clinical symptoms in clinically asymptomatic individuals who have the HD mutation. The capacity to control for the effect of repeat length on age of onset has facilitated the search for other genetic factors and for environmental factors that modify age of disease onset [45]. However, neither individual sequence differences at the *HTT* locus nor sequence differences elsewhere in the genome (e.g., in *GRIK2*) seem to play a major role [45]. Thus, while not yet successful, these efforts will now benefit from increasingly powerful genetic and neurobiological tools and could lead to novel therapeutic strategies.

The *HTT* gene is large, consisting of 67 exons and spanning 180 kb. Exon 1 contains the CAG repeat. The expansion does not have a major effect on gene expression, so that the presumption has been that pathogenesis occurs through a gain-of-function mechanism. Most investigations have focused on the role of the mutant protein, which contains a string of glutamine residues encoded by the exon 1 CAG repeat and has neurotoxic properties. Recent studies have explored the potential toxicity of the CAG repeat in the RNA transcript [46–48], and other lines of investigation have examined the effect of the mutation on normal huntingtin function [49, 50]. So far, nonspecific neuroprotective agents such as coenzyme Q and remacemide have proven ineffective in clinical trials. Many groups are attempting to identify therapeutic targets based on specific pathways implicated in pathogenesis (e.g., misfolding of mutant protein, loss of BDNF function, impaired autophagy) [51–54]. As an alternative to therapeutic approaches that target individual mechanisms, suppression of expression of the mutant *HTT* allele has the considerable theoretical advantage of simultaneously preventing activation of most of these pathways. It is clearly possible to design siRNA or oligonucleotides that knock down *HTT* expression [55–60]. However, these approaches face numerous hurdles [61]: – off-target inhibition of other genes, immunostimulation, lack of specificity for the mutant allele, the need to target large regions of the brain, and clinically feasible delivery mechanisms.

Genetic Choreas Most Similar to HD

Huntington's Disease-Like 2 (HDL2): The Disease Most Similar to HD

HDL2, discovered and genetically defined in 2001 based on an index family in the southeastern United States, is a rare, autosomal dominant neurodegenerative disorder, clinically nearly indistinguishable from HD [62, 63], and characterized, like HD, by midlife onset; marked motor, emotional, and cognitive disturbances; and a relentless progression to death. While there have been too few reported cases to establish details of the phenotype with certainty, there appears to be one form of the disorder characterized by prominent chorea, as in prototypical HD. A second form is characterized by a more parkinsonian presentation, with prominent bradykinesia and dystonia but little chorea, similar to the Westphal variation of HD. Whether this distinction is related to repeat length remains uncertain. Acanthocytes have been found in some, but not all, HDL2 patients [64].

Both disorders are characterized by marked cortical and striatal neurodegeneration, with indistinguishable images on routine neuroimaging. Pathologically, neuronal protein aggregates are readily detectable in both diseases. The ultrastructure of HD and HDL2 aggregates appear similar, and both types stain with anti-ubiquitin antibodies and with antibodies thought to be specific for expanded polyglutamine tracts [65]. The pattern of aggregate distribution in HD and HDL2 also overlaps, with a higher density in the cortex and amygdala than in the striatum and a very low density in the cerebellum and midbrain [65, 66]. Aggregates in HDL2 are more frequent in the upper cortical layers II/III than in HD, while aggregates have been detected in the pons and medulla in HD but not in HDL2 [65, 66].

While relatively uncommon, cases of HDL2 have been detected in multiple countries among individuals of likely African descent, including most recently Brazil and Venezuela [67, 68]. In South Africa, HDL2 is as common among individuals of African descent as HD [69].

HDL2 is caused by a CTG/CAG expansion on chromosome 16q24.3. Normal alleles contain 6–28 triplets, while pathogenic repeats range from 40 to 59 triplets [69]. The clinical, neuropathological, and genetic similarities of HDL2 to HD suggested that the HDL2 mutation would be translated into an expanded polyglutamine repeat. Paradoxically, however, the only well-documented gene at the HDL2 locus is *junctophilin-3* (*JPH3*), in which the repeat is in the CTG orientation and falls within the alternatively spliced exon 2. This exon is not included in the primary transcript that encodes the *JPH3* protein product, though at least four JPH3 splice variants contain exon 2A. On the sense strand, in *JPH3*, the repeat alternatively encodes polyalanine and polyleucine or falls within 3′ UTR. On the antisense strand, a small open reading frame (ORF) contains the repeat in the CAG orientation. HDL2 pathogenesis remains enigmatic. Three non-mutually exclusive mechanisms have been implicated: (1) loss of expression of *JPH3* protein, potentially related to RNA sequestration [70]; (2) toxic expression of a *JPH3* transcript with an expanded CUG repeat [71]; and (3) toxic expression, from the strand antisense to

JPH3, of a cryptic transcript containing a CAG repeat and encoding polyglutamine, a hypothesis supported by evidence in mouse models [72], but not in human post-mortem HDL2 brains [70].

The only reliable method for distinguishing HDL2 from HD is by genetic testing. The disease should be suspected in any individual of African ancestry with a family history of an HD-like disorder that has not been genetically identified. Whether HDL2 will eventually be detected in individuals with no African ancestry remains an open question.

Other Autosomal Dominant Disorders That May Be Mistaken for Huntington's Disease

SCA17, caused by a CAG repeat expansion in TATA box-binding protein (*TBP*) [73], is characterized by a heterogeneous phenotype, with chorea or choreoathetosis present in 36 % of cases [74], sometimes as the key presenting symptoms. However, unlike HD, cerebellar ataxia (and corresponding pathological changes in the cerebellum) is the most frequent presenting sign and is an almost universal feature of the disease. Dementia and psychiatric symptoms are also common, and patients may frequently exhibit parkinsonism, pyramidal signs, and epilepsy. Overall, it has been estimated that 1 % of HD-like cases can be accounted for by SCA17. Disease onset has been detected from age 3 to 75, with a reported mean age of onset of 34.6 years. Normal alleles are thought to range from 25 to 40 triplets (a combination of CAA and CAG codons, encoding one of the longest stretches of polyglutamine in the human proteome); alleles from 41 to 48 have reduced penetrance [75, 76], with full penetrance in alleles greater than 48 repeats [77]. The longest published repeat is 66 triplets [78]. Other types of spinocerebellar ataxias (e.g., SCAs 1, 2, and 3, see below) may also present with chorea as the main presentation.

Dentatorubropallidoluysian atrophy (DRPLA) is a similar autosomal dominant disorder caused by a CAG repeat expansion (in this case in the gene atrophin-1) [79]. Typical clinical features in adults include ataxia, chorea and choreoathetosis, dementia, and psychiatric disorders; chorea may be a sufficiently dominant presenting symptom that HD is on the list of differential diagnoses [80]. Mean age of onset is about 30 years of age. Repeat range is ~6–35 triplets in normal subjects, with 48–93 triplets causing disease. DRPLA is predominantly a disease affecting individuals of Japanese ancestry [81], but a few cases have been reported in non-Japanese pedigrees [82].

Benign Hereditary Chorea (BHC)

The classic presenting feature of BHC, an autosomal dominant disorder typically beginning in childhood, is nonprogressive chorea in relative isolation. However, the chorea can be severe, and at times the phenotype can include, sometimes variably within the same family, dystonia, ataxia, myoclonus, cognitive impairment, and short stature [83, 84]. The primary known cause of BHC is mutation of thyroid transcription factor 1 (*TITF-1*) [85–87], also known as *NKX2.1*. However, individuals and pedigrees with similar presentations do not have mutations in this gene, indicating genetic heterogeneity [88]. The chorea, paradoxically, has been reported to respond to both down-tuning of dopaminergic transmission or to L-dopa [89], presumably reflecting pathological heterogeneity.

Nondominant Disorders That Phenotypically Closely Resemble HD

Chorea-Acanthocytosis

Chorea-acanthocytosis (ChAc), originally referred to as Levine-Critchley syndrome, is another disorder prominently affecting the basal ganglia and with prominent chorea, often presenting in young adults along with orolingual dystonia, and not infrequently with psychiatric disturbances, tics, and parkinsonism [90]. The disease progresses over 10–20 years, with occasional unexplained sudden deaths. The distinguishing features, which if present readily distinguish ChAc from HD, are an autosomal recessive pattern of inheritance, temporal lobe seizures (developing during the course of the disease in almost half of patients, but responsive to treatment), and a sensorimotor neuropathy which can be quite severe and even dominate the clinical presentation [91]. Other characteristic features include elevated creatine kinase and liver enzymes. Acanthocytes, which gave the disease its name, are not an inevitable finding [92]. Postmortem examination has revealed neuronal loss, accompanied by gliosis, most prominently in the head of the caudate, but also in other basal ganglia structures including the putamen, globus pallidus, and substantia nigra.

ChAc is caused by mutations in splice variant 1A of *VPSA13*, a large gene of 73 exons found on chromosome 9q21 [93]. Mutations have been detected throughout VPSA13, so that genetic testing typically requires sequencing and is not widely available. The pathogenesis of ChAc remains poorly understood. The protein product of *VPSA131A*, chorein, participates in actin polymerization, suggesting that the mutant protein may destabilize cell structure, explaining the formation of acanthocytic erythrocytes [94]. Chorein levels in erythrocytes provide an alternative method of disease diagnosis [95], though this measurement remains a research tool.

McLeod Syndrome

McLeod neuroacanthocytosis is readily distinguishable from HD and other choreas in families of sufficient size due to X-linked inheritance and multisystem manifestations. McLeod syndrome prototypically presents in men of middle age with parkinsonism, dystonia, and chorea. The cognitive and psychiatric features present in most basal ganglia disorders may occur, but are not a universal finding [96]. Some patients may have orolingual dystonia suggestive of ChAc [97]. Also as in ChAc, peripheral sensorimotor neuropathy with absent deep tendon reflexes is common, as are seizures. A key feature of the disease, present in a majority of patients and requiring close clinical attention, is cardiomyopathy [98]. Generalized muscle weakness and atrophy is a variable finding [99]. Serum creatine phosphokinase is almost always elevated, and other markers associated with myopathy may also be abnormal. The hematologic manifestations involve acanthocytosis (as in ChAc this is not invariable) and hemolysis [100], stemming from loss of expression of the Kx erythrocyte antigen and Kell blood group antigens [101].

McLeod syndrome is caused by mutations of *XK* on Xp21.1, leading to loss of expression or dysfunctional Xk protein. This protein probably functions as part of the membrane transport system [102], with systemic manifestations correlated to its widespread expression [102–104]. While most affected individuals are men, affected women have been reported, probably a result of X-inactivation [105, 106]. Variability of clinical presentation exists within families [107], and some families have a mild phenotype, probably from point mutations that do not lead to complete absence of protein [108, 109].

Hereditary Iron Accumulation Diseases Featuring Chorea

The group of disorders, referred to as neurodegeneration with brain iron accumulation (NBIA), are typified, and readily identified, by MRI findings of basal ganglia iron deposits. Neuroferritinopathy, the only known autosomal dominant form of NBIA, is caused by mutations in *FTL*, encoding the ferritin light chain, located on 9q13.3 [110]. Movement abnormalities, typically beginning in mid-adulthood, include chorea, dystonia, and parkinsonism; cognitive impairment is occasionally present [111–113]. Aceruloplasminemia is an autosomal recessive NBIA disorder presenting in adulthood caused by mutation of *CP*, resulting in the instability or dysfunction of its protein product, ceruloplasmin. The effect is impaired iron transport. Phenotypically, the disease is characterized by the systemic effects of iron deposition, notably retinal degeneration and diabetes mellitus [114, 115], and later by ataxia, dystonia, chorea, and parkinsonism. Cognitive impairment is often an early feature [116] and may progress to marked dementia. In addition to MRI and genetic testing, the disease is also indicated by decreased levels of ceruloplasmin. Important neuropathological features include neurons and astrocytes carrying excess iron found in the cerebellum, basal ganglia, and cortex [114, 115]. At least seven other very rare autosomal recessive and one X-linked dominant NBIAs have been described, usually characterized by childhood-onset dystonia and parkinsonism (for further discussion of NBIA disorders, see Chap. 13 Wiethoff & Houlden)

Hereditary Paroxysmal Disorders Characterized by Chorea and Other Dyskinesias

Chorea may occur in an episodic manner as a manifestation of any of the group of disorders referred to as the paroxysmal dyskinesias, which are characterized by attacks lasting seconds to hours of abnormal movements of various types. In some disorders abnormal movements are precipitated by sudden movements (e.g., exercise, yawning, talking, or hyperventilation). Because chorea in almost any context may wax and wane, either spontaneously or in response to internal or external stress, paroxysmal chorea may not be readily distinguishable from typical chorea, and differential diagnosis will likely require attention to other clinical factors and, for definitive diagnosis, genetic testing. In some autosomal dominant cases, the disease is caused by mutations in *proline-rich transmembrane protein 2* (*PRRT2*), which may have a role in neurotransmitter release [117, 118]. Other clinical features include hemiplegic migraine, infantile convulsions, and episodic ataxia [119–121]. Paroxysmal non-kinesigenic dyskinesia is similarly characterized by attacks of abnormal movements, spontaneous or brought on by a somewhat different set of stressors (caffeine, alcohol, stress, fatigue, etc.). The autosomal dominant familial form is caused by mutations in *MR-1*, encoding myofibrillogenesis regulator 1, on chromosome 2q33 [122–124]. Chorea and other abnormal movements following prolonged exertion, referred to as paroxysmal exertional dyskinesia, may form part of a variable multisystem autosomal dominant syndrome caused by mutations in *SLC2A1* (formerly *GLUT1*), a gene encoding glucose transporter 1 [125–128]. The disease may be quite severe, with marked developmental delays and seizures, in addition to dystonia and chorea. Of interest, a ketogenic diet is at times helpful. The pathogenesis of the disease was originally thought to stem from glucose-mediated energy deficits, but recent investigations have suggested a more complex pathobiology [129]. For further discussion of the paroxysmal disorders, see Chap. 10 Brockmann et al).

Disorders in Which Chorea Is Likely to Accompany Other Distinguishing Phenotypic Features

In addition to SCA17, in which chorea is common and at times a predominant symptom, chorea can be observed in other dominant SCAs, particularly SCAs 1, 2, and 3. In these disorders chorea is typically a secondary symptom; thus, these diseases are rarely confused with HD or other disorders in which chorea is primary [130]. Huntington's disease-like 3, a recessive condition defined on the basis of one consanguineous family [131], presents with chorea, dystonia, dysarthria, cognitive impairment, and seizures, and cortical and caudate atrophy by imaging. Huntington's disease-like 1 (HDL1) is a familial prion disease, with mutations of *PRNP* found in one Swedish family [132, 133] characterized by mid-adult onset, with psychiatric manifestations, cognitive decline, dysarthria, myoclonus, ataxia, chorea, and occasionally seizures, with progression over 1–2 decades. The mutation is an octapeptide repeat insertion, which has been reported in 3 other families with different phenotypes. Furthermore, various metabolic disorders (including Wilson's disease) may present with chorea, but other distinguishing phenotypic features are typically present. Tables 8.1 and 8.2 include several other potentially relevant disorders.

Table 8.1 Molecular features of autosomal dominant choreiform disorders

Diagnosis	Gene	Location	Protein product	Mutation	Useful tests	Movement disorder	Other neurological features	Usual age of onset
HD	*HD/IT15*	4p15	Huntingtin	Expanded CAG repeats	–	Chorea, dystonia, parkinsonism	Ataxia, seizures (juvenile onset)	Inv. related to repeats
HDL1	*PRNP*	20p12	Prion protein	192 nucleotide insertion	–	Chorea, rigidity	Seizures (variable)	20–40 years
HDL2	*JPH*	16q24.3	Junctophilin-3	Expanded CAG/ CTG repeats	Acanthocytosis+/–	Chorea, dystonia parkinsonism	Hyperreflexia	Inv. related to repeats
Spinocerebellar ataxia 1	*SC1*	6p23	Ataxin-1	Expanded CAG repeats	–	Chorea, dystonia	Ataxia, eye movement abnormalities, peripheral neuropathy	Inv. related to repeats
Spinocerebellar ataxia 2	*SCA2*	12q24	Ataxin-2	Expanded CAG repeats	–	Chorea, dystonia, parkinsonism, tremor	Ataxia, eye movement abnormalities, peripheral neuropathy	Inv. related to repeats
Spinocerebellar ataxia 3	*MJD1*	14q32.1	Ataxin-3	Expanded CAG repeats	–	Chorea, dystonia parkinsonism	Ataxia, eye movement abnormalities, peripheral neuropathy	Inv. related to repeats
Spinocerebellar ataxia 17	*TBP*	6q.27	TATA box-binding protein	Expanded CAA/ CAG repeats	–	Chorea, dystonia parkinsonism	Ataxia, hyperreflexia	Inv. related to repeats

DRPLA	*DRPLA*	12p13.31	Atrophin-1	Expanded CAG repeats	–	Chorea, myoclonus	Ataxia, seizures	Inv. related to repeats
Benign hereditary chorea	*TITF-1* (*NKX2.1*) *other*	14q13.1	Thyroid transcription factor 1; other	Transversions, deletions, substitutions	–	Chorea	Mild ataxia	Childhood
Neuroferritinopathy	*FTL*	19q13.3	Ferritin light chain	Adenine insertion	Serum ferritin	Chorea, dystonia, parkinsonism	Spasticity, rigidity	40–55 years
Paroxysmal exertional dyskinesia	*SLC2A1*	1p34.2	Glucose transporter GLUT1	Deletion, missense	Low CSF/serum glucose ratio	Chorea, dystonia	Seizures	Childhood

Reproduced with permission from Walker RH, "Chorea: Differential diagnosis and treatment" in *Continuum*: *Movement Disorders*, ed. Espay A, © American Academy of Neurology

Abbreviations: *DPRLA* dentatorubropallidoluysian atrophy, *HD* Huntington's disease, *HDL2* Huntington's disease-like 2, *inv* inversely

Table 8.2 Molecular features of autosomal recessive, X-linked, and mitochondrial choreiform disorders

Diagnosis	Inheritance	Gene	Location	Protein product	Mutation	Useful tests	Movement disorder	Other neurological features	Usual age of onset
Chorea-acanthocytosis	AR	*VPS13*	9q21	Chorein	Many	Acanth; CK, LFTs; chorein Western blot	Chorea, dystonia, parkinsonism, od	Seizures, pn self-mutilation	20–50 years
PLAN	AR	*PLA2G6*	22q12-q13	Phospholipase A	Many	–	Chorea, dystonia	Ataxia	Childhood
Aceruloplasminemia	AR	*CP*	3q23	Ceruloplasmin	Nonsense	Ceruloplasmin, glucose	Chorea, dystonia	Ataxia, retinal degeneration	30–50 years
Wilson's disease	AR	*ATP7B*	13q14.3	Copper-transporting ATPase 2	Many	Ceruloplasmin	Coarse tremor, dystonia, parkinsonism	Psychiatric disease	6–55 years
HDL3	AR	*NK*	4p15.3	NK	NK	–	Chorea, dystonia	Seizures, spasticity, ataxia	Childhood
Infantile bilateral striatal necrosis	AR, mitochondrial	*NK*	19q13.32-13.41, mitochondrial	–	–	–	Chorea	Dysarthria, pendular nystagmus, oa	Infancy
Ataxia-telangiectasia	AR	*ATM*	11q22.3	Serine-protein kinase ATM	Many	Alpha-fetoprotein	Chorea	Ataxia, oculomotor apraxia, dysarthria	Early childhood
Ataxia with oculomotor apraxia I	AR	*APTX*	9p13.3	Aprataxin	Many	Hypoalbuminemia, high cholesterol	Chorea, dystonia	Ataxia, oculomotor apraxia, pn	Childhood

Ataxia with oculomotor apraxia 2	AR	*SETX*	9q34	Senataxin	Truncation	Alpha-fetoprotein, high cholesterol	Chorea, dystonia	Ataxia, oculomotor apraxia, pn	Childhood
Friedreich's ataxia	AR	*Frataxin*	9p13	Frataxin	Trinucleotide expansions, deletion	–	Dystonia, chorea	Ataxia, spasticity, myoclonus	Childhood
Non-ketotic hyperglycinemia	AR	Several	Several	Glycine cleavage enzymes	Many	Glycine	Encephalopathy, chorea	Ataxia, ophthalmoplegia	Child/adult
Recessive hereditary methemoglobinemia type II	AR	*DIA1*	22q13-qter	NADPH-cytochrome *b5* reductase	Many	Methemoglobin	Chorea, dystonia	Encephalopathy	Child/adult
Beta-ketothiolase deficiency	AR	*ACAT1/T2*	11q22.3	Mitochondrial acetoacetyl-CoA thiolase	Various	Urinary organic acids	Chorea, myoclonus	Ataxia, developmental delay	Childhood
Pyruvate dehydrogenase deficiency	AR/X-linked	Several	Several	PDH; various subunits	Various	Lactate, pyruvate	Chorea, dystonia, parkinsonism	Encephalopathy, seizures, pn, ataxia	Child/adult
McLeod syndrome	X-linked recessive	*XK*	Xp21	XK	Deletions, missense, insertions	Acanth; Kx, Kell ags; CK, LFTs	Chorea, dystonia, parkinsonism, od	Seizures, pn, myopathy	40–70 years
Lubag	X-linked recessive	*DYT3*	Xq13.1	Multiple transcript system	Missense, deletions	–	Dystonia, chorea parkinsonism, tremor, myoclonus	–	10–40 years

(continued)

Table 8.2 (continued)

Diagnosis	Inheritance	Gene	Location	Protein product	Mutation	Useful tests	Movement disorder	Other neurological features	Usual age of onset
Lesch-Nyhan syndrome	X-linked recessive	*HPRT*	Xq26-27	Hypoxanthine phosphoribosyl-transferase	Many	Hyperuricemia	Chorea, dystonia	Spasticity, self-mutilation	Infancy
Leigh syndrome	Mitochondrial	Many	Many	Many	Many	Elevated lactate/pyruvate	Chorea, dystonia	Hypotonia, cn, ataxia, seizures	Infancy

Reproduced with permission from Walker RH, "Chorea: Differential diagnosis and treatment" in *Continuum*: *Movement Disorders*, ed. Espay A, © American Academy of Neurology

Abbreviations: *acanth* acanthocytosis, *AR* autosomal recessive, *cn* cranial neuropathy, *HDL3* Huntington's disease-like 3, *NK* not known, *oa* optic atrophy, *od* orofacial dyskinesias, *PKAN* pantothenate kinase-associated neurodegeneration, *pn* peripheral neuropathy

Conclusion

Chorea is a feature of many familial conditions. While HD remains the most likely diagnosis in those cases with a clear autosomal dominant inheritance, other diagnoses need to be considered. The availability of genetic testing now greatly aids the diagnostic process, though as always, a careful history and examination will greatly narrow the likely possibilities.

References

1. Huntington G. On chorea. Med Surg Report Philadelphia. 1872;26:317–21.
2. Bates G, Tabrizi S, Jones L. Huntington's disease. 4th ed. Oxford/New York: Oxford University Press; 2014.
3. Ross CA, Pantelyat A, Kogan J, Brandt J. Determinants of functional disability in Huntington's disease: role of cognitive and motor dysfunction. Mov Disord. 2014;29:1351–8.
4. Hoth KF, Paulsen JS, Moser DJ, Tranel D, Clark LA, Bechara A. Patients with Huntington's disease have impaired awareness of cognitive, emotional, and functional abilities. J Clin Exp Neuropsychol. 2007;29:365–76.
5. Warby SC, Visscher H, Collins JA, Doty CN, Carter C, Butland SL, et al. HTT haplotypes contribute to differences in Huntington disease prevalence between Europe and East Asia. Eur J Hum Genet. 2011;19:561–6.
6. Nakashima K, Watanabe Y, Kusumi M, Nanba E, Maeoka Y, Nakagawa M, et al. Epidemiological and genetic studies of Huntington's disease in the San-in area of Japan. Neuroepidemiology. 1996;15:126–31.
7. Masuda N, Goto J, Murayama N, Watanabe M, Kondo I, Kanazawa I. Analysis of triplet repeats in the huntingtin gene in Japanese families affected with Huntington's disease. J Med Genet. 1995;32:701–5.
8. Adachi Y, Nakashima K. Population genetic study of Huntington's disease–prevalence and founder's effect in the San-in area, western Japan. Nihon Rinsho. 1999;57:900–4.
9. van der Burg JM, Bjorkqvist M, Brundin P. Beyond the brain: widespread pathology in Huntington's disease. Lancet Neurol. 2009;8:765–74.
10. Martin B, Golden E, Keselman A, Stone M, Mattson MP, Egan JM, et al. Therapeutic perspectives for the treatment of Huntington's disease: treating the whole body. Histol Histopathol. 2008;23:237–50.
11. Cai H, Cong WN, Ji S, Rothman S, Maudsley S, Martin B. Metabolic dysfunction in Alzheimer's disease and related neurodegenerative disorders. Curr Alzheimer Res. 2012;9:5–17.
12. Aziz NA, Pijl H, Frolich M, Snel M, Streefland TC, Roelfsema F, et al. Systemic energy homeostasis in Huntington's disease patients. J Neurol Neurosurg Psychiatry. 2010;81:1233–7.
13. Squitieri F, Gellera C, Cannella M, Mariotti C, Cislaghi G, Rubinsztein DC, et al. Homozygosity for CAG mutation in Huntington disease is associated with a more severe clinical course. Brain. 2003;126:946–55.
14. Wang SC, Lee-Chen GJ, Wang CK, Chen CM, Tang LM, Wu YR. Markedly asymmetrical parkinsonism as a leading feature of adult-onset Huntington's disease. Mov Disord. 2004;19:854–6.
15. Hobbs NZ, Henley SM, Ridgway GR, Wild EJ, Barker RA, Scahill RI, et al. The progression of regional atrophy in premanifest and early Huntington's disease: a longitudinal voxel-based morphometry study. J Neurol Neurosurg Psychiatry. 2010;81:756–63.

16. Aylward EH, Nopoulos PC, Ross CA, Langbehn DR, Pierson RK, Mills JA, et al. Longitudinal change in regional brain volumes in prodromal Huntington disease. J Neurol Neurosurg Psychiatry. 2011;82:405–10.
17. Reading SA, Dziorny AC, Peroutka LA, Schreiber M, Gourley LM, Yallapragada V, et al. Functional brain changes in presymptomatic Huntington's disease. Ann Neurol. 2004;55: 879–83.
18. Biglan KM, Ross CA, Langbehn DR, Aylward EH, Stout JC, Queller S, et al. Motor abnormalities in premanifest persons with Huntington's disease: the PREDICT-HD study. Mov Disord. 2009;24:1763–72.
19. Bechtel N, Scahill RI, Rosas HD, Acharya T, van den Bogaard SJ, Jauffret C, et al. Tapping linked to function and structure in premanifest and symptomatic Huntington disease. Neurology. 2010;75:2150–60.
20. Rupp J, Dzemidzic M, Blekher T, Bragulat V, West J, Jackson J, et al. Abnormal error-related antisaccade activation in premanifest and early manifest Huntington disease. Neuropsychology. 2011;25:306–18.
21. Duff K, Paulsen J, Mills J, Beglinger LJ, Moser DJ, Smith MM, et al. Mild cognitive impairment in prediagnosed Huntington disease. Neurology. 2010;75:500–7.
22. Goodman AO, Rogers L, Pilsworth S, McAllister CJ, Shneerson JM, Morton AJ, et al. Asymptomatic sleep abnormalities are a common early feature in patients with Huntington's disease. Curr Neurol Neurosci Rep. 2011;11:211–7.
23. Rosenblatt A. Neuropsychiatry of Huntington's disease. Dialogues Clin Neurosci. 2007;9: 191–7.
24. Anderson KE, Louis ED, Stern Y, Marder KS. Cognitive correlates of obsessive and compulsive symptoms in Huntington's disease. Am J Psychiatry. 2001;158:799–801.
25. Papoutsi M, Labuschagne I, Tabrizi SJ, Stout JC. The cognitive burden in Huntington's disease: pathology, phenotype, and mechanisms of compensation. Mov Disord. 2014;29: 673–83.
26. Craufurd D, Thompson JC, Snowden JS. Behavioral changes in Huntington disease. Neuropsychiatry Neuropsychol Behav Neurol. 2001;14:219–26.
27. Deng YP, Albin RL, Penney JB, Young AB, Anderson KD, Reiner A. Differential loss of striatal projection systems in Huntington's disease: a quantitative immunohistochemical study. J Chem Neuroanat. 2004;27:143–64.
28. Albin RL, Reiner A, Anderson KD, Dure LST, Handelin B, Balfour R, et al. Preferential loss of striato-external pallidal projection neurons in presymptomatic Huntington's disease. Ann Neurol. 1992;31:425–30.
29. Starr PA, Kang GA, Heath S, Shimamoto S, Turner RS. Pallidal neuronal discharge in Huntington's disease: support for selective loss of striatal cells originating the indirect pathway. Exp Neurol. 2008;211:227–33.
30. Thu DC, Oorschot DE, Tippett LJ, Nana AL, Hogg VM, Synek BJ, et al. Cell loss in the motor and cingulate cortex correlates with symptomatology in Huntington's disease. Brain. 2010;133:1094–110.
31. La Spada AR, Wilson EM, Lubahn DB, Harding AE, Fischbeck KH. Androgen receptor gene mutations in X-linked spinal and bulbar muscular atrophy. Nature. 1991;352:77–9.
32. Kenney C, Powell S, Jankovic J. Autopsy-proven Huntington's disease with 29 trinucleotide repeats. Mov Disord. 2007;22:127–30.
33. Groen JL, de Bie RM, Foncke EM, Roos RA, Leenders KL, Tijssen MA. Late-onset Huntington disease with intermediate CAG repeats: true or false? J Neurol Neurosurg Psychiatry. 2010;81:228–30.
34. Andrich J, Arning L, Wieczorek S, Kraus PH, Gold R, Saft C. Huntington's disease as caused by 34 CAG repeats. Mov Disord. 2008;23:879–81.
35. Rubinsztein DC, Leggo J, Coles R, Almqvist E, Biancalana V, Cassiman JJ, et al. Phenotypic characterization of individuals with 30-40 CAG repeats in the Huntington disease (HD) gene reveals HD cases with 36 repeats and apparently normal elderly individuals with 36-39 repeats. Am J Hum Genet. 1996;59:16–22.

36. Shelbourne PF, Keller-McGandy C, Bi WL, Yoon SR, Dubeau L, Veitch NJ, et al. Triplet repeat mutation length gains correlate with cell-type specific vulnerability in Huntington disease brain. Hum Mol Genet. 2007;16:1133–42.
37. Aronin N, Chase K, Young C, Sapp E, Schwarz C, Matta N, et al. CAG expansion affects the expression of mutant Huntingtin in the Huntington's disease brain. Neuron. 1995;15: 1193–201.
38. Nahhas F, Garbern J, Feely S, Feldman GL. An intergenerational contraction of a fully penetrant Huntington disease allele to a reduced penetrance allele: interpretation of results and significance for risk assessment and genetic counseling. Am J Med Genet A. 2009;149A: 732–6.
39. Duyao M, Ambrose C, Myers R, Novelletto A, Persichetti F, Frontali M, et al. Trinucleotide repeat length instability and age of onset in Huntington's disease. Nat Genet. 1993;4: 387–92.
40. Myers RH, MacDonald ME, Koroshetz WJ, Duyao MP, Ambrose CM, Taylor SA, et al. De novo expansion of a (CAG)n repeat in sporadic Huntington's disease. Nat Genet. 1993;5:168–73.
41. Andresen JM, Gayan J, Djousse L, Roberts S, Brocklebank D, Cherny SS, et al. The relationship between CAG repeat length and age of onset differs for Huntington's disease patients with juvenile onset or adult onset. Ann Hum Genet. 2007;71:295–301.
42. Rosas HD, Reuter M, Doros G, Lee SY, Triggs T, Malarick K, et al. A tale of two factors: what determines the rate of progression in Huntington's disease? A longitudinal MRI study. Mov Disord. 2011;26:1691–7.
43. Ravina B, Romer M, Constantinescu R, Biglan K, Brocht A, Kieburtz K, et al. The relationship between CAG repeat length and clinical progression in Huntington's disease. Mov Disord. 2008;23:1223–7.
44. Rosenblatt A, Kumar BV, Mo A, Welsh CS, Margolis RL, Ross CA. Age, CAG repeat length, and clinical progression in Huntington's disease. Mov Disord. 2012;27:272–6.
45. Gusella JF, MacDonald ME. Huntington's disease: the case for genetic modifiers. Genome Med. 2009;1:80.
46. Wojciechowska M, Krzyzosiak WJ. CAG repeat RNA as an auxiliary toxic agent in polyglutamine disorders. RNA Biol. 2011;8:565–71.
47. Rudnicki DD, Margolis RL, Pearson CE, Krzyzosiak WJ. Diced triplets expose neurons to RISC. PLoS Genet. 2012;8:e1002545.
48. Fiszer A, Krzyzosiak WJ. RNA toxicity in polyglutamine disorders: concepts, models, and progress of research. J Mol Med (Berl). 2013;91:683–91.
49. Zuccato C, Valenza M, Cattaneo E. Molecular mechanisms and potential therapeutical targets in Huntington's disease. Physiol Rev. 2010;90:905–81.
50. Schulte J, Littleton JT. The biological function of the Huntingtin protein and its relevance to Huntington's disease pathology. Curr Trends Neurol. 2011;5:65–78.
51. Wild EJ, Tabrizi SJ. Targets for future clinical trials in Huntington's disease: what's in the pipeline? Mov Disord. 2014;29:1434–45.
52. Martin DD, Ladha S, Ehrnhoefer DE, Hayden MR. Autophagy in Huntington disease and huntingtin in autophagy. Trends Neurosci. 2015;38:26–35.
53. Cortes CJ, La Spada AR. The many faces of autophagy dysfunction in Huntington's disease: from mechanism to therapy. Drug Discov Today. 2014;19:963–71.
54. Appl T, Kaltenbach L, Lo DC, Terstappen GC. Targeting mutant huntingtin for the development of disease-modifying therapy. Drug Discov Today. 2012;17:1217–23.
55. Yu D, Pendergraff H, Liu J, Kordasiewicz HB, Cleveland DW, Swayze EE, et al. Single-stranded RNAs use RNAi to potently and allele-selectively inhibit mutant huntingtin expression. Cell. 2012;150:895–908.
56. Sah DW, Aronin N. Oligonucleotide therapeutic approaches for Huntington disease. J Clin Invest. 2011;121:500–7.
57. Pfister EL, Kennington L, Straubhaar J, Wagh S, Liu W, DiFiglia M, et al. Five siRNAs targeting three SNPs may provide therapy for three-quarters of Huntington's disease patients. Curr Biol. 2009;19:774–8.

58. Munroe SH, Zhu J. Overlapping transcripts, double-stranded RNA and antisense regulation: a genomic perspective. Cell Mol Life Sci. 2006;63:2102–18.
59. Kordasiewicz HB, Stanek LM, Wancewicz EV, Mazur C, McAlonis MM, Pytel KA, et al. Sustained therapeutic reversal of Huntington's disease by transient repression of huntingtin synthesis. Neuron. 2012;74:1031–44.
60. Hu J, Matsui M, Gagnon KT, Schwartz JC, Gabillet S, Arar K, et al. Allele-specific silencing of mutant huntingtin and ataxin-3 genes by targeting expanded CAG repeats in mRNAs. Nat Biotechnol. 2009;27:478–84.
61. Aronin N. Target selectivity in mRNA silencing. Gene Ther. 2006;13:509–16.
62. Margolis RL, O'Hearn E, Rosenblatt A, Willour V, Holmes SE, Franz ML, et al. A disorder similar to Huntington's disease is associated with a novel CAG repeat expansion. Ann Neurol. 2001;50:373–80.
63. Schneider SA, Marshall KE, Xiao J, LeDoux MS. JPH3 repeat expansions cause a progressive akinetic-rigid syndrome with severe dementia and putaminal rim in a five-generation African-American family. Neurogenetics. 2012;13:133–40.
64. Walker RH, Rasmussen A, Rudnicki D, Holmes SE, Alonso E, Matsuura T, et al. Huntington's disease–like 2 can present as chorea-acanthocytosis. Neurology. 2003;61:1002–4.
65. Rudnicki DD, Pletnikova O, Vonsattel JP, Ross CA, Margolis RL. A comparison of huntington disease and huntington disease-like 2 neuropathology. J Neuropathol Exp Neurol. 2008;67:366–74.
66. Greenstein PE, Vonsattel JP, Margolis RL, Joseph JT. Huntington's disease like-2 neuropathology. Mov Disord. 2007;22:1416–23.
67. Rodrigues GG, Walker RH, Brice A, Cazeneuve C, Russaouen O, Teive HA, et al. Huntington's disease-like 2 in Brazil–report of 4 patients. Mov Disord. 2008;23:2244–7.
68. Paradisi I, Ikonomu V, Arias S. Huntington disease-like 2 (HDL2) in Venezuela: frequency and ethnic origin. J Hum Genet. 2013;58:3–6.
69. Margolis RL, Holmes SE, Rosenblatt A, Gourley L, O'Hearn E, Ross CA, et al. Huntington's Disease-like 2 (HDL2) in North America and Japan. Ann Neurol. 2004;56:670–4.
70. Seixas AI, Holmes SE, Takeshima H, Pavlovich A, Sachs N, Pruitt JL, et al. Loss of junctophilin-3 contributes to Huntington disease-like 2 pathogenesis. Ann Neurol. 2012;71:245–57.
71. Rudnicki DD, Holmes SE, Lin MW, Thornton CA, Ross CA, Margolis RL. Huntington's disease–like 2 is associated with CUG repeat-containing RNA foci. Ann Neurol. 2007;61:272–82.
72. Wilburn B, Rudnicki DD, Zhao J, Weitz TM, Cheng Y, Gu X, et al. An antisense CAG repeat transcript at JPH3 locus mediates expanded polyglutamine protein toxicity in Huntington's disease-like 2 mice. Neuron. 2011;70:427–40.
73. Koide R, Kobayashi S, Shimohata T, Ikeuchi T, Maruyama M, Saito M, et al. A neurological disease caused by an expanded CAG trinucleotide repeat in the TATA-binding protein gene: a new polyglutamine disease? Hum Mol Genet. 1999;8:2047–53.
74. Stevanin G, Brice A. Spinocerebellar ataxia 17 (SCA17) and Huntington's disease-like 4 (HDL4). Cerebellum. 2008;7:170–8.
75. Nolte D, Sobanski E, Wissen A, Regula JU, Lichy C, Muller U. Spinocerebellar ataxia type 17 associated with an expansion of 42 glutamine residues in TATA-box binding protein gene. J Neurol Neurosurg Psychiatry. 2010;81:1396–9.
76. Nanda A, Jackson SA, Schwankhaus JD, Metzer WS. Case of spinocerebellar ataxia type 17 (SCA17) associated with only 41 repeats of the TATA-binding protein (TBP) gene. Mov Disord. 2007;22:436.
77. Toyoshima Y, Yamada M, Onodera O, Shimohata M, Inenaga C, Fujita N, et al. SCA17 homozygote showing Huntington's disease-like phenotype. Ann Neurol. 2004;55:281–6.
78. Maltecca F, Filla A, Castaldo I, Coppola G, Fragassi NA, Carella M, et al. Intergenerational instability and marked anticipation in SCA-17. Neurology. 2003;61:1441–3.
79. Koide R, Ikeuchi T, Onodera O, Tanaka H, Igarashi S, Endo K, et al. Unstable expansion of CAG repeat in hereditary dentatorubral-pallidoluysian atrophy (DRPLA). Nat Genet. 1994;6:9–13.

80. Ikeuchi T, Onodera O, Oyake M, Koide R, Tanaka H, Tsuji S. Dentatorubral-pallidoluysian atrophy (DRPLA): close correlation of CAG repeat expansions with the wide spectrum of clinical presentations and prominent anticipation. Semin Cell Biol. 1995;6:37–44.
81. Tsuji S. Dentatorubral-pallidoluysian atrophy. Handb Clin Neurol. 2012;103:587–94.
82. Burke JR, Wingfield MS, Lewis KE, Roses AD, Lee JE, Hulette C, et al. The Haw River syndrome: dentatorubropallidoluysian atrophy (DRPLA) in an African-American family. Nat Genet. 1994;7:521–4.
83. Gras D, Jonard L, Roze E, Chantot-Bastaraud S, Koht J, Motte J, et al. Benign hereditary chorea: phenotype, prognosis, therapeutic outcome and long term follow-up in a large series with new mutations in the TITF1/NKX2-1 gene. J Neurol Neurosurg Psychiatry. 2012;83: 956–62.
84. Armstrong MJ, Shah BB, Chen R, Angel MJ, Lang AE. Expanding the phenomenology of benign hereditary chorea: evolution from chorea to myoclonus and dystonia. Mov Disord. 2011;26:2296–7.
85. Breedveld GJ, van Dongen JW, Danesino C, Guala A, Percy AK, Dure LS, et al. Mutations in TITF-1 are associated with benign hereditary chorea. Hum Mol Genet. 2002;11:971–9.
86. Devos D, Vuillaume I, de Becdelievre A, de Martinville B, Dhaenens CM, Cuvellier JC, et al. New syndromic form of benign hereditary chorea is associated with a deletion of TITF-1 and PAX-9 contiguous genes. Mov Disord. 2006;21:2237–40.
87. Willemsen MA, Breedveld GJ, Wouda S, Otten BJ, Yntema JL, Lammens M, et al. Brain-Thyroid-Lung syndrome: a patient with a severe multi-system disorder due to a de novo mutation in the thyroid transcription factor 1 gene. Eur J Pediatr. 2005;164:28–30.
88. Bauer P, Kreuz FR, Burk K, Saft C, Andrich J, Heilemann H, et al. Mutations in TITF1 are not relevant to sporadic and familial chorea of unknown cause. Mov Disord. 2006;21:1734–7.
89. Asmus F, Horber V, Pohlenz J, Schwabe D, Zimprich A, Munz M, et al. A novel TITF-1 mutation causes benign hereditary chorea with response to levodopa. Neurology. 2005;64:1952–4.
90. Dobson-Stone C, Rampoldi L, Bader B, Velayos BA, Walker RH, Danek A, et al. Chorea-acanthocytosis. GeneReviews® [Internet]. Seattle (WA): University of Washington; 2002: 1993–2015.
91. Neutel D, Miltenberger-Miltenyi G, Silva I, de Carvalho M. Chorea-acanthocytosis presenting as motor neuron disease. Muscle Nerve. 2012;45:293–5.
92. Sorrentino G, De Renzo A, Miniello S, Nori O, Bonavita V. Late appearance of acanthocytes during the course of chorea-acanthocytosis. J Neurol Sci. 1999;163:175–8.
93. Rampoldi L, Dobson-Stone C, Rubio JP, Danek A, Chalmers RM, Wood NW, et al. A conserved sorting-associated protein is mutant in chorea-acanthocytosis. Nat Genet. 2001;28:119–20.
94. Foller M, Hermann A, Gu S, Alesutan I, Qadri SM, Borst O, et al. Chorein-sensitive polymerization of cortical actin and suicidal cell death in chorea-acanthocytosis. FASEB J. 2012;26: 1526–34.
95. Dobson-Stone C, Velayos-Baeza A, Filippone LA, Westbury S, Storch A, Erdmann T, et al. Chorein detection for the diagnosis of chorea-acanthocytosis. Ann Neurol. 2004;56: 299–302.
96. Jung HH, Danek A, Walker RH, Frey BM, Gassner C. McLeod neuroacanthocytosis syndrome. GeneReviews® [Internet]. Seattle (WA): University of Washington; 2004: 1993–2015.
97. Gantenbein AR, Damon-Perriere N, Bohlender JE, Chauveau M, Latxague C, Miranda M, et al. Feeding dystonia in McLeod syndrome. Mov Disord. 2011;26:2123–6.
98. Danek A, Rubio JP, Rampoldi L, Ho M, Dobson-Stone C, Tison F, et al. McLeod neuroacanthocytosis: genotype and phenotype. Ann Neurol. 2001;50:755–64.
99. Hewer E, Danek A, Schoser BG, Miranda M, Reichard R, Castiglioni C, et al. McLeod myopathy revisited: more neurogenic and less benign. Brain. 2007;130:3285–96.
100. Klempir J, Roth J, Zarubova K, Pisacka M, Spackova N, Tilley L. The McLeod syndrome without acanthocytes. Parkinsonism Relat Disord. 2008;14:364–6.

101. Allen Jr FH, Krabbe SM, Corcoran PA. A new phenotype (McLeod) in the Kell blood-group system. Vox Sang. 1961;6:555–60.
102. Ho M, Chelly J, Carter N, Danek A, Crocker P, Monaco AP. Isolation of the gene for McLeod syndrome that encodes a novel membrane transport protein. Cell. 1994;77:869–80.
103. Jung HH, Russo D, Redman C, Brandner S. Kell and XK immunohistochemistry in McLeod myopathy. Muscle Nerve. 2001;24:1346–51.
104. Russo D, Wu X, Redman CM, Lee S. Expression of Kell blood group protein in nonerythroid tissues. Blood. 2000;96:340–6.
105. Jung HH, Hergersberg M, Kneifel S, Alkadhi H, Schiess R, Weigell-Weber M, et al. McLeod syndrome: a novel mutation, predominant psychiatric manifestations, and distinct striatal imaging findings. Ann Neurol. 2001;49:384–92.
106. Ueyama H, Kumamoto T, Nagao S, Masuda T, Sugihara R, Fujimoto S, et al. A novel mutation of the McLeod syndrome gene in a Japanese family. J Neurol Sci. 2000;176:151–4.
107. Walker RH, Jung HH, Tison F, Lee S, Danek A. Phenotypic variation among brothers with the McLeod neuroacanthocytosis syndrome. Mov Disord. 2007;22:244–8.
108. Jung HH, Hergersberg M, Vogt M, Pahnke J, Treyer V, Rothlisberger B, et al. McLeod phenotype associated with a XK missense mutation without hematologic, neuromuscular, or cerebral involvement. Transfusion. 2003;43:928–38.
109. Walker RH, Danek A, Uttner I, Offner R, Reid M, Lee S. McLeod phenotype without the McLeod syndrome. Transfusion. 2007;47:299–305.
110. Curtis AR, Fey C, Morris CM, Bindoff LA, Ince PG, Chinnery PF, et al. Mutation in the gene encoding ferritin light polypeptide causes dominant adult-onset basal ganglia disease. Nat Genet. 2001;28:350–4.
111. Mir P, Edwards MJ, Curtis AR, Bhatia KP, Quinn NP. Adult-onset generalized dystonia due to a mutation in the neuroferritinopathy gene. Mov Disord. 2005;20:243–5.
112. Crompton DE, Chinnery PF, Bates D, Walls TJ, Jackson MJ, Curtis AJ, et al. Spectrum of movement disorders in neuroferritinopathy. Mov Disord. 2005;20:95–9.
113. Kubota A, Hida A, Ichikawa Y, Momose Y, Goto J, Igeta Y, et al. A novel ferritin light chain gene mutation in a Japanese family with neuroferritinopathy: description of clinical features and implications for genotype-phenotype correlations. Mov Disord. 2009;24:441–5.
114. Xu X, Pin S, Gathinji M, Fuchs R, Harris ZL. Aceruloplasminemia: an inherited neurodegenerative disease with impairment of iron homeostasis. Ann N Y Acad Sci. 2004;1012:299–305.
115. Miyajima H. Aceruloplasminemia, an iron metabolic disorder. Neuropathology. 2003;23:345–50.
116. McNeill A, Pandolfo M, Kuhn J, Shang H, Miyajima H. The neurological presentation of ceruloplasmin gene mutations. Eur Neurol. 2008;60:200–5.
117. Chen WJ, Lin Y, Xiong ZQ, Wei W, Ni W, Tan GH, et al. Exome sequencing identifies truncating mutations in PRRT2 that cause paroxysmal kinesigenic dyskinesia. Nat Genet. 2011;43:1252–5.
118. Lee HY, Huang Y, Bruneau N, Roll P, Roberson ED, Hermann M, et al. Mutations in the gene PRRT2 cause paroxysmal kinesigenic dyskinesia with infantile convulsions. Cell Rep. 2012;1:2–12.
119. Cloarec R, Bruneau N, Rudolf G, Massacrier A, Salmi M, Bataillard M, et al. PRRT2 links infantile convulsions and paroxysmal dyskinesia with migraine. Neurology. 2012;79:2097–103.
120. Gardiner AR, Bhatia KP, Stamelou M, Dale RC, Kurian MA, Schneider SA, et al. PRRT2 gene mutations: from paroxysmal dyskinesia to episodic ataxia and hemiplegic migraine. Neurology. 2012;79:2115–21.
121. Marini C, Conti V, Mei D, Battaglia D, Lettori D, Losito E, et al. PRRT2 mutations in familial infantile seizures, paroxysmal dyskinesia, and hemiplegic migraine. Neurology. 2012;79:2109–14.
122. MacDonald ME, Barnes G, Srinidhi J, Duyao MP, Ambrose CM, Myers RH, et al. Gametic but not somatic instability of CAG repeat length in Huntington's disease. J Med Genet. 1993;30:982–6.

123. Rainier S, Thomas D, Tokarz D, Ming L, Bui M, Plein E, et al. Myofibrillogenesis regulator 1 gene mutations cause paroxysmal dystonic choreoathetosis. Arch Neurol. 2004;61:1025–9.
124. Shen Y, Lee HY, Rawson J, Ojha S, Babbitt P, Fu YH, et al. Mutations in PNKD causing paroxysmal dyskinesia alters protein cleavage and stability. Hum Mol Genet. 2011;20: 2322–32.
125. Perez-Duenas B, Prior C, Ma Q, Fernandez-Alvarez E, Setoain X, Artuch R, et al. Childhood chorea with cerebral hypotrophy: a treatable GLUT1 energy failure syndrome. Arch Neurol. 2009;66:1410–4.
126. Schneider SA, Paisan-Ruiz C, Garcia-Gorostiaga I, Quinn NP, Weber YG, Lerche H, et al. GLUT1 gene mutations cause sporadic paroxysmal exercise-induced dyskinesias. Mov Disord. 2009;24:1684–8.
127. Suls A, Dedeken P, Goffin K, Van Esch H, Dupont P, Cassiman D, et al. Paroxysmal exercise-induced dyskinesia and epilepsy is due to mutations in SLC2A1, encoding the glucose transporter GLUT1. Brain. 2008;131:1831–44.
128. Weber YG, Storch A, Wuttke TV, Brockmann K, Kempfle J, Maljevic S, et al. GLUT1 mutations are a cause of paroxysmal exertion-induced dyskinesias and induce hemolytic anemia by a cation leak. J Clin Invest. 2008;118:2157–68.
129. Marin-Valencia I, Good LB, Ma Q, Duarte J, Bottiglieri T, Sinton CM, et al. Glut1 deficiency (G1D): epilepsy and metabolic dysfunction in a mouse model of the most common human phenotype. Neurobiol Dis. 2012;48:92–101.
130. Perlman SL. Spinocerebellar degenerations. Handb Clin Neurol. 2011;100:113–40.
131. Kambouris M, Bohlega S, Al-Tahan A, Meyer BF. Localization of the gene for a novel autosomal recessive neurodegenerative Huntington-like disorder to 4p15.3. Am J Hum Genet. 2000;66:445–52.
132. Moore RC, Xiang F, Monaghan J, Han D, Zhang Z, Edstrom L, et al. Huntington disease phenocopy is a familial prion disease. Am J Hum Genet. 2001;69:1385–8.
133. Xiang F, Almqvist EW, Huq M, Lundin A, Hayden MR, Edstrom L, et al. A Huntington disease-like neurodegenerative disorder maps to chromosome 20p. Am J Hum Genet. 1998; 63:1431–8.

Chapter 9
Genetics of Tourette Syndrome

Jessica B. Lennington, Gianfilippo Coppola, and Thomas V. Fernandez

Abstract Tourette syndrome (TS) is a developmental neuropsychiatric disorder that is characterized by vocal and motor tics and is estimated to affect 0.2–1 % of the population. Despite evidence for a substantial genetic contribution toward disease risk, identification and replication of associations between genetic variants and TS have been challenging. Rare mutations in several genes have been identified, yet it is unclear whether these genes or their biological pathways play a role in the majority of TS cases. Similar to other complex neuropsychiatric disorders, it is likely that multiple variations in multiple genes, both within the individual and the population, may act together with environmental factors to confer risk. Centralized consortia are collecting larger patient cohorts required to identify candidate genes and biological pathways for TS. Recent profiling of gene expression in the striatum, a brain region highly implicated in TS, indicates downregulation of GABAergic and cholinergic interneurons and shows overlap with gene networks implicated by rare structural genetic variants. Together, integrated analyses of common and rare sequence and structural variation, transcriptomic variation, and bioinformatic analyses of convergent gene networks and pathways may elucidate the genetic etiology of TS.

Keywords Tourette syndrome • Copy number variation (CNV) • Genome-wide association study (GWAS) • Next-generation sequencing • Transcriptome analysis

J.B. Lennington, PhD
Child Study Center, Yale University School of Medicine, New Haven, CT 06520, USA

G. Coppola, PhD
Child Study Center, Yale School of Medicine, New Haven, CT 06520, USA

T.V. Fernandez, MD (✉)
Child Study Center and Psychiatry, Yale University School of Medicine, New Haven, CT 06519, USA
e-mail: thomas.fernandez@yale.edu

S.A. Schneider, J.M.T. Brás (eds.), *Movement Disorder Genetics*,
DOI 10.1007/978-3-319-17223-1_9

Introduction

Tic disorders are estimated to affect 4–20 % of the general population and in some cases are accompanied by debilitating physical and social stress [1]. Gilles de la Tourette syndrome, or Tourette syndrome (TS), was first described in the late 1800s and is currently diagnosed in approximately 0.2–1 % of the population, following childhood onset of chronic motor and vocal tics [2, 3]. While there is great variation in the presentation of discrete tics, symptoms generally wax and wane, are exacerbated by stress and illness, and are greatly reduced or eliminated by adulthood in the majority of patients [4–6].

Twin studies indicate a significant genetic contribution to TS, with co-diagnosis of TS, or concordance, occurring in 8 % of dizygotic twins (who share about 50 % of their DNA) versus 53 % of monozygotic twins (who share all of their DNA) [7–9]. Furthermore, family aggregation studies are consistent with this idea that genes play a major role. Overall, there is a tenfold increase in the risk for recurrence of TS in first-degree relatives compared to the general population [3, 10–12].

Given this rationale for a genetic contribution to TS etiology, various study designs and methodologies have been employed over the last few decades to examine the broad spectrum of genetic variation. Approaches include segregation and linkage analyses, candidate gene association studies, genome-wide association studies (GWAS), rare variant studies (including chromosomal alteration mapping, parametric linkage, and copy number variation [CNV] analysis), and transcriptome analyses. Ultimately, larger patient cohorts and more deliberate efforts to conduct integrated analyses across multiple methods may assist in the discovery of convergent molecular pathways responsible for the production of tics, opening our awareness to novel treatment targets.

Segregation and Linkage Analyses

Early pedigree analyses to clarify how genes might be contributing to TS proposed that most or all of TS could be explained by the inheritance of mutations in one gene; that is, these studies proposed a single-gene autosomal dominant inheritance pattern with partial penetrance [13–16]. Based on this hypothesis, early parametric linkage focused on studying large multigenerational pedigrees. However, despite intensive discovery efforts, no single TS gene locus was identified and confirmed based on this simple inheritance hypothesis [9, 17–23]. In retrospect, an underestimation of the population prevalence of TS and an under appreciation for the high rate of bilineal inheritance (both parents with tics or TS having an affected child) [24–26] contributed to this mischaracterization.

With this failure came a realization that the transmission of TS is likely to be complex, wherein the interplay of multiple gene variants along with environmental factors may act together to confer risk [9, 27, 28]. Subsequently, different linkage strategies were employed that allowed for genetic heterogeneity within and among families. Nonparametric linkage studies have suggested multiple potential gene loci, including those on chromosome 2p [29], 4q [30, 31], 5q [31], 7q [32], 8p [30], 11q24 [33], 17q [31, 34], and at several other genetic markers (D5S1981, D5S2050, D10S591, D10S189, D13S217, and D14S288) [18, 29]. However, none of these studies converged on a single region or led to the identification of an altered transcript, further highlighting the genetic heterogeneity and complexity of TS. More recent studies in psychiatry and other areas of medicine have emphasized the need for alternate genetic discovery approaches in addition to much larger sample cohorts, especially in the face of such heterogeneity, in order to identify risk alleles that are common in the population [35, 36].

Candidate Gene Association Studies

A large number of studies following early linkage analyses in TS tested hypotheses of differential allele frequencies in TS versus the general population. These studies typically used a case-control design, assessing single nucleotide polymorphisms (SNPs) in candidate genes that were selected based on known gene functions and the theoretical plausibility of their relationship to TS pathology. For example, SNP frequencies in the dopamine receptor (e.g., *DRD2*, *DRD3*, *DRD4*), dopamine transporter (*DAT*, *SLC6A3*), and dopamine catabolizing (*COMT*) genes have been examined based on the long-standing recognition that TS symptoms are sometimes alleviated with medications that block dopamine neurotransmission [37–45]. Other candidate genes investigated for association include noradrenergic transcripts (*ADRA1C*, *ADRA2A*, *ADRA2C*) [46, 47], tyrosine hydroxylase [48], several serotonergic genes (*TPH2*, *5HT3*, *5HTTLR*) [44, 49, 50], and monoamine oxidase A (*MAO-A*) [38]. Most recently, a study investigating two common SNPs and one rare coding variant in the serotonin transporter (*SLC6A4*) found evidence for association of both the common and rare gain-of-function single nucleotide allele variants in TS versus controls, a finding which requires replication in other cohorts [51].

Similar to other areas of medicine, candidate gene association studies in TS have generally not yielded significant reproducible findings [35]. Reasons for this shortcoming include (1) a low a priori probability that a selected candidate allele will be associated, given millions of SNPs and a limited understanding of the underlying biology of TS; (2) a combination of small effect sizes for common SNPs and relatively small sample sizes in candidate gene association studies; and (3) failure to adequately control for occult population stratification effects, whereby any differences in ancestry between cases and controls can yield a false-positive result that is unlikely to be reproduced [35, 52].

Genome-Wide Association Studies

The aforementioned difficulties with candidate gene association studies as well as timely advancements in microarray genotyping technologies facilitated a shift to focusing on genome-wide association studies (GWAS) as another approach for studying complex disorders. GWAS permits simultaneous testing of common SNPs for association across the genome. While this method detects SNPs with small individual effect sizes, the genome-wide scope can theoretically detect many associated variants which, in aggregate, can explain a large proportion of disease susceptibility [53]. GWAS have been widely used to identify potential genetic risk factors in many complex disorders, with varying degrees of success [54, 55].

In the first TS GWAS of 1,285 cases and 4,964 ancestry-matched controls, no individual locus reached the accepted statistical threshold for significance of $p<5\times10^{-8}$ [56]. However, the top signals were collectively enriched for functional gene variants associated with brain gene expression levels. Further study suggested that the large majority of TS heritability could be captured by GWAS [57], suggesting that larger cohorts may lead to the discovery of definitive TS risk genes. Additional, larger-scale sample collection and a second GWAS analysis in TS is currently underway. Meanwhile, a subsequent analysis in 609 independent TS cases and 610 ancestry-matched controls genotyped 42 SNPs from the TS GWAS (using an inclusion criteria of $p<10^{-3}$). One of these SNPs (rs2060546), closest to *NTN4* (*netrin-4 precursor*) on chromosome 12q22, achieved statistical significance for association and significantly predicted case-control status, suggesting that many of the variants underlying the top GWAS peaks may represent true TS risk alleles [58].

Rare Variation Studies

In TS and other complex disorders, the various approaches reviewed above have so far yielded only suggestive evidence for common variants conferring small increments of risk. As a result, there has been a steadily increasing focus on examining the contribution of rare variation to complex disease. Like modern common variant studies, these rare variant studies conceptualize TS as a highly complex and heterogeneous disorder. While any discovered association carrying large effects may represent only a small fraction of the total population risk, it has the potential to reveal important biological functions that may be more generally relevant to TS pathogenesis.

Cytogenetic Abnormalities

Analyses of de novo and rare segregating chromosomal alterations in TS families have revealed a number of potential candidate regions, including in 2p21-p23, 3p21.3, 6q16, 7q22-q31, 7q35-36, 8q21.4, 9pter, 13q31, 17p11, and 18q22 [36,

59–66]. Several of these loci have pointed to potential candidate genes, including *IMMP2L* (*mitochondrial inner membrane protease subunit 2*) on chromosome 7q31.1 [62, 67, 68], *CNTNAP2* (*contactin-associated protein-like 2*) on chromosome 7q35-36.1 [36], *NLGN4X* (*neuroligin 4, X-linked*) on Xp22.3 [69], and *DPP6* (*dipeptidyl aminopeptidase-like protein 6*) on chromosome 7p36.2 [66].

A few notable points of convergence have emerged from reports of cytogenetic rearrangements in TS. First, three patients have been described with rearrangements involving chromosome 7q31 and *IMMP2L* [32, 60, 62, 67]; recently, an excess of intragenic deletions in this gene was reported in 188 Danish TS patients versus controls [70]. Second, three separate studies reported rearrangements in chromosome 18q22, with break points mapping within 5 Mb of one another [60, 61, 63]. Third, a chromosomal rearrangement described by Verkerk et al. [36] involved an insertion of chromosome 2p21-p23 at chromosome 7q35-36 that disrupted *CNTNAP2*; the inserted region of chromosome 2p overlaps a region underlying a subsequent genome-wide significant linkage peak [29].

Furthermore, three studies of cytogenetic abnormalities are notable because they implicate regions identified in other neurodevelopmental disorders. First, Verkerk et al. [36] reported a complex rearrangement shared by a father with TS and his affected children, disrupting *CNTNAP2*, a gene implicated in autism spectrum disorders (ASD), intellectual disability, and schizophrenia [71–77]. Second, Lawson-Yuen et al. [69] report a deletion in *NLGN4X*, shared by a mother and two affected sons; neuroligin 4 genes have previously been associated with ASD [78–80]. Finally, Prontera et al. [66] report a deletion in the first exon of *DPP6*, a gene implicated in the pathogenesis of ASD, in a boy and his father with TS.

SLITRK1

In 2005, Abelson et al. reported a de novo inversion of chromosome 13 in a TS proband [59]. The gene *SLITRK1* (*Slit and Trk-like, Family Member 1*) mapped within 350 kb of one of the inversion breakpoints on 13q31. Sequence analysis of this gene in 174 unrelated European TS probands identified a single nucleotide deletion that occurred in one TS subject and another with a diagnosis of trichotillomania (TTM). In addition, two independent occurrences of a very rare single base change (var321) were identified in a highly conserved region of the *SLITRK1* 3'UTR that corresponds to the binding site for the microRNA hsa-miR-189. Screening for this variant in more than 4,000 controls yielded a significant association with TS ($p=0.0056$).

While in vitro [81] and mouse knockout [82] studies of *SLITRK1* are consistent with what is known about the neuropathology and phenotype of TS, genetic studies attempting to confirm the initial *SLITRK1* association have yielded both positive [83, 84] and negative [56, 85–90] association findings. It is clear that further studies involving much larger TS cohorts and employing the latest genomic technologies will be needed to clarify the contribution of variation in and around *SLITRK1* toward TS disease risk.

HDC

As described above, initial linkage studies of large pedigrees failed to identify a single gene mutation that explained most TS risk. Subsequent parametric linkage analyses concentrated on studying smaller families to identify rare gene alleles of large effect. Rather than identifying a gene variant which would explain the etiology of most TS cases, this approach looks at "outlier families" to identify rare variants that can help to shed light on some aspect of the underlying biology of TS.

The first study of this type to identify a rare mutation within a linkage interval that accounted for the statistical results was one by Ercan-Sencicek et al. [91]. In a two-generation family with 9 members affected with TS, a region on chromosome 15 was identified that reached the maximum theoretical statistical (LOD) score. A heterozygous loss-of-function point mutation was identified in the gene *HDC* (*histidine decarboxylase*) in all affected family members, resulting in a truncated protein lacking key segments of the active domain. HDC is the rate-limiting enzyme in histamine biosynthesis, suggesting that histaminergic neurotransmission may underlie the pathophysiology of TS in this family.

Normally, histamine receptors in the central nervous system regulate the release of histamine as well as other neurotransmitters including dopamine [92, 93]. Histamine H2 and H3 receptors are enriched in the striatum and cortex, brain regions previously implicated in TS [94]. Furthermore, histamine modulates functional connectivity in the striatum, increasing feed-forward inhibition and suppressing excitatory drive [95]. More recent work has established that mice lacking one or both *Hdc* genes functionally recapitulate the TS-associated mutation in humans, showing increased stereotypies when administered dopamine agonists, general behavioral phenotypes similar to TS patients, and disrupted dopamine neurotransmission and dopamine receptors in the basal ganglia [96, 97]. A study of copy number variation [98] and a European family-based association study [99] lend further support to a "histamine hypothesis" of TS. Encouraged by all of these findings, a clinical trial of a histamine receptor (H3)- modulating compound is currently underway in TS patients (ClinicalTrials.gov ID: NCT01904773).

Copy Number Variation

Over the past decade, the development and widespread adoption of high-resolution microarray technologies that can detect submicroscopic structural variation have led to the realization that extensive copy number variation (CNV) is present throughout the genome of all individuals [100–103]. Studies in ASD and schizophrenia have demonstrated an increased burden of rare CNVs, particularly those that are de novo and overlap with genes [104–107].

In the first study to report on the contribution of CNVs in TS, there was no significant difference in CNV burden between 111 cases and 73 controls. The authors hypothesized potential overlap of risk among TS, ASD, and schizophrenia based on their findings of rare recurrent CNVs in *NRXN1* (*neurexin 1*) and *CTNNA3* (*catenin, alpha 3*) [108].

A subsequent study of rare CNVs in 460 TS and 1,131 control subjects found that genes mapping within rare CNV regions overlap with those previously identified in ASD, but not schizophrenia or intellectual disability [98]. Furthermore, pathway analyses revealed an enrichment of genes involved in histamine neurotransmission, and a large, likely pathogenic, de novo CNV was identified that disrupted multiple gamma-aminobutyric (GABA) receptor genes, providing additional support of recent findings regarding the involvement of histaminergic and GABAergic neurotransmission in the etiology of TS [91, 97, 109–111]. While rare CNV burden differences between TS and controls were not statistically significant in this study, there was a trend toward an increased burden of de novo rare exonic CNVs in 148 TS and 436 control parent-child trios ($p=0.07$) [98], providing impetus for studies currently underway to examine de novo CNV burden differences in larger TS cohorts.

Two recent CNV studies have also supported the idea that some TS risk loci overlap with ASD and other neurodevelopmental disorders. The first examined 210 TS cases and 285 controls from Latin American populations and identified two additional CNVs overlapping *NRXN1* [112]. This study also reported an excess of large (>500 kb) CNVs in cases, a finding previously unreported in TS. Most recently, a cross-disorder CNV study of 1,086 TS, 1,613 OCD, and 1,789 control subjects reported a 3.3-fold higher burden of large deletions within regions previously known to harbor recurrent, pathogenic CNVs in subjects with other neurodevelopmental disorders. While no global CNV burden was detected for either disorder and no individual locus was significant on its own, five subjects harbored large deletions within 16p13.11, including three with OCD, one with OCD and CT, and one with TS in the absence of OCD [113].

Genome-Wide Sequencing

Genome-wide "next-generation" sequencing (exome and whole-genome) is providing an unprecedented opportunity to investigate genetic variation that is both common and rare, sequence and structural, in large numbers of individuals. Application of this methodology to TS individuals and parent-child trios is underway by TS genetic consortia and will likely increase in scope as technology costs continue to fall. To date, two studies utilizing next-generation sequencing in TS have been published. In one, exome sequencing in ten members of a three-generation pedigree with 7 affected by TS or chronic tics found three novel, nonsynonymous single nucleotide variants in three genes (*MRPL3*, *DNAJC13*, *OFCC1*) that segregated with the chronic tic phenotype and fell within linkage peaks approaching the maximum LOD score [114]. The other study used whole-genome sequencing and array CGH to map the breakpoints of an apparently balanced translocation involving chromosomes 6q16 and 22p13 that was previously identified by cytogenetics and FISH in a male patient with TS and OCD. This study found a 400 kb deletion on chromosome 6q16 affecting three genes (*GPR63*, *NDUFA4*, *KLHL32*) and overlapping a region previously implicated in an ASD case report [64].

Transcriptome Analysis

Whole transcriptome analysis compares gene expression patterns between cases and controls, providing another route for researchers to gain insight into the molecular mechanisms underlying TS. Several groups attempted to analyze the transcriptome of TS patients by microarray technology, three investigating blood [115–117] and two studying *postmortem* putamen brain tissue [118]. In the first brain tissue study [118], ten genes were nominally differentially expressed in TS versus controls, implicating proteins in the protein tyrosine phosphatase (PTP) family. Natural killer cell cytotoxicity and antigen presentation were implicated by 13 genes, found nominally differentially expressed by exon microarray in TS blood samples [115]. In another study of blood samples from TS patients, GABA- and acetylcholine-related genes were found to be correlated with tic severity and/or were alternatively spliced [116]. Finally, communication between innate and adaptive immune cell pathways was implicated by a pathway analysis of the 376 exons found nominally differentially expressed in a third study of TS blood samples [119].

In a more recent study using RNA sequencing technology (RNAseq), the putamen and caudate regions of nine postmortem TS brains and nine matched normal control brains were investigated [111]. The authors demonstrated a convergence of results from differential gene expression, gene co-expression network analyses, and CNVs previously implicated in TS [98], strongly implicating disrupted basal ganglia interneuron function in the pathophysiology of severe, persistent TS. Interestingly, they also found a significant increase in immune and inflammatory transcripts that appear to be endogenous to the central nervous system. Specifically, this study reported significantly altered expression levels in 1,131 genes. The upregulated transcripts strongly implicated inflammatory response and immune cell development and trafficking signatures, including TNFa, IL6, and IL-12, found altered in a previous blood study [120]. The downregulated transcripts implicated broad dysfunction in several subpopulations of interneurons, including cholinergic interneurons (implicated by genes involved in acetylcholine neurotransmitter synthesis and transport, cholinergic receptors, and homeodomain genes critical for the development of forebrain cholinergic neurons [121–123]) and striatal GABAergic interneurons. The transcriptome results were consistent with immunocytochemical findings [111]. These interneuron classes are widely implicated in other neuropsychiatric disorders [124].

In this study, the authors also exploited weighted gene co-expression network analysis (WGCNA) [125], identifying ten modules of co-expressed genes with altered expression pattern in TS versus controls. Two of the modules (*turquoise* and

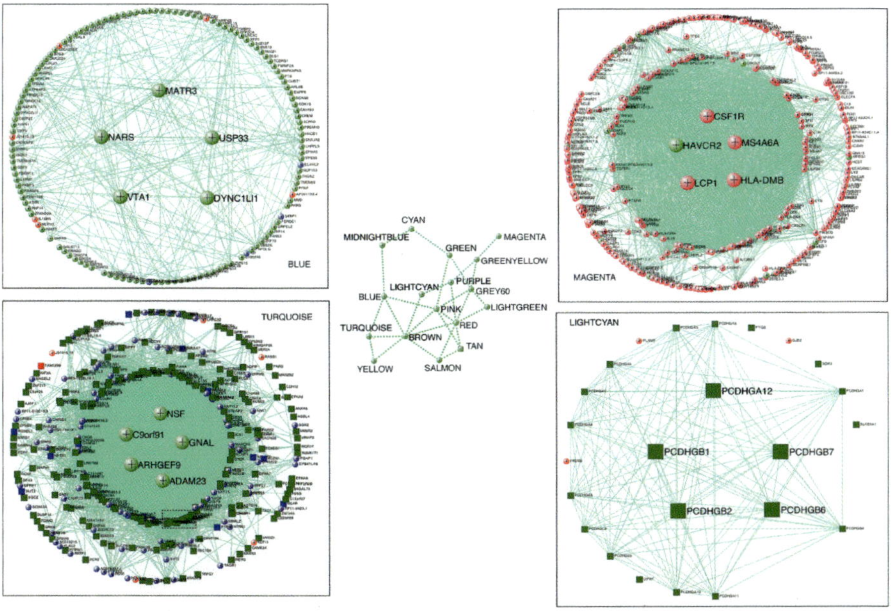

Fig. 9.1 Graphical representation of the WGCNA network. The center of the figure shows the overall network where the nodes (*green circles*) are modules and the edges are significant correlations (correlation *p*-value <0.05 and correlation coefficient >0.5) between the first principal component of the gene expression values. *Top left*: blue module. *Top right*: magenta module. *Bottom right*: lightcyan module. *Bottom left*: turquoise module. *Circles*: network genes. *Large circles*: top five genes with highest intra-modular connectivity (hubs). *Squares*: network genes overlapping with CNV genes. *Red*: upregulated genes. *Blue*: downregulated genes. Concentric circle arrangement in the case of the turquoise (*bottom left*) and magenta (*top right*) modules reflects intra-modular connectivity: genes closer to the center have higher intra-modular connectivity than genes further away from the center (Reproduced with permission from Lennington et al. [111])

blue; see Fig. 9.1) contain multiple genes involved in the function of striatal interneurons, providing the first confirmation that cholinergic and GABAergic interneurons may be functionally immature or missing in TS, consistent with immunohistochemical findings [109–111]. The *magenta* module suggested increased expression of genes related to microglia cell-type categories and immune-related pathways (see Fig. 9.1). Interestingly, peripheral immunological changes in TS patients have been reported previously [120, 126–129]. Additional modules contained genes related to cell adhesion, astrocyte-related metabolic pathways, and protocadherin-gamma molecules (light cyan; see Fig. 9.1) [111].

Analysis of the distribution of the differentially expressed genes within the modules revealed a bias toward more central, highly interconnected genes for the *magenta* (microglia/immune) module and in the opposite direction for the other relevant modules, toward more peripheral, less interconnected genes (Fig. 9.1).

Finally, the authors integrated their network analysis with a list of genes intersecting rare CNVs from one of the studies described above [98], to identify genetic alterations as potential causative factors of the changes observed at transcriptome level. Interestingly, they found significant overlap between the subset of TS-specific genes and the *turquoise* and *light cyan* modules, respectively, with more peripheral (i.e., low-connectivity) and more central (i.e., high-connectivity) genes (Fig. 9.1). The lack of overlap between the *magenta* module (microglia/immune) and the CNV genes was somewhat surprising, given the widespread perturbation in gene expression levels, which also included many hub genes. Taken together with the reported lack of correlation between the *magenta* and the *turquoise* and/or *light cyan* modules, these findings may suggest that the immunological alterations are either not pathophysiologically dependent on the other alterations or that a previous relationship might have existed developmentally, but was lost as a consequence of disease [111].

Summary and Future Directions

As can be said for all genetically complex disorders, the process of gene discovery in TS to date has been challenging. Despite strong evidence that genes contribute to the disorder, there have been a considerable number of gene discovery efforts that have yet to account for a significant proportion of disease etiology. Nevertheless, there is reason for optimism given emerging evidence for the contribution of specific genes and biological pathways from rare variation and gene expression studies in TS (see Table 9.1) and given significant progress being made in other neuropsychiatric and neurodevelopmental disorders, particularly ASD and schizophrenia. Large-scale studies in both of these disorders have resulted in dramatic advances in the understanding of their respective genomic architectures, signaling a good prognosis for the future of TS genetics research.

Whether the field focuses on the identification of rare mutations, common polymorphisms, gene expression changes, or all three, it is abundantly clear that large patient cohorts will be an essential requirement to identify relevant genes and to minimize the risk for false-positive findings. Over the last decade, the Tourette Syndrome Association International Consortium for Genetics (TSAICG), consisting of 14 different collaborative sites, has been working to collect larger samples of TS subjects. Using this collection and additional samples from other collaborating investigators, the TSAICG completed the first GWAS of TS [56], described above, and has recently undertaken a second TS GWAS in 3,000 cases and 5,000 ancestry-matched controls (http://www.findtsgenes.org/). The analyses of these data are nearing completion and should help identify common and rare genetic variants that increase the risk for TS. Once these genes are characterized, there is optimism that subsequent research will elucidate the biological processes that are important for the development of TS.

In 2011, a second consortium, the Tourette International Collaborative Genetics (TIC Genetics; http://tic-genetics.org/) study, was established, with the aims of collecting clinical data and biomaterials (DNA, transformed cell lines, RNA) from TS

Table 9.1 Tourette syndrome gene candidates, organized according to neurotransmitter class and functional categories (A-I) Type of study used in reference(s)

Gene	Description	Site	References	A	B	C	D	E	F	G	H	I
Histamine signaling			[98]						•			
HDC	Histidine decarboxylase	15q21.2	[91, 94, 96–99]					•				
GABAergic signaling			[98]						•		•	•
GAD1	Glutamate decarboxylase 1	2q31	[111]								•	
GABRA1	Gamma-aminobutyric acid (GABA) A receptor, alpha 1	5q34	[111]								•	
GABRG2	Gamma-aminobutyric acid (GABA) G receptor, gamma 2	5q34	[111]								•	
GABRA3	Gamma-aminobutyric acid (GABA) A receptor, alpha 3	Xq28	[111]								•	
NOS1	Nitric oxide synthase 1	12q24.2	[111]								•	
NPY	Neuropeptide Y	7p15.1	[111]								•	
NPY2R	Neuropeptide Y receptor Y2	4q31	[111]								•	
Cholinergic signaling												
CHAT	Choline acetyltransferase	10q11.2	[10, 91, 111]								•	•
CHRM2	Cholinergic receptor, muscarinic 2	7q33	[111]								•	
GBX2	Gastrulation brain homeobox2	2q37.2	[111]								•	
NTRK1	Neurotrophic tyrosine kinase, receptor type 1	1q21-22	[111]								•	
SLC18A3	VACHT; Solute carrier family 18 (vesicular acetylcholine transporter), member 3	10q11.23	[111]								•	

(continued)

Table 9.1 (continued)

Gene	Description	Site	References	A	B	C	D	E	F	G	H	I
SLC5A7	CHT1; Solute carrier family 5 (sodium/choline cotransporter), member 7	2q12	[111]								•	
Monoamine signaling												
DRD1	Dopamine receptor D1	5q35	[111]; neg findings [43]								•	
DRD2	Dopamine receptor D2	11q23	[40]		•							
DRD4	Dopamine receptor D4	11q15	[37–39]; neg findings [41, 42]		•							
DRD5	Dopamine receptor D5	4p16	[111]								•	
HTR2C	Serotonin receptor 2C	Xq23	[111]								•	
MAOA	Monoamine oxidase A	Xp11.3	[38]		•						•	
TPH2	Tryptophan hydroxylase 2	12q21.1	[50]		•							
SLC6A3	DAT; Solute carrier family 6 (neurotransmitter transporter), member 3	5p15.3	[41, 45]		•							
SLC6A4	SERT; Solute carrier family 6 (neurotransmitter transporter), member 4	17q	[51]		•							
Other neuronal signaling, axon guidance, etc												
CNTNAP2	Contactin-associated protein like-2	7q35-36.1	[29, 36]				•					
DNAJC13	DNAJ homolog, subfamily C, member 12	3q21-23	[108]							•		
GPR63	G protein-coupled receptor 63	6q16.1	[64]							•		
NLGN4X	Neuroligin 4, X-linked	Xp22.3	[69]				•					
NTN4	Netrin 4	12q22	[58]			•						
SLITRK1	SLIT and NTRK-like family, member 1	13q31.1	[59, 83, 84]; neg findings [56, 85–90]					•				

				A	B	C	D	E	F	G	H	I
SLITRK5	SLIT and NTRK-like family, member 5	13q31.2	[111]								•	
Bioenergetics/ metabolism												
IMMP2L	Mitochondrial inner membrane protease subunit 2	17q31.1	[32, 60, 62, 65, 67, 68, 70]				•					
MRPL3	Mitochondrial ribosomal protein L3	3q21-23	[108]							•		
NDUFA4	NADH dehydrogenase 1 alpha subcomplex, 4, 9kDa	7p21.3	[64]							•		
Immune-related genes			[111]								•	
IL6	Interleukin 6	7p15-21	[1, 11, 119]								•	•
IL12	Interleukin 12	3q25	[1, 11, 119]								•	•
TNFa	Tumor necrosis factor	6p21.3	[1, 11, 119]								•	•
Other genes												
DPP6	Dipeptidyl aminopeptidase-like protein 6	7p36.2	[66]					•				
KLHL32	Kelch-like family member 32	6q16.1	[64]							•		
OFCC1	Orofacial cleft 1 candidate 1	6p24.3	[108]							•		

A Linkage; *B* Gene Association; *C* GWAS; *D* Cytogenetic Abnormalities; *E* Rare Variation; *F* CNV; *G* Genome Wide Sequencing; *H* Transcriptome Analysis (Striatum); *I* Evaluation of patient blood/tissue patients and their family members. Recruitment is from more than twenty sites in the USA, Europe, and South Korea, and these materials are part of a sharing repository of the National Institute for Mental Health (NIMH) Center for Collaborative Genetic Studies on Mental Disorders. Data and biomaterials will be made available to the widest possible research community to hasten the identification of causal genetic factors and facilitate better understanding and treatment of TS [130]. Both consortia, TSAICG and TIC Genetics, are currently working closely to plan complementary analyses and to combine existing data for analyses of larger TS data sets.

Finally, a large consortium of TS investigators in the European Union is conducting a parallel, longitudinal study of 1,000 TS subjects, with a plan to complete a third GWAS in the near future (http://www.emtics.eu/).

There is great hope that the efforts of these groups and their research will elucidate novel cellular and molecular mechanisms that may not have been previously hypothesized to be important for the etiology of TS. Recent discovery of rare mutations in the histamine neurotransmission pathway led to a current clinical trial of an H3-modulating compound, serving as one example of how such a process might proceed from gene discovery to the development of new intervention strategies. In the end, the continued generosity of patients and their families participating in research, the sharing of biomaterials across the scientific community, and the effective collaboration among scientists, patients, families, and research-funding institutions will all be critical to success. There is reason for great optimism that the pace of genetic discovery in TS will accelerate and inform intervention strategies that will alleviate suffering endured by those with TS and related disorders.

Acknowledgments This work is supported by the Brain and Behavior Research Foundation (NARSAD) to GC, by the National Institute of Mental Health (NIMH) T32 Fellowship for post-doctoral training in childhood neuropsychiatric disorders, Award Number MH018268 to JBL, and by NIMH Award Number K08MH099424 to TVF.

References

1. Cubo E. Review of prevalence studies of tic disorders: methodological caveats. Tremor Other Hyperkinet Mov (N Y). 2012;2: http://www.ncbi.nlm.nih.gov/pubmed/?term=23440028
2. Bitsko RH, Holbrook JR, Visser SN, Mink JW, Zinner SH, Ghandour RM, et al. A National Profile of Tourette syndrome, 2011–2012. J Dev Behav Pediatr. 2014;35(5):317–22.
3. Robertson MM. The prevalence and epidemiology of Gilles de la Tourette syndrome. Part 1: the epidemiological and prevalence studies. J Psychosom Res. 2008;65(5):461–72.
4. Bloch MH, Peterson BS, Scahill L, Otka J, Katsovich L, Zhang HP, et al. Adulthood outcome of tic and obsessive-compulsive symptom severity in children with Tourette syndrome. Arch Pediatr Adolesc Med. 2006;160(1):63–9.
5. Leckman JF, Zhang HP, Vitale A, Lahnin F, Lynch K, Bondi C, et al. Course of tic severity in Tourette syndrome: the first two decades. Pediatrics. 1998;102(1):14–9.
6. Lin HQ, Yeh CB, Peterson BS, Scahill L, Grantz H, Findley DB, et al. Assessment of symptom exacerbations in a longitudinal study of children with Tourette's syndrome or obsessive-compulsive disorder. J Am Acad Child Adolesc Psychiatry. 2002;41(9):1070–7.

7. Hyde TM, Aaronson BA, Randolph C, Rickler KC, Weinberger DR. Relationship of birth weight to the phenotypic expression of Gilles de la Tourette's syndrome in monozygotic twins. Neurology. 1992;42(3 Pt 1):652–8.
8. Price RA, Kidd KK, Cohen DJ, Pauls DL, Leckman JF. A twin study of Tourette syndrome. Arch Gen Psychiatry. 1985;42(8):815–20.
9. Walkup JT, LaBuda MC, Singer HS, Brown J, Riddle MA, Hurko O. Family study and segregation analysis of Tourette syndrome: evidence for a mixed model of inheritance. Am J Hum Genet. 1996;59(3):684–93.
10. Pauls DL, Raymond CL, Stevenson JM, Leckman JF. A family study of Gilles de la Tourette syndrome. Am J Hum Genet. 1991;48(1):154–63.
11. Centers for Disease Control and Prevention. Prevalence of diagnosed Tourette syndrome in persons aged 6-17 years – United States, 2007. MMWR Morb Mortal Wkly Rep. 2009; 58(21):581–5.
12. Robertson MM, Eapen V, Cavanna AE. The international prevalence, epidemiology, and clinical phenomenology of Tourette syndrome: a cross-cultural perspective. J Psychosom Res. 2009;67(6):475–83.
13. Baron M, Shapiro E, Shapiro A, Rainer JD. Genetic-analysis of Tourette syndrome suggesting major gene effect. Am J Hum Genet. 1981;33(5):767–75.
14. Curtis D, Robertson MM, Gurling HMD. Autosomal dominant gene Transmission in a large Kindred with Gilles-De-La-Tourette syndrome. Brit J Psychiat. 1992;160:845–9.
15. Kidd KK, Pauls DL. Genetic hypotheses for Tourette syndrome. Adv Neurol. 1982;35:243–9.
16. Pauls DL, Leckman JF. The inheritance of Gilles de la Tourette's syndrome and associated behaviors. Evidence for autosomal dominant transmission. N Engl J Med. 1986;315(16): 993–7.
17. Barr CL, Wigg KG, Kurlan R, Pakstis AJ, Kidd KK, Pauls D, et al. Genome scan for linkage to Gilles de la Tourette syndrome. Am J Hum Genet. 1999;65(4):A242-A.
18. Curtis D, Brett P, Dearlove AM, McQuillin A, Kalsi G, Robertson MM, et al. Genome scan of Tourette syndrome in a single large pedigree shows some support for linkage to regions of chromosomes 5, 10 and 13. Psychiatr Genet. 2004;14(2):83–7.
19. Heutink P, Vandewetering BJM, Breedveld GJ, Oostra BA. Genetic-study on Tourette syndrome in the Netherlands. Adv Neurol. 1992;58:167–72.
20. Mcmahon WM, Leppert M, Filloux F, Vandewetering BJM, Hasstedt S. Tourette symptoms in 161 related family members. Adv Neurol. 1992;58:159–65.
21. Pakstis AJ, Heutink P, Pauls DL, Kurlan R, Vandewetering BJM, Leckman JF, et al. Progress in the search for genetic-linkage with Tourette syndrome – an exclusion map covering more than 50-percent of the autosomal genome. Am J Hum Genet. 1991;48(2):281–94.
22. Pauls DL, Pakstis AJ, Kurlan R, Kidd KK, Leckman JF, Cohen DJ, et al. Segregation and linkage analyses of Tourette's syndrome and related disorders. J Am Acad Child Adolesc Psychiatry. 1990;29(2):195–203.
23. Verkerk AJMH, Cath DC, van der Linde HC, Both J, Heutink P, Breedveld G, et al. Genetic and clinical analysis of a large Dutch Gilles de la Tourette family. Mol Psychiatr. 2006; 11(10):954–64.
24. Hanna PA, Janjua FN, Contant CF, Jankovic J. Bilineal transmission in Tourette syndrome. Neurology. 1999;53(4):813–8.
25. Kurlan R, Eapen V, Stern J, McDermott MP, Robertson MM. Bilineal transmission in Tourette's syndrome families. Neurology. 1994;44(12):2336–42.
26. McMahon WM, van de Wetering BJM, Filloux F, Betit K, Coon H, Leppert M. Bilineal transmission and phenotypic variation of Tourette's disorder in a large pedigree. J Am Acad Child Adolesc Psychiatry. 1996;35(5):672–80.
27. Hasstedt SJ, Leppert M, Filloux F, Vandewetering BJM, Mcmahon WM. Intermediate inheritance of Tourette syndrome, assuming assortative mating. Am J Hum Genet. 1995;57(3):682–9.
28. Seuchter SA, Hebebrand J, Klug B, Knapp M, Lehmkuhl G, Poustka F, et al. Complex segregation analysis of families ascertained through Gilles de la Tourette syndrome. Genet Epidemiol. 2000;18(1):33–47.

29. Tourette Syndrome Association International Consortium for Genetics. Genome scan for Tourette disorder in affected-sibling-pair and multigenerational families. Am J Hum Genet. 2007;80(2):265–72.
30. Tourette Syndrome Association International Consortium for Genetics. A complete genome screen in sib pairs affected by Gilles de la Tourette syndrome. Am J Hum Genet. 1999;65(5):1428–36.
31. Zhang HP, Leckman JF, Pauls DL, Tsai CP, Kidd KK, Campos MR, et al. Genomewide scan of hoarding in sib pairs in which both sibs have Gilles de la Tourette syndrome. Am J Hum Genet. 2002;70(4):896–904.
32. Kroisel PM, Petek E, Emberger W, Windpassinger C, Wladika W, Wagner K. Candidate region for Gilles de la Tourette syndrome at 7q31. Am J Med Genet. 2001;101(3):259–61.
33. Miranda DM, Wigg K, Feng Y, Sandor P, Barr CL. Association study between Gilles de la Tourette Syndrome and two genes in the Robo-Slit pathway located in the chromosome 11q24 linked/associated region. Am J Med Genet Part B Neuropsychiatr Genet Off Publ Int Soc Psychiatr Genet. 2008;147B(1):68–72.
34. Paschou P, Feng Y, Pakstis AJ, Speed WC, DeMille MM, Kidd JR, et al. Indications of linkage and association of Gilles de la Tourette syndrome in two independent family samples: 17q25 is a putative susceptibility region. Am J Hum Genet. 2004;75(4):545–60.
35. Altshuler D, Daly MJ, Lander ES. Genetic mapping in human disease. Science. 2008; 322(5903):881–8.
36. Verkerk AJMH, Mathews CA, Joosse M, Eussen BHJ, Heutink P, Oostra BA, et al. CNTNAP2 is disrupted in a family with Gilles de la Tourette syndrome and obsessive compulsive disorder. Genomics. 2003;82(1):1–9.
37. Cruz C, Camarena B, King N, Páez F, Sidenberg D, de la Fuente JR, et al. Increased prevalence of the seven-repeat variant of the dopamine D4 receptor gene in patients with obsessive-compulsive disorder with tics. Neurosci Lett. 1997;231(1):1–4.
38. Díaz-Anzaldúa A, Joober R, Rivière JB, Dion Y, Lespérance P, Richer F, et al. Tourette syndrome and dopaminergic genes: a family-based association study in the French Canadian founder population. Mol Psychiatry. 2004;9(3):272–7.
39. Grice D, Leckman J, Pauls D, Kurlan R, Kidd K, Pakstis A, et al. Linkage disequilibrium between an allele at the dopamine D4 receptor locus and Tourette syndrome, by the transmission-disequilibrium test. Am J Hum Genet. 1996;59(3):644–52.
40. Herzberg I, Valencia-Duarte AV, Kay VA, White DJ, Müller H, Rivas IC, et al. Association of DRD2 variants and Gilles de la Tourette syndrome in a family-based sample from a South American population isolate. Psychiatr Genet. 2010;20(4):179–83.
41. Tarnok Z, Ronai Z, Gervai J, Kereszturi E, Gadoros J, Sasvari-Szekely M, et al. Dopaminergic candidate genes in Tourette syndrome: association between tic severity and 3' UTR polymorphism of the dopamine transporter gene. Am J Med Genet B Neuropsychiatr Genet. 2007;144B(7):900–5.
42. Barr CL, Wigg KG, Zovko E, Sandor P, Tsui LC. No evidence for a major gene effect of the dopamine D4 receptor gene in the susceptibility to Gilles de la Tourette syndrome in five Canadian families. Am J Med Genet. 1996;67(3):301–5.
43. Chou IC, Tsai CH, Lee CC, Kuo HT, Hsu YA, Li CI, et al. Association analysis between Tourette's syndrome and dopamine D1 receptor gene in Taiwanese children. Psychiat Genet. 2004;14(4):219–21.
44. Cavallini MC, Di Bella D, Catalano M, Bellodi L. An association study between 5-HTTLPR polymorphism, COMT polymorphism, and Tourette's syndrome. Psychiatry Res. 2000; 97(2–3):93–100.
45. Yoon D, Rippel C, Kobets A, Morris C, Lee J, Williams P, et al. Dopaminergic polymorphisms in Tourette syndrome: association with the DAT gene (SLC6A3). Am J Med Genet B Neuropsychiatr Genet. 2007;144B(5):605–10.
46. Chou IC, Tsai CH, Wan L, Hsu YA, Tsai FJ. Association study between Tourette's syndrome and polymorphisms of noradrenergic genes (ADRA2A, ADRA2C). Psychiat Genet. 2007;17(6):359.

47. Xu C, Ozbay F, Wigg K, Shulman R, Tahir E, Yazgan Y, et al. Evaluation of the genes for the adrenergic receptors alpha 2A and alpha 1C and Gilles de la Tourette Syndrome. Am J Med Genet B Neuropsychiatr Genet. 2003;119B(1):54–9.
48. Comings DE, Gade R, Muhleman D, Sverd J. No association of a tyrosine hydroxylase gene tetranucleotide repeat polymorphism in autism, Tourette syndrome, or ADHD. Biol Psychiatry. 1995;37(7):484–6.
49. Brett P, Curtis D, Robertson M, Gurling H. Exclusion of the 5-HT1A serotonin neuroreceptor and tryptophan oxygenase genes in a large British kindred multiply affected with Tourette's syndrome, chronic motor tics, and obsessive-compulsive behavior. Am J Psychiatry. 1995;152(3):437–40.
50. Mössner R, Müller-Vahl KR, Döring N, Stuhrmann M. Role of the novel tryptophan hydroxylase-2 gene in Tourette syndrome. Mol Psychiatry. 2007;12(7):617–9.
51. Moya PR, Wendland JR, Rubenstein LM, Timpano KR, Heiman GA, Tischfield JA, et al. Common and rare alleles of the serotonin transporter gene, SLC6A4, associated with Tourette's disorder. Mov Disord Off J Mov Disord Soc. 2013;28(9):1263–70.
52. Manolio TA, Collins FS, Cox NJ, Goldstein DB, Hindorff LA, Hunter DJ, et al. Finding the missing heritability of complex diseases. Nature. 2009;461(7265):747–53.
53. Lee SH, Wray NR, Goddard ME, Visscher PM. Estimating missing heritability for disease from genome-wide association studies. Am J Hum Genet. 2011;88(3):294–305.
54. Hindorff L, MacArthur J, Morales J, Junkins H, Hall P, Klemm A, et al. A catalog of published genome-wide association studies [August 1, 2014]. Available from: http://www.genome.gov/gwastudies.
55. Manolio TA. Genomewide association studies and assessment of the risk of disease. New Engl J Med. 2010;363(2):166–76.
56. Scharf JM, Yu D, Mathews CA, Neale BM, Stewart SE, Fagerness JA, et al. Genome-wide association study of Tourette's syndrome. Mol Psychiatr. 2013;18(6):721–8.
57. Davis LK, Yu D, Keenan CL, Gamazon ER, Konkashbaev AI, Derks EM, et al. Partitioning the heritability of Tourette syndrome and obsessive compulsive disorder reveals differences in genetic architecture. PLoS Genet. 2013;9(10):e1003864.
58. Paschou P, Yu D, Gerber G, Evans P, Tsetsos F, Davis LK, et al. Genetic association signal near NTN4 in Tourette syndrome. Ann Neurol. 2014;76(2):310–5.
59. Abelson JF, Kwan KY, O'Roak BJ, Baek DY, Stillman AA, Morgan TM, et al. Sequence variants in SLITRK1 are associated with Tourette's syndrome. Science. 2005;310(5746):317–20.
60. Boghosian-Sell L, Comings DE, Overhauser J. Tourette syndrome in a pedigree with a 7;18 translocation: identification of a YAC spanning the translocation breakpoint at 18q22.3. Am J Hum Genet. 1996;59(5):999–1005.
61. Cuker A, State MW, King RA, Davis N, Ward DC. Candidate locus for Gilles de la Tourette syndrome/obsessive compulsive disorder/chronic tic disorder at 18q22. Am J Med Genet A. 2004;130A(1):37–9.
62. Petek E, Windpassinger C, Vincent JB, Cheung J, Boright AP, Scherer SW, et al. Disruption of a novel gene (IMMP2L) by a breakpoint in 7q31 associated with Tourette syndrome. Am J Hum Genet. 2001;68(4):848–58.
63. State MW, Greally JM, Cuker A, Bowers PN, Henegariu O, Morgan TM, et al. Epigenetic abnormalities associated with a chromosome 18(q21-q22) inversion and a Gilles de la Tourette syndrome phenotype. Proc Natl Acad Sci U S A. 2003;100(8):4684–9.
64. Hooper SD, Johansson AC, Tellgren-Roth C, Stattin EL, Dahl N, Cavelier L, et al. Genome-wide sequencing for the identification of rearrangements associated with Tourette syndrome and obsessive-compulsive disorder. BMC Med Genet. 2012;13:123.
65. Shelley BP, Robertson MM, Turk J. An individual with Gilles de la Tourette syndrome and Smith-Magenis microdeletion syndrome: is chromosome 17p11.2 a candidate region for Tourette syndrome putative susceptibility genes? J Intellect Disabil Res JIDR. 2007;51(Pt 8):620–4.
66. Prontera P, Napolioni V, Ottaviani V, Rogaia D, Fusco C, Augello B, et al. DPP6 gene disruption in a family with Gilles de la Tourette syndrome. Neurogenetics. 2014;15:237–42.

67. Patel C, Cooper-Charles L, McMullan DJ, Walker JM, Davison V, Morton J. Translocation breakpoint at 7q31 associated with tics: further evidence for IMMP2L as a candidate gene for Tourette syndrome. Eur J Hum Genet. 2011;19(6):634–9.
68. Petek E, Schwarzbraun T, Noor A, Patel M, Nakabayashi K, Choufani S, et al. Molecular and genomic studies of IMMP2L and mutation screening in autism and Tourette syndrome. Mol Genet Genomics MGG. 2007;277(1):71–81.
69. Lawson-Yuen A, Saldivar JS, Sommer S, Picker J. Familial deletion within NLGN4 associated with autism and Tourette syndrome. Eur J Hum Genet. 2008;16(5):614–8.
70. Bertelsen B, Melchior L, Jensen LR, Groth C, Glenthoj B, Rizzo R, et al. Intragenic deletions affecting two alternative transcripts of the IMMP2L gene in patients with Tourette syndrome. Eur J Hum Genet EJHG. 2014;22:1283–9.
71. Alarcon M, Abrahams BS, Stone JL, Duvall JA, Perederiy JV, Bomar JM, et al. Linkage, association, and gene-expression analyses identify CNTNAP2 as an autism-susceptibility gene. Am J Hum Genet. 2008;82(1):150–9.
72. Arking DE, Cutler DJ, Brune CW, Teslovich TM, West K, Ikeda M, et al. A common genetic variant in the neurexin superfamily member CNTNAP2 increases familial risk of autism. Am J Hum Genet. 2008;82(1):160–4.
73. Bakkaloglu B, O'Roak BJ, Louvi A, Gupta AR, Abelson JE, Morgan TM, et al. Molecular cytogenetic analysis and resequencing of Contactin Associated Protein-Like 2 in autism spectrum disorders. Am J Hum Genet. 2008;82(1):165–73.
74. Friedman JI, Vrijenhoek T, Markx S, Janssen IM, Van der Vliet WA, Faas BHW, et al. CNTNAP2 gene dosage variation is associated with schizophrenia and epilepsy. Mol Psychiatr. 2008;13(3):261–6.
75. Penagarikano O, Abrahams BS, Herman EI, Winden KD, Gdalyahu A, Dong H, et al. Absence of CNTNAP2 leads to epilepsy, neuronal migration abnormalities, and core autism-related deficits. Cell. 2011;147(1):235–46.
76. Strauss KA, Puffenberger EG, Huentelman MJ, Gottlieb S, Dobrin SE, Parod JM, et al. Recessive symptomatic focal epilepsy and mutant contactin-associated protein-like 2. New Engl J Med. 2006;354(13):1370–7.
77. Zweier C, de Jong EK, Zweier M, Orrico A, Ousager LB, Collins AL, et al. CNTNAP2 and NRXN1 are mutated in autosomal-recessive Pitt-Hopkins-like mental retardation and determine the level of a common synaptic protein in Drosophila. Am J Hum Genet. 2009;85(5): 655–66.
78. Jamain S, Quach H, Betancur C, Rastam M, Colineaux C, Gillberg IC, et al. Mutations of the X-linked genes encoding neuroligins NLGN3 and NLGN4 are associated with autism. Nat Genet. 2003;34(1):27–9.
79. Laumonnier F, Bonnet-Brilhault F, Gomot M, Blanc R, David A, Moizard MP, et al. X-linked mental retardation and autism are associated with a mutation in the NLGN4 gene, a member of the neuroligin family. Am J Hum Genet. 2004;74(3):552–7.
80. Marshall CR, Noor A, Vincent JB, Lionel AC, Feuk L, Skaug J, et al. Structural variation of chromosomes in autism spectrum disorder. Am J Hum Genet. 2008;82(2):477–88.
81. Stillman AA, Krsnik Z, Sun JH, Rasin MR, State MW, Sestan N, et al. Developmentally regulated and evolutionarily conserved expression of SLITRK1 in brain circuits implicated in Tourette syndrome. J Comp Neurol. 2009;513(1):21–37.
82. Katayama K, Yamada K, Ornthanalai VG, Inoue T, Ota M, Murphy NP, et al. Slitrk1-deficient mice display elevated anxiety-like behavior and noradrenergic abnormalities. Mol Psychiatr. 2010;15(2):177–84.
83. Karagiannidis I, Rizzo R, Tarnok Z, Wolanczyk T, Hebebrand J, Nothen MM, et al. Replication of association between a SLITRK1 haplotype and Tourette syndrome in a large sample of families. Mol Psychiatr. 2012;17(7):665–8.
84. Miranda DM, Wigg K, Kabia EM, Feng Y, Sandor P, Barr CL. Association of SLITRK1 to Gilles de la Tourette syndrome. Am J Med Genet B. 2009;150B(4):483–6.
85. Chou IC, Wan L, Liu SC, Tsai CH, Tsai FJ. Association of the Slit and Trk-like 1 gene in Taiwanese patients with Tourette syndrome. Pediatr Neurol. 2007;37(6):404–6.

86. Deng H, Le WD, Xie WJ, Jankovic J. Examination of the SLITRK1 gene in Caucasian patients with Tourette syndrome – clinical commentary. Acta Neurol Scand. 2006;114(6): 400–2.
87. Keen-Kim D, Mathews CA, Reus VI, Lowe TL, Herrera LD, Budman CL, et al. Overrepresentation of rare variants in a specific ethnic group may confuse interpretation of association analyses. Hum Mol Genet. 2006;15(22):3324–8.
88. Scharf JM, Moorjani P, Fagerness J, Platko JV, Illmann C, Galloway B, et al. Lack of association between SLITRK1var321 and Tourette syndrome in a large family-based sample. Neurology. 2008;70(16 Pt 2):1495–6.
89. Zimprich A, Hatala K, Riederer F, Stogmann E, Aschauer HN, Stamenkovic M. Sequence analysis of the complete SLITRK1 gene in Austrian patients with Tourette's disorder. Psychiatr Genet. 2008;18(6):308–9.
90. Yasmeen S, Melchior L, Bertelsen B, Skov L, Mol Debes N, Tumer Z. Sequence analysis of SLITRK1 for var321 in Danish patients with Tourette syndrome and review of the literature. Psychiatr Genet. 2013;23(3):130–3.
91. Ercan-Sencicek AG, Stillman AA, Ghosh AK, Bilguvar K, O'Roak BJ, Mason CE, et al. L-histidine decarboxylase and Tourette's syndrome. New Engl J Med. 2010;362(20):1901–8.
92. Ferrada C, Ferre S, Casado V, Cortes A, Justinova Z, Barnes C, et al. Interactions between histamine H3 and dopamine D2 receptors and the implications for striatal function. Neuropharmacology. 2008;55(2):190–7.
93. Munzar P, Tanda G, Justinova Z, Goldberg SR. Histamine H3 receptor antagonists potentiate methamphetamine self-administration and methamphetamine-induced accumbal dopamine release. Neuropsychopharmacol. 2004;29(4):705–17.
94. Haas HL, Sergeeva OA, Selbach O. Histamine in the nervous system. Physiol Rev. 2008;88(3):1183–241.
95. Ellender TJ, Huerta-Ocampo I, Deisseroth K, Capogna M, Bolam JP. Differential modulation of excitatory and inhibitory striatal synaptic transmission by histamine. J Neurosci. 2011; 31(43):15340–51.
96. Kubota Y, Ito C, Sakurai E, Sakurai E, Watanabe T, Ohtsu H. Increased methamphetamine-induced locomotor activity and behavioral sensitization in histamine-deficient mice. J Neurochem. 2002;83(4):837–45.
97. Castellan Baldan L, Williams KA, Gallezot JD, Pogorelov V, Rapanelli M, Crowley M, et al. Histidine decarboxylase deficiency causes Tourette syndrome: parallel findings in humans and mice. Neuron. 2014;81(1):77–90.
98. Fernandez TV, Sanders SJ, Yurkiewicz IR, Ercan-Sencicek AG, Kim YS, Fishman DO, et al. Rare copy number variants in Tourette syndrome disrupt genes in histaminergic pathways and overlap with autism. Biol Psychiatry. 2012;71(5):392–402.
99. Karagiannidis I, Dehning S, Sandor P, Tarnok Z, Rizzo R, Wolanczyk T, et al. Support of the histaminergic hypothesis in Tourette syndrome: association of the histamine decarboxylase gene in a large sample of families. J Med Genet. 2013;50(11):760–4.
100. Conrad DF, Pinto D, Redon R, Feuk L, Gokcumen O, Zhang Y, et al. Origins and functional impact of copy number variation in the human genome. Nature. 2010;464(7289):704–12.
101. Iafrate AJ, Feuk L, Rivera MN, Listewnik ML, Donahoe PK, Qi Y, et al. Detection of large-scale variation in the human genome. Nat Genet. 2004;36(9):949–51.
102. Redon R, Ishikawa S, Fitch KR, Feuk L, Perry GH, Andrews TD, et al. Global variation in copy number in the human genome. Nature. 2006;444(7118):444–54.
103. Sebat J, Lakshmi B, Troge J, Alexander J, Young J, Lundin P, et al. Large-scale copy number polymorphism in the human genome. Science. 2004;305(5683):525–8.
104. Pinto D, Pagnamenta AT, Klei L, Anney R, Merico D, Regan R, et al. Functional impact of global rare copy number variation in autism spectrum disorders. Nature. 2010;466(7304): 368–72.
105. Sanders SJ, Ercan-Sencicek AG, Hus V, Luo R, Murtha MT, Moreno-De-Luca D, et al. Multiple recurrent De Novo CNVs, including duplications of the 7q11.23 Williams syndrome region, are strongly associated with autism. Neuron. 2011;70(5):863–85.

106. Sebat J, Lakshmi B, Malhotra D, Troge J, Lese-Martin C, Walsh T, et al. Strong association of de novo copy number mutations with autism. Science. 2007;316(5823):445–9.
107. Xu B, Roos JL, Levy S, van Rensburg EJ, Gogos JA, Karayiorgou M. Strong association of de novo copy number mutations with sporadic schizophrenia. Nat Genet. 2008;40(7):880–5.
108. Sundaram SK, Huq AM, Wilson BJ, Chugani HT. Tourette syndrome is associated with recurrent exonic copy number variants. Neurology. 2010;74(20):1583–90.
109. Kalanithi PSA, Zheng W, Kataoka Y, DiFiglia M, Grantz H, Saper CB, et al. Altered parvalbumin-positive neuron distribution in basal ganglia of individuals with Tourette syndrome. Proc Natl Acad Sci U S A. 2005;102(37):13307–12.
110. Kataoka Y, Kalanithi PSA, Grantz H, Schwartz ML, Saper C, Leckman JF, et al. Decreased number of parvalbumin and cholinergic interneurons in the striatum of individuals with Tourette syndrome. J Comp Neurol. 2010;518(3):277–91.
111. Lennington JB, Coppola G, Kataoka-Sasaki Y, Fernandez TV, Palejev D, Li Y, et al. Transcriptome analysis of the human striatum in Tourette syndrome. Biol Psychiatry. 2014:24. pii: S0006–3223(14)00551–4. doi: 10.1016/j.biopsych.2014.07.018. [Epub ahead of print]
112. Nag A, Bochukova EG, Kremeyer B, Campbell DD, Muller H, Valencia-Duarte AV, et al. CNV analysis in Tourette syndrome implicates large genomic rearrangements in COL8A1 and NRXN1. PLoS One. 2013;8(3):e59061.
113. McGrath LM, Yu DM, Marshall C, Davis LK, Thiruvahindrapuram B, Li BB, et al. Copy number variation in obsessive-compulsive disorder and Tourette syndrome: a cross-disorder study. J Am Acad Child Adolesc Psychiatry. 2014;53(8):910–9.
114. Sundaram SK, Huq AM, Sun Z, Yu W, Bennett L, Wilson BJ, et al. Exome sequencing of a pedigree with Tourette syndrome or chronic tic disorder. Ann Neurol. 2011;69(5):901–4.
115. Lit L, Gilbert DL, Walker W, Sharp FR. A subgroup of Tourette's patients overexpress specific natural killer cell genes in blood: a preliminary report. Am J Med Genet Part B Neuropsychiatr Genet Off Publ Int Soc Psychiatr Genet. 2007;144B(7):958–63.
116. Tian Y, Gunther JR, Liao IH, Liu D, Ander BP, Stamova BS, et al. GABA- and acetylcholine-related gene expression in blood correlate with tic severity and microarray evidence for alternative splicing in Tourette syndrome: a pilot study. Brain Res. 2011;1381:228–36.
117. Tian Y, Liao IH, Zhan X, Gunther JR, Ander BP, Liu D, et al. Exon expression and alternatively spliced genes in Tourette syndrome. Am J Med Genet Part B Neuropsychiatr Genet Off Publ Int Soc Psychiatr Genet. 2011;156B(1):72–8.
118. Hong JJ, Loiselle CR, Yoon DY, Lee O, Becker KG, Singer HS. Microarray analysis in Tourette syndrome postmortem putamen. J Neurol Sci. 2004;225(1–2):57–64.
119. Tian Y, Apperson ML, Ander BP, Liu D, Stomova BS, Jickling GC, et al. Differences in exon expression and alternatively spliced genes in blood of multiple sclerosis compared to healthy control subjects. J Neuroimmunol. 2011;230(1–2):124–9.
120. Leckman JF, Katsovich L, Kawikova I, Lin H, Zhang H, Kronig H, et al. Increased serum levels of interleukin-12 and tumor necrosis factor-alpha in Tourette's syndrome. Biol Psychiatry. 2005;57(6):667–73.
121. Zhao Y, Marin O, Hermesz E, Powell A, Flames N, Palkovits M, et al. The LIM-homeobox gene Lhx8 is required for the development of many cholinergic neurons in the mouse forebrain. Proc Natl Acad Sci U S A. 2003;100(15):9005–10.
122. Mori T, Yuxing Z, Takaki H, Takeuchi M, Iseki K, Hagino S, et al. The LIM homeobox gene, L3/Lhx8, is necessary for proper development of basal forebrain cholinergic neurons. Eur J Neurosci. 2004;19(12):3129–41.
123. Chen L, Chatterjee M, Li JY. The mouse homeobox gene Gbx2 is required for the development of cholinergic interneurons in the striatum. J Neurosci. 2010;30(44):14824–34.
124. Marin O. Interneuron dysfunction in psychiatric disorders. Nat Rev Neurosci. 2012;13(2): 107–20.
125. Langfelder P, Horvath S. WGCNA: an R package for weighted correlation network analysis. BMC bioinformatics. 2008;9:559.

126. Morshed SA, Parveen S, Leckman JF, Mercadante MT, Bittencourt Kiss MH, Miguel EC, et al. Antibodies against neural, nuclear, cytoskeletal, and streptococcal epitopes in children and adults with Tourette's syndrome, Sydenham's chorea, and autoimmune disorders. Biol Psychiatry. 2001;50(8):566–77.
127. Murphy TK, Storch EA, Turner A, Reid JM, Tan J, Lewin AB. Maternal history of autoimmune disease in children presenting with tics and/or obsessive-compulsive disorder. J Neuroimmunol. 2010;229(1–2):243–7.
128. Kawikova I, Leckman JF, Kronig H, Katsovich L, Bessen DE, Ghebremichael M, et al. Decreased numbers of regulatory T cells suggest impaired immune tolerance in children with Tourette syndrome: a preliminary study. Biol Psychiatry. 2007;61(3):273–8.
129. Bos-Veneman NG, Olieman R, Tobiasova Z, Hoekstra PJ, Katsovich L, Bothwell AL, et al. Altered immunoglobulin profiles in children with Tourette syndrome. Brain Behav Immun. 2011;25(3):532–8.
130. Dietrich A, Fernandez TV, King RA, State MW, Tischfield JA, Hoekstra PJ, et al. The Tourette International Collaborative Genetics (TIC Genetics) study, finding the genes causing Tourette syndrome: objectives and methods. Eur Child Adolesc Psychiatry. 2015;24:141–51.

Chapter 10
Genetics of Paroxysmal Dyskinesia

Knut Brockmann and Hendrik Rosewich

Abstract Paroxysmal dyskinesias (PxDs) constitute a clinically and genetically heterogeneous group of rare conditions characterized by recurrent brief episodes of abnormal involuntary movements. PxDs may present with episodic choreic, ballistic, athetoid features or any mixture of dystonic symptoms. Current classification of PxDs based on different precipitating factors recognizes three subtypes including paroxysmal kinesigenic (PKD), nonkinesigenic (PNKD), and exercise-induced (PED) dyskinesia. Neurological examination between the attacks is usually normal in these subtypes. However, PxDs occur as a distinct feature of complex chronic neurological disorders, comprising Glut1 deficiency syndrome, MCT8 deficiency (Allen-Herndon-Dudley syndrome), and ATP1A3-related conditions (alternating hemiplegia of childhood; rapid-onset dystonia-parkinsonism). Alliance of meticulous phenotyping with state-of-the-art methods of molecular genetics resulted in new insights concerning the genetic causes of PxDs.

Keywords Paroxysmal kinesigenic dyskinesia • Paroxysmal nonkinesigenic dyskinesia • Paroxysmal exercise-induced dyskinesia • *PRRT2* • Glut1 deficiency syndrome • *ATP1A3*

K. Brockmann, MD (✉)
Interdisciplinary Pediatric Center for Children with Developmental Disabilities and Severe Chronic Disorders, University Medical Center, Georg August University Göttingen, Göttingen 37075, Germany
e-mail: kbrock@med.uni-goettingen.de

H. Rosewich, MD
Division of Pediatric Neurology, Department of Pediatrics and Adolescent Medicine, University Medical Center Göttingen, Georg August University, Göttingen 37099, Germany

Department of Pediatrics and Pediatric Neurology, University Medical Center Göttingen, Georg August University, Göttingen, Germany

S.A. Schneider, J.M.T. Brás (eds.), *Movement Disorder Genetics*,
DOI 10.1007/978-3-319-17223-1_10

Introduction

Paroxysmal dyskinesias (PxDs) constitute a clinically and genetically heterogeneous group of rare conditions characterized by recurrent brief episodes of abnormal involuntary movements. PxDs present with episodic choreic, ballistic, athetoid features or any mixture of dystonic symptoms. Neurological examination between the attacks is usually normal. On the other hand, PxDs are seen in more complex chronic neurological disorders comprising glucose transport protein type 1 deficiency syndrome (Glut1-DS), Allan-Herndon-Dudley syndrome (monocarboxylate transporter 8 deficiency), alternating hemiplegia of childhood (AHC), and various other conditions.

Classification of Paroxysmal Dyskinesias (PxDs)

Based on the European Federation of Neurological Societies current scheme, dystonia in general may be classified by etiology, by age at onset, or by distribution of affected body parts [1]. In this scheme, paroxysmal dystonia/dyskinesias (PxDs) constitute a subtype of primary dystonia. Similar to classification of dystonia at large, systematization of PxDs is "complex and not entirely satisfactory" [2].

While early denominations focused largely on the duration of attacks [3], the current classification of PxDs is based on the difference of precipitating factors. Three subtypes are recognized including paroxysmal nonkinesigenic (PNKD), kinesigenic (PKD), and exercise-induced (PED) dyskinesia [4–6]. Idiopathic (genetic, primary) PxDs are discriminated from symptomatic (acquired, secondary) PxDs, depending on the etiology [7]. In idiopathic PxDs, familial as well as sporadic cases are observed. According to the current conventional definition, there are no abnormal findings on neurological examination between the attacks in idiopathic (genetic, primary) PxDs. The clinical diagnosis is based upon history and occasionally upon personal observation or videotaping of an attack. The presence of baseline neurological defects has been thought to be a distinguishing feature between primary and symptomatic (acquired, secondary) PxDs [7]. Symptomatic PxDs are typically accompanied by neurological symptoms discernable between the paroxysms. These interictal features may comprise intellectual disability, epilepsy, and persistent movement disorders.

However, during the last decade evidence has evolved indicating that several genetic conditions with prominent persistent neurological defects are accompanied by PxDs as well. PxDs were recognized to be part of multifaceted genetic disorders with marked baseline neurological defects [8]. Thus, we propose a classification of PxDs which separates "pure" from "complicated" PxDs, similar to the widely accepted classification of hereditary spastic paraplegia. In pure PxDs, the neurological examination between the attacks is normal. In complicated PxDs, the episodic dyskinesias are embedded in persisting neurological abnormalities evident on physical examination between the attacks. Pure PxDs are of genetic origin in general, while complicated PxDs may arise in genetic as well as in acquired conditions.

Furthermore, based on recent discoveries of genetic causes of different subtypes of pure PxDs, it has been recognized that there is no consistent genotype-phenotype correlation in these conditions. Each subtype of pure PxDs (PNKD, PKD, and PED) displays genetic heterogeneity, as many affected patients do not carry a mutation in one of the presently discovered genes. On the other hand, the phenotypic spectra of mutations in *PRRT2*, *SLC2A1*, and *MR1* keep expanding, thus indicating marked pleiotropy of these molecular alterations [9].

Table 10.1 summarizes clinical and genetic features of pure and complicated genetic PxDs.

Paroxysmal hypnogenic dyskinesia (PHD), delineated as a further subtype in former classifications [5] and characterized by attacks of dyskinesia occurring primarily during sleep, is now generally recognized as autosomal dominant nocturnal frontal lobe epilepsy.

Paroxysmal Dyskinesia with Normal Interepisodic Findings (Pure PxDs)

Paroxysmal Nonkinesigenic Dyskinesia (PNKD)

Familial paroxysmal nonkinesigenic dyskinesia (PNKD), first described in 1940 by Mount and Reback, was originally designated familial paroxysmal choreoathetosis [10]. In PNKD, involuntary movements comprising any combination of chorea, athetosis, and ballism occur spontaneously in recurrent episodes without a trigger such as sudden movement or physical exertion. The dyskinetic paroxysms involve the limbs, face, and trunk. Consciousness is preserved. Some patients report premonitory sensations, mainly focal limb paresthesia. Caffeine, alcohol, sleep deprivation, and emotional stress may reduce the threshold of these paroxysms. Duration of attacks is longer than in PKD and ranges from minutes to hours. Interepisodic neurological examination does not reveal any abnormalities. Most cases are familial following an autosomal dominant pattern of inheritance. While all types of PNKD share these characteristics in common, they display clinical variety with respect to age of onset, precipitating factors, paroxysmal symptoms, and response to medication as well as genetic heterogeneity.

Genetics of PNKD

MR1

As early as 1996, a first PNKD gene had been mapped to the long arm of chromosome 2. Almost 20 years later, the gene was identified, when in 2004 two independent research groups discovered heterozygous mutations in the myofibrillogenesis regulator gene (*MR1*) in several families with PNKD [11, 12]. Penetrance is reduced, as single family members carried a mutation but were free of PNKD.

Table 10.1 Clinical and genetic features of paroxysmal dyskinesias

Disorder (abbreviation)	OMIM	Clinical hallmarks	Inheritance	Gene	Location	Remarks
Pure PxDs (normal interepisodic findings)						
PNKD						
Paroxysmal nonkinesigenic dyskinesia (PNKD)	#118800	Onset in early childhood	AD	*MF1*	2q35	
		Precipitation by caffeine, alcohol				
		Duration of attacks 10 min to few hrs				
Paroxysmal nonkinesigenic dyskinesia and generalized epilepsy (GEPD)	#609446	Onset in early childhood	AD	*KCNMA1*	10q22	One family reported
		Absences, GTCS				
Paroxysmal nonkinesigenic dyskinesia	%611147	PNKD affecting hands and feet	AD	?	2q31	One family reported
PKD						
Paroxysmal kinesigenic dyskinesia (PKD)	#128200	Onset age 6–15 yrs		*PRRT2*	16p11.2	Allelism with BFIS, ICCA, hemiplegic migraine, others. Genetic heterogeneity
		Sudden movements trigger attacks				
		Duration of attacks seconds to 1 min				
		Response to CPZ, PHT				
PED						
Paroxysmal exercise-induced dyskinesia (PED)	#612126	PED without epilepsy or learning difficulties	AD	*SLC2A1*	1p34.2	DYT18, mild variant of GLUT1-DS
Rolandic epilepsy with PED and writer's cramp (RE-PED-WC)	%608105	Rolandic seizures and PED peaking in childhood, writer's cramp persisting.	AR	?	16p12-11.2	One family reported. Similarity with ICCA

Infantile paroxysmal dyskinesia						
Transient paroxysmal dystonia of infancy	–	Onset in first months of life	Sporadic	?	?	Infantile variant of PKD?
		Opisthotonus, (a) symmetrical dyskinesia of arms, cessation within first years of life, normal development				
Benign paroxysmal torticollis of infancy	–	Onset in first year of life	Sporadic	?	?	*CACNA1A* or *PRRT2* mutations reported in few cases
		Paroxysmal tilting of head, vomiting, duration hours to days, persisting during sleep, cessation by 3–5 years of age				Family history of migraine
Complicated PxDs (embedded in chronic and complex neurological conditions)						
Glucose transport protein type 1 deficiency syndrome (GLUT1-DS)	#606777	Wide phenotypic variability from infantile epileptic encephalopathy to adult-onset absence seizures	AD	*SLC2A1*	1p34.2	Reduced CSF glucose level, reduced CSF/blood glucose ratio
		PED in many patients				
Paroxysmal exercise induced (PED) with or without epilepsy and/or hemolytic anemia	#612126	PED with or without epilepsy, learning difficulties	AD	*SLC2A1*	1p34.2	DYT18, part of GLUT1-DS

(continued)

Table 10.1 (continued)

Disorder (abbreviation)	OMIM	Clinical hallmarks	Inheritance	Gene	Location	Remarks
Paroxysmal choreoathetosis and progressive spastic paraplegia	#601042	PKD/PED, onset in childhood	AD	*SLC2A1*	1p34.2	DYT9, part of GLUT1-DS
		Spastic paraplegia				
		Cognitive impairment				
Alternating hemiplegia of childhood (AHC)	#614820	Onset before age 18 mo	AD	*ATP1A3*	19q13.2	Phenotypic spectrum with RDP (DYT12)
		Paroxysmal hemidystonia, hemiplegia triggered by emotional, physical stress				
		Baseline DD/ID, ataxia, dystonia				
Monocarboxylate transporter 8 (MCT8) deficiency, Allan-Herndon-Dudley syndrome	#300523	Severe intellectual disability	XD	*SLC16A2*	Xq13.2	Increased serum triiodothyronine (FT3)
		Hypotonia, later spasticity, ataxia				
		Elongated face, bitemporal narrowing				
		PKD in some patients, triggered by passive movements				

Adapted and modified from Brockmann [8]. With kind permission from Springer Science and Business Media

Abbreviations: *AD* autosomal dominant, *BFIS* benign familial infantile seizures, *CBZ* carbamazepine, *CNS* central nervous system, *DD/ID* developmental delay/intellectual disability, *DYT9* dystonia 9, *DYT12* dystonia 12, *DYT18* dystonia 18, *ICCA* infantile convulsions and choreoathetosis, *GTCS* generalized tonic-clonic seizure, *hrs* hours, *min* minute, *mo* months, *OMIM* Online Mendelian Inheritance in Man, *PHT* phenytoin, *RDP* rapid-onset dystonia-parkinsonism, *XD* X-linked dominant, *yrs* years

The *MR1* (alternatively designated *PNKD*) gene on chromosome 2q35 contains 12 exons and encodes for a protein with three isoforms (MR1L, MR1M, and MR1S) with different cellular distribution and presumably distinct biological functions. The CNS-specific isoform MR1L consists of 385 amino acids and is localized mainly on the cell membrane. However, details of its function are not yet known [11, 12]. Studies of the subcellular localization of both wild-type and mutant MR1 isoforms pointed to a novel disease mechanism involving the mitochondrial targeting sequence [13]. Investigations of the stability, cellular localization, and enzymatic activity of the PNKD protein in cultured cells and transgenic animals indicated that *MR1* mutations disrupt protein processing in vivo resulting in an impairment of cellular redox status due to reduced glutathione levels [14].

Subsequently *MR1* mutations were confirmed in further kindreds with PNKD. A large study included 49 patients with PNKD from eight families carrying *MR1* mutations and compared them with 22 patients from six kindreds with clinical diagnosis of PKND but without *MR1* mutations [15]. In kindreds with *MR1* mutations, penetrance was calculated as 98 %. In patients with *MR1* mutations, onset of attacks was in infancy or early childhood, attacks were precipitated by consumption of either alcohol or caffeine, and PNKD showed positive response to benzodiazepines or sleep. In contrast, patients with PNKD who did not carry an *MR1* mutation showed a broader variation in their age of onset, triggering factors, paroxysmal features, and response to medication [15].

To date, a total of 73 patients from 13 families with MR1 mutations have been reported (reviewed in [9]). In a small number of patients, PxDs were triggered by prolonged exercise, thus linking *MR1* mutations with PED.

KCNMA1

In a large kindred with 16 individuals (10 males, 6 females) who were affected by PNKD ($n=7$), generalized epileptic seizures (absence, generalized tonic-clonic) ($n=4$), or both ($n=5$), the locus was mapped to chromosome 10q22 (generalized epilepsy and paroxysmal dyskinesia, GEPD, OMIM #609446). The region identified by linkage analysis contained two genes encoding ion channels, and a missense mutation was detected in one of them, the *KCNMA1* gene. This gene encodes for the pore-forming α-subunit of the BK channel, a calcium-sensitive potassium channel [16]. To date, no further patients with this disorder were reported.

Locus 2q31

Autosomal dominantly inherited PNKD was observed in a Canadian family with 10 affected members (8 females, 2 males) over three generations [17]. PNKD involved the hands and feet symmetrically, with a duration ranging between 2 and 10 min. The attacks were not triggered by movement, exercise, alcohol, caffeine, or excitement. Onset was variable, ranging from 1 to 77 years. Genetic analysis of the *MR1* gene was normal in these patients. A locus was identified on chromosome 2q31 [17] and termed PNKD2 (OMIM %611147), although its report dated slightly later than the discovery of *KCNMA1*-associated PNKD.

PRRT2 and *SLC2A1*

Few patients with mutations of the *PRRT2* or the *SLC2A1* gene experience PNKD. They are discussed in more details below.

Paroxysmal Kinesigenic Dyskinesia (PKD)

In 1967 Kertesz was the first to describe a condition then termed paroxysmal kinesigenic choreoathetosis [18]. Later designated paroxysmal kinesigenic dyskinesia (PKD), and alternatively called episodic kinesigenic dyskinesia (EKD), this subtype has now been recognized as the most common form of PxDs. Attacks consist of choreatic, ballistic, and mixed dystonic symptoms with unilateral, bilateral, or alternating appearance. Involvement of the face may result in dysarthria or anarthria. However, consciousness is preserved, and the attacks are not painful. Mean age at onset is 10 years, with a range from 1 to 40 years [9]. PKD episodes are precipitated by sudden movements like initiation of standing, walking, or running. Attacks are short, with duration ranging from a few seconds to a minute. An aura is reported by a subset of patients. Aura symptoms comprise paresthesias, numbness, tingling sensations, or a feeling of muscular tension in the limb that immediately afterward would display the dyskinesia. Some patients learn to prevent the episode by slowing down their movement. Attacks recur frequently with most patients having up to 20 attacks daily, up to 100 episodes per day in puberty, and marked decrease in frequency after age 20 years.

In a large series of 121 patients, about two thirds had a family history of PKD [19]. Sporadic occurrence is observed more frequently in males than in females [19, 20].

Neurological examination is normal in primary PKD. Neuroimaging and laboratory studies may help in ruling out secondary PKD caused by multiple sclerosis, cerebral vascular disorder, or traumatic brain injury.

Genetics of PKD

The combination of familial PKD with benign familial infantile convulsions (BFIS) in the same family or even the same patient had been recognized for a long time [21]. Linkage studies in kindreds with the infantile convulsions and choreoathetosis (ICCA) syndrome and in families with PKD mapped the locus for both disorders to the pericentric region of chromosome 16 [22–24]. Thus, allelism of these conditions was suggested. Further studies narrowed down the critical region for PKD/ICCA. However, conventional genetic methods including linkage and haplotype analysis as well as Sanger sequencing of more than 150 genes located around the critical region in chromosome 16 were not able to identify the associated gene [25]. Only with the advent of whole-exome sequencing it was possible to demonstrate heterozygous mutations in *PRRT2* as a cause of PKD [26–29]. The *PRRT2* gene consists of four exons and encodes the proline-rich transmembrane protein 2. This protein comprises 340 amino acids and two putative transmembrane domains. Numerous reports subsequently confirmed that *PRRT2* mutations are the major cause of both, PKD and BFIS [30–35]. Most of these mutations are truncating and are predicted to result in haploinsufficiency. A recent review analyzed clinical features of 374 patients with *PRRT2* mutations reported in the literature [9].

Phenotypic Spectrum of PRRT2-Related Disorders

Heterozygous *PRRT2* changes are found with high prevalence in familial PKD, BFIS, and ICCA and somewhat less often in sporadic patients. The detection of *PRRT2* mutations in episodic neurological disorders prompted molecular analysis of this gene in similar conditions. This resulted in a remarkable unfolding of the clinical phenotypes of *PRRT2* mutations, which were discovered in patients with migraine, hemiplegic migraine, episodic ataxia, febrile seizures, sporadic infantile convulsions, and paroxysmal torticollis – as sole presentation or in various combinations [36–47].

Homozygous *PRRT2* mutations were detected in two families with more severe clinical features comprising intellectual disability, episodic ataxia, and infantile seizures [48, 49].

However, *PRRT2* mutations are not a common cause of infantile epileptic encephalopathies (IEE). In a cohort of 220 patients with IEE, neither the frequent c.649-650insC mutation nor any other pathogenic variants in *PRRT2* were found [50].

The function of the proline-rich transmembrane protein 2 is hardly understood at present. Evidence for an interaction with synaptosomal-associated protein 25 (SNAP-25) indicates an involvement in the release of neurotransmitters from synaptic vesicles at the presynaptic membrane [51]. An imbalance in the release of excitatory and inhibitory transmitters may result in episodic neurological features including seizures and PKD. Further research is needed to clarify the function of PRRT2 in detail.

While there is now evidence that mutations of the *PRRT2* gene are the major cause of PKD, genetic heterogeneity in this most frequent subtype of PxDs is suggested by several studies [52, 53].

Paroxysmal Dystonia of Infancy

The term transient paroxysmal dystonia of infancy designates a rare condition observed in infants aged 1–7 months with brief frequently recurring episodes of opisthotonus or symmetrical or asymmetrical dyskinesia of the upper limbs [54–56]. Frequency of episodes usually decreases, and complete resolution of paroxysms is observed over the first years of life. Development is unimpaired. Paroxysms may be precipitated by certain movements or positions. Thus, this condition may present an infantile variant of PKD. The cause is unknown, and *PRRT2* mutations are not yet on record.

Benign Paroxysmal Torticollis of Infancy

Benign paroxysmal torticollis of infancy is characterized by recurrent episodes of cervical dystonia. A recent report concerned 10 patients and reviewed 103 cases described in the literature [57]. Onset is during the 1st year of life. Paroxysmal tilting of the head may be accompanied by vomiting, signs of discomfort, pallor, ataxia, limb dystonia, tortipelvis, and gaze abnormalities. Torticollis may concern the same side or alternate sides with successive episodes. Attacks last from several hours to a few days and typically persist during sleep. Paroxysms usually dissolve by age 3–5 years. Search for triggering factors was largely negative. Many patients show early gross and fine motor delay of mild to moderate severity, which may persist in a few cases. A family history of migraine is frequent, and there is obviously a relationship to benign paroxysmal vertigo as well as to paroxysmal dystonia of infancy [57, 58]. In a few patients with benign paroxysmal torticollis mutations of the CACNA1A gene encoding for a neuronal calcium channel were detected [59]. In addition, a *PRRT2* mutation was found in a patient with transient infantile paroxysmal torticollis [41]. Further studies will clarify whether *CACNA1A* and *PRRT2* mutations significantly account for infantile paroxysmal torticollis or paroxysmal dystonia.

Paroxysmal Exercise-Induced Dyskinesia (PED)

The term paroxysmal exercise-induced dyskinesia (PED) designates a rare subtype of PxDs with phenotypical and genetic heterogeneity. In PED, episodes of dyskinesia are by definition triggered by prolonged exercise. Additional precipitating factors were reported in some patients comprising passive movements, exposure to cold, or electric nerve stimulation [60, 61].

Duration of episodes ranges from a few minutes to several hours, largely shorter than in PNKD, but clearly longer than in PKD. Frequency of episodes depends on the extent of sustained physical exercise and the individual threshold for a PED. A compilation of reports of approximately nine families and 20 sporadic patients with PED was provided by Suls et al. [62].

PED may constitute the only clinical symptom without any accompanying clinical features between the attacks [61]. On the other hand, PED may occur together with epilepsy, as reported in several patients and families [60, 63, 64]. PED was observed in association with rolandic epilepsy and writer's cramp (RE-PED-WC,

OMIM %608105) [65] and with migraine [66]. Moreover, PED may be embedded in a more complex chronic neurological condition. PED was reported as a presenting symptom of young-onset Parkinson's disease [67, 68]. The genes associated with these disorders are not yet identified.

Genetics of PED

At present, mutations in the *SLC2A1* gene encoding for glucose transport protein type 1 (GLUT1) are considered the major cause of PED in both sporadic patients and affected families (DYT18, OMIM #612126) [62, 69, 70]. PED has been recognized to be part of the phenotypic spectrum of GLUT1 deficiency syndrome (GLUT1-DS) and in fact had been mentioned in this context earlier [71]. Most patients with PED due to *SLC2A1* mutations present with complex interepisodic neurological features. A recent review of 41 mostly sporadic patients with *SLC2A1-related* PxDs attributed exercise as precipitating factor in 95.2 % and reported concomitant disturbances in 65.8 % [9]. Therefore, this condition is addressed in more detail in the next chapter. Possibly, particularly the mono- or oligosymptomatic GLUT1-DS patients with PED as the prominent feature will go undiagnosed in many cases.

Paroxysmal Dyskinesia Embedded in Chronic Neurological Conditions (Complicated PxDs)

PxDs are occasionally incorporated in a chronic and complex neurological disease. Only for a few of these conditions detailed phenotypic description and elucidation of the genetic basis has been achieved to date.

Glucose Transport Protein Type 1 Deficiency Syndrome (GLUT1-DS)

A continuous maintenance of glucose provides the main energy supply for the mammalian brain. Transfer of hydrophilic glucose across the lipophilic blood-brain barrier is facilitated by the glucose transport protein type 1 (GLUT1). Heterozygous mutations of the *SLC2A1* gene encoding GLUT1 impair glucose transport into the brain. Most reported mutations occurred *de novo*; in familial cases, the disorder is inherited following an autosomal dominant trait. The classic phenotype was designated GLUT1 deficiency syndrome (GLUT1-DS, OMIM #606777) and comprises marked motor and mental developmental delay, epilepsy with onset in the 1st year of life, deceleration of head growth resulting in secondary microcephaly, and a mixed movement disorder with spasticity, dystonia, and ataxia. Lowered glucose levels in CSF (hypoglycorrhachia) and a reduced ratio of the glucose concentrations in CSF and serum are the clinical laboratory hallmarks. Therapy with ketogenic diet provides ketone bodies as alternative energy source for the brain and results in marked improvement of seizures and movement disorder. The effect on cognitive impairment is less impressive.

Marked variability of the clinical phenotype of GLUT1-DS has been recognized over the last years. A carbohydrate-responsive phenotype with clinical features aggravated by fasting and improving after carbohydrate intake and movement disorders such as intermittent ataxia with mild learning difficulties or predominant dystonia, but without epilepsy, were observed [72, 73]. In a study of 57 patients with GLUT1-DS, nonepileptic paroxysmal events were found in 28 % of cases. These attacks included episodes of ataxia, parkinsonian features, weakness, and nonkinesigenic dyskinesias [74].

The present expansion of the phenotypic spectrum of GLUT1-DS includes recognition of familial and sporadic PED caused by *SLC2A1* mutations. Whereas a subset of patients displayed PED as the sole neurological feature or showed just mild clumsiness or dysdiadochokinesis as interepisodic findings, many patients had additional epilepsy or cognitive impairment (ranging from learning difficulties to moderate intellectual disability) or both (DYT18, OMIM #612126) [62, 69, 70]. Attacks may present with choreoathetotic movements or stiffening and cramps. In our experience, many patients with GLUT1-DS are affected by PED triggered by walking or running, but not all patients complain spontaneously about this symptom, as they learned to alleviate the dyskinesias by taking a rest or eating sweets. Apart from sustained exertion, precipitating factors include stress, fasting, anxiety, and sleep deprivation. Duration of attacks ranges from 5 min to several hours, but most PED last for about 30 min. Frequency ranges from several times a day to occasional episodes over a year [9, 62]. Ketogenic diet proved effective in many patients, if they adhere to the diet. Some patients rely on eating sweets or sugar to ease the paroxysms. Good response of PED to medication with acetazolamide was observed in a single patient with GLUT1-DS [75].

Few patients with *SLC2A1* mutations experience PxDs without exertion or any other precipitating factors; some others have PxDs triggered by fasting, stress, or anxiety. These PxDs may therefore be classified as PNKD.

Reevaluation of the clinical presentation in a large kindred with PED and progressive spastic paraplegia resulted in the detection of a heterozygous *SLC2A1* mutation [76]. This condition had been originally reported as paroxysmal choreoathetosis/spasticity and designated DYT9 (OMIM #601042) or alternatively termed "choreoathetosis/spasticity, episodic" (CSE) [77]. An *SLC2A1* mutation was demonstrated in monozygotic twins with PED and progressive spastic paraparesis, but not in 139 patients with hereditary spastic paraplegia without PxDs [76].

Allan-Herndon-Dudley Syndrome (AHDS)

Based on recognition of the monocarboxylate transporter type 8 (MCT8) as a thyroid hormone transporter, a candidate gene approach resulted in the discovery of mutations in the *SLC16A2* gene on chromosome Xq13.2 encoding for MCT8 in males with intellectual disability and a peculiar pattern of thyroid hormone concentrations in serum (OMIM #300523) [78, 79]. Clinical features in these patients comprise proximal muscular hypotonia with poor head control in infancy, generalized muscular hypotrophy, marked developmental delay with severe intellectual disability and inability to communicate, spasticity with joint contractures and scoliosis evolving during childhood or young adulthood, inability to stand or walk in many patients, ataxia in those who ambulate, dysarthria or complete absence of speech, elongated face with bitemporal narrowing, and microcephaly or normal head circumference.

Subsequent reappraisal of clinical and laboratory features of large kindreds with a special type of X-linked mental retardation (Allan-Herndon-Dudley syndrome, AHDS) originally described in 1944 [80] demonstrated that AHDS is in fact caused by MCT8 deficiency [81]. To date, more than 70 different *SLC16A2* mutations in about 200 patients from approximately 100 families of diverse ethnic background have been reported [82]. A characteristic pattern of thyroid hormone concentrations in blood including elevated serum T_3, low reverse T_3, low normal to reduced T_4, and normal or slightly elevated thyrotropin (TSH) levels is found in obviously all patients as a laboratory hallmark of this condition.

SLC16A2 mutations compromise transmembrane uptake of triiodothyronine (T_3) from the blood into the neurons. Thus, AHDS patients have neuronal hypothyroidism despite elevated FT_3 levels in the blood. However, details of the emergence of the clinical presentation are not yet understood.

In a subset of affected boys, PxDs were observed. As these attacks were precipitated by passive movements like changing of their clothes or diapers, the episodes were classified as PKD [83, 84]. Interestingly, PxDs are known to occur in other conditions with disordered thyroid hormone metabolism, including endemic cretinism and hyperthyroidism [83].

The special paroxysmal features of PKD observed in one patient with a proven *SLC16A2* mutation [83] showed impressive similarity with hemidystonic attacks seen in alternating hemiplegia of childhood.

Alternating Hemiplegia of Childhood (AHC)

Alternating hemiplegia of childhood (AHC) represents a prototype of a complex chronic neurological disorder with PxDs as a clinical hallmark. AHC is a rare, largely sporadic disorder; the prevalence is estimated to be one in 1,000,000 people.

The clinical presentation of AHC includes paroxysmal and nonparoxysmal manifestations. The nonparoxysmal symptoms take a progressive course in most cases, but a more favorable outcome is observed in a subset of patients. Paroxysmal manifestations occur as PxDs in most patients, although episodes of flaccid paresis without dyskinesia dominate in some cases. Frequent episodes of hemidystonia or hemiplegia accompanied by other paroxysmal symptoms including nystagmus, anarthria, dysphagia, hypersalivation, and seizures are highly characteristic [85, 86]. Hemiplegic and hemidystonic attacks typically shift from one side of the body to the other and may merge to quadriplegia. By definition onset of the paroxysmal manifestations is within the first 18 months of life. Duration of attacks ranges from a few minutes to several days, and episodes recur from repeatedly within a day to several times a month. The attacks are typically provoked by physical or emotional stressors, most commonly emotional triggers such as excitement. Physical triggers include hypo- or hyperthermia, respiratory tract infections, and bright light. Characteristically all paroxysmal symptoms dissolve on falling asleep, and induction of sleep is a major therapeutic measure to bring severe attacks to an end. Paroxysmal manifestations prevail throughout life, but in most patients will diminish in frequency and duration over the years.

In most patients interepisodic features appear after a course of months or years. These nonparoxysmal manifestations comprise global developmental delay, learning difficulties or intellectual disability, ataxia, dysarthria, dystonia, and occasionally pyramidal tract signs. Most patients are severely handicapped after a course of several years [85–88].

Extensive laboratory investigations and neuroimaging studies failed to provide any conclusive finding indicating the pathomechanism or a candidate gene. Sporadic occurrence in almost all cases precluded linkage mapping as an approach to identify the causative gene.

Genetics of AHC

The use of whole-exome sequencing enabled several independent research groups to demonstrate heterozygous *de novo* mutations in the *ATP1A3* gene as the cause of AHC (OMIM # 614820) [88–90]. *ATP1A3* mutations were detected in 74 % (82 of 105) of patients with the clinical diagnosis of AHC in one study [89]. Two smaller studies found a mutation in each of 24 and 8 clinically well-characterized AHC cases, respectively [88, 90].

ATP1A3 encodes for the α_3-subunit of the Na^+/K^+-ATPase, a transmembrane ion pump generating transmembrane electrical and chemical gradients of sodium and potassium. Generation of these gradients constitutes a basic process in cellular physiology and is a prerequisite for the electrical excitability of nerve and muscle cells. Thus, a considerable part of the energy consumption of the mammalian brain is due to the Na^+/K^+-ATPase.

The large catalytic α-subunit of the Na^+/K^+-ATPase contains the binding sites for ATP, cations, and cardiac glycosides. Among the four α-isoforms with different expression patterns known in mammals, the α_1-isoform is ubiquitously expressed while the α_2- and α_3-isoforms are expressed in brain. The α_2-isoform is found in the hippocampus, astrocytes, and oligodendrocytes. The α_3-isoform is abundantly and selectively expressed in the neurons of various brain structures, comprising basal ganglia, hippocampus, and cerebellum [91]. Nonuniform expression of the Na^+/K^+-ATPase isoforms points to a neuron-specific role of the α_3-isoform. As a hypothesis it was suggested that in neurons background ionic homeostasis is maintained by α_1-Na/K-ATPase, thus playing the role of "housekeeping" transporter, whereas the α_3-isoform serves as a "reserve" transporter activated only when Na^+ concentration is high, as it is the case following repeated action potentials [92]. This assumption would match with the clinical observation of stressing events precipitating paroxysmal manifestations of AHC and with dyskinesia as a clinical feature related to the highly energy-dependent basal ganglia.

To date, mutations only in *ATP1A2* and *ATP1A3*, the genes encoding the α_2- and α_3-isoforms, were found to be associated with neurological disease in humans. Autosomal dominantly inherited heterozygous *ATP1A2* mutations were demonstrated in patients with familial hemiplegic migraine [93] and in familial basilar migraine [94].

Phenotypic Spectrum of ATP1A3-Related Disorders

Already in 2004 heterozygous mutations of *ATP1A3* were linked with a rare disorder called rapid-onset dystonia-parkinsonism (RDP, DYT12, OMIM #128235) [95]. This condition was clinically first described in 1993 [96]. RDP is characterized by abrupt onset of dystonia and parkinsonism with bradykinesia and gait instability. Dystonia is asymmetric, and bulbar symptoms including dysarthria and dysphagia are prominent. Onset of symptoms is typically triggered by physical or emotional stressors and occurs within a time span ranging from 1 h to a few weeks. Onset is largely in the 2nd and 3rd decade of life. Some patients showed a subsequent slow improvement over several months followed by a 2nd abrupt deterioration of dystonia and parkinsonian features. To date, about 50 patients worldwide with heterozygous missense mutations of the *ATP1A3* gene were reported. Inheritance is autosomal dominant with reduced penetrance in familial cases, and a number of sporadic *de novo* mutations were observed [97].

Whether AHC and RDP represent distinct clinical phenotypes [98] or different manifestations along a clinical spectrum [99] of *ATP1A3*-related disorders remains a matter of debate. Major clinical features shared in common by both conditions comprise strikingly asymmetric dystonia, a rostrocaudal (face to arm to leg) gradient of involvement, pronounced signs of brainstem dysfunction such as dysphagia, dysarthria or even anarthria, and hypomimia. Triggering of onset by physical and emotional stress constitutes a further mutual peculiarity. On the other hand, both phenotypes clearly differ in their chronologic evolution of symptoms: while RDP is a mono- or biphasic condition, AHC is a polyphasic disorder with frequently recurring attacks. Several patients reported recently exhibit intermediate features, and in a number of cases diagnosed as having RDP, recurrent episodes of dyskinesia superimposed on the baseline movement disorder were described [100–103].

18q23 Deletion Syndrome

The 18q23 deletion syndrome comprises congenital malformations, motor and mental developmental delay, autism, seizures, short stature, and hearing loss. In a 7-month-old infant with the karyotype 46,XX, del(18)(q21.3-ter), PxDs were reported. Paroxysmal dystonic posturing occurred in clusters with increased muscle tone, flexion of the right arm, and stretching of the other limbs [104].

References

1. Albanese A, Asmus F, Bhatia KP, Elia AE, Elibol B, Filippini G, et al. EFNS guidelines on diagnosis and treatment of primary dystonias. Eur J Neurol. 2011;18(1):5–18.
2. Charlesworth G, Bhatia KP, Wood NW. The genetics of dystonia: new twists in an old tale. Brain. 2013;136(Pt 7):2017–37.
3. Lance JW. Familial paroxysmal dystonic choreoathetosis and its differentiation from related syndromes. Ann Neurol. 1977;2(4):285–93.
4. Bhatia KP. Paroxysmal dyskinesias. Mov Disord. 2011;26(6):1157–65.
5. Demirkiran M, Jankovic J. Paroxysmal dyskinesias: clinical features and classification. Ann Neurol. 1995;38(4):571–9.
6. Weber YG, Lerche H. Genetics of paroxysmal dyskinesias. Curr Neurol Neurosci Rep. 2009;9(3):206–11.
7. Blakeley J, Jankovic J. Secondary paroxysmal dyskinesias. Mov Disord. 2002;17(4):726–34.
8. Brockmann K. Episodic movement disorders: from phenotype to genotype and back. Curr Neurol Neurosci Rep. 2013;13(10):379.
9. Erro R, Sheerin UM, Bhatia KP. Paroxysmal dyskinesias revisited: a review of 500 genetically proven cases and a new classification. Mov Disord. 2014;25.
10. Mount LA, Reback S. Familial paroxysmal choreoathetosis: preliminary report on a hitherto undescribed clinical syndrome. Arch Neurol Psychiatry. 1940;44(4):841–7.
11. Lee HY, Xu Y, Huang Y, Ahn AH, Auburger GW, Pandolfo M, et al. The gene for paroxysmal non-kinesigenic dyskinesia encodes an enzyme in a stress response pathway. Hum Mol Genet. 2004;13(24):3161–70.
12. Rainier S, Thomas D, Tokarz D, Ming L, Bui M, Plein E, et al. Myofibrillogenesis regulator 1 gene mutations cause paroxysmal dystonic choreoathetosis. Arch Neurol. 2004;61(7):1025–9.
13. Ghezzi D, Viscomi C, Ferlini A, Gualandi F, Mereghetti P, DeGrandis D, et al. Paroxysmal non-kinesigenic dyskinesia is caused by mutations of the MR-1 mitochondrial targeting sequence. Hum Mol Genet. 2009;18(6):1058–64.
14. Shen Y, Lee HY, Rawson J, Ojha S, Babbitt P, Fu YH, et al. Mutations in PNKD causing paroxysmal dyskinesia alters protein cleavage and stability. Hum Mol Genet. 2011;20(12):2322–32.
15. Bruno MK, Lee HY, Auburger GW, Friedman A, Nielsen JE, Lang AE, et al. Genotype-phenotype correlation of paroxysmal nonkinesigenic dyskinesia. Neurology. 2007;68(21):1782–9.

16. Du W, Bautista JF, Yang H, Diez-Sampedro A, You SA, Wang L, et al. Calcium-sensitive potassium channelopathy in human epilepsy and paroxysmal movement disorder. Nat Genet. 2005;37(7):733–8.
17. Spacey SD, Adams PJ, Lam PC, Materek LA, Stoessl AJ, Snutch TP, et al. Genetic heterogeneity in paroxysmal nonkinesigenic dyskinesia. Neurology. 2006;66(10):1588–90.
18. Kertesz A. Paroxysmal kinesigenic choreoathetosis. An entity within the paroxysmal choreoathetosis syndrome. Description of 10 cases, including 1 autopsied. Neurology. 1967;17(7):680–90.
19. Bruno MK, Hallett M, Gwinn-Hardy K, Sorensen B, Considine E, Tucker S, et al. Clinical evaluation of idiopathic paroxysmal kinesigenic dyskinesia: new diagnostic criteria. Neurology. 2004;63(12):2280–7.
20. Houser MK, Soland VL, Bhatia KP, Quinn NP, Marsden CD. Paroxysmal kinesigenic choreoathetosis: a report of 26 patients. J Neurol. 1999;246(2):120–6.
21. Watanabe K, Yamamoto N, Negoro T, Takaesu E, Aso K, Furune S, et al. Benign complex partial epilepsies in infancy. Pediatr Neurol. 1987;3(4):208–11.
22. Swoboda KJ, Soong B, McKenna C, Brunt ER, Litt M, Bale Jr JF, et al. Paroxysmal kinesigenic dyskinesia and infantile convulsions: clinical and linkage studies. Neurology. 2000;55(2):224–30.
23. Szepetowski P, Rochette J, Berquin P, Piussan C, Lathrop GM, Monaco AP. Familial infantile convulsions and paroxysmal choreoathetosis: a new neurological syndrome linked to the pericentromeric region of human chromosome 16. Am J Hum Genet. 1997;61(4):889–98.
24. Tomita H, Nagamitsu S, Wakui K, Fukushima Y, Yamada K, Sadamatsu M, et al. Paroxysmal kinesigenic choreoathetosis locus maps to chromosome 16p11.2-q12.1. Am J Hum Genet. 1999;65(6):1688–97.
25. Kikuchi T, Nomura M, Tomita H, Harada N, Kanai K, Konishi T, et al. Paroxysmal kinesigenic choreoathetosis (PKC): confirmation of linkage to 16p11-q21, but unsuccessful detection of mutations among 157 genes at the PKC-critical region in seven PKC families. J Hum Genet. 2007;52(4):334–41.
26. Chen WJ, Lin Y, Xiong ZQ, Wei W, Ni W, Tan GH, et al. Exome sequencing identifies truncating mutations in PRRT2 that cause paroxysmal kinesigenic dyskinesia. Nat Genet. 2011;43(12):1252–5.
27. Lee HY, Huang Y, Bruneau N, Roll P, Roberson ED, Hermann M, et al. Mutations in the novel protein PRRT2 cause paroxysmal kinesigenic dyskinesia with infantile convulsions. Cell Rep. 2012;1(1):2–12.
28. Li J, Zhu X, Wang X, Sun W, Feng B, Du T, et al. Targeted genomic sequencing identifies PRRT2 mutations as a cause of paroxysmal kinesigenic choreoathetosis. J Med Genet. 2012;49(2):76–8.
29. Wang JL, Cao L, Li XH, Hu ZM, Li JD, Zhang JG, et al. Identification of PRRT2 as the causative gene of paroxysmal kinesigenic dyskinesias. Brain. 2011;134(Pt 12):3493–501.
30. Friedman J, Olvera J, Silhavy JL, Gabriel SB, Gleeson JG. Mild paroxysmal kinesigenic dyskinesia caused by PRRT2 missense mutation with reduced penetrance. Neurology. 2012;79(9):946–8.
31. Heron SE, Grinton BE, Kivity S, Afawi Z, Zuberi SM, Hughes JN, et al. PRRT2 mutations cause benign familial infantile epilepsy and infantile convulsions with choreoathetosis syndrome. Am J Hum Genet. 2012;90(1):152–60.
32. Liu Q, Qi Z, Wan XH, Li JY, Shi L, Lu Q, et al. Mutations in PRRT2 result in paroxysmal dyskinesias with marked variability in clinical expression. J Med Genet. 2012;49(2):79–82.
33. Meneret A, Grabli D, Depienne C, Gaudebout C, Picard F, Durr A, et al. PRRT2 mutations: a major cause of paroxysmal kinesigenic dyskinesia in the European population. Neurology. 2012;79(2):170–4.
34. Ono S, Yoshiura K, Kinoshita A, Kikuchi T, Nakane Y, Kato N, et al. Mutations in PRRT2 responsible for paroxysmal kinesigenic dyskinesias also cause benign familial infantile convulsions. J Hum Genet. 2012;57(5):338–41.
35. van Vliet R, Breedveld G, de Rijk-van AJ, Brilstra E, Verbeek N, Verschuuren-Bemelmans C, et al. PRRT2 phenotypes and penetrance of paroxysmal kinesigenic dyskinesia and infantile convulsions. Neurology. 2012;79(8):777–84.

36. Cloarec R, Bruneau N, Rudolf G, Massacrier A, Salmi M, Bataillard M, et al. PRRT2 links infantile convulsions and paroxysmal dyskinesia with migraine. Neurology. 2012;79(21):2097–103.
37. Dale RC, Gardiner A, Antony J, Houlden H. Familial PRRT2 mutation with heterogeneous paroxysmal disorders including paroxysmal torticollis and hemiplegic migraine. Dev Med Child Neurol. 2012;54(10):958–60.
38. Gardiner AR, Bhatia KP, Stamelou M, Dale RC, Kurian MA, Schneider SA, et al. PRRT2 gene mutations: from paroxysmal dyskinesia to episodic ataxia and hemiplegic migraine. Neurology. 2012;79(21):2115–21.
39. Heron SE, Dibbens LM. Role of PRRT2 in common paroxysmal neurological disorders: a gene with remarkable pleiotropy. J Med Genet. 2013;50(3):133–9.
40. Labate A, Tarantino P, Palamara G, Gagliardi M, Cavalcanti F, Ferlazzo E, et al. Mutations in PRRT2 result in familial infantile seizures with heterogeneous phenotypes including febrile convulsions and probable SUDEP. Epilepsy Res. 2013;104(3):280–4.
41. Marini C, Conti V, Mei D, Battaglia D, Lettori D, Losito E, et al. PRRT2 mutations in familial infantile seizures, paroxysmal dyskinesia, and hemiplegic migraine. Neurology. 2012;79(21):2109–14.
42. Mink JW. Defining and refining the phenotype of PRRT2 mutations. Dev Med Child Neurol. 2013;55(4):297.
43. Riant F, Roze E, Barbance C, Meneret A, Guyant-Marechal L, Lucas C, et al. PRRT2 mutations cause hemiplegic migraine. Neurology. 2012;79(21):2122–4.
44. Scheffer IE, Grinton BE, Heron SE, Kivity S, Afawi Z, Iona X, et al. PRRT2 phenotypic spectrum includes sporadic and fever-related infantile seizures. Neurology. 2012;79(21):2104–8.
45. Schubert J, Paravidino R, Becker F, Berger A, Bebek N, Bianchi A, et al. PRRT2 mutations are the major cause of benign familial infantile seizures. Hum Mutat. 2012;33(10):1439–43.
46. Sheerin UM, Stamelou M, Charlesworth G, Shiner T, Spacey S, Valente EM, et al. Migraine with aura as the predominant phenotype in a family with a PRRT2 mutation. J Neurol. 2013;260(2):656–60.
47. Specchio N, Terracciano A, Trivisano M, Cappelletti S, Claps D, Travaglini L, et al. PRRT2 is mutated in familial and non-familial benign infantile seizures. Eur J Paediatr Neurol. 2013;17(1):77–81.
48. Labate A, Tarantino P, Viri M, Mumoli L, Gagliardi M, Romeo A, et al. Homozygous c.649dupC mutation in PRRT2 worsens the BFIS/PKD phenotype with mental retardation, episodic ataxia, and absences. Epilepsia. 2012;53(12):e196–9.
49. Najmabadi H, Hu H, Garshasbi M, Zemojtel T, Abedini SS, Chen W, et al. Deep sequencing reveals 50 novel genes for recessive cognitive disorders. Nature. 2011;478(7367):57–63.
50. Heron SE, Ong YS, Yendle SC, McMahon JM, Berkovic SF, Scheffer IE, et al. Mutations in PRRT2 are not a common cause of infantile epileptic encephalopathies. Epilepsia. 2013;54(5):e86–9.
51. Stelzl U, Worm U, Lalowski M, Haenig C, Brembeck FH, Goehler H, et al. A human protein-protein interaction network: a resource for annotating the proteome. Cell. 2005;122(6):957–68.
52. Spacey SD, Valente EM, Wali GM, Warner TT, Jarman PR, Schapira AH, et al. Genetic and clinical heterogeneity in paroxysmal kinesigenic dyskinesia: evidence for a third EKD gene. Mov Disord. 2002;17(4):717–25.
53. Valente EM, Spacey SD, Wali GM, Bhatia KP, Dixon PH, Wood NW, et al. A second paroxysmal kinesigenic choreoathetosis locus (EKD2) mapping on 16q13-q22.1 indicates a family of genes which give rise to paroxysmal disorders on human chromosome 16. Brain. 2000;123(Pt 10):2040–5.
54. Angelini L, Rumi V, Lamperti E, Nardocci N. Transient paroxysmal dystonia in infancy. Neuropediatrics. 1988;19(4):171–4.
55. Deonna TW, Ziegler AL, Nielsen J. Transient idiopathic dystonia in infancy. Neuropediatrics. 1991;22(4):220–4.

56. Willemse J. Benign idiopathic dystonia with onset in the first year of life. Dev Med Child Neurol. 1986;28(3):355–60.
57. Rosman NP, Douglass LM, Sharif UM, Paolini J. The neurology of benign paroxysmal torticollis of infancy: report of 10 new cases and review of the literature. J Child Neurol. 2009; 24(2):155–60.
58. Cohen HA, Nussinovitch M, Ashkenasi A, Straussberg R, Kauschanksy A, Frydman M. Benign paroxysmal torticollis in infancy. Pediatr Neurol. 1993;9(6):488–90.
59. Vila-Pueyo M, Gené GG, Flotats-Bastardes M, Elorza X, Sintas C, Valverde MA, et al. A loss-of-function CACNA1A mutation causing benign paroxysmal torticollis of infancy. Eur J Paediatr Neurol. 2014;18(3):430–3.
60. Bhatia KP, Soland VL, Bhatt MH, Quinn NP, Marsden CD. Paroxysmal exercise-induced dystonia: eight new sporadic cases and a review of the literature. Mov Disord. 1997;12(6):1007–12.
61. Plant GT, Williams AC, Earl CJ, Marsden CD. Familial paroxysmal dystonia induced by exercise. J Neurol Neurosurg Psychiatry. 1984;47(3):275–9.
62. Suls A, Dedeken P, Goffin K, Van Esch H, Dupont P, Cassiman D, et al. Paroxysmal exercise-induced dyskinesia and epilepsy is due to mutations in SLC2A1, encoding the glucose transporter GLUT1. Brain. 2008;131(Pt 7):1831–44.
63. Guerrini R, Sanchez-Carpintero R, Deonna T, Santucci M, Bhatia KP, Moreno T, et al. Early-onset absence epilepsy and paroxysmal dyskinesia. Epilepsia. 2002;43(10):1224–9.
64. Kamm C, Mayer P, Sharma M, Niemann G, Gasser T. New family with paroxysmal exercise-induced dystonia and epilepsy. Mov Disord. 2007;22(6):873–7.
65. Guerrini R, Bonanni P, Nardocci N, Parmeggiani L, Piccirilli M, De Fusco M, et al. Autosomal recessive rolandic epilepsy with paroxysmal exercise-induced dystonia and writer's cramp: delineation of the syndrome and gene mapping to chromosome 16p12-11.2. Ann Neurol. 1999;45(3):344–52.
66. Munchau A, Valente EM, Shahidi GA, Eunson LH, Hanna MG, Quinn NP, et al. A new family with paroxysmal exercise induced dystonia and migraine: a clinical and genetic study. J Neurol Neurosurg Psychiatry. 2000;68(5):609–14.
67. Bozi M, Bhatia KP. Paroxysmal exercise-induced dystonia as a presenting feature of young-onset Parkinson's disease. Mov Disord. 2003;18(12):1545–7.
68. Bruno MK, Ravina B, Garraux G, Hallett M, Ptacek L, Singleton A, et al. Exercise-induced dystonia as a preceding symptom of familial Parkinson's disease. Mov Disord. 2004;19(2):228–30.
69. Schneider SA, Paisan-Ruiz C, Garcia-Gorostiaga I, Quinn NP, Weber YG, Lerche H, et al. GLUT1 gene mutations cause sporadic paroxysmal exercise-induced dyskinesias. Mov Disord. 2009;24(11):1684–8.
70. Weber YG, Storch A, Wuttke TV, Brockmann K, Kempfle J, Maljevic S, et al. GLUT1 mutations are a cause of paroxysmal exertion-induced dyskinesias and induce hemolytic anemia by a cation leak. J Clin Invest. 2008;118(6):2157–68.
71. Wang D, Pascual JM, Yang H, Engelstad K, Jhung S, Sun RP, et al. Glut-1 deficiency syndrome: clinical, genetic, and therapeutic aspects. Ann Neurol. 2005;57(1):111–8.
72. Brockmann K. The expanding phenotype of GLUT1-deficiency syndrome. Brain Dev. 2009;31(7):545–52.
73. Leen WG, Klepper J, Verbeek MM, Leferink M, Hofste T, van Engelen BG, et al. Glucose transporter-1 deficiency syndrome: the expanding clinical and genetic spectrum of a treatable disorder. Brain. 2010;133(Pt 3):655–70.
74. Pons R, Collins A, Rotstein M, Engelstad K, De Vivo DC. The spectrum of movement disorders in Glut-1 deficiency. Mov Disord. 2010;25(3):275–81.
75. Anheim M, Maillart E, Vuillaumier-Barrot S, Flamand-Rouviere C, Pineau F, Ewenczyk C, et al. Excellent response to acetazolamide in a case of paroxysmal dyskinesias due to GLUT1-deficiency. J Neurol. 2011;258(2):316–7.
76. Weber YG, Kamm C, Suls A, Kempfle J, Kotschet K, Schule R, et al. Paroxysmal choreoathetosis/spasticity (DYT9) is caused by a GLUT1 defect. Neurology. 2011;77(10):959–64.

77. Auburger G, Ratzlaff T, Lunkes A, Nelles HW, Leube B, Binkofski F, et al. A gene for autosomal dominant paroxysmal choreoathetosis/spasticity (CSE) maps to the vicinity of a potassium channel gene cluster on chromosome 1p, probably within 2 cM between D1S443 and D1S197. Genomics. 1996;31(1):90–4.
78. Dumitrescu AM, Liao XH, Best TB, Brockmann K, Refetoff S. A novel syndrome combining thyroid and neurological abnormalities is associated with mutations in a monocarboxylate transporter gene. Am J Hum Genet. 2004;74(1):168–75.
79. Friesema EC, Grueters A, Biebermann H, Krude H, von Moers A, Reeser M, et al. Association between mutations in a thyroid hormone transporter and severe X-linked psychomotor retardation. Lancet. 2004;364(9443):1435–7.
80. Allan W, Herndon CN, Dudley FC. Some examples of the inheritance of mental deficiency: apparently sex-linked idiocy and microcephaly. Am J Ment Defic. 1944;48:325–34.
81. Schwartz CE, May MM, Carpenter NJ, Rogers RC, Martin J, Bialer MG, et al. Allan-Herndon-Dudley syndrome and the monocarboxylate transporter 8 (MCT8) gene. Am J Hum Genet. 2005;77(1):41–53.
82. Fu J, Refetoff S, Dumitrescu AM. Inherited defects of thyroid hormone-cell-membrane transport: review of recent findings. Curr Opin Endocrinol Diabetes Obes. 2013;20(5):434–40.
83. Brockmann K, Dumitrescu AM, Best TT, Hanefeld F, Refetoff S. X-linked paroxysmal dyskinesia and severe global retardation caused by defective MCT8 gene. J Neurol. 2005; 252(6):663–6.
84. Gika AD, Siddiqui A, Hulse AJ, Edward S, Fallon P, McEntagart ME, et al. White matter abnormalities and dystonic motor disorder associated with mutations in the SLC16A2 gene. Dev Med Child Neurol. 2010;52(5):475–82.
85. Aicardi J, Bourgeois M, Goutieres F, editors. Alternating hemiplegia of childhood: Clinical findings and diagnostic criteria. New York: Raven; 1995.
86. Bourgeois M, Aicardi J, Goutieres F. Alternating hemiplegia of childhood. J Pediatr. 1993;122(5 Pt 1):673–9.
87. Panagiotakaki E, Gobbi G, Neville B, Ebinger F, Campistol J, Nevsimalova S, et al. Evidence of a non-progressive course of alternating hemiplegia of childhood: study of a large cohort of children and adults. Brain. 2010;133(Pt 12):3598–610.
88. Rosewich H, Thiele H, Ohlenbusch A, Maschke U, Altmuller J, Frommolt P, et al. Heterozygous de-novo mutations in ATP1A3 in patients with alternating hemiplegia of childhood: a whole-exome sequencing gene-identification study. Lancet Neurol. 2012;11(9): 764–73.
89. Heinzen EL, Swoboda KJ, Hitomi Y, Gurrieri F, Nicole S, de Vries B, et al. De novo mutations in ATP1A3 cause alternating hemiplegia of childhood. Nat Genet. 2012;44(9):1030–4.
90. Ishii A, Saito Y, Mitsui J, Ishiura H, Yoshimura J, Arai H, et al. Identification of ATP1A3 mutations by exome sequencing as the cause of alternating hemiplegia of childhood in Japanese patients. PLoS One. 2013;8(2):e56120.
91. Palmgren MG, Nissen P. P-type ATPases. Annu Rev Biophys. 2011;40:243–66.
92. Dobretsov M, Stimers JR. Neuronal function and alpha3 isoform of the Na/K-ATPase. Front Biosci. 2005;10:2373–96.
93. De Fusco M, Marconi R, Silvestri L, Atorino L, Rampoldi L, Morgante L, et al. Haploinsufficiency of ATP1A2 encoding the Na+/K+ pump alpha2 subunit associated with familial hemiplegic migraine type 2. Nat Genet. 2003;33(2):192–6.
94. Ambrosini A, D'Onofrio M, Grieco GS, Di Mambro A, Montagna G, Fortini D, et al. Familial basilar migraine associated with a new mutation in the ATP1A2 gene. Neurology. 2005; 65(11):1826–8.
95. de Carvalho AP, Sweadner KJ, Penniston JT, Zaremba J, Liu L, Caton M, et al. Mutations in the Na+/K+ –ATPase alpha3 gene ATP1A3 are associated with rapid-onset dystonia parkinsonism. Neuron. 2004;43(2):169–75.
96. Dobyns WB, Ozelius LJ, Kramer PL, Brashear A, Farlow MR, Perry TR, et al. Rapid-onset dystonia-parkinsonism. Neurology. 1993;43(12):2596–602.

97. Brashear A, Dobyns WB, de Carvalho AP, Borg M, Frijns CJ, Gollamudi S, et al. The phenotypic spectrum of rapid-onset dystonia-parkinsonism (RDP) and mutations in the ATP1A3 gene. Brain. 2007;130(Pt 3):828–35.
98. Heinzen EL, Arzimanoglou A, Brashear A, Clapcote SJ, Gurrieri F, Goldstein DB, et al. Distinct neurological disorders with ATP1A3 mutations. Lancet Neurol. 2014;13(5): 503–14.
99. Ozelius LJ. Clinical spectrum of disease associated with ATP1A3 mutations. Lancet Neurol. 2012;11(9):741–3.
100. Anselm IA, Sweadner KJ, Gollamudi S, Ozelius LJ, Darras BT. Rapid-onset dystonia-parkinsonism in a child with a novel atp1a3 gene mutation. Neurology. 2009;73(5):400–1.
101. Brashear A, Mink JW, Hill DF, Boggs N, McCall WV, Stacy MA, et al. ATP1A3 mutations in infants: a new rapid-onset dystonia-Parkinsonism phenotype characterized by motor delay and ataxia. Dev Med Child Neurol. 2012;54(11):1065–7.
102. Pittock SJ, Joyce C, O'Keane V, Hugle B, Hardiman MO, Brett F, et al. Rapid-onset dystonia-parkinsonism: a clinical and genetic analysis of a new kindred. Neurology. 2000;55(7):991–5.
103. Rosewich H, Ohlenbusch A, Huppke P, Schlotawa L, Baethmann M, Carrilho I, et al. The expanding clinical and genetic spectrum of ATP1A3-related disorders. Neurology. 2014; 82(11):945–55.
104. Ishikawa N, Kobayashi Y, Fujii Y, Kobayashi M. Paroxysmal periodic dystonic postures in an infant with 18q23 deletion syndrome. Neuropediatrics. 2013;44(3):163–6.

Chapter 11
Genetics of Dominant Ataxias

Mario Manto and Daniele Marmolino

Abstract Dominant ataxias represent a clinically and genetically heterogeneous group of hereditary disorders comprising autosomal dominant spinocerebellar ataxias (ADCAs, SCAs) and episodic ataxias (EAs). From the clinical point of view, patients with ADCA exhibit a progressive cerebellar syndrome, either isolated or in combination with extra-cerebellar deficits. EAs are characterized by recurrent episodes of dizziness and ataxia, occurring either in a context of interictal neurological deficits or not. Current genetic classification includes 32 SCA loci (numbered from SCA1 to SCA36, plus dentatorubropallidoluysian atrophy DRPLA) and 7 EA loci (numbered from EA1 to EA7). A group of 12 ADCAs are related to an expansion of CAG repeats (polyglutaminopathies) or to repeats outside the coding region. Disease progression and severity are correlated with the repeat size. Anticipation is due to an instability of the expanded allele during transmission. The other ADCAs are due to conventional gene mutations. Overall, the causative gene is identified in about 60 % of dominant ataxias. There is still no cure for this group of disabling degenerative diseases. Current management is symptomatic.

Keywords Cerebellum • Ataxias • Genes • Dominant • Polyglutamine • Episodic ataxias • Atrophy

The terminology of "ataxia" designates a lack of coordination and balance. Ataxia may be consecutive to a disorder affecting the cerebellum, its afferences and/or its efferences, or the peripheral nerves (the so-called sensory ataxias). Numerous disorders can cause ataxia of cerebellar origin, including sporadic and genetic diseases [1, 2]. This chapter will focus on cerebellar ataxias with a dominant transmission. These rare disorders have an estimated prevalence of 3–4/100,000 individuals [3]. Autosomal recessive ataxias and X-linked ataxias are not discussed in this chapter.

M. Manto, MD, PhD (✉)
Neurologie, FNRS, ULB-Erasme, Bruxelles 1070, Belgium
e-mail: mmanto@ulb.ac.be

D. Marmolino, PhD
Parkinson Disease Area, UCB Pharma S.A., Braine-l'Alleud 1420, Belgium

S.A. Schneider, J.M.T. Brás (eds.), *Movement Disorder Genetics*,
DOI 10.1007/978-3-319-17223-1_11

Classification of Dominant Ataxias

Autosomal dominant spinocerebellar ataxias (ADCAs) were initially classified on the basis of clinical and neuropathological features. Patients were grouped according to the clinical phenotype: presence of a cerebellar syndrome which was pure or associated with brainstem signs, extrapyramidal deficits, signs of peripheral nerve involvement, or retinal deficits. The dominantly inherited pattern was pointed out by Pierre Marie [4]. Neuropathological classification has considered a pattern of olivopontocerebellar atrophy (OPCA) and the cerebellar cortical atrophy (CCA) type, in addition to the cerebello-olivary degeneration of Holmes [5–8]. However, these terms have encompassed both sporadic and genetic ataxias, causing some confusion. The classification of Greenfield [9] has considered predominantly spinal ataxias (such as Friedreich ataxia and hereditary spastic paraplegias), predominantly cerebellar ataxias, and spinocerebellar ataxias involving extra-cerebellar regions. Again, this classification was ambiguous if analyzed from a genetic standpoint, because several modes of transmission were gathered in the same groups of disorders.

The works of Harding clarified greatly the classification of dominant ataxias [10–12]. This author underlined the limits of the neuropathological classification. For instance, she pointed out that patients within the same family fall in distinct neuropathological groups. She suggested a new classification which took into account the clinical presentation, the mode of inheritance, and the presumed biological causes. ADCAs were divided into four types:

1. ADCA type I: cerebellar ataxia "plus" (presence of extra-cerebellar deficits, such as ophthalmoplegia, optic atrophy, cognitive deficits, and extrapyramidal signs)
2. ADCA type II: cerebellar ataxia with visual deficits due to pigmentary retinal degeneration (ophthalmoplegia, dementia, and extrapyramidal deficits may occur)
3. ADCA type III: pure cerebellar syndrome usually starting after the third decade
4. ADCA type IV: cerebellar ataxia with mental retardation, deafness, and myoclonus

The current classification is based on genetics and considers three groups:

1. The spinocerebellar ataxias (SCAs)
2. Dentatorubropallidoluysian atrophy (DRPLA)
3. Episodic ataxias (EAs)

SCAs and DRPLA are progressive disorders characterized by a cerebellar syndrome which may be associated with noticeable extra-cerebellar deficits. The most common SCAs are SCA1, SCA2, SCA3 (Machado–Joseph disease (MJD)), and SCA6 [3]. The incidence and prevalence of the various SCAs varies according to the geographical region of the world. It is important to note that the phenotype of SCAs may vary greatly within the same family and between families. The main clinical feature of EAs is the recurrent aspect of ataxia (crises or attacks of ataxia). Table 11.1 lists the main clinical signs in the various SCAs.

Table 11.1 Clinical phenotype of SCAs

Pure cerebellar syndrome	SCA5, SCA6, SCA11, SCA26		
Cerebellar ataxia combined with extra-cerebellar deficits ("ataxia plus")	Cognitive deficits and/or behavioral symptoms	SCA1, SCA2, SCA3, SCA10, SCA12, SCA13, SCA14, SCA17, SCA19, SCA21, SCA27, DRPLA	
	Seizures	SCA10, SCA17, DRPLA	
	Oculomotor deficits and/or involvement of eyes	Downbeat nystagmus	SCA6
		Ocular dyskinesia	SCA10
		Slow saccades	SCA1, SCA2, SCA3, SCA7, SCA28
		Ophthalmoplegia	SCA1, SCA2, SCA3, SCA28, SCA30
		Retinopathy	SCA7
	Pyramidal deficits	SCA1, SCA2, SCA3, SCA4, SCA7, SCA8, SCA10, SCA11, SCA12, SCA13, SCA14, SCA15, SCA28, SCA30	
	Movement disorders	Dystonia	SCA3, SCA14, SCA17
		Parkinsonism	SCA1, SCA2, SCA3, SCA12, SCA17, SCA21
		Tremor	SCA8, SCA12, SCA16, SCA19, SCA20
		Dyskinesias	SCA27
		Chorea	SCA1, SCA17, DRPLA
		Myoclonic jerks	SCA2, SCA14, SCA19, DRPLA
	Peripheral neuropathy	SCA1, SCA2, SCA3, SCA4, SCA6, SCA8, SCA27, SCA12, SCA18, SCA22, SCA25	

Adapted from Manto [1]

Establishing the Diagnosis of Dominant Ataxias

Establishing the diagnosis of hereditary ataxia requires:

1. A detailed neurological examination and detection of typical clinical signs including:
   (a) Poorly coordinated gait and finger/hand movements
   (b) Dysarthria (incoordination of speech)
   (c) Eye movement abnormalities such as nystagmus, abnormal ocular saccades, and ophthalmoplegia

2. Brain imaging studies (especially MRI studies)
3. Documentation of the hereditary nature of the disease:
   (a) Positive family history of ataxia
   (b) Identification of an ataxia-causing mutation
   (c) To recognize a clinical phenotype characteristic of a genetic form of ataxia
4. Exclusion of nongenetic causes of ataxia.

Diagnosis

The diagnostic thus relies on the family history, the clinical presentation, the neuroimaging pattern, and the genetic tests. Overall, the genetic tests are currently successful in about 60 % of SCAs (see below). Time should be devoted to construct the family tree in order to determine the mode of inheritance. Families with a history of a predominant cerebellar syndrome during successive generations have a high likelihood to present a SCA when both sexes are affected. Anticipation (discussed below) is an additional argument. However, the family tree may be difficult to set when the other members of the family cannot be examined (following death, for instance) or in case of no apparent symptom in some family members (patients at a presymptomatic stage). The variable penetrance and a possible false paternity or adoption also need to be taken into account. The ethnic and geographical background is also a clue for the diagnosis.

Additional tests may be valuable for the differential diagnosis. Neurophysiological studies such as nerve conduction velocities (NCV) and visual-evoked potentials (VEP) are useful to determine the presence of a peripheral neuropathy and optical nerve disease, respectively. Motor-evoked potentials (MEP) confirm the involvement of the corticospinal tract, especially in SCA1. The presence of periodic leg movements (PLM) during sleep is detected by polysomnography.

Brain Imaging

Brain MRI is noninvasive and is considered as a technique of choice to assess the anatomy of the brain in dominant ataxias (Fig. 11.1). It is important to exclude other causes of ataxia which could mimic a degenerative disorder (brain tumor, stroke, malformation, immune disease, etc.). Although brain MRI may be totally normal at the beginning of the symptoms, it becomes a sensitive tool to quantify atrophy as the disorder evolves with time. The main morphological patterns are the following:

- A pattern of pure cerebellar atrophy (in particular in SCA6).
- A pattern of OPCA with atrophy of the cerebellum and brainstem (typical for SCA1, SCA2, SCA3, and SCA7). The atrophy can extend to the upper segments of the spinal cord.
- A pattern of global brain atrophy (for instance, in DRPLA).

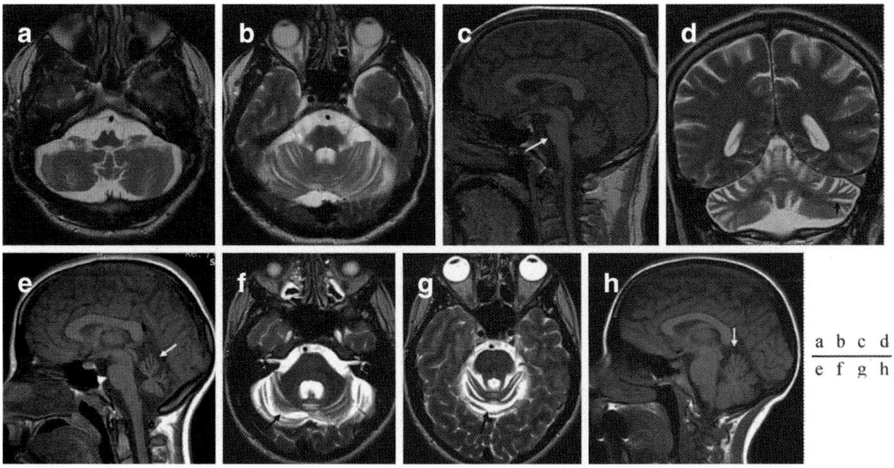

Fig. 11.1 Brain imaging in SCAs. (**a–c**) Brain MRI in a 52-year-old man presenting a SCA2. Atrophy of the medulla, pons, and cerebellum on T2-weighted axial images (**a**, **b**). Flattening of the pons on T1-weighted sagittal image (**c**; see *white arrow*). Atrophy of the cerebellar cortex on coronal T2-weighted image (*black arrow*, **d**) in a 44-year-old man with a SCA2. Atrophy of the vermis (*white arrow*) and slight flattening of the pons (*arrowhead*) in a 23-year-old woman presenting a SCA8 (**e**; T1-weighted sagittal image). The atrophy of the cerebellar cortex is well identified on T2-weighted axial images in this patient (**f–g**; *black arrows*). Slight atrophy of the upper vermis in a patient presenting EA2 (**h**; sagittal T1-weighted image; *white arrow*)

Some findings may be very suggestive of a given SCA. Dentate nuclei calcifications are observed in SCA20.

Volumetric studies are now available as routine procedures and allow to quantify the degree of regional atrophy and the progression with time.

Differential Diagnosis

Differential diagnosis of hereditary ataxia includes:

Acquired, nongenetic causes of ataxia: alcoholism, vitamin deficiencies, multiple sclerosis, cerebrovascular disease, primary or metastatic tumors, and paraneoplastic diseases associated with occult carcinoma of the ovary, breast, or lung and the idiopathic degenerative disease multiple system atrophy (MSA). An acquired cause of ataxia should be considered in all cases of ataxia.

Molecular Genetic Testing of SCAs

ADCAs are associated to mutations that include nucleotide expansions occurring in either expressed or non-expressed regions of the gene, point mutations, duplications, and deletions. The normal size of CAG repeat allele and of the full-penetrance disease-causing CAG expansion varies among the disorders (for reviews, see GeneReviews.org). Today, 50–60 % of the dominant hereditary ataxias can be identified with accurate and specific molecular genetic testing. This is the case for SCA1, SCA2, SCA3, SCA6, SCA7, SCA8, SCA10, SCA12, SCA17, and DRPLA. These disorders are characterized by CAG repeats within the coding region of the genes, translating into an elongated polyglutamine tract in the protein. Molecular genetic tests for CAG repeat length are highly specific and sensitive diagnostic tools, and further they are commercially available. However, pursuing tests for multiple genes simultaneously may seem less optimal than serial genetic testing, but their cost is decreasing. Molecular genetic testing results more specific than MRI findings in the hereditary ataxias and guidelines for genetic testing of hereditary ataxia have been published [13]. Testing is also available for some autosomal dominant forms of SCA that are not associated with repeat expansions (SCA5, SCA13, SCA14, SCA15, SCA27, SCA28, and 16q22-linked SCA). Interpretation of results can be an issue in the same case and should be done with caution, and the following aspects should be taken into account:

- The exact range for the abnormal repeat expansion has not been fully established for many of these disorders.
- In some cases, there may be an overlap between the upper range of normal values and the lower range of abnormal CAG repeat size. Such alleles are classified as mutable normal or reduced penetrance. Mutable normal alleles do not cause disease themselves but can expand during the genetic transmission to a reduced or fully penetrant allele. In a few words, children of an individual carrying a mutable normal allele have increased risk of inheriting a disease-causing allele. Therefore, interpretation of results in which the CAG repeat length is at the interface between the allele categories mutable normal/reduced penetrance and reduced penetrance/disease-causing results can be difficult. In such cases, a consultation with the testing laboratory should be considered.
- SCA2, SCA7, SCA8, and SCA10 mutations may present with extremely large CAG expansions in length, only detectable by Southern blot analysis. For these disorders, a test of apparent homozygosity (detection of a single allele by PCR analysis) should be associated to the clinical findings, the family history, and the age of onset of symptoms (to determine whether Southern blot analysis is needed).

The Risk for Family Members

Generally autosomal dominant ataxia patients have an affected parent, although in some cases the family history is negative. For example, family history may not be obvious because of:

- An early death of a parent or a late-onset disorder
- A failure to recognize autosomal dominant ataxia in family members
- A reduced penetrance of the mutant allele in an asymptomatic parent or a de novo mutation

The risk to siblings depends on the genetic status of the proband's parents. If one of the proband's parents has a mutant allele, the risk for the sibs of inheriting the mutant allele is 50 %. Individuals with autosomal dominant ataxia have a 50 % chance of transmitting the mutant allele to each child.

Related Genetic Counseling Issues

At-risk asymptomatic adult can be tested for autosomal dominant cerebellar ataxia after identification of a specific disorder and mutation in their family. Such testing should be performed in the context of formal genetic counseling and will remain a predictive testing and not a diagnostic testing. The test will not predict the age of onset, the severity, the type of symptoms, or the rate of progression. However, molecular genetic testing of asymptomatic individuals younger than 18 years who are at risk for adult-onset disorders for which no effective treatment exists is not considered appropriate. Concern exists regarding the potential unhealthy adverse effects that such information may have on family dynamics, the risk of discrimination and stigmatization in the future, and the anxiety that such information may cause. For more information, see the recommendations of the *National Society of Genetic Counselors resolution on genetic testing of children* and the *American Society of Human Genetics* and *American College of Medical Genetics points*.

New Genetic Technologies

Looking for the exact genetic mutation in patients with a cerebellar ataxia may be difficult, time consuming, and costly. The relatively uniform phenotype of many patients with cerebellar ataxia makes it difficult to decide which gene should be investigated first. Since conventional testing is expensive, many genes that are rarely involved in disease causation may not be tested. Thus, the development of novel technologies such as exome capture and next-generation DNA sequencing (NGS) is very interesting to screen the whole coding part of the genome in one experiment at reduced costs. This has been demonstrated to be a powerful diagnostic approach in the case of ataxia and Charcot–Marie–Tooth disease, which is a similarly heterogeneous disease [14]. The costs for this test decreased dramatically over the last year (it is about 1,000 USD). However, limitations need to be considered, in particular in the diagnosis of ataxia. In fact, currently NGS has a poor ability to sequence stretches of repetitive DNA such as the polyglutamine repeats.

Recently, systems biology approach based on whole-transcriptome gene expression analysis has been used to address the possible relationships among known SCA genes, predict their functions, identify overlapping pathways, and provide a framework for candidate gene discovery. Published results showed that two cerebellar gene coexpression modules were statistically enriched in SCA transcripts and contained established granule and Purkinje cell markers, respectively. One module includes genes involved in the ubiquitin–proteasome system and contains SCA genes usually associated with a complex phenotype, while the other module encloses many genes important for calcium homeostasis and signaling and contains SCA genes associated mostly with pure ataxia [15].

DNA Banking

DNA banking is the storage of DNA (generally from white blood cells) for possible future use. Because it is likely that testing methodology will improve in the future, consideration should be given to banking DNA of affected individuals with dominant ataxias.

Prenatal Testing

Prenatal diagnosis for some of the hereditary ataxias is possible by analyzing fetal DNA (from chorionic villus sampling at about 10–12 weeks' gestation or amniocentesis, usually performed at about 15–18 weeks' gestation) for disease-causing mutations. The disease-causing allele(s) of an affected family member must be identified before prenatal testing. Although most centers would consider decisions about prenatal testing to be the choice of the parents, discussion regarding the purpose of the testing should be considered, like pregnancy termination rather than early diagnosis. Preimplantation genetic diagnosis may also be available when the disease-causing mutation has been identified.

Genetics of SCAs and DRPLA

Historically, SCA1 was linked to chromosome 6 in 1977. SCA1 was identified as the first disorder associated with a trinucleotide repeat expansion [16]. Current numbering of SCAs is based on the chronological order of the gene discovery.

Table 11.2 lists the SCAs and their respective locus, and Table 11.3 provides the normal repeat range, the intermediate repeat range, and the pathological repeat range. A number of 32 genetic loci have been discovered:

- SCA1 to SCA8.
- SCA9 is not attributed.
- SCA10 to SCA15/16 (SCA15 and SCA16 are identical).
- SCA17 to SCA23 (SCA22 is an allelic variant of SCA19).
- SCA24 is not attributed.

Table 11.2 Loci of the SCAs

Disease	Chromosomal locus (mutation)	MIM number (http://www.omim.org)
SCA1	6p23 (CAG expansion)	164400
SCA2	12q24.1 (CAG expansion)	183090
SCA3	14q24.3-q31 (CAG expansion)	607407
SCA4	16q22.1	600223
SCA5	11q13 (point mutations, in-frame deletions)	600224
SCA6	19p13 (CAG expansion)	601011
SCA7	3p14-p21.1 (CAG expansion)	164500
SCA8	13q21 (CTG–CAG expansion)	608768
SCA10	22q13 (ATTCT expansion)	603516
SCA11	15q14-21.3 (point mutations, insertions, deletions)	604432
SCA12	5q31-q33 (CAG expansion)	604326
SCA13	19q13.3-q13.4 (point mutations)	605259
SCA14	19q13.4-qter (point mutations)	605361
SCA15	3p26-p25 (point mutations, deletions)	606658
SCA17	6q27 (CAG expansion)	607136
SCA18	7q22-q32	607458
SCA19	1p21-q21	607346
SCA20	11p13-q11 (duplication)	608687
SCA21	7p21.3-p15.1	607454
SCA22	1p21-q23	607346
SCA23	20p13-12.3 (point mutations)	610245
SCA25	2p15-p21	608703
SCA26	19p13.3	609306
SCA27 (FGF14)	13q34 (point mutations)	609307
SCA28	18p11.22-q11.2 (point mutations)	610246
SCA29	3p26	117360
SCA30	4q34-q35	613371
SCA31	16q22.1 ($TGGAA_n$ repeat)	117210
SCA32	7q32-q33	613909
SCA35	20p13 (point mutations)	613908
SCA36	20p13 (point mutations)	614153
DRPLA	12p13.31 (CAG expansion)	125370

- SCA25 to SCA28.
- SCA29 is an allelic variant of SCA15.
- SCA30 to SCA32.
- SCA35 to SCA36.
- DRPLA.

On the basis of the genetic mutation, three groups of SCAs can be considered (Fig. 11.2).

Table 11.3 Ranges of repeats in SCAs

Disease	Normal range	Intermediate range	Pathological range
SCA1	6–35	35–39	39–83
SCA2	14–31	31–34	34–77
SCA3	12–44	44–52	52–86
SCA6	4–18	18–20	20–33
SCA7	7–19	19–37	37 to >400
SCA8	15–50	50–80	80 to >1,300
SCA10	10–29	280–800	800–4,500
SCA12	4–32	32–51	51–78
SCA17	25–42	42–49	49–66
SCA31	1.2–2.0 kb		2.5–3.8 kb
SCA36	3–8		1,500–2,500
DRPLA	3–35	35–48	48–93

Adapted from Taroni et al. [17].

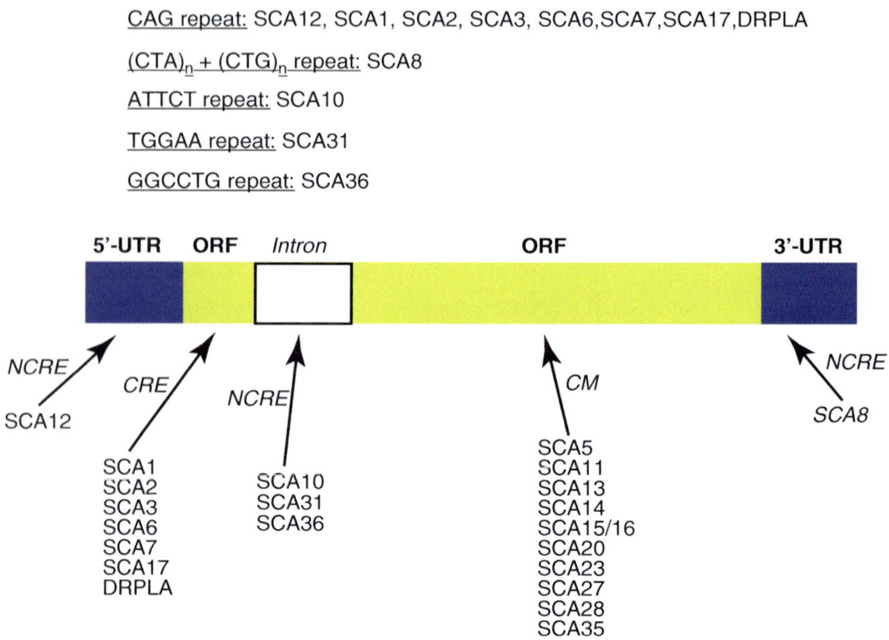

Fig. 11.2 Mutations in SCAs. *NCRE* noncoding repeat expansions, *CRE* coding repeat expansions, *CM* conventional mutations (missense, in-frame deletions, frameshift, nonsense, duplication)

Due to Repeat Expansion

This group is characterized by a CAG repeat expansion within the coding or non-coding parts of the relevant genes [18]. This includes SCA1, SCA2, SCA3, SCA6, SCA7, SCA17, and DRPLA. Because the CAG codon codes for glutamine (Q), the mutation results in the production of mutant protein characterized by a polyQ (polyglutamine, hence the terminology of polyglutaminopathies). Genotype–phenotype correlations of these disorders are well described [3] with the disease manifesting above a threshold of CAG repeats. The proteins are named ataxin-1 (ATXN1) for SCA1, ATXN2 for SCA2, ATXN3 for SCA3, ATXN7 for SCA7, and atrophin-1 for DRPLA. In SCA6, the mutation involves the calcium channel CACNA1A and in SCA17 the TATA-binding protein (TBP). Three important features are found in this group: (a) there is an inverse relationship between the number of CAG repeats and the age of onset of the clinical deficits, (b) the age of onset is characterized by anticipation, (c) and above a certain threshold in terms of number of CAG repeats, a full penetrance of the disorder occurs. It should be noted that CAG expansions are also found in two disorders usually not classified within ataxias: spinobulbar muscular atrophy (SBMA) and Huntington's disease (HD).

Due to Repeat Expansion Outside the Protein-Coding Region

This group includes SCA8, SCA10, SCA12, SCA31, and SCA36. There is some debate about SCA8 expansion because large repeats have been found in controls or patients with other diseases [19]. The repeat is a CTG triplet. SCA10 is characterized by a repeat expansion of the pentanucleotide ATTCT in intron 9 of the ATXN10 gene. An RNA-mediated toxicity has been proposed for both SCA8 and SCA10. In SCA12, the triplet expansion (CAG) affects the promoter of the PPP2R2B gene. For SCA31, another pentanucleotide (TGGAA) is expanded in an intron shared by the genes BEAN and TK2. SCA36 is due to an expansion of a hexanucleotide GGCCTG in the intron 1 of the NOP56 gene [20]. The pathogenesis is presumed to be due to a gain-of-function toxicity of the expanded RNA, along with a drop in the transcription of miRNA.

Due to Conventional Mutations

A minority of the dominant ataxia syndromes (SCA type 5, 11, 13, 14, 15, 20, 23, 27, 28, and 35) are caused by conventional mutations (deletions, duplications, nonsense, missense, splice). Conventional mutations have been reported to be up to 6 % of all dominant ataxia in France, with repeat expansions accounting for 45 % with the remaining 48 % being genetically undiagnosed [21]. Genotype–phenotype correlations were difficult to determine due to the limited number of families. A correlation between the degree of functional impairment and the severity of the phenotype has been demonstrated by functional analysis of potassium channels (EA1, SCA13) and calcium channels (SCA6, EA2). These disorders often have a "purer" cerebellar phenotype (ADCAIII), with a slower rate of progression when compared to SCAs due to repeat expansions.

SCA5 is caused by a mutation in the SPTBN2 gene, which encodes the B3 spectrin [22]. A pure cerebellar syndrome with onset between 15 and 50 years has been described in the presence of missense and in-frame deletions. In 1994, 56 affected individuals have been reported for the first time over ten generations. SCA5 has also been reported in French and German pedigrees [23].

SCA11 is caused by stop mutations, frameshift insertions, or deletions in the TTBK2 gene, resulting in a pure cerebellar syndrome with normal life expectancy [24]. The disease was initially reported in British families. Subsequently, pathogenic variants in TTBK2 have been reported in French and German families [25].

SCA13 is caused by missense mutations in KCNC3 encoding for a voltage-gated potassium channel [26]. The disease was initially reported in French and Filipino families. Different missense mutations correlate with a wide phenotypic spectrum. In the case of the childhood-onset form, two variants from European and Filipino families have been associated to the disease: (g.10693G>A p.Arg423His) and (g. 10767 T>C p.Phe448Leu) [27]. In SCA13, motor and mental developmental delay is a common feature. Two missense mutations have been reported. The p.Phe448Leu variant is associated to a more severe phenotype. The p.Arg423His variant has also been described in a Caucasian family in the United States.

SCA14 is caused by mutations in PRKCG [28] and is associated with a variable ataxic phenotype, including myoclonus, dystonia, or peripheral neuropathy. The onset is usually in adulthood, and patients carry in most case mutations (missense) in exons 4, 5, 10, and 18. SCA14 has been described in many families from Europe, Japan, and Australia [29].

SCA15/16 is caused by heterozygous deletions of the 5′ part of the ITPR1 gene [30]. A missense mutation (c.1480G>A p.V494I) has also been reported. The ITPR1 protein is highly expressed in cerebellar Purkinje cells and is an important modulator of intracellular calcium signaling. SCA15/16 is characterized by a mild cerebellar ataxia with slow disease progression. SCA15 was identified in 1.8 % of patients in French families [31]. SCA15/16 also shares a locus with SCA29, raising the hypothesis that they could be allelic disorders.

SCA20 is due to a 260 kb duplication in a region comprising >12 genes at 11q12 [32]. It was originally described in an Australian family. Disease characteristics include dysphonia and spasmodic cough (bulbar symptoms) and dentate nucleus calcifications.

SCA21 has been reported in a French family [33]. The age of onset is variable. Oculomotor deficits are mild. Patients may exhibit akinesia and tendon hyporeflexia. A mild cognitive impairment may be observed.

SCA23 is due to missense mutations of PDYN [34], which encodes prodynorphin protein, an opioid neuropeptide precursor. This causes a relatively pure cerebellar syndrome with a late onset (43–73 years) and slow progression. The disease has been reported in a single Dutch ataxia family [35].

SCA27 is caused by missense and nonsense mutations in the fibroblast growth factor 14 (FGF14). The gene was identified in Dutch families and is associated with early-onset ataxia [36], plus cognitive deficits, head/limb tremor, and dyskinesia that can be exacerbated by stress or exercise. There is a normal life expectancy. Most affected patients are unable to walk by the seventh to eighth decade. The disease has also been reported in a German ataxia patient.

SCA28 is caused by a mutation in AFG3L2, which encodes a metalloprotease located in the mitochondria [37]. Missense mutations have been reported. They are commonly located in the proteolytic domain of the protein with a mutation hotspot in exons 15–16. SCA28 has a typically early onset between 12 and 36 years and is characterized by a slowly progressive cerebellar ataxia with ophthalmoparesis and lower limb hyperreflexia. The disease is estimated to account for 1.5 % of European ADCA cases [38].

SCA35 is caused by mutations in the cerebral transglutaminase TGM6 and was the first dominant ataxia gene to be identified through exome sequencing [39]. Missense mutations were reported in two Chinese families in which a late-onset cerebellar syndrome with upper motor neuron involvement was reported. There is a moderate rate of progression. Patients use a wheelchair about 20 years after disease onset.

Anticipation

Anticipation is one of the main features of polyglutaminopathies. It designates the tendency of symptoms to start earlier and with a more severe phenotype [40]. Anticipation is related to changes in the size of the repeat expansion during transmission. Expanded alleles are unstable, with a trend towards an increase of CAG repeats (intergenerational elongation of the expansion). The instability is higher for paternal expansions, because the trends towards expansion are greater during spermatogenesis. Anticipation may be particularly marked in SCA7 and DRPLA, so that the disease can manifest in children before the parents develop symptoms. SCA2 is also characterized by anticipation, although to a lesser degree. There is threshold of 35–40 triplets beyond which the polyglutamine adopts an abnormal conformation, with a tendency to form aggregates and to interact with other proteins [40]. Unlike polyglutaminopathies, a phenomenon of contraction of the ATTCT repeat may be observed in SCA10, in particular for paternal transmission.

Prevalence

The prevalence of these disorders is not exactly known. ADCAs in the Netherlands are estimated to be at around 3:100,000 [41], and the prevalence of individual subtypes of ADCA may vary from region to region, because of founder effects. DRPLA was found to be more common in Japan and rare in North America, while SCA3 is much more common in Portugal, Japan, and Germany than in the United Kingdom [42–44]. SCA2 is relatively common in Korea. Further, SCA3 was originally described in Portuguese families from the Azores and called Machado–Joseph disease. A recent study found evidence of frequency variation between different regions in Japan [45].

Pathogenesis of SCAs

The concept of a toxic effect of polyglutamine expansion is now widely accepted (gain of function), but the intimate mechanisms of the toxicity are still not established. The polyQ tract adopts an impaired conformation (misfolding of the protein) and forms aggregates. These neuronal intranuclear inclusions are a major feature of the following polyglutaminopathies: SCA1, SCA3, SCA7, SCA17, and DRPLA. In SCA2, aggregates occur in the cytoplasm of neurons, whereas they are located in perinuclear regions in SCA6. It is interesting to note that one of the most vulnerable neurons in the cerebellum of SCA patients is the Purkinje cell. However, these neurons do not contain aggregates of proteins. Some consider that this indicates a possible dissociation between neuronal toxicity and the process of aggregation. The mutant proteins may interact with transcription factors such as senseless/Gfi1 by increasing its degradation, for instance, in SCA1 [46]. In case of the Purkinje cell, the mutant protein would impair the functions of ROR-alpha, known to play critical roles for the cerebellar cortex. Transcriptional dysregulation and proteasome inhibition would both contribute to the pathogenesis of polyglutaminopathies. There is a colocalization between the ubiquitin and the nuclear inclusions, suggesting a failure in the attempt to remove the misfolded proteins. There is also a colocalization with heat-shock proteins (HSPs) such as HSP70, HSP40, and CHIp. This is interpreted as an attempt of the cell to transform the misfolded protein in soluble components [47].

Natural Course and Follow-Up of SCAs

SCAs are characterized by a slow worsening of symptoms. The average disease duration in polyglutaminopathies is between 15 and 30 years [40]. A clinical scale called SARA has been designed for SCAs and can be used to monitor the clinical progression of the deficits [48]. Score ranges from 0 (no ataxia) to a maximum of 40. The ICARS (international cooperative ataxia rating scale) scale and the BARS (brief ataxia rating scale) scale can be used also. The extra-cerebellar deficits can be monitored using the INAS inventory (inventory for non-ataxia symptoms; 30 items) [49].

Table 11.4 Symptomatic therapies in SCAs

Seizures	Antiepileptic drugs
Psychiatric manifestations	Psychotropic medications
Tremor	Primidone, gabapentin, propranolol Deep brain stimulation (DBS) in selected cases
Restless legs syndrome	Dopamine agonists
Extrapyramidal deficits	Levodopa, dopamine agonists, amantadine
Spasticity	Baclofen, tizanidine
Muscle cramps	Magnesium, quinine

Therapies of SCAs

There is still no medication which reverts the natural course of SCAs. Table 11.4 shows the symptomatic treatments. Tandospirone and buspirone might improve slightly postural deficits, and acetazolamide may improve ataxia in SCA6 at the beginning of the disease [50]. The positive effects with the amino acid acetyl-DL-leucine acting on vestibular circuits need to be confirmed in a placebo-controlled trial [51]. Therapies under investigation aim to increase the clearance of proteins, to perform gene silencing, to modulate the transcription, or to decrease the expression of a mutated allele [52].

Regular physical therapy, speech/language therapy (which likely decreases the risk of swallowing difficulties), and occupational therapy are recommended. Intensive coordination training (3 × 1 h/week) improves motor activities [53]. Assisting devices (sticks, strollers) may be helpful in selected cases.

Episodic Ataxias

The episodic ataxias are monogenic disorders, also considered as a group of heterogeneous channel disorders. They are characterized by attacks of ataxia, which may be associated with a range of other neurological manifestations including myokymia, migraine, seizures, or chorea. The recurrent episodes of ataxia are often associated with vertigo and dizziness. The absence of impaired consciousness is very suggestive. Usually, the beginning and the end of the attack are clearly identified by the patients.

Eight episodic ataxia syndromes have been described: EA 1–7 and episodic ataxia with paroxysmal choreoathetosis and spasticity (CSE). EA 1 and 2 are the most common and best characterized of these. The genes for EA 1, 2, 5, and 6 (Table 11.5) have been identified with linkage loci mapped in EA 3, 7, and CSE. Episodic ataxia is rare with a combined incidence of <1:100,000.

Table 11.5 Episodic ataxias

EA	Gene (locus)	Mutation	Age of onset (years)
EA1	KCNA1 (12p13)	Point mutations	2–15
EA2	CACNA1A (19p13)[a]	Point mutations Deletions	1–30
EA3	? (1q42)	–	1–42
EA4	? (?)	–	20–60
EA5	CACNB4 (2q22-23)	Point mutations	3–19
EA6	SLC1A3 (5p13)	Point mutations	<20
EA7	? (19q13)	–	13–19

[a]Allelic to SCA6 and FHM (familial hemiplegic migraine)

EA1

Patients exhibit brief attacks of ataxia. They show an ictal dysarthria and typical interictal myokymia (continuous muscle unit activity) especially in the face or the hands. The episodes last from a few seconds to a few minutes, often triggered by stress, exercise (kinesigenic), or startle. Between the episodes, there is usually no ataxia or nystagmus. EA1 is primarily due to missense mutations in KCNA1 [54] although truncated mutations have been reported. The degree of channel impairment correlates with the severity of the phenotype. Mutations associated with severe phenotypes that may be poorly responsive to treatment or are associated with seizures or neuromyotonia show the most significant impairment of potassium channel function.

Patients usually benefit from a therapy with acetazolamide (500 mg/day). The drug reduces the number of attacks. Side effects include numbness, loss of appetite, loss of concentration, and kidney stones. Myokymia may be reduced with clonazepam, carbamazepine, or valproic acid.

EA2

This is the most common EA. The attacks are usually longer as compared to EA1, lasting from hours to days. An interictal nystagmus is commonly observed, and 50 % of the patients complain of headaches and nausea, sometimes with a misdiagnosis of migraine. The triggering factors are usually emotions, exercise, and fatigue. With time, patients develop an interictal mild ataxic syndrome that may mimic a SCA. Vermian atrophy is often detected on MRI (see Fig. 11.1). EA2 is due to a range of mutations in CACNA1A [55], which include missense, nonsense, aberrant splicing, and nucleotide insertions and deletions.

EA2 is allelic with FHM type 1 (migraine, hemiplegia, interictal nystagmus, and progressive ataxia) and SCA6 [56]. Most of the mutations that cause EA2 disrupt the open reading frame, whereas FHM is caused primarily by missense mutations. Acetazolamide (500 mg/day) is very effective. Aminopyridines may be effective also [57].

EA3

This EA has been reported in Canada. Episodes of ataxia, vertigo, and tinnitus last a few minutes [58]. Patients exhibit interictal myokymia. Acetazolamide reduces the number of attacks.

EA4

EA4 was reported in US families. It is also called periodic vestibulocerebellar ataxia (PATX). Patients exhibit attacks of ataxia and vertigo lasting a few hours. They show interictal ataxia and gaze-evoked nystagmus. Ocular pursuit is abnormal. Patients do not respond to acetazolamide.

EA5

EA5 has been described in a single French-Canadian family that was heterozygous for a missense mutation in the beta4-subunit of the calcium channel Cav2.1. Clinical presentation may be similar to EA2 (missense mutation), but mutations may present with a phenotype of generalized epilepsy or juvenile myoclonic epilepsy (heterozygous nonsense mutation) [59]. The precise functional effects of this mutation are not clear as the same mutation was identified in a German family with generalized epilepsy but no ataxia.

EA6

The disorder was initially reported in a child showing episodic ataxia, epilepsy, alternating hemiplegia, and migraine [60]. A de novo mutation was identified in the SLC1A3 gene, which results in complete loss of function of the protein EAAT1, a glutamate transporter localized to astrocytes. A Dutch family has been reported with the p.C186S variant that resulted in a milder phenotype without the manifestations of seizures or alternating hemiplegia [61]. Acetazolamide is effective to reduce symptoms.

Table 11.6 Differential diagnosis of EAs

Disease	Triggering factor
Hartnup disease (SLC6A19 gene – 5p15.33)	Sunlight exposure
	Fasting
	Emotion
	Intake of sulfonamides
Maple syrup urine disease (19q13.2, 7q31)	Intake of branched-chain amino acids
Deficiencies in urea cycle enzymes	Protein loads
	Valproate intake

EA7

In EA7, exertion or excitement provokes ataxia, vertigo, and weakness. Deficits last a few hours to a few days [62].

Differential Diagnosis

Table 11.6 lists the differential diagnosis of EAs.

Conclusion

With an expanding and aging population, the genetic cerebellar ataxias are becoming an increasingly important problem from the healthcare standpoint. The recent genetic progresses have significantly increased our understanding of these clinically heterogeneous disorders, allowing to dissect and better stratify the ataxias. Still, about 40 % of these patients remain with an undetermined etiology. The availability of novel genetic technologies to both research and diagnostic laboratories will facilitate a further rapid progress in this field. In the near future, a greater efficiency in diagnosis and the identification of many new forms of ataxia are therefore expected. The challenges for the future will be the complete understanding of the pathogenetic mechanisms in order to develop new therapies that will ultimately halt or reverse the degeneration and therefore the ataxia.

References

1. Manto MU. Cerebellar disorders. A practical approach to diagnosis and management. Cambridge: Cambridge University Press; 2010.
2. Manto M, Marmolino D. Cerebellar ataxias. Curr Opin Neurol. 2009;22:419–29.

3. Schöls L, Bauer P, Schmidt T, Schulte T, Riess O. Autosomal dominant cerebellar ataxias: clinical features, genetics, and pathogenesis. Lancet Neurol. 2004;3:291–304.
4. Marie P. Sur l'hérédoataxie cérébelleuse. Sem Med Paris. 1893;13:444–7.
5. Menzel P. Beitrag zur kenntniss der hereditären ataxie und kleinhirnatrophie. Arch Psychiatr Nervenkr. 1891;22:160–90.
6. Déjerine JJ, Thomas A. L'atrophie olivo-ponto-cérébelleuse. Nouv Iconogr Salpétr. 1900;13:330–70.
7. Holmes G. An attempt to classify cerebellar disease, with a note on Marie's hereditary cerebellar ataxia. Brain. 1907;30:545–67.
8. Marie P, Foix C, Alajouanine T. De l'atrophie cérébelleuse tardive à prédominance corticale. Rev Neurol. 1922;38:1082–111.
9. Greenfield JG. The spino-cerebellar degenerations. Oxford: Blackwell; 1954.
10. Harding AE. Classification of the hereditary ataxias and paraplegias. Lancet. 1983;1:1151–5.
11. Harding AE. The clinical features and classification of the late onset autosomal dominant cerebellar ataxias. A study of 11 families, including descendants of the 'the Drew family of Walworth'. Brain. 1982;105:1–28.
12. Harding AE. The hereditary ataxias and related disorders. Edinburgh: Churchill Livingstone; 1984.
13. Gasser T, Finsterer J, Baets J, et al. EFNS guidelines on the molecular diagnosis of ataxias and spastic paraplegias. Eur J Neurol. 2010;17:179–88.
14. Montenegro G, Powell E, Huang J, et al. Exome sequencing allows for rapid gene identification in a Charcot-Marie-Tooth family. Ann Neurol. 2011;69:464–70.
15. Bettencourt C, Ryten M, Forabosco P, Schorge S, Hersheson J, Hardy J, Houlden H, United Kingdom Brain Expression Consortium. Insights from cerebellar transcriptomic analysis into the pathogenesis of ataxia. JAMA Neurol. 2014;71:831–9.
16. Orr HT, Chung M, Banfi S, et al. Expansion of an unstable trinucleotide CAG repeat in spinocerebellar ataxia type 1. Nat Genet. 1993;4:221–6.
17. Taroni F, Chiapparani L, Mariotti C. Autosomal dominant spinocerebellar ataxias and episodic ataxias. In: Manto M, Gruol D, Schmahmann J, Koibuchi N, Rossi F, editors. Handbook of the cerebellum and cerebellar disorders. Dordrecht: Springer; 2013. p. 2193–267.
18. Duenas AM, Goold R, Giunti P. Molecular pathogenesis of spinocerebellar ataxias. Brain. 2006;129:1357–70.
19. Worth PF, Houlden H, Giunti P, Davis MB, Wood NW. Large, expanded repeats in SCA8 are not confined to patients with cerebellar ataxia. Nat Genet. 2000;24:214–5.
20. Kobayashi H, Abe K, Matsuura T, Ikeda Y, Hitomi T, Akechi Y, Habu T, Liu W, Okuda H, Koizumi A. Expansion of intronic GGCCTG hexanucleotide repeat in NOP56 causes SCA36, a type of spinocerebellar ataxia accompanied by motor neuron involvement. Am J Hum Genet. 2011;89:121–30.
21. Durr A, Forlani S, Cazeneuve C, et al. Conventional mutations are associated with a different phenotype than polyglutamine expansions in spinocerebellar ataxias. Eur J Hum Genet. 2009; 17:335.
22. Ikeda Y, Dick KA, Weatherspoon MR, Gincel D, Armbrust KR, Dalton JC, Stevanin G, Dürr A, Zühlke C, Bürk K, Clark HB, Brice A, et al. Spectrin mutations cause spinocerebellar ataxia type 5. Nat Genet. 2006;38:184–90.
23. Zühlke C, Bernard V, Dalski A, Lorenz P, Mitulla B, Gillessen-kaesbach G, Burk K. Screening of the SPTBN2 (SCA5) gene in German SCA patients. J Neurol. 2007;254:1649–52.
24. Houlden H, Johnson J, Gardner-Thorpe C, Lashley T, Hernandez D, Worth P, Singleton AB, Hilton DA, Holton J, Revesz T, Davis MB, Giunti P, Wood NW. Mutations in TTBK2, encoding a kinase implicated in tau phosphorylation, segregate with spinocerebellar ataxia type 11. Nat Genet. 2007;39:1434–6.
25. Bauer P, Stevanin G, Beetz C, Synofzik M, Schmitz-Hübsch T, Wüllner U, Berthier E, Ollagnon-Roman E, Riess O, Forlani S, Mundwiller E, Durr A, Schols L, Brice A. Spinocerebellar ataxia type 11 (SCA11) is an uncommon cause of dominant ataxia among French and German kindreds. J Neurol Neurosurg Psychiatry. 2010;81:1229–32.

26. Figueroa KP, Minassian NA, Stevanin G, Waters M, Garibyan V, Forlani S, Strzelczyk A, Bürk K, Brice A, Dürr A, Papazian DM, Pulst SM. KCNC3: phenotype, mutations, channel biophysics-a study of 260 familial ataxia patients. Hum Mutat. 2010;31:191–6.
27. Figueroa KP, Waters MF, Garibyan V, Bird TD, Gomez CM, Ranum LP, Minassian NA, Papazian DM, Pulst SM. Frequency of KCNC3 DNA variants as causes of spinocerebellar ataxia 13 (SCA13). PloS One. 2011;6:17811.
28. Yabe I, Sasaki H, Chen DH, Raskind WH, Bird TD, Yamashita I, Tsuji S, Kikuchi S, Tashiro K. Spinocerebellar ataxia type 14 caused by a mutation in protein kinase C gamma. Arch Neurol. 2003;60:1749–51.
29. Klebe S, Durr A, Rentschler A, Hahn-Barma V, Abele M, Bouslam N, Schöls L, Jedynak P, Forlani S, Denis E, Dussert C, et al. New mutations in protein kinase C gamma associated with spinocerebellar ataxia type 14. Ann Neurol. 2005;58:720–9.
30. van de Leemput J, Chandran J, Knight MA, Holtzclaw LA, Scholz S, Cookson MR, Houlden H, Gwinn-Hardy K, Fung HC, Lin X, Hernandez D, Simon-Sanchez J, et al. Deletion at ITPR1 underlies ataxia in mice and spinocerebellar ataxia 15 in humans. PLoS Genet. 2007;3:108.
31. Marelli C, van deLeemput J, Johnson J, Tison F, Thauvin-Robinet C, Picard F, Tranchant C, Hernandez D, Huttin B, Boulliat MD, Iban Sangla MD. SCA15 due to large ITPR1 deletions in a cohort of 333 white families with dominant ataxia. Arch Neurol. 2011;68:637–43.
32. Knight MA, Gardner RJ, Bahlo M, Matsuura T, Dixon JA, Forrest SM, Storey E. Dominantly inherited ataxia and dysphonia with dentate calcification: spinocerebellar ataxia type 20. Brain. 2004;127:1172–81.
33. Devos D, Schraen-Maschke S, Vuillaume I, Dujardin K, Nazé P, Willoteaux C, Destée A, Sablonnière B. Clinical features and genetic analysis of a new form of spinocerebellar ataxia. Neurology. 2001;56:234–8.
34. Bakalkin G, Watanabe H, Jezierska J, Depoorter C, Verschuuren-Bemelmans C, Bazov I, Artemenko K, Yakovleva T, Dooijes D, Van de Warrenburg B, Zubarev R, Kremer B, et al. Prodynorphin mutations cause the neurodegenerative disorder spinocerebellar ataxia type 23. Am J Hum Genet. 2010;87:593–603.
35. Schicks J, Synofzik M, Beetz C, Schiele F, Schöls L. Mutations in the PDYN gene (SCA23) are not a frequent cause of dominant ataxia in Central Europe. Clin Genet. 2011;80:503–4.
36. Brusse E, de Koning I, Maat-Kievit A, Oostra B, Heutink P, van Swieten J. Spinocerebellar ataxia associated with a mutation in the fibroblast growth factor 14 gene (SCA27): a new phenotype. Mov Disord. 2006;21:396–401.
37. Di Bella D, Lazzaro F, Brusco A, Plumari M, Battaglia G, Pastore A, Finardi A, Cagnoli C, Tempia F, Frontali M, Veneziano L, Sacco T, et al. Mutations in the mitochondrial protease gene AFG3L2 cause dominant hereditary ataxia SCA28. Nat Genet. 2010;42:313–21.
38. Cagnoli C, Stevanin G, Brussino A, Barberis M, Mancini C, Margolis R, Holmes S, Nobili M, Forlani S, Padovan S, Pappi P, Zaros C, et al. Missense mutations in the AFG3L2 proteolytic domain account for ~ 1.5 % of European autosomal dominant cerebellar ataxias. Hum Mutat. 2010;31:1117–24.
39. Wang JL, Yang X, Xia K, Hu ZM, Weng L, Jin X, Jiang H, Zhang P, Shen L, Guo JF, Li N, Li YR, et al. TGM6 identified as a novel causative gene of spinocerebellar ataxias using exome sequencing. Brain. 2010;133:3510–8.
40. Rüb U, Schöls L, Paulson H, Auburger G, Kermer P, Jen JC, Seidel K, Korf HW, Deller T. Clinical features, neurogenetics and neuropathology of the polyglutamine spinocerebellar ataxias type 1, 2, 3, 6 and 7. Prog Neurobiol. 2013;104:38–66.
41. van de Warrenburg BP, Sinke RJ, Verschuuren-Bemelmans CC, et al. Spinocerebellar ataxias in the Netherlands: prevalence and age at onset variance analysis. Neurology. 2002;58:702–8.
42. Silveira I, Miranda C, Guimarães L, et al. Trinucleotide repeats in 202 families with ataxia: a small expanded (CAG)n allele at the SCA17 locus. Arch Neurol. 2002;59:623–9.
43. Watanabe H, Tanaka F, Matsumoto M, et al. Frequency analysis of autosomal dominant cerebellar ataxias in Japanese patients and clinical characterization of spinocerebellar ataxia type 6. Clin Genet. 1998;53:13–9.

44. Kim JY, Park SS, Joo SI, Kim JM, Jeon BS. Molecular analysis of Spinocerebellar ataxias in Koreans: frequencies and reference ranges of SCA1, SCA2, SCA3, SCA6, and SCA7. Mol Cells. 2001;12:336–41.
45. Matsumura R, Futamura N, Ando N, Ueno S. Frequency of spinocerebellar ataxia mutations in the Kinki district of Japan. Acta Neurol Scand. 2003;107:38–41.
46. Zoghbi HY, Orr HT. Pathogenic mechanisms of a polyglutamine-mediated neurodegenerative disease, spinocerebellar ataxia type 1. J Biol Chem. 2009;284:7425–9.
47. Dickey CA, Patterson C, Dickson D, Petrucelli L. Brain CHIP: removing the culprits in neurodegenerative disease. Trends Mol Med. 2007;13:32–8.
48. Schmitz-Hübsch T, du Montcel ST, Baliko L, Berciano J, Boesch S, Depondt C, Giunti P, Globas C, Infante J, Kang JS, Kremer B, Mariotti C, Melegh B, Pandolfo M, Rakowicz M, Ribai P, Rola R, Schöls L, Szymanski S, van de Warrenburg BP, Dürr A, Klockgether T, Fancellu R. Scale for the assessment and rating of ataxia: development of a new clinical scale. Neurology. 2006;66:1717–20.
49. Schmitz-Hübsch T, Fimmers R, Rakowicz M, Rola R, Zdzienicka E, Fancellu R, Mariotti C, Linnemann C, Schöls L, Timmann D, Filla A, Salvatore E, Infante J, Giunti P, Labrum R, Kremer B, van de Warrenburg BP, Baliko L, Melegh B, Depondt C, Schulz J, du Montcel ST, Klockgether T. Responsiveness of different rating instruments in spinocerebellar ataxia patients. Neurology. 2010;74:678–84.
50. Jen JC, Yue Q, Karrim J, Nelson SF, Baloh RW. Spinocerebellar ataxia type 6 with positional vertigo and acetazolamide responsive episodic ataxia. J Neurol Neurosurg Psychiatry. 1998;65:565–8.
51. Strupp M, Teufel J, Habs M, Feuerecker R, Muth C, van de Warrenburg BP, Klopstock T, Feil K. Effects of acetyl-DL-leucine in patients with cerebellar ataxia: a case series. J Neurol. 2013;260:2556–61.
52. Underwood BR, Rubinsztein DC. Spinocerebellar ataxias caused by polyglutamine expansions: a review of therapeutic strategies. Cerebellum. 2008;7:215–21.
53. Ilg W, Synofzik M, Brötz D, Burkard S, Giese MA, Schöls L. Intensive coordinative training improves motor performance in degenerative cerebellar disease. Neurology. 2009;73:1823–30.
54. Browne D, Gancher S, Nutt J, Brunt ERP, Smith E, Kramer P, Litt M. Episodic ataxia/myokymia syndrome is associated with point mutations in the human potassium channel gene, KCNA1. Nat Genet. 1994;8:136–40.
55. Ophoff RA, Terwindt GM, Vergouwe MN, van Eijk R, Oefner PJ, Hoffman SM, Lamerdin JE, Mohrenweiser HW, Bulman DE, Ferrari M, Haan J, Lindhout D, van Ommen GJ, Hofker MH, Ferrari MD, Frants RR. Familial hemiplegic migraine and episodic ataxia type-2 are caused by mutations in the Ca2+ channel gene CACNL1A4. Cell. 1996;87:543–52.
56. Ducros A, Denier C, Joutel A, Cecillon M, Lescoat C, Vahedi K, Darcel F, Vicaut E, Bousser MG, Tournier-Lasserve E. The clinical spectrum of familial hemiplegic migraine associated with mutations in a neuronal calcium channel. N Engl J Med. 2001;345:17–24.
57. Ilg W, Bastian AJ, Boesch S, Burciu RG, Celnik P, Claaßen J, Feil K, Kalla R, Miyai I, Nachbauer W, Schöls L, Strupp M, Synofzik M, Teufel J, Timmann D. Consensus paper: management of degenerative cerebellar disorders. Cerebellum. 2014;13:248–68.
58. Steckley JL, Ebers GC, Cader MZ, McLachlan RS. An autosomal dominant disorder with episodic ataxia, vertigo, and tinnitus. Neurology. 2001;57:1499–502.
59. Escayg A, De Waard M, Lee DD, Bichet D, Wolf P, Mayer T, Johnston J, Baloh R, Sander T, Meisler MH. Coding and noncoding variation of the human calcium-channel beta4-subunit gene CACNB4 in patients with idiopathic generalized epilepsy and episodic ataxia. Am J Hum Genet. 2000;66:1531–9.
60. Jen JC, Wan J, Palos TP, Howard BD, Baloh RW. Mutation in the glutamate transporter EAAT1 causes episodic ataxia, hemiplegia, and seizures. Neurology. 2005;65:529–34.
61. de Vries B, Mamsa H, Stam AH, Wan J, Bakker SL, Vanmolkot KR, Haan J, Terwindt GM, Boon EM, Howard BD, Frants RR, Baloh RW, Ferrari MD, Jen JC, van den Maagdenberg AM. Episodic ataxia associated with EAAT1 mutation C186S affecting glutamate reuptake. Arch Neurol. 2009;66:97–101.
62. Kerber KA, Jen JC, Lee H, Nelson SF, Baloh RW. A new episodic ataxia syndrome with linkage to chromosome 19q13. Arch Neurol. 2007;64:749–52.

Chapter 12
Genetics of Recessive Ataxias

Stephan Klebe and Mathieu Anheim

Abstract Autosomal recessive cerebellar ataxias (ARCA) comprise a heterogeneous group of rare and most often complex hereditary neurodegenerative diseases. In the last few years, an acceleration of new ARCA gene discovery, including microarrays and next-generation sequencing, has occurred. These techniques have also led to the description of mutations in known genes associated with unusual phenotypes and the demonstration that there is a continuum between ARCA and other neurodegenerative disorders. An ARCA should be considered in patients (1) with an age at onset before 30 years, (2) with other affected siblings, and (3) if consanguinity in the family is known. According to pathophysiological principles, the ARCA might be associated with further neurological, especially neuropathy, and extra-neurological symptoms. Thus, results of electromyography are of interest for the classification of ARCA as well as for the etiological investigation. Similarly, another key point is whether there is clear cerebellar atrophy on brain MRI or not. However, both electromyography and MRI may be normal at the onset of the disease and should be repeated later in such cases. Several common pathophysiological pathways for ARCA have been described so far, including mitochondrial dysfunction, DNA repair deficiency, abnormal protein folding, and degradation, paroxysmal disorders. The following chapter classifies ARCA according to an absence or involvement of the peripheral nervous system in: (1) ARCA with pure sensory neuropathy, (2) ARCA with motor and sensory polyneuropathy, and (3) ARCA without polyneuropathy.

Keywords ARCA • Friedreich ataxia • Ataxia telangiectasia • AOA1 • AOA2

S. Klebe, MD (✉)
Department of Neurology, University Hospital Würzburg, Würzburg 97082, Germany
e-mail: Klebe_S@ukw.de

M. Anheim, MD, PhD
Movement Disorders Unit, Department of Neurology, University Hospital of Strasbourg, Strasbourg 67098, France

S.A. Schneider, J.M.T. Brás (eds.), *Movement Disorder Genetics*,
DOI 10.1007/978-3-319-17223-1_12

Introduction

Autosomal recessive cerebellar ataxias (ARCA) comprise a heterogeneous group of rare and most often complex hereditary neurodegenerative diseases [1]. The first symptoms of ARCA are subtle, with an age at onset (AAO) before 30 years for the majority of patients. ARCA persistently and gradually worsen over the years, leading to major disability in most patients after a mean disease duration of 10 years (Table 12.1). The foremost affected structures of the central nervous system are the cerebellum and/or the spinocerebellar tract and the posterior column of the spinal cord. Hence the principal clinical sign is cerebellar dysfunction and/or sensory ataxia. According to the pathophysiological principles, the ARCA might be associated with further neurological and extra-neurological symptoms. Thus the treatment of ARCA is not only limited to movement disorder specialists but requires close interaction between several medical disciplines as well as supporting treatment by speech therapy, occupational therapy, and physiotherapy. Regarding associated neurological symptoms, the peripheral nervous system is frequently affected in terms of polyneuropathy. Another common neurological overlap exists between ARCA and hereditary spastic paraplegias (HSP), in which an upper motor neuron syndrome (UMN) is the leading clinical feature. As for any other hereditary disease, the elicitation of family history is a crucial step in ARCA diagnosis. It is important to identify putative autosomal dominant pedigrees, as the autosomal dominant spinocerebellar ataxias (SCA) are frequently caused by polyglutamine and non-polyglutamine expansions that might be missed in sequencing diagnostic strategies. It is often more difficult to clinically and genetically assess patients without family history or without reliable information. An ARCA should be considered in patients (1) with an AAO before 30 years, (2) with other affected siblings (sisters and/or brothers), and (3) if consanguinity in the family is known. However, patients with an AAO >30 years are frequently reported in ARCA, especially for Friedreich ataxia (FRDA). According to the geographic origin of the patients and the number of siblings, the ARCA could also appear as sporadic ataxia. In these sporadic cases, ARCA is essentially a diagnosis of exclusion. The most frequent ARCA is FRDA, but in the last few years, an acceleration of gene discovery consecutive to the development of new technologies, including microarrays and next-generation sequencing (NGS), has occurred. These technologies, which respectively allow detection of copy number variations and small variants present all over the genome, have completely revolutionized the strategies used for gene identification; in particular, the analysis of small families and sporadic cases at an individual scale is now possible. These techniques have led to the identification of many new ARCA genes in which mutations are extremely rare and account for only a few families worldwide. Another consequence of the use of NGS in clinical practice is the description of mutations in known genes associated with unusual phenotypes and the demonstration that there is a continuum between ARCA and other neurodegenerative disorders. Examples for recently discovered ARCA genes are the ataxias with oculomotor apraxia (AOA1; *APTX*; AOA2; *SETX*) [2, 3]; ARSACS (*SACS*) [4]; autosomal recessive cerebellar ataxia types 1–3 (ARCA1 (*SYNE1*) [5], ARCA2 (*ADCK3*)

Table 12.1 Autosomal recessive ataxias according to the classification of autosomal recessive spinocerebellar ataxia (SCAR)

SCAR (OMIM)	Disease	Gene (OMIM)
SCAR1 (606002)	AOA2	SETX (608465)
SCAR2 (213200)	CPDIII	–
SCAR3 (271250)	SCABD	–
SCAR4 (607317)	SCASI	–
SCAR5 (606937)	CAMOS	ZNF592 (613624)
SCAR6 (608029)	–	–
SCAR7 (609270)	–	TPP1 (607998)
SCAR8 (610743)	ARCA1	SYNE1 (608441)
SCAR9 (612016)	ARCA2	ADCK3 (606980)
SCAR10 (613728)	ARCA3	ANO10 (613726)
SCAR11 (614229)	–	SYT14 (610949)
SCAR12 (614322)	–	WWOX (605131)
SCAR13 (614831)	–	GRM1 (604473)
SCAR14 (615386)	SPARCA1	SPTBN2 (604985)
SCAR15 (615705)	Salih ataxia	KIAA0226 (613516)
SCAR16 (615768)	–	STUB1 (607207)
SCAR17 (616217)	–	CWF19L1 (616120)

OMIM Online Mendelian Inheritance in Man®, *AOA* ataxia with oculomotor apraxia, *CPO III* cerebelloparenchymal disorder III, *SCABD* spinocerebellar ataxia with blindness and deafness, *SCASI* spinocerebellar ataxia with saccadic intrusions, *CAMOS* cerebellar ataxia with mental retardation, optic atrophy, and skin abnormalities, *ARCA* autosomal recessive ataxia, *SPARCA1* spectrin-associated autosomal recessive ataxia

[6], ARCA3 (*ANO10*) [7]); ataxia with peripheral neuropathy, hearing loss, ataxia, retinitis pigmentosa, and cataract (PHARC, *ABHD12*) [8]; Salih ataxia (*KIAA0226*) [9]; SCAR16 (STUB1) [10]; and Boucher–Neuhauser/Gordon Holmes Syndrome (*PNPLA6*) [11].

In patients with the suspected diagnosis of an ARCA, the available laboratory testing for biomarkers of several ARCA subtypes should be performed (ataxia telangiectasia (AT), AOA2, ataxia with vitamin E deficiency (AVED), ARCA3 (ANO10), Refsum disease, cerebrotendinous xanthomatosis (CTX), Niemann–Pick type C disease (NPC), Wilson disease, abetalipoproteinemia (ABL), ARCA2, ARCA3) – particularly as a treatment exists for some of these metabolic disorders. Several common pathophysiological pathways for ARCA have been described so far, including mitochondrial dysfunction, DNA repair deficiency, abnormal protein folding and degradation, paroxysmal disorders, and recently identified pathologies like a disorder of the endocannabinoid metabolism [8]. Several attempts to classify ARCA have been made according to the transmission (autosomal recessive spinocerebellar ataxias = SCAR) (Fig. 12.1; Table 12.1), while certain ARCA were subsumed due to the clinical picture (spastic ataxia = SPAX) (Fig. 12.1; Table 12.2).

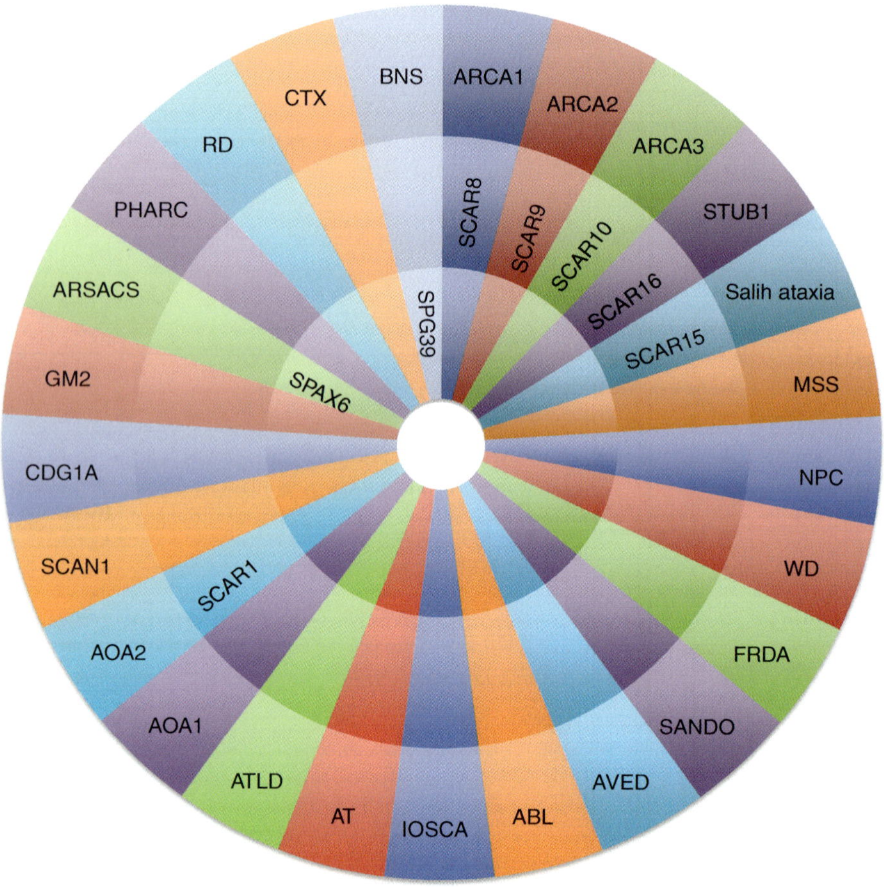

Fig. 12.1 Association between the ARCA, SCAR, and SPAX classifications. SPG39: hereditary spastic paraplegia type 39 is allelic with mutations in the *PNPLA6* gene, causing BNS

Table 12.2 Spastic ataxias according to the spastic ataxia (SPAX) classification

SPAX gene (OMIM)	Gene (OMIM)	Transmission
SPAX1 (108600)	VAMP1 (185880)	AD
SPAX2 (611302)	KIF1C (603060)	AR
SPAX3 (611390)	MARS2 (609728)	AR
SPAX4 (614672)	MTPAP (613669)	AR
SPAX5 (614672)	AFG3L2[a] (604581)	AR

OMIM Online Mendelian Inheritance in Man®, *AD* autosomal dominant, *AR* autosomal recessive
[a]Allelic to SCA28

However, the ARCA classification is confusing because of similarity to other neurodegenerative movement disorders such as HSP. The reason why some HSP are not classified as SPAX and *vice versa* is not obvious.

In the following chapter, the ARCA are classified according to their associated pathology in the peripheral nervous system. Three different groups are presented (Table 12.3): (1) ARCA with pure sensory neuropathy, (2) ARCA with motor and sensory polyneuropathy, and (3) ARCA without polyneuropathy.

ARCA with Pure Sensory Neuropathy

Friedreich Ataxia (FRDA)

FRDA is the most common ARCA in Europe, the Middle East, the Indian subcontinent, and North Africa [12, 13]. Its prevalence is estimated to be 1/25,000–1/50,000 in Caucasians, with a carrier frequency of 1/60–1/100 [12, 14]. The most common abnormality in >95 % of FRDA patients is a GAA trinucleotide repeat expansion in intron 1 of the *FXN* gene, which leads to a loss of function of the corresponding protein frataxin [15]. The penetrance of FRDA is complete when both alleles have full-penetrance GAA repeat (≥70 GAA trinucleotides) or in compound heterozygous patients with a GAA repeat expansion on one allele and a *FXN* pathogenic variant in the other. Frataxin is an iron-binding protein, predominately located in the mitochondria. The loss of function of frataxin results in mitochondrial respiratory chain dysfunction and elevated oxidative stress [16]. The mean AAO is between 10 and 15 years [17], but AAO of 2 years and over 70 years has been described [18]. The AAO is inversely correlated with the length of GAA repeats [18, 19]. Disease progression depends on the time since diagnosis, the AAO (faster progression if AAO ≤14 years [19]) and the GAA repeat length. The phenotype is dominated by a mixed cerebellar and sensory (proprioceptive)

Table 12.3 ARCA according to the associated involvement of the peripheral nervous system

Disease (OMIM)	AAO (mean)	Symptoms	Biological abnormalities	Gene (OMIM)	Protein
Ataxia without neuropathy (*Pure cerebellar ataxia, possibly associated with other symptoms*)					
ARCA1 (610743)	Late onset: 32 y (17–46 y)	Pure cerebellar ataxia, late onset, tendon reflexes⇑	–	SYNE1 (608441)	SYNE1
ARCA2 (612016)	4 y (1–11 y)	Epilepsy, myoclonus, mental retardation, stroke-like syndromes, tendon reflexes⇑	Muscle and/or fibroblasts: Lactate ⇑ CoQ10 (⇓)	ADCK3 (CABC1) (606980)	ADCK3
ARCA3 (613728)	23 y (6–43 y)	Cerebellar ataxia, UMN	Blood: AFP (⇑) Skin/muscle biopsy, blood: CoQ10 (⇓)	ANO10 (613726)	ANO10
STUB1 (615768)	8 months–49 y	Cerebellar ataxia, UMN, intellectual deficiencies, hypogonadism	–	STUB1 (607207)	CHIP
Salih ataxia (615705)	<7 y	Epilepsy, mental retardation	–	KIAA0226 (613516)	Rundataxin
MSS (248800)	Since birth	Bilateral congenital cataract, myopathy, developmental delay	Blood: Creatine kinase ⇑	SIL1 (608005)	SIL1
NPC (257220)	2–30 y	Supranuclear ophthalmoplegia, splenomegaly, dystonia, cognitive deficits	Leucocytes and/or fibroblasts: Chitotriosidase⇑ Oxysterol ⇑ Skin biopsy: Filipin test	NPC1/NPC2 (607623/601015)	NPC1/NPC2
Wilson disease (277900)	5–35 y	Hepatopathy, dystonia, tremor, parkinsonism, Kayser–Fleischer rings, hemolytic anemia, osteoporosis, protein-losing nephropathy	Serum: Ceruloplasmin⇓, copper⇓ 24-h urine: Copper⇑	ATP7B (606882)	Copper-transporting ATPase

Ataxia with pure sensory neuropathy					
FRDA (229300)	16 y (2–60 y)	Most frequent ARCA, square wave jerks, sensory neuropathy, UMN, no or only discrete cerebellar atrophy	–	FXN (606829)	Frataxin
SANDO (607459)	20–60 y	Ophthalmoparesis, sensory neuropathy, dysarthria, ptosis, myoclonia	–	POLG/Twinkle (174763/606075)	Polymerase gamma/ twinkle
AVED (277460)	17 y (2–50 y)	Friedreich-like phenotype, retinitis pigmentosa, sometimes head tremor	Vitamin E⇓⇓	Alpha-TTP (600415)	Alpha-TTP
ABL (200100)	Malabsorption: since birth Neurological symptoms: childhood–adolescence	Friedreich-like phenotype Vomiting, diarrhea, neonatal steatorrhea	Blood: Cholesterol⇓, triglycerides⇓ Vitamin A, D, E, K⇓ Abetalipoproteinemia Acanthocytosis	MTP (157147)	MTP
IOSCA (–)	≈1 y		–	C10ORF2 (Twinkle) (606075)	Twinkle
Cerebellar ataxia with motor and sensory polyneuropathy					
AT (208900)	≈2–3 y (most often < 5 y)	Telangiectasias, oculomotor apraxia, predisposition to cancer and infections, increased radiosensitivity choreodystonic movements	Blood: AFP⇑ Immunoglobulin deficit Chromosome translocation	ATM (607585)	ATM
ATLD (604391)	1–6 y	Oculomotor apraxia, choreodystonic movements, increased radiosensitivity	Blood: AFP normal	MRE11 (600814)	MRE11

(continued)

Table 12.3 (continued)

Disease (OMIM)	AAO (mean)	Symptoms	Biological abnormalities	Gene (OMIM)	Protein
AOA1 (208920)	7 y (1–20 y)	Hypometric saccades, choreodystonic movements, severe motor and sensory polyneuropathy	Blood: LDL⇑ Cholesterol⇑ Albumin⇓ Sometimes: CoQ10⇓	APTX (606350)	Aprataxin
AOA2 (606002)	15 y (7–25 y)	Oculomotor apraxia, strabismus	Blood: AFP⇑	SETX (608465)	Senataxin
SCAN1 (607250)	13–15 y	Axonal neuropathy	Blood: LDL (⇑) Cholesterol (⇑) Albumin (⇓)	TDP1 (607198)	Tyrosyl-DNA-phosphodiesterase
CDG1A (212065)	Congenital	Mental retardation, retinitis pigmentosa, spinal and thoracic deformities, epilepsy, cerebellar atrophy	Disturbed serum transferrin by isoelectric focusing	PMM2 (601785)	Phosphomannomutase
GM2 gangliosidoses with late onset (272800/268800)	15–45 y	Spastic paraplegia, dystonia, epilepsy, cognitive disturbance, psychosis, EMG with evidence of anterior horn cell involvement	Hexosaminidase A deficiency (Tay–Sachs) Hexosaminidase A + B deficiency (Sandhoff)	HEXA (Tay–Sachs)/ HEXB (Sandhoff) (606869/606873)	HEXA (Tay–Sachs) or HEXB (Sandhoff)
ARSACS (270550)	2–12 y	Spastic ataxia, RNFL thickening, axonal and demyelinating polyneuropathy	–	SACS (604490)	Sacsin
PHARC (612674)	15 y (4–37 y)	Demyelinating polyneuropathy, hearing loss, ataxia, retinitis pigmentosa, cataract, UMN	–	ABHD12 (613599)	ABHD12
RD (266500)	7 months–50 y	Demyelinating polyneuropathy, hearing loss, ataxia, retinitis pigmentosa, cardiac manifestation	Blood: Phytanic acid⇑	PhyH/PEX7 (602026/601757)	Phytanoyl-CoA hydroxylase/PEX7

CXT (213700)	Childhood	Spastic ataxia, dementia and/or mental retardation, tendon xanthomas, chronic diarrhea, early cataract	Blood: Cholestanol⇑ Bile acid⇑⇑	CYP27A1 (606530)	Sterol 27 hydroxylase
BNS (212840/215470)	1–30 y	Spastic ataxia, chorioretinal dystrophy, hypogonadotropic hypogonadism, intellectual deficiency, sensorimotor axonal neuropathy	–	PNPLA6 (603197)	PNPLA6

OMIM Online Mendelian Inheritance in Man®, *AAO* age at onset, *y* years, *ARCA* autosomal recessive ataxias, *UMN* upper motor neuron syndrome, *RNFL* retinal nerve fiber layer, *ARCA* autosomal recessive ataxia, *MSS* Marinesco–Sjögren syndrome, *NPC* Niemann–Pick type C disease, *FRDA* Friedreich ataxia, *SANDO* sensory ataxia neuropathy dysarthria and ophthalmoplegia, *IOSCA* infantile-onset spinocerebellar ataxia, *AVED* ataxia with vitamin E deficiency, *ABL* abetalipoproteinemia, *AT* ataxia telangiectasia, *ATLD* ataxia telangiectasia-like disorder, *AOA* ataxia with oculomotor apraxia, *SCAN1* spinocerebellar ataxia with axonal neuropathy, *CDG1A* congenital disorder of glycosylation type 1a, *ARSACS* autosomal recessive spastic ataxia of Charlevoix–Saguenay, *PHARC* polyneuropathy, hearing loss, ataxia, retinitis pigmentosa, and cataract, *RD* Refsum disease, *CTX* cerebrotendinous xanthomatosis, *BNS* Boucher–Neuhauser/Gordon Holmes ataxia. The sensory part of the ataxia is due to an affected dorsal column and a sensory polyneuropathy that can be seen in nerve conduction studies and the weak or absent tendon reflexes. A number of different neurological symptoms could be associated with FRDA: cerebellar dysarthria, UMN, auditory neuropathy, oculomotor manifestations (fixation instability, square wave jerks, seldom nystagmus), dysphagia, and optic atrophy. Rarely, psychiatric manifestations including cognitive impairment, depression, emotional liability, and schizophrenia-like psychosis are described [20, 21]. The most life-threatening, extra-neurological manifestation is hypertrophic cardiomyopathy (60 % of cases) that usually develops after the neurological symptoms. A correlation between the severity of neurological symptoms and cardiac involvement has not been found [22]. Other extra-neurological symptoms are diabetes mellitus type 1 (30 % of cases) and skeletal deformities (foot deformities, scoliosis). MRI scans reveal thinning of the cervical spinal cord and might also show signal abnormalities in the posterior and lateral columns [1]. It should be noted that cerebellar atrophy is not usually evident on brain CT or MRI imaging, especially early in the disease course (Fig. 12.2) [12, 23]. Several clinical types of FRDA have been described, like Friedreich ataxia with retained reflexes (FARR) [24, 25] despite the sensory polyneuropathy and late-onset Friedreich ataxia (LOFA) [26] or very late-onset Friedreich ataxia (vLOFA) [27, 28], with an AAO over 25 and over 40 years, respectively, as well as an FRDA dominated by spastic paraplegia [29].

The treatment of FRDA is so far based on physiotherapy, occupational therapy, and speech therapy. Several attempts that have addressed mitochondrial pathogenesis have been promising, but without striking success [13]. A substance with some potential is idebenone, which is structurally related to coenzyme Q_{10}. A number of double blind, placebo-controlled, and open-label trials have tested the clinical efficacy of idebenone (dosage 5–45 mg/kg per day) on neurological and cardiac symptoms in FRDA patients [30–34]. However, the studies led to conflicting results regarding cardiac and neurological outcome, and idebenone is currently not generally recommended in the treatment of FRDA. The same applies to erythropoietin (EPO); several open-label studies reported frataxin upregulation after EPO exposure, but no clinical efficacy has been shown [35, 36].

Ataxia with Vitamin E Deficiency (AVED)

The phenotype of AVED is very similar to FRDA progressive with a progressive sensory and cerebellar ataxia. AVED patients might also present cardiomyopathy, but less commonly than with FRDA. In most cases, the AAO is <20 years, with a slower disease progression than FRDA. Decreased visual acuity or retinitis pigmentosa may manifest early in the disease course. Interestingly, head tremor or titubation might be evocative for the diagnosis of an AVED, which resembles a dystonic head tremor. Electrophysiological studies show an axonal sensory neuropathy [37].

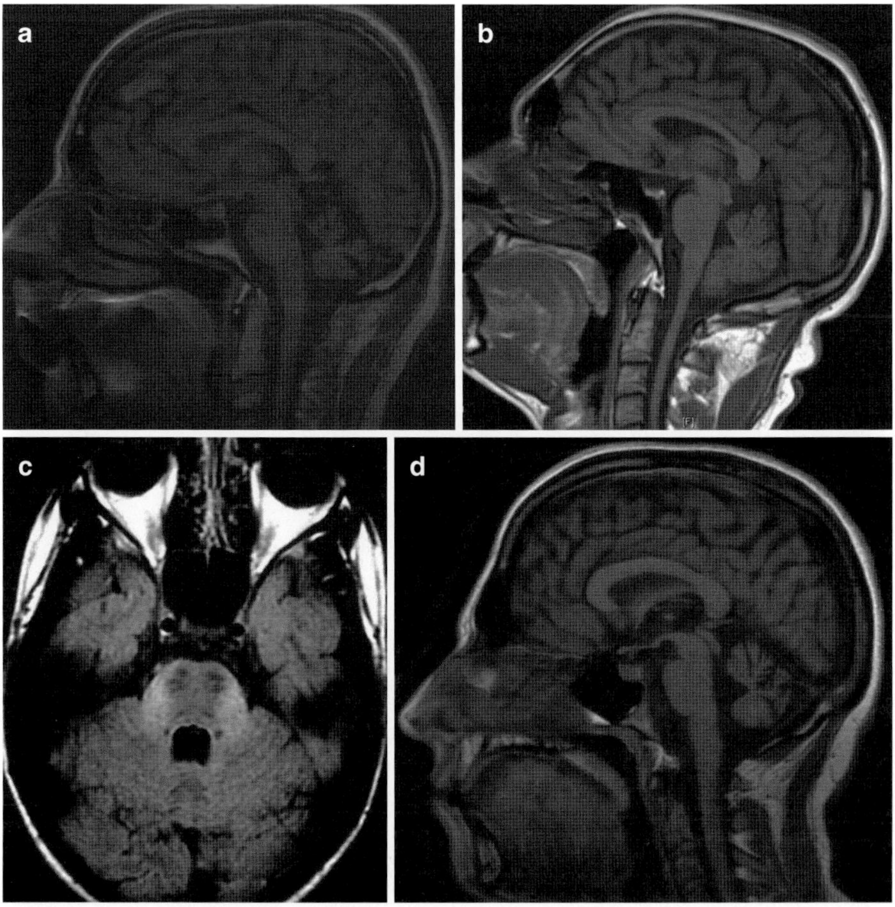

Fig. 12.2 Cerebellar MRI imaging of different ARCA. (**a**) Ataxia with oculomotor apraxia type 2 (AOA2) with marked cerebellar atrophy; (**b**) Friedreich ataxia without obvious cerebellar atrophy; (**c**) autosomal recessive spastic ataxia of Charlevoix–Saguenay (ARSACS) with linear hypointensities in the pons; (**d**) Niemann–Pick type C disease (NPC): marked cerebellar atrophy

AVED is the second most common ARCA after FRDA in North Africa due to a founder effect (744delA frameshift mutation) [38], but many patients have been reported elsewhere including Europe, North America, and Japan [39]. The laboratory hallmark is the low plasma level of vitamin E (<2.5 mg/l; normal, 5–20 mg/l). The identification of mutations in the TTPA gene confirms the disease. *TTPA* encodes for the α-tocopherol transfer protein that is implicated in the incorporation of vitamin E into circulating lipoproteins. The mutation results in a reduced delivery of vitamin E to the central nervous system (CNS). The therapy is based on a daily intake of 800–2,000 mg vitamin E, resulting in slower disease progression and probably a slight improvement of neurological symptoms.

Abetalipoproteinemia (ABL)

ABL, or Bassen–Kornzweig disease, is caused by an error of lipoprotein metabolism due to mutations in the microsomal triglyceride transfer protein gene (*MTP*) [40]. MTP plays a role in assembly or secretion of plasma lipoproteins that contain apolipoprotein B [37]. The clinical features therefore consist of a malabsorption syndrome due to a reduction of the lipid-soluble vitamins A, D, E, and K, cholesterol, and triglycerides, the absence of apolipoprotein B, and elevated serum transaminases with hepatomegaly due to hepatic steatosis [41]. ABL is a rare ARCA that usually starts in the perinatal period with diarrhea and vomiting and an insufficient gain in weight [42]. In the peripheral blood film acanthocytes and in the ophthalmological examination, retinitis pigmentosa might be found. The neurological symptoms often appear later in childhood and adolescence and comprise hyporeflexia, reduced proprioception, and vibratory sensation, muscle weakness, mild sensory neuropathy in the EMG, and a Friedreich-like ataxia, especially when the patients are not supplemented with vitamin E [43, 44]. The treatment for ABL is based on dietary modification and replacement of lipid-soluble vitamins (Table 12.4) [43].

Infantile-Onset Spinocerebellar Ataxia (IOSCA)

IOSCA is a rare ARCA that has initially been described in Finland [45] but recently also in Turkey [46], Korea [47], and England [48]. Between 1 and 2 years of life, following a normal period after birth, patients develop progressive ataxia, hypotonia, loss of deep tendon reflexes, myopathy, and athetosis [47, 49]. Signs of advanced disease include ophthalmoplegia, optic atrophy, epilepsy, and sensory axonal neuropathy [47, 49, 50]; sensory–motor neuropathy has been reported recently [47]. Extra-neurological symptoms might comprise elevated transaminases, sensorineural hearing loss, and female hypogonadism [49]. MRI images have revealed high-signal-intensity areas around the fourth ventricle, the superior cerebellar peduncle, the dentate nuclei, and the symmetric cerebellar cortical atrophy [47, 49]. IOSCA is due to mutations in the nuclear-encoded C10ORF2 gene (*Twinkle*). *Twinkle* encodes for a mitochondrial DNA (mtDNA) helicase responsible for the maintenance of mtDNA. Besides the autosomal recessive transmitted IOSCA, heterozygous mutations of *Twinkle* are associated with autosomal dominant progressive external ophthalmoplegia (adPEO) [51, 52]. A phenotypic overlap between adPEO and ataxia in patients with a heterozygous twinkle mutation has been described [50].

Table 12.4 Recommended intake of lipid-soluble vitamins in ABL [43]

Vitamin	Daily dosage
E	2,400–12,000 IU
A	100–400 IU/kg
D	1,000 mg
K	1,000 mg

Sensory Ataxic Neuropathy, Dysarthria, and Ophthalmoparesis (SANDO)

SANDO is frequently caused by homozygous or compound heterozygous mutation in the nuclear-encoded DNA polymerase gamma gene (POLG). Together with the *Twinkle* protein, the mitochondrial DNA polymerase gamma is responsible for mtDNA replication and repair in the mitochondria of eukaryotic cells. The phenotype of POLG mutations is variable and contains SANDO, spinocerebellar ataxia with epilepsy, Alpers syndrome (hepatocerebral mitochondrial depletion syndrome), mitochondrial recessive ataxia syndrome (MIRAS), myoclonic epilepsy myopathy sensory ataxia (MEMSA), mitochondrial neurogastrointestinal encephalopathy syndrome (MNGIE), PEO (autosomal dominant and recessive), and others [53–57].

SANDO is dominated by a mixed progressive cerebellar and sensory (proprioceptive) ataxia due to a predominantly sensory axonal neuropathy. The AAO is highly variable, between 15 and 60 years. Epileptic seizures, myoclonia, ophthalmoplegia, extrapyramidal symptoms, a myopathy with ragged red fibers, psychiatric phenomena, and liver failure are infrequently associated with SANDO [53, 58]. Besides *POLG*, mutations in *Twinkle* are known to cause the SANDO phenotype [50]. Cerebral MRI in SANDO patients reveals high-signal, sometimes "stroke-like" lesions in different brain regions such as the occipital lobes, deep cerebellar nuclei, thalamus, and basal ganglia [53, 58].

ARCA with Cerebellar Ataxia and Motor and Sensory Polyneuropathy

In this subgroup, ARCA with sensorimotor axonal neuropathy are summarized. The phenotype of cerebellar ataxia is variable and associated with oculocephalic dissociation or oculomotor apraxia (OMA) (AT, ATLD, AOA1, AOA2) or UMN (ARSACS, CTX, PHARC) (Table 12.3). Pathophysiologically, this group frequently contains DNA repair and/or cell cycle control mechanisms. Biomarkers exist for most of these entities, such as alpha-fetoprotein (AFP) (AT, AOA2, and to some extent AOA1), albumin (AOA1), and cholesterol (AOA1).

Ataxia Telangiectasia (AT)

AT commonly starts in early childhood (usually before age five). In certain populations, AT is the second most common ARCA but is much less common than FRDA with an estimated prevalence of 1–2.5/100,000 [12, 37]. OMA appears in a high proportion of patients [59]. Severe choreodystonic movements occur in

90 % of AT patients. The EMG might reveal an axonal motor and sensory polyneuropathy [60]. Brain MRI shows cerebellum atrophy. AT should be taken into account if patients develop oculocutaneous telangiectasias (conjunctivae, ears, mouth cavity) and disturbed endocrinological functions (stunted growth in puberty, delayed secondary sexual characteristics, infertility, type 2 diabetes). The cerebellar symptoms are progressive, and the patients are wheelchair bound around the age of 10 years. The lifespan is reduced due to malignancies or respiratory failure, but some patients survive until the fourth decade of life [37]. Laboratory tests show in almost every case an increase of AFP (200–300 ng/ml; normal <7 ng/ml) and immunoglobulin A and G deficiency. AT patients have an increased risk of recurrent infections (especially sinopulmonary and bronchopulmonary), malignancies (mainly hematological), and enhanced radiosensitivity. Recently, a less severe phenotypic variant with a milder disease course and a later AAO has been reported [59]. The presenting features in these patients were extrapyramidal disorder and choreatic movements [59]. In contrast to the classic phenotype, no immunodeficiency, less frequent endocrinological disturbances, but also a high risk for malignancies were noted [59]. The differences between the classic AT phenotype and these variants are explained by different mutations resulting in preserved small amounts of the responsible *ATM* gene. *ATM* encodes a P13kinase (ATM protein) that is involved in DNA repair and/or cell cycle control. In addition to the mutated ATM gene, rearrangements of chromosome 7 and 14 appear in 5–15 % of AT patients [37]. A few observational treatment studies have suggested that betamethasone is effective in AT patients [61–64]. Very recently, a multicenter, single-arm, open-label, phase II clinical trial with long-lasting monthly delivery of low doses of dexamethasone over 6 months led to an improvement of the International Cooperative Ataxia Rating Scale as primary outcome parameter [65].

Ataxia Telangiectasia-Like Disorder (ATLD)

The phenotype of the very rare ATLD comprises cerebellar ataxia with OMA, choreodystonic movements (mainly of the face and upper extremities), and peripheral neuropathy [66, 67]. ATLD is characterized by later onset and a slower progression than AT [68]. Nevertheless ATLD frequently starts in early childhood with cerebellar atrophy on MRI imaging. As for AT, increased radiosensitivity and increased levels of chromosome aberrations in lymphocytes are known. However, the terminology "AT-like" disorder is confusing, as ATLD has no raised AFP nor reduced immunoglobulin levels. For the cancer prone, conflicting results exist [66, 69–71]. ATLD is caused by mutations in the *MRE11* gene that codes for a protein with nuclease and intrinsic DNA-binding activity responsible for DNA repair.

Ataxia–Oculomotor Apraxia (AOA1 and AOA2)

The AAO of AOA1 is frequently from early childhood to adolescence (mean 7 years) [72], but AOA1 patients with a later AAO up to 40 years have been reported [73, 74]. AOA1 is the most frequent ARCA in Japan and is diagnosed in about 10 % of ARCA with an AAO less than 25 years in Europe [72]. The dominant clinical findings are cerebellar ataxia, mental retardation, and motor and sensory polyneuropathy [72, 75, 76]. The phenotype might also comprise choreodystonic movements (maybe only in early disease stages) and muscle weakness [72]. The OMA has been seen in more than two-thirds of patients [72]. The motor and sensory polyneuropathy can be particularly severe and might mimic Charcot–Marie–Tooth disease [72]. The time until wheelchair dependency ranges from 5 to 20 years [72]. Reduced levels of albumin and elevated levels of cholesterol in the serum, and decreased muscle CoQ10 levels in some cases, have been reported as biomarkers. The serum AFP is normal [72, 74, 76–78]. AOA1 patients show marked cerebellar atrophy in MRI [12, 72] and are generally confined to a wheelchair at around 18 years. The causative gene APTX and its protein aprataxin are ubiquitously expressed [2, 79]. APTX acts in an RNA–DNA damage response [80, 81].

AOA2 is genetically defined by mutations in the *SETX* gene, which codes for senataxin implicated in the DNA repair pathway and may also be a nuclear RNA helicase with a role in the splicing machinery [3]. The main features of AOA2 are cerebellar ataxia and axonal sensory–motor neuropathy, infrequently accompanied by UMN and/or choreodystonic movements [82, 83]. OMA is only observed in approximately half of the patients [84]; in some studies, OMA is even absent despite a sufficient number of patients [85]. The MRI reveals a marked cerebellar or pontocerebellar atrophy (Fig. 12.2). During the disease course, most AOA2 patients show elevated serum levels of AFP up to 30 ng/ml. In comparison to AOA1, a later AAO (usually between 10 and 25 years) and a better functional prognosis are observed in AOA2. Interestingly, besides AOA2 missense mutations in *SETX* can cause an autosomal dominant form of juvenile amyotrophic lateral sclerosis (ALS4) [86, 87].

Spinocerebellar Ataxia with Axonal Neuropathy (SCAN1)

SCAN1 is an extremely rare disease with a late-childhood onset (13–15 years) due to mutations in *TDP1* [88]. *TDP1* encodes for tyrosyl-DNA phosphodiesterase 1 (TDP1), a DNA repair enzyme that is involved in correction of the DNA. The clinical phenotype is characterized by cerebellar ataxia, cerebellar atrophy especially of the vermis in the MRI, and axonal sensory–motor neuropathy [89]. OMA or extraneurological manifestations are so far not known. Laboratory tests might reveal hypercholesterolemia and low levels of albumin in the serum [89].

Congenital Disorder of Glycosylation Type 1a (PMM2-CDG)

PMM2-CDG could be the cause of an ARCA, with an AAO between 3 and 10 years, mental retardation (IQ 40–70), retinitis pigmentosa, joint contractures, skeletal deformities, epilepsy, and motor and sensory polyneuropathy. In teenagers and adults, primary ovarian insufficiency, growth retardation, coagulation anomalies, and thrombotic events can complicate the phenotype [90]. PMM2-CDG is diagnosed by transferrin isoform analysis to determine the number of sialylated N-linked oligosaccharide residues linked to serum transferrin. These findings may lead to a molecular analysis of the *PMM2* gene coding phosphomannomutase. The brain MRI shows frequently cerebellar atrophy, sometimes associated with a mild atrophy of the pons.

Autosomal Recessive Spastic Ataxia of Charlevoix–Saguenay (ARSACS)

For a long time, ARSACS was thought to be a subtype of early-onset ataxia limited to the Quebec region due to founder mutations from a French ancestor. After the discovery of *SACS* as the responsible gene, ARSACS [4] is recognized worldwide as an important cause of inherited ataxia [91] and is now the second most common ARCA behind FRDA [92]. In most patients, ARSACS starts early in life (between 2 and 10 years), but onset from adulthood up to 40 years has been reported [93]. The clinical phenotype may imitate progressive spastic paraplegia in early disease stages, followed by cerebellar ataxia and axonal demyelinating motor and sensory polyneuropathy [92, 94]. Around 40 years of age, most patients are wheelchair bound. The classical ARSACS phenotype of spastic ataxia and polyneuropathy is sometimes associated with mental retardation, retinal striations in funduscopy, and hypertrophy of the retinal nerve fiber layer if optical coherence tomography is used [95]. However, unusual phenotypes lacking spasticity and/or polyneuropathy with ARSACS mutations have also been reported, especially outside Quebec [96–98]. Brain MRI demonstrates a cerebellar atrophy mainly of superior cerebellar vermis, linear pontine T2 hypointensities (Fig. 12.2), and bilateral FLAIR–T2 hyperintensities of the lateral pons when merging into the middle cerebellar peduncles (MCP), as well as thickening of the MCP. The *SACS* gene codes for sacsin, which is highly expressed in neurons, including Purkinje cells, and probably regulates the Hsp70 chaperone machinery [99].

Refsum Disease (**RD)**

RD is a peroxisomal disorder due to mutations of *PhyH* (encoding phytanoyl-CoA hydroxylase) or of *PEX7* (coding the peroxisome targeting signal 2 receptor). The first symptoms of RD appear between 7 months ("classic" RD) to over 50 years ("adult" RD). The clinical phenotype of RD is a variable combination of cerebellar ataxia, motor and sensory polyneuropathy, deafness, ataxia, anosmia, ichthyosis, and cardiac manifestations (cardiomyopathy, arrhythmias) [100, 101]. Nearly all patients have increased phytanic acid in the serum and/or other tissues, with elevated protein levels without pleocytosis in the cerebrospinal fluid. A lifelong dietary restriction of phytanic acid intake (avoidance of milk products, ruminant meat, fish, fat, green vegetables) that is optimally installed before irreversible symptoms appear can lead to a normal life. The daily intake of phytanic acid should be reduced from the usual level of 50 mg/day to less than 5 mg/day. In severe or rapidly worsening clinical conditions, plasmapheresis or lipapheresis is useful [102, 103].

Cerebrotendinous Xanthomatosis (CTX)

CTX is an inherited disorder of bile acid metabolism. There is a remarkable mean diagnostic delay of up to 16 years [104] in CTX patients that present their first symptoms in their late teens [105]. Clinical symptoms of the CNS comprise neurological (cerebellar ataxia, UMN, dystonia, palatal myoclonus) and psychiatric features (intellectual disability, dementia, behavioral changes, depression, agitation, hallucination, suicide attempts). The EMG reveals an axonal demyelinating motor and sensory polyneuropathy. Multiorgan, non-neurological manifestations have been described (i.e., tendon xanthomas, childhood-onset cataracts, infantile-onset diarrhea, premature atherosclerosis, osteoporosis, pulmonary insufficiency). MRI reveals cerebellar atrophy, white matter signal alterations, symmetric hyperintensities in the dentate nuclei, and a reduced brain volume [106]. The plasma cholestanol concentration, urine bile concentration and plasma bile concentration are dramatically increased. CTX is caused by mutations in the CYP27A1 gene coding for the mitochondrial enzyme sterol 27-hydroxylase. A replacement should be started as early as possible. The therapy is based on bile acid supplementation and administration of HMG-CoA reductase inhibitors, which lead to restoration of the bile acid synthesis by reducing plasma cholestanol levels and eliminating bile acid [107, 108].

GM2 Gangliosidoses *with Late Onset*: Tay–Sachs Disease (*GM2 Gangliosidosis, Type 1*) *and Sandhoff Disease* (*GM2 Gangliosidosis, Type 2*) *with Late Onset*

GM2 gangliosidoses belong to the lysosomal storage diseases. The neurological symptoms of GM2 gangliosidosis with late onset (between 15 and 45 years) usually start with spastic paraplegia, dystonia, cerebellar ataxia with cerebellar atrophy, epilepsy, cognitive deterioration, parkinsonism, neurobehavioral manifestations, and affection of anterior horn cells. Mutations in the *HEXA* gene cause Tay–Sachs disease, leading to the absence of beta-hexosaminidase A (HEX A) enzymatic activity in the serum, whereas the activity of the beta-hexosaminidase B (HEX B) isoenzyme is normal or elevated. Sandhoff disease is caused by mutations in the *HEXB*, resulting in disturbed activity of beta-hexosaminidase A and beta-hexosaminidase B.

Peripheral Neuropathy, Hearing Loss, Ataxia with Cerebellar Atrophy, Retinitis Pigmentosa, and Cataract (PHARC)

PHARC is a recently reported slowly progressive, "Refsum-like" disease [109] with an AAO from early childhood to the fourth decade of life [8]. Clinically, patients are affected by a sensory–motor neuropathy (more often demyelinating), hearing loss, ataxia with cerebellar atrophy, retinitis pigmentosa, cataracts, and UMN [8]. Patients from Europe, the Middle East, the USA, and Algeria have been reported so far [8, 110]. MRI shows cerebellar atrophy in some cases and is described as normal in others [8, 110]. PHARC is caused by mutations in *ABHD12* that encodes the a/b-hydrolase 12 enzyme implicated in the endocannabinoid metabolism [8]. Only a couple of *ABCD12* mutations have been reported in the literature so far [8, 110–112].

Boucher–Neuhauser/Gordon Holmes Syndrome (BNS)

BNS is defined as early-onset ataxia, hypogonadotropic hypogonadism (including primary amenorrhea in females), and chorioretinal dystrophy (Boucher–Neuhauser syndrome) or brisk reflexes (Gordon Holmes syndrome). The major cause of BNS was recently reported in European and South American patients with mutations in the *PNPLA6* gene [11]. The predominant phenotype of patients with *PNPLA6* mutations is cerebellar ataxia, UMN, hypogonadism, chorioretinal dystrophy, and sensorimotor axonal neuropathy [11]. The presenting symptoms are variable and could either be ophthalmologic or neurologic. The AAO ranges from 1 to 30 years [11, 113]. The brain MRI shows an atrophic pons and cerebellum, as well as a small pituitary gland. Formerly, mutations in *PNPLA6* gene were described as hereditary spastic paraplegia type 39 (SPG39) in two families with spastic paraplegia and distal muscle wasting [114]. *PNPLA6* encodes the patatin-like, phospholipase domain-containing protein 6 implicated in the de-esterification of membrane phosphatidylcholine into fatty acids and glycerophosphocholine.

ARCA Without Neuropathy

This group of ARCA describes cerebellar ataxias without changes in nerve conduction studies but commonly associated with other neurological or extra-neurological manifestations.

Autosomal Recessive Ataxia Type 1 (ARCA1)

Similar to ARSACS, ARCA1 was first discovered in families originating from a Quebec region (Beauce and Bas-St-Laurent) [5, 115]. Recently, ARCA1 has been reported in patients of Brazilian, French, and Japanese origin [116, 117]. In contrast to most other forms of ARCA, ARCA1 has a later mean AAO of 32 years (17–46 years) with cerebellar ataxia and increased tendon reflexes in some cases [5]. The MRI shows diffuse pure cerebellar atrophy. ARCA1 is caused by mutations in the *SYNE1* gene coding the SNYE1 protein. SYNE1 mutations have also been detected in Emery–Dreifuss muscular dystrophy [118]. SYNE1 is a spectrin, which is expressed in multiple tissues probably implicated in the cerebellar architecture. It also plays a role in neuromuscular junctions.

Autosomal Recessive Ataxia Type 2 (ARCA2)

ARCA2 is caused by mutations in the *ADCK3* gene. ADCK3 encodes for a mitochondrial kinase that is implicated in the metabolism of coenzyme Q_{10} [6]. The AAO ranges from childhood up to 19 years [119]. Recent studies noted the broad phenotypic spectrum of ARCA2 patients. Cerebellar ataxia appears in most patients, but dystonia, myoclonus, choreatic movements, UMN, intellectual deficiency, and, to a lesser extent, epilepsy might be the first symptoms [119]. The disease course is slowly progressive, as most patients are still ambulatory even after a disease duration of >20 years [119]. In some patients with a more severe disease course, stroke-like episodes including typical MRI changes have been noted [119, 120]. Fibroblasts, lymphoblast, or muscle biopsy might uncover coenzyme Q_{10} deficiency [6, 119]. Therefore, treatment with ubidecarenone or idebenone has been undertaken in ARCA2 patients but with no effect in most patients. However, clinical and/or electrophysiological improvement was seen in several patients [119, 121].

Autosomal Recessive Ataxia Type 3 (ARCA3)

ARCA3, due to mutations in the *ANO10* gene, was discovered recently in several European and West Indian pedigrees [7, 121, 122]. *ANO10* codes for a member of a family of putative calcium-activated chloride channels. The mean AAO of ARCA3 patients was 21 years (6–43 years) with a slow disease progression. The phenotype comprises cerebellar ataxia associated with marked cerebellar atrophy in the MRI and UMN. The laboratory showed mildly increased AFP levels and, as in ARCA2, a coenzyme Q_{10} deficiency in some patients [121, 122].

STUB1 Mutations

Mutations in the *STUB1* gene were first discovered in China [10, 123] and later confirmed in families of German, Belgium, Turkish, Middle Eastern, and Sri Lankan origin with ARCA or spastic paraplegia by whole exome sequencing [124–126]. *STUB1* encodes CHIP (C-terminus of heat shock protein 70-interacting protein) that has two different functions, with a role in ubiquitination and as an E3 ligase. The AAO varies between 8 months and 49 years [125]. Cerebellar ataxia is often associated with UMN (not in all cases), intellectual deficiencies, and a hypogonadism that resembles a Gordon Holmes syndrome [10, 123–126]. However other genes such as *PNPLA6*, *RNF216*, or *OTUD4* might also cause hereditary cerebellar ataxia with hypogonadism. MRI analyses have shown severe cerebellar atrophy and a distinct thinning of the anterior part of the corpus callosum in some cases [125].

Salih Ataxia

Salih ataxia is caused by mutations in the *KIAA0226* gene that codes for rundataxin. Only one Saudi Arabian family has been identified yet, with an early AAO between 2 and 7 years. The phenotype shows a progressive cerebellar ataxia, mental retardation, and epilepsy in several family members [127].

Marinesco–Sjögren Syndrome (MSS)

The symptoms of MSS frequently comprise bilateral congenital cataracts, cerebellar ataxia, intellectual disability, and progressive muscle weakness due to myopathy with elevated serum levels of creatine kinase. These key features might be associated with short stature, hypergonadotropic hypogonadism [128], strabismus, and optic atrophy [129, 130]. In most patients, mutations in the *SIL1* gene (coding the SIL1 protein) have been described in several European countries, Egypt, and Asia [131]. A loss of SIL1 protein function results in an accumulation of unfolded proteins in the endoplasmic reticulum [132]. However, several patients with the MSS phenotype have been reported to lack SIL1 mutations [133]. Patients without SIL1 mutations are clinically indistinguishable to SIL1 mutation carriers [130]. First symptoms appear after birth, including bilateral cataracts and delayed motor development. The ability to walk independently is only reached in some patients. Cerebellar atrophy is not an obligatory finding in MSS patients [134] but often seen [130]. Low vitamin E levels in an Italian family have recently been reported [135].

Niemann–Pick Type C Disease (NPC)

NPC is a lipid storage disorder. The clinical hallmark of NPC is the combination of ataxia, choreodystonic movements, vertical supranuclear gaze palsy, and cognitive and psychiatric impairment. These conditions can be associated with myoclonus, cataplexy (episodes of sudden loss of muscle tone), and splenomegaly. In patients for whom NPC is suspected, elevated chitotriosidase and oxysterol levels in the serum and filipin staining in fibroblast provide diagnostic clues [136]. The MRI frequently discovers a brain and/or cerebellar atrophy (Fig. 12.2), whereas the EMG is normal. The disease is confirmed by mutations in *NPC1* or *NPC2*. Miglustat is a treatment option in NPC patients, to stabilize or slow disease progression [136, 137].

Wilson Disease (WD)

WD or hepatolenticular degeneration is characterized by disturbed copper metabolism, with the consequence of hepatic, ophthalmological, and neurological symptoms. Clinically, WD consists of cerebellar ataxia, extrapyramidal symptoms (dystonia, parkinsonism), tremor, psychiatric manifestations, dementia, hemolytic anemia, osteoporosis, tubulointerstitial nephropathy, and Kayser–Fleischer rings of the eye. Serum specimens of WD patients present low ceruloplasmin and low copper (but high non-ceruloplasmin-bound copper). The copper in the 24-h urine is increased.

T2-weighted MRI imaging might reveal hyperintense lesions involving bilateral thalami, midbrain, and pons. These midbrain hyperintensities form the "face of the giant panda" sign [138, 139]. In addition, a generalized brain atrophy and/or cerebellar atrophy might exist. WD is caused by mutations in *ATP7B*, encoding a copper ATPase transporter. The treatment of WD is based on increasing copper urinary excretion by, for example, penicillamine.

References

1. Fogel BL, Perlman S. Clinical features and molecular genetics of autosomal recessive cerebellar ataxias. Lancet Neurol. 2007;6:245–57.
2. Date H, Onodera O, Tanaka H, et al. Early-onset ataxia with ocular motor apraxia and hypoalbuminemia is caused by mutations in a new HIT superfamily gene. Nat Genet. 2001;29:184–8.
3. Moreira MC, Klur S, Watanabe M, et al. Senataxin, the ortholog of a yeast RNA helicase, is mutant in ataxia-ocular apraxia 2. Nat Genet. 2004;36:225–7.
4. Engert JC, Berube P, Mercier J, et al. ARSACS, a spastic ataxia common in northeastern Quebec, is caused by mutations in a new gene encoding an 11.5-kb ORF. Nat Genet. 2000;24:120–5.

5. Gros-Louis F, Dupre N, Dion P, et al. Mutations in SYNE1 lead to a newly discovered form of autosomal recessive cerebellar ataxia. Nat Genet. 2007;39:80–5.
6. Lagier-Tourenne C, Tazir M, Lopez LC, et al. ADCK3, an ancestral kinase, is mutated in a form of recessive ataxia associated with coenzyme Q10 deficiency. Am J Hum Genet. 2008;82:661–72.
7. Vermeer S, Hoischen A, Meijer RP, et al. Targeted next-generation sequencing of a 12.5 Mb homozygous region reveals ANO10 mutations in patients with autosomal-recessive cerebellar ataxia. Am J Hum Genet. 2010;87:813–9.
8. Fiskerstrand T, H'Mida-Ben Brahim D, Johansson S, et al. Mutations in ABHD12 cause the neurodegenerative disease PHARC: an inborn error of endocannabinoid metabolism. Am J Hum Genet. 2010;87:410–7.
9. Assoum M, Salih MA, Drouot N, Hnia K, Martelli A, Koenig M. The Salih ataxia mutation impairs Rubicon endosomal localization. Cerebellum. 2013;12:835–40.
10. Shi Y, Wang J, Li JD, et al. Identification of CHIP as a novel causative gene for autosomal recessive cerebellar ataxia. PLoS One. 2013;8:e81884.
11. Synofzik M, Gonzalez MA, Lourenco CM, et al. PNPLA6 mutations cause Boucher-Neuhauser and Gordon Holmes syndromes as part of a broad neurodegenerative spectrum. Brain. 2014;137:69–77.
12. Anheim M, Fleury M, Monga B, et al. Epidemiological, clinical, paraclinical and molecular study of a cohort of 102 patients affected with autosomal recessive progressive cerebellar ataxia from Alsace, Eastern France: implications for clinical management. Neurogenetics. 2010;11:1–12.
13. Schulz JB, Boesch S, Burk K, et al. Diagnosis and treatment of Friedreich ataxia: a European perspective. Nat Rev Neurol. 2009;5:222–34.
14. Cossee M, Schmitt M, Campuzano V, et al. Evolution of the Friedreich's ataxia trinucleotide repeat expansion: founder effect and permutations. Proc Natl Acad Sci U S A. 1997;94:7452–7.
15. Campuzano V, Montermini L, Molto MD, et al. Friedreich's ataxia: autosomal recessive disease caused by an intronic GAA triplet repeat expansion. Science. 1996;271:1423–7.
16. Santos R, Lefevre S, Sliwa D, Seguin A, Camadro JM, Lesuisse E. Friedreich ataxia: molecular mechanisms, redox considerations, and therapeutic opportunities. Antioxid Redox Signal. 2010;13:651–90.
17. Delatycki MB, Paris DB, Gardner RJ, et al. Clinical and genetic study of Friedreich ataxia in an Australian population. Am J Med Genet. 1999;87:168–74.
18. Durr A, Cossee M, Agid Y, et al. Clinical and genetic abnormalities in patients with Friedreich's ataxia. N Engl J Med. 1996;335:1169–75.
19. Metz G, Coppard N, Cooper JM, et al. Rating disease progression of Friedreich's ataxia by the International Cooperative Ataxia Rating Scale: analysis of a 603-patient database. Brain. 2013;136:259–68.
20. Chan YC. Aripiprazole treatment for psychosis associated with Friedreich's ataxia. Gen Hosp Psychiatry. 2005;27:372.
21. White M, Lalonde R, Botez-Marquard T. Neuropsychologic and neuropsychiatric characteristics of patients with Friedreich's ataxia. Acta Neurol Scand. 2000;102:222–6.
22. Weidemann F, Rummey C, Bijnens B, et al. The heart in Friedreich ataxia: definition of cardiomyopathy, disease severity, and correlation with neurological symptoms. Circulation. 2012;125:1626–34.
23. Mascalchi M, Salvi F, Piacentini S, Bartolozzi C. Friedreich's ataxia: MR findings involving the cervical portion of the spinal cord. AJR Am J Roentgenol. 1994;163:187–91.
24. Coppola G, De Michele G, Cavalcanti F, et al. Why do some Friedreich's ataxia patients retain tendon reflexes? A clinical, neurophysiological and molecular study. J Neurol. 1999;246:353–7.
25. Armani M, Zortea M, Pastorello E, et al. Friedreich's ataxia: clinical heterogeneity in two sisters. Neurol Sci. 2006;27:140–2.
26. Bhidayasiri R, Perlman SL, Pulst SM, Geschwind DH. Late-onset Friedreich ataxia: phenotypic analysis, magnetic resonance imaging findings, and review of the literature. Arch Neurol. 2005;62:1865–9.

27. Patel PI, Dimachkie MM. Atypical friedreich ataxia with a very late onset and an unusual limited GAA repeat. Arch Neurol. 2000;57:1380–2.
28. Bidichandani SI, Garcia CA, Patel PI, Dimachkie MM. Very late-onset Friedreich ataxia despite large GAA triplet repeat expansions. Arch Neurol. 2000;57:246–51.
29. de Bot ST, Willemsen MA, Vermeer S, Kremer HP, van de Warrenburg BP. Reviewing the genetic causes of spastic-ataxias. Neurology. 2012;79:1507–14.
30. Lynch DR, Perlman SL, Meier T. A phase 3, double-blind, placebo-controlled trial of idebenone in friedreich ataxia. Arch Neurol. 2010;67:941–7.
31. Di Prospero NA, Baker A, Jeffries N, Fischbeck KH. Neurological effects of high-dose idebenone in patients with Friedreich's ataxia: a randomised, placebo-controlled trial. Lancet Neurol. 2007;6:878–86.
32. Di Prospero NA, Sumner CJ, Penzak SR, Ravina B, Fischbeck KH, Taylor JP. Safety, tolerability, and pharmacokinetics of high-dose idebenone in patients with Friedreich ataxia. Arch Neurol. 2007;64:803–8.
33. Hausse AO, Aggoun Y, Bonnet D, et al. Idebenone and reduced cardiac hypertrophy in Friedreich's ataxia. Heart. 2002;87:346–9.
34. Ribai P, Pousset F, Tanguy ML, et al. Neurological, cardiological, and oculomotor progression in 104 patients with Friedreich ataxia during long-term follow-up. Arch Neurol. 2007;64:558–64.
35. Mariotti C, Fancellu R, Caldarazzo S, et al. Erythropoietin in Friedreich ataxia: no effect on frataxin in a randomized controlled trial. Mov Disord. 2012;27:446–9.
36. Mariotti C, Nachbauer W, Panzeri M, Poewe W, Taroni F, Boesch S. Erythropoietin in Friedreich ataxia. J Neurochem. 2013;126 Suppl 1:80–7.
37. Palau F, Espinos C. Autosomal recessive cerebellar ataxias. Orphanet J Rare Dis. 2006;1:47.
38. Ouahchi K, Arita M, Kayden H, et al. Ataxia with isolated vitamin E deficiency is caused by mutations in the alpha-tocopherol transfer protein. Nat Genet. 1995;9:141–5.
39. Cavalier L, Ouahchi K, Kayden HJ, et al. Ataxia with isolated vitamin E deficiency: heterogeneity of mutations and phenotypic variability in a large number of families. Am J Hum Genet. 1998;62:301–10.
40. Narcisi TM, Shoulders CC, Chester SA, et al. Mutations of the microsomal triglyceride-transfer-protein gene in abetalipoproteinemia. Am J Hum Genet. 1995;57:1298–310.
41. Collins JC, Scheinberg IH, Giblin DR, Sternlieb I. Hepatic peroxisomal abnormalities in abetalipoproteinemia. Gastroenterology. 1989;97:766–70.
42. Kohlschutter A. Abetalipoproteinemia. In: Klockgether T, editor. Handbook of ataxia disorders. New York: Marcel Dekker; 2000. p. 205–21.
43. Zamel R, Khan R, Pollex RL, Hegele RA. Abetalipoproteinemia: two case reports and literature review. Orphanet J Rare Dis. 2008;3:19.
44. Muller DP, Lloyd JK, Wolff OH. The role of vitamin E in the treatment of the neurological features of abetalipoproteinaemia and other disorders of fat absorption. J Inherit Metab Dis. 1985;8 Suppl 1:88–92.
45. Koskinen T, Sainio K, Rapola J, Pihko H, Paetau A. Sensory neuropathy in infantile onset spinocerebellar ataxia (IOSCA). Muscle Nerve. 1994;17:509–15.
46. Dundar H, Ozgul RK, Yalnizoglu D, et al. Identification of a novel Twinkle mutation in a family with infantile onset spinocerebellar ataxia by whole exome sequencing. Pediatr Neurol. 2012;46:172–7.
47. Park MH, Woo HM, Hong YB, et al. Recessive C10orf2 mutations in a family with infantile-onset spinocerebellar ataxia, sensorimotor polyneuropathy, and myopathy. Neurogenetics. 2014;15:171–82.
48. Hartley JN, Booth FA, Del Bigio MR, Mhanni AA. Novel Autosomal Recessive c10orf2 Mutations Causing Infantile-Onset Spinocerebellar Ataxia. Case Rep Pediatr. 2012;2012:303096.
49. Hakonen AH, Isohanni P, Paetau A, Herva R, Suomalainen A, Lonnqvist T. Recessive Twinkle mutations in early onset encephalopathy with mtDNA depletion. Brain. 2007;130:3032–40.

50. Hudson G, Deschauer M, Busse K, Zierz S, Chinnery PF. Sensory ataxic neuropathy due to a novel C10Orf2 mutation with probable germline mosaicism. Neurology. 2005;64:371–3.
51. Van Hove JL, Cunningham V, Rice C, et al. Finding twinkle in the eyes of a 71-year-old lady: a case report and review of the genotypic and phenotypic spectrum of TWINKLE-related dominant disease. Am J Med Genet A. 2009;149A:861–7.
52. Fratter C, Gorman GS, Stewart JD, et al. The clinical, histochemical, and molecular spectrum of PEO1 (Twinkle)-linked adPEO. Neurology. 2010;74:1619–26.
53. Tchikviladze M, Gilleron M, Maisonobe T, et al. A diagnostic flow chart for POLG-related diseases based on signs sensitivity and specificity. J Neurol Neurosurg Psychiatry. 2014 (Epub ahead of print).
54. Menezes MP, Ouvrier RA. Peripheral neuropathy associated with mitochondrial disease in children. Dev Med Child Neurol. 2012;54:407–14.
55. Mancuso M, Filosto M, Bellan M, et al. POLG mutations causing ophthalmoplegia, sensorimotor polyneuropathy, ataxia, and deafness. Neurology. 2004;62:316–8.
56. Winterthun S, Ferrari G, He L, et al. Autosomal recessive mitochondrial ataxic syndrome due to mitochondrial polymerase gamma mutations. Neurology. 2005;64:1204–8.
57. Milone M, Benarroch EE, Wong LJ. POLG-related disorders: defects of the nuclear and mitochondrial genome interaction. Neurology. 2011;77:1847–52.
58. Tzoulis C, Engelsen BA, Telstad W, et al. The spectrum of clinical disease caused by the A467T and W748S POLG mutations: a study of 26 cases. Brain. 2006;129:1685–92.
59. Verhagen MM, Abdo WF, Willemsen MA, et al. Clinical spectrum of ataxia-telangiectasia in adulthood. Neurology. 2009;73:430–7.
60. Woods CG, Taylor AM. Ataxia telangiectasia in the British Isles: the clinical and laboratory features of 70 affected individuals. Q J Med. 1992;82:169–79.
61. Zannolli R, Buoni S, Betti G, et al. A randomized trial of oral betamethasone to reduce ataxia symptoms in ataxia telangiectasia. Mov Disord. 2012;27:1312–6.
62. Buoni S, Zannolli R, Sorrentino L, Fois A. Betamethasone and improvement of neurological symptoms in ataxia-telangiectasia. Arch Neurol. 2006;63:1479–82.
63. Broccoletti T, Del Giudice E, Amorosi S, et al. Steroid-induced improvement of neurological signs in ataxia-telangiectasia patients. Eur J Neurol. 2008;15:223–8.
64. Broccoletti T, Del Giudice E, Cirillo E, et al. Efficacy of very-low-dose betamethasone on neurological symptoms in ataxia-telangiectasia. Eur J Neurol. 2011;18:564–70.
65. Chessa L, Leuzzi V, Plebani A, et al. Intra-erythrocyte infusion of dexamethasone reduces neurological symptoms in ataxia telangiectasia patients: results of a phase 2 trial. Orphanet J Rare Dis. 2014;9:5.
66. Delia D, Piane M, Buscemi G, et al. MRE11 mutations and impaired ATM-dependent responses in an Italian family with ataxia-telangiectasia-like disorder. Hum Mol Genet. 2004;13:2155–63.
67. Stewart GS, Maser RS, Stankovic T, et al. The DNA double-strand break repair gene hMRE11 is mutated in individuals with an ataxia-telangiectasia-like disorder. Cell. 1999;99:577–87.
68. Taylor AM, Groom A, Byrd PJ. Ataxia-telangiectasia-like disorder (ATLD)-its clinical presentation and molecular basis. DNA Repair (Amst). 2004;3:1219–25.
69. Uchisaka N, Takahashi N, Sato M, et al. Two brothers with ataxia-telangiectasia-like disorder with lung adenocarcinoma. J Pediatr. 2009;155:435–8.
70. Fernet M, Gribaa M, Salih MA, Seidahmed MZ, Hall J, Koenig M. Identification and functional consequences of a novel MRE11 mutation affecting 10 Saudi Arabian patients with the ataxia telangiectasia-like disorder. Hum Mol Genet. 2005;14:307–18.
71. Oba D, Hayashi M, Minamitani M, et al. Autopsy study of cerebellar degeneration in siblings with ataxia-telangiectasia-like disorder. Acta Neuropathol. 2010;119:513–20.
72. Le Ber I, Moreira MC, Rivaud-Pechoux S, et al. Cerebellar ataxia with oculomotor apraxia type 1: clinical and genetic studies. Brain. 2003;126:2761–72.
73. Criscuolo C, Mancini P, Menchise V, et al. Very late onset in ataxia oculomotor apraxia type I. Ann Neurol. 2005;57:777.

74. Criscuolo C, Mancini P, Sacca F, et al. Ataxia with oculomotor apraxia type 1 in Southern Italy: late onset and variable phenotype. Neurology. 2004;63:2173–5.
75. Anheim M, Tranchant C, Koenig M. The autosomal recessive cerebellar ataxias. N Engl J Med. 2012;366:636–46.
76. Castellotti B, Mariotti C, Rimoldi M, et al. Ataxia with oculomotor apraxia type1 (AOA1): novel and recurrent aprataxin mutations, coenzyme Q10 analyses, and clinical findings in Italian patients. Neurogenetics. 2011;12:193–201.
77. Le Ber I, Dubourg O, Benoist JF, et al. Muscle coenzyme Q10 deficiencies in ataxia with oculomotor apraxia 1. Neurology. 2007;68:295–7.
78. Quinzii CM, Lopez LC, Naini A, DiMauro S, Hirano M. Human CoQ10 deficiencies. Biofactors. 2008;32:113–8.
79. Moreira MC, Barbot C, Tachi N, et al. Homozygosity mapping of Portuguese and Japanese forms of ataxia-oculomotor apraxia to 9p13, and evidence for genetic heterogeneity. Am J Hum Genet. 2001;68:501–8.
80. Tumbale P, Williams JS, Schellenberg MJ, Kunkel TA, Williams RS. Aprataxin resolves adenylated RNA-DNA junctions to maintain genome integrity. Nature. 2014;506:111–5.
81. Moreira MC, Barbot C, Tachi N, et al. The gene mutated in ataxia-ocular apraxia 1 encodes the new HIT/Zn-finger protein aprataxin. Nat Genet. 2001;29:189–93.
82. Anheim M, Monga B, Fleury M, et al. Ataxia with oculomotor apraxia type 2: clinical, biological and genotype/phenotype correlation study of a cohort of 90 patients. Brain. 2009;132:2688–98.
83. Anheim M, Fleury MC, Franques J, et al. Clinical and molecular findings of ataxia with oculomotor apraxia type 2 in 4 families. Arch Neurol. 2008;65:958–62.
84. Le Ber I, Bouslam N, Rivaud-Pechoux S, et al. Frequency and phenotypic spectrum of ataxia with oculomotor apraxia 2: a clinical and genetic study in 18 patients. Brain. 2004;127:759–67.
85. Duquette A, Roddier K, McNabb-Baltar J, et al. Mutations in senataxin responsible for Quebec cluster of ataxia with neuropathy. Ann Neurol. 2005;57:408–14.
86. Chen YZ, Hashemi SH, Anderson SK, et al. Senataxin, the yeast Sen1p orthologue: characterization of a unique protein in which recessive mutations cause ataxia and dominant mutations cause motor neuron disease. Neurobiol Dis. 2006;23:97–108.
87. Chen YZ, Bennett CL, Huynh HM, et al. DNA/RNA helicase gene mutations in a form of juvenile amyotrophic lateral sclerosis (ALS4). Am J Hum Genet. 2004;74:1128–35.
88. El-Khamisy SF, Saifi GM, Weinfeld M, et al. Defective DNA single-strand break repair in spinocerebellar ataxia with axonal neuropathy-1. Nature. 2005;434:108–13.
89. Takashima H, Boerkoel CF, John J, et al. Mutation of TDP1, encoding a topoisomerase I-dependent DNA damage repair enzyme, in spinocerebellar ataxia with axonal neuropathy. Nat Genet. 2002;32:267–72.
90. Monin ML, Mignot C, De Lonlay P, et al. 29 French adult patients with PMM2-congenital disorder of glycosylation: outcome of the classical pediatric phenotype and depiction of a late-onset phenotype. Orphanet J Rare Dis. 2014;9:207.
91. Duquette A, Brais B, Bouchard JP, Mathieu J. Clinical presentation and early evolution of spastic ataxia of Charlevoix-Saguenay. Mov Disord. 2013;28:2011–4.
92. Synofzik M, Soehn AS, Gburek-Augustat J, et al. Autosomal recessive spastic ataxia of Charlevoix Saguenay (ARSACS): expanding the genetic, clinical and imaging spectrum. Orphanet J Rare Dis. 2013;8:41.
93. Baets J, Deconinck T, Smets K, et al. Mutations in SACS cause atypical and late-onset forms of ARSACS. Neurology. 2010;75:1181–8.
94. Vermeer S, Meijer RP, Pijl BJ, et al. ARSACS in the Dutch population: a frequent cause of early-onset cerebellar ataxia. Neurogenetics. 2008;9:207–14.
95. Yu-Wai-Man P, Pyle A, Griffin H, Santibanez-Korev M, Horvath R, Chinnery PF. Abnormal retinal thickening is a common feature among patients with ARSACS-related phenotypes. Br J Ophthalmol. 2014;98:711–3.
96. Gerwig M, Kruger S, Kreuz FR, Kreis S, Gizewski ER, Timmann D. Characteristic MRI and funduscopic findings help diagnose ARSACS outside Quebec. Neurology. 2010;75:2133.

97. Gregianin E, Vazza G, Scaramel E, et al. A novel SACS mutation results in non-ataxic spastic paraplegia and peripheral neuropathy. Eur J Neurol. 2013;20:1486–91.
98. Shimazaki H, Takiyama Y, Sakoe K, Ando Y, Nakano I. A phenotype without spasticity in sacsin-related ataxia. Neurology. 2005;64:2129–31.
99. Parfitt DA, Michael GJ, Vermeulen EG, et al. The ataxia protein sacsin is a functional co-chaperone that protects against polyglutamine-expanded ataxin-1. Hum Mol Genet. 2009;18:1556–65.
100. Horn MA, van den Brink DM, Wanders RJ, et al. Phenotype of adult Refsum disease due to a defect in peroxin 7. Neurology. 2007;68:698–700.
101. Jansen GA, Ofman R, Ferdinandusse S, et al. Refsum disease is caused by mutations in the phytanoyl-CoA hydroxylase gene. Nat Genet. 1997;17:190–3.
102. Harari D, Gibberd FB, Dick JP, Sidey MC. Plasma exchange in the treatment of Refsum's disease (heredopathia atactica polyneuritiformis). J Neurol Neurosurg Psychiatry. 1991;54:614–7.
103. Dickson N, Mortimer JG, Faed JM, Pollard AC, Styles M, Peart DA. A child with Refsum's disease: successful treatment with diet and plasma exchange. Dev Med Child Neurol. 1989;31:92–7.
104. Pilo-de-la-Fuente B, Jimenez-Escrig A, Lorenzo JR, et al. Cerebrotendinous xanthomatosis in Spain: clinical, prognostic, and genetic survey. Eur J Neurol. 2011;18:1203–11.
105. Nie S, Chen G, Cao X, Zhang Y. Cerebrotendinous xanthomatosis: a comprehensive review of pathogenesis, clinical manifestations, diagnosis, and management. Orphanet J Rare Dis. 2014;9:179.
106. Guerrera S, Stromillo ML, Mignarri A, et al. Clinical relevance of brain volume changes in patients with cerebrotendinous xanthomatosis. J Neurol Neurosurg Psychiatry. 2010;81:1189–93.
107. Verrips A, Wevers RA, Van Engelen BG, et al. Effect of simvastatin in addition to chenodeoxycholic acid in patients with cerebrotendinous xanthomatosis. Metabolism. 1999;48:233–8.
108. Moghadasian MH, Salen G, Frohlich JJ, Scudamore CH. Cerebrotendinous xanthomatosis: a rare disease with diverse manifestations. Arch Neurol. 2002;59:527–9.
109. Fiskerstrand T, Knappskog P, Majewski J, Wanders RJ, Boman H, Bindoff LA. A novel Refsum-like disorder that maps to chromosome 20. Neurology. 2009;72:20–7.
110. Nishiguchi KM, Avila-Fernandez A, van Huet RA, et al. Exome sequencing extends the phenotypic spectrum for ABHD12 mutations: from syndromic to nonsyndromic retinal degeneration. Ophthalmology. 2014;121:1620–7.
111. Chen DH, Naydenov A, Blankman JL, et al. Two novel mutations in ABHD12: expansion of the mutation spectrum in PHARC and assessment of their functional effects. Hum Mutat. 2013;34:1672–8.
112. Eisenberger T, Slim R, Mansour A, et al. Targeted next-generation sequencing identifies a homozygous nonsense mutation in ABHD12, the gene underlying PHARC, in a family clinically diagnosed with Usher syndrome type 3. Orphanet J Rare Dis. 2012;7:59.
113. Synofzik M, Kernstock C, Haack TB, Schols L. Ataxia meets chorioretinal dystrophy and hypogonadism: Boucher-Neuhauser syndrome due to PNPLA6 mutations. J Neurol Neurosurg Psychiatry. 2014 (Epub ahead of print).
114. Rainier S, Bui M, Mark E, et al. Neuropathy target esterase gene mutations cause motor neuron disease. Am J Hum Genet. 2008;82:780–5.
115. Dupre N, Gros-Louis F, Chrestian N, et al. Clinical and genetic study of autosomal recessive cerebellar ataxia type 1. Ann Neurol. 2007;62:93–8.
116. Noreau A, Bourassa CV, Szuto A, et al. SYNE1 mutations in autosomal recessive cerebellar ataxia. JAMA Neurol. 2013;70:1296–331.
117. Izumi Y, Miyamoto R, Morino H, et al. Cerebellar ataxia with SYNE1 mutation accompanying motor neuron disease. Neurology. 2013;80:600–1.
118. Zhang Q, Bethmann C, Worth NF, et al. Nesprin-1 and –2 are involved in the pathogenesis of Emery Dreifuss muscular dystrophy and are critical for nuclear envelope integrity. Hum Mol Genet. 2007;16:2816–33.

119. Mignot C, Apartis E, Durr A, et al. Phenotypic variability in ARCA2 and identification of a core ataxic phenotype with slow progression. Orphanet J Rare Dis. 2013;8:173.
120. Mollet J, Delahodde A, Serre V, et al. CABC1 gene mutations cause ubiquinone deficiency with cerebellar ataxia and seizures. Am J Hum Genet. 2008;82:623–30.
121. Balreira A, Boczonadi V, Barca E, et al. ANO10 mutations cause ataxia and coenzyme Q(1)(0) deficiency. J Neurol. 2014;261:2192–8.
122. Renaud M, Anheim M, Kamsteeg EJ, et al. Autosomal recessive cerebellar ataxia type 3 due to ANO10 mutations: delineation and genotype-phenotype correlation study. JAMA Neurol. 2014;71:1305–10.
123. Shi CH, Schisler JC, Rubel CE, et al. Ataxia and hypogonadism caused by the loss of ubiquitin ligase activity of the U box protein CHIP. Hum Mol Genet. 2014;23:1013–24.
124. Synofzik M, Schule R, Schulze M, et al. Phenotype and frequency of STUB1 mutations: next-generation screenings in Caucasian ataxia and spastic paraplegia cohorts. Orphanet J Rare Dis. 2014;9:57.
125. Heimdal K, Sanchez-Guixe M, Aukrust I, et al. STUB1 mutations in autosomal recessive ataxias - evidence for mutation-specific clinical heterogeneity. Orphanet J Rare Dis. 2014;9:146.
126. Depondt C, Donatello S, Simonis N, et al. Autosomal recessive cerebellar ataxia of adult onset due to STUB1 mutations. Neurology. 2014;82:1749–50.
127. Assoum M, Salih MA, Drouot N, et al. Rundataxin, a novel protein with RUN and diacylglycerol binding domains, is mutant in a new recessive ataxia. Brain. 2010;133:2439–47.
128. Skre H, Berg K. Linkage studies on Marinesco-Sjogren syndrome and hypergonadotropic hypogonadism. Clin Genet. 1977;11:57–66.
129. Dotti MT, Bardelli AM, De Stefano N, et al. Optic atrophy in Marinesco-Sjogren syndrome: an additional ocular feature. Report of three cases in two families. Ophthalmic Paediatr Genet. 1993;14:5–7.
130. Goto M, Okada M, Komaki H, et al. A nationwide survey on Marinesco-Sjogren syndrome in Japan. Orphanet J Rare Dis. 2014;9:58.
131. Takahata T, Yamada K, Yamada Y, et al. Novel mutations in the SIL1 gene in a Japanese pedigree with the Marinesco-Sjogren syndrome. J Hum Genet. 2010;55:142–6.
132. Zhao L, Longo-Guess C, Harris BS, Lee JW, Ackerman SL. Protein accumulation and neurodegeneration in the woozy mutant mouse is caused by disruption of SIL1, a cochaperone of BiP. Nat Genet. 2005;37:974–9.
133. Senderek J, Krieger M, Stendel C, et al. Mutations in SIL1 cause Marinesco-Sjogren syndrome, a cerebellar ataxia with cataract and myopathy. Nat Genet. 2005;37:1312–4.
134. Reinhold A, Scheer I, Lehmann R, et al. MR imaging features in Marinesco-Sjogren syndrome: severe cerebellar atrophy is not an obligatory finding. AJNR Am J Neuroradiol. 2003;24:825–8.
135. Aguglia U, Annesi G, Pasquinelli G, et al. Vitamin E deficiency due to chylomicron retention disease in Marinesco-Sjogren syndrome. Ann Neurol. 2000;47:260–4.
136. Mengel E, Klunemann HH, Lourenco CM, et al. Niemann-Pick disease type C symptomatology: an expert-based clinical description. Orphanet J Rare Dis. 2013;8:166.
137. Lyseng-Williamson KA. Miglustat: a review of its use in Niemann-Pick disease type C. Drugs. 2014;74:61–74.
138. Liebeskind DS, Wong S, Hamilton RH. Faces of the giant panda and her cub: MRI correlates of Wilson's disease. J Neurol Neurosurg Psychiatry. 2003;74:682.
139. Singh P, Ahluwalia A, Saggar K, Grewal CS. Wilson's disease: MRI features. J Pediatr Neurosci. 2011;6:27–8.

Chapter 13
Genetics of NBIA Disorders

Sarah Wiethoff, Kailash P. Bhatia, and Henry Houlden

Abstract Neurodegeneration with brain iron accumulation (NBIA) or pallidopyramidal disorders comprise several clinical and genetic entities. The presence of increased regional, nonphysiological aging-associated brain iron is often seen as their unifying characteristic even though its occurrence in the course of disease can be highly variable or absent. The clinical phenotype of this group consists of an early-onset movement disorder with a core combination of dystonia, parkinsonism, and pyramidal signs. Ataxia, axonal neuropathy, and cognitive decline can also occur but are less frequent. Iron accumulation or abnormal basal ganglia signal seen on MRI remains an important hallmark of this group of disorders when present. Neuropathologically, NBIA disorders usually cause widespread axonal spheroids in the CNS (and at times peripheral nerves) and accumulation of iron in the basal ganglia; they can further be subgrouped by the neuropathological presence of Lewy bodies, TDP-43 pathology, or tau pathology.

Even though recently there have been a number of advances in elucidating the pathophysiology of NBIA disorders, treatment usually remains symptomatic. Certain clinical presentations can point towards a specific genetic defect, and genetic tests usually make for the final confirmation of the disease. This review gives an overview about the genetic defects that lead to the different phenotypes of NBIA disorders, revealing overlap as well as important phenotypic presentations that can direct genetic testing. Where possible it provides information about (symptomatic) treatment options and their outcomes and finally discusses the upcoming challenges and future hopes in the field.

Keywords NBIA • Pallidopyramidal disorders • Neurodegeneration with brain iron accumulation • Genetics • iPSC • Movement disorders

---

S. Wiethoff, MD
Department of Molecular Neuroscience, Institute of Neurology, University College London, London, UK

K.P. Bhatia, MD, DM, FRCP
Sobell Department, University College London/Institute of Neurology, London WC1N 3BG, UK

H. Houlden, MD, MRCP, PhD (✉)
Department of Molecular Neuroscience, Institute of Neurology, University College London, London, UK
e-mail: h.houlden@ucl.ac.uk

S.A. Schneider, J.M.T. Brás (eds.), *Movement Disorder Genetics*,
DOI 10.1007/978-3-319-17223-1_13

Introduction

Neurodegeneration with brain iron accumulation (NBIA) or pallidopyramidal disorders comprise several clinical and genetic entities. The presence of increased, nonaging-associated regional brain iron stores is often seen as their unifying characteristic (e.g., for review [1, 2]) even though its occurrence in the course of disease can be highly variable and might even remain absent in certain genetically confirmed NBIA disorders [3–6]. The most prevalent clinical symptoms are severe and progressive dystonia, spasticity, parkinsonism, and dysarthria. The phenotypic variety in terms of manifestation and progression can be limitless, but prominent iron accumulation detectable on MRI remains – despite of its caveats – an important hallmark of the diagnostic workup [7, 8]. Certain clinical presentations can point towards groups of specific genetic defects [9, 10], and genetic tests usually make for the final confirmation of the disease in most of the cases where neuropathology is unavailable during lifetime.

Neuropathological findings in NBIA most commonly comprise axonal spheroids in predominantly central nerves alongside a variable quantity of iron accumulation in the basal ganglia; see Fig. 13.1 [11, 12].

In compliance with its heterogeneous nature, alpha-synuclein and Lewy body pathology [11, 13, 14] and TDP-43 and tau pathology [15–18] have additionally been observed for some subtypes of NBIA (for summary and overview, see Table 13.1).

Despite ongoing advances in elucidating its various pathophysiologies, the treatment of NBIA disorders to date essentially remains symptomatic. NBIA disorders can be inherited in autosomal dominant, autosomal recessive, and x-linked fashion. Up to now, at least ten genes are known to be associated with neurodegeneration with brain iron accumulation, nine of which will be discussed in more detail in separate sections below. The genetic underpinnings of the disease which are in the focus of this review are as heterogeneous as its clinical phenotypes [19].

Firstly, NBIA disorders can be caused by mutations in genes with a direct link to iron metabolism. The most famous examples thereof are mutations in the ferroxidase encoding gene ceruloplasmin (*CP*) leading to aceruloplasminemia [20, 21] or pathogenic mutations in the gene ferritin light polypeptide (*FTL*) that lead to hereditary ferritinopathies as this gene encodes the light subunit of the ferritin protein responsible for iron storage and release [22–25]. Secondly, most of the disease-associated mutations in NBIA impair genes in phospho- and sphingolipid metabolic pathways [26], mitochondrial or lysosomal activity [27, 28], and the mechanisms linking those to iron metabolism are less clear. Finally, the ultimate hope in studying NBIA disorders is to use this presence of overlapping clinical features and molecular/biological pathways in order to identify new therapeutic alleys, not only for these rare disorders but also for more common disorders as Parkinson's disease (PD) and dystonia that share elements of pathophysiology.

This review gives an overview about the distinct genetic defects that lead to the different, yet overlapping, phenotypes of NBIA disorders, highlights important phenotypic presentations that direct genetic testing where possible, provides

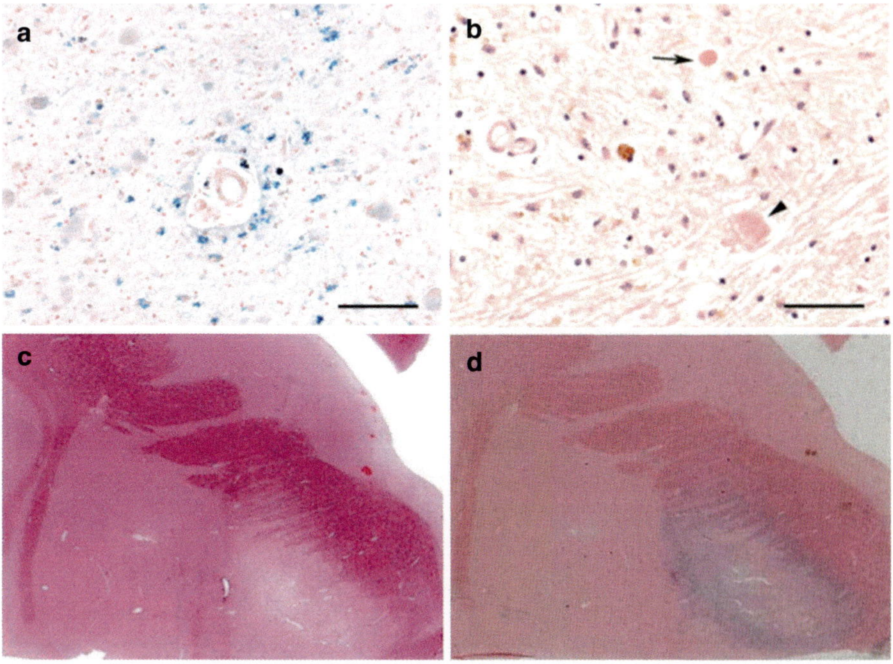

Fig. 13.1 Neuropathological hallmarks of pantothenate kinase-associated neurodegeneration (PKAN), representative of NBIA. (**a**) Typical Perl's stained iron deposits in the globus pallidus of a *PANK2*-positive case. Scale: 200 µm, low magnification. (**b**) Typical presence of smaller neuroaxonal spheroids (*arrow*) and large degenerating neurons (*arrowhead*) in the globus pallidus of a *PANK2*-positive case. Hemosiderin in the background, scale: 50 µm (**a**, **b**, reproduced with permission from Kruer et al. [7], by permission of Oxford University Press). (**c**, **d**) Section through the basal ganglia in *PANK2*-positive case, hematoxylin and eosin (H&E) stain with pale area representing neuronal loss (**c**) and typical Perl' s stain with blue representing excess iron (**d**) (**c**, **d**, Images courtesy of Prof. T. Revesz and Dr. A. Li, Queen Square Brain Bank, UCL)

information about treatment options when present, and discusses remaining controversies of this highly dynamic field of neurodegeneration.

Pantothenate Kinase-Associated Neurodegeneration (PKAN)

PKAN, also recognized under the acronym NBIA1, accounts for about 35–50 % of NBIA cases [29]. However, there is a possibility of overestimation depending on the cases screened and possibly confounding selection bias. It has an estimated worldwide prevalence of about 1:1,000,000 with regional higher prevalences (e.g. Dominican Republic) due to founder effects. It was formerly assessed under the name Hallervorden-Spatz syndrome (HSS) – a terminology that has been

Table 13.1 Overview of NBIA conditions, genes, MRI findings, and neuropathology in order of appearance throughout the chapter

Condition (acronym)	Synonym(s)	Gene	Cytogenetic band (Ensembl)	MRI features and areas of highest iron density	Inclusion type additional to iron and predominant region	Additional neuropathological findings
PKAN	NBIA1	*PANK2*	20p13	Iron deposits with highest density in GP, "eye-of-the-tiger" sign	Tau or none	Spheroid bodies throughout CNS, focussed in GP,variable involvement of putamen and internal capsule. Tau pathology possible. Only occasional peripheral manifestation
PLAN	NBIA2, PARK14	*PLA2G6*	22q13.1	Area of highest iron in GP, milder SN involvement. Cerebral and cerebellar atrophy possible	Alpha-synucleinopathy with cortically widespread Lewy bodies, additional tau pathology	Central and peripheral neuroaxonal spheroids. Widespread cortical alpha-synuclein-positive stainings, Lewy body pathology. Additional presence of tau. Neurodegeneration in brainstem, cerebellum, optic pathway, and spinal cord

MPAN	NBIA4, SPG43	*C19orf12*	19q12	Iron deposits in GP and SN	Alpha-synucleinopathy with cortically widespread Lewy bodies, additional tau pathology	Neuronal loss, axonal spheroids, iron deposits in globus pallidus and substantia nigra, Lewy bodies, Lewy neurites in globus pallidus, neurofibrillatory tangles, and tau-positive inclusions. Loss of myelin: pyramidal tracts, optic nerve
BPAN	NBIA5, formerly: SENDA syndrome	*WDR45*	Xp11.23	Specific substantia nigra hyperintensity with central hypointensity on T1, iron accumulation in GP and SN, mild cerebellar atrophy and white matter changes possible	Tau (personal communication)	Widespread tangles and threads, distribution and neuronal autophagy-associated markers under current observation
FAHN	SPG35	*FA2H*	16q23.1	Iron deposits with focus in GP. White matter changes. Thin corpus callosum	Not known yet	No human brain data. Peripheral nerve biopsy: decrease of myelinated nerve fibers. Animal models with cerebellar abnormalities, demyelination, profound axonal loss throughout CNS

(continued)

Table 13.1 (continued)

Condition (acronym)	Synonym(s)	Gene	Cytogenetic band (Ensembl)	MRI features and areas of highest iron density	Inclusion type additional to iron and predominant region	Additional neuropathological findings
Kufor-Rakeb disease	PARK9	*ATP13A2*	1p36.13	Atrophy of GP and pyramids. More generalized brain atrophy in later disease course. Highest iron content mostly in putamen and caudate	Not known yet – clinically and genetically significant overlap with lipofuscinoses	Widespread neuronal and glial lipofuscinosis sparing white matter, whorled lamellar inclusions in electron microscopy in one *ATP13A2*-positive NCL case. Peripheral nerve biopsy: cytoplasmic inclusion bodies
Neuroferritinopathy	NBIA3, hereditary ferritinopathy, FTL	*FTL*	19q13.33	Iron deposits in SN > caudate, GP, red nuclei, and putamen. Cystic necrosis in basal ganglia and bilateral pallidum	Tau	Spherical inclusions positive for ferritin staining in cerebellum, posterior putamen, and other iron-rich areas; spheroids and neurofilaments immunoreactive to ubiquitin and tau. Additional hepatic iron deposits possible

Aceruloplasminemia	–	*CP*	3q25.1	T2-weighted MRI with marked hypointensity of thalami, basal ganglia-nuclei, dentate. Most prominent iron deposits in basal ganglia, dentate nuclei > thalami, cerebral and cerebellar cortices	No alpha-synucleinopathy. Additional iron deposits in internal organs (mainly pancreas/liver).	Purkinje cell loss in cerebellum. Globular structures in astrocytes > neurons. No alpha-synuclein reactivity. Positivity to anti-4-hydroxynonenal andanti-ubiquitinantibodies
CoPAN	NBIA6	*COASY*	17q21.2	"Eye-of-the-tiger"-like MRI in 1 subject, 2nd subject: isolated involvement of neostriatum preceded evidence of typical pallida iron content increase	Not known yet	Not known yet

abandoned due to the unethical implications of these researchers under the Nazi regime but can still be found sporadically for historic reasons [30].

Clinically, PKAN can be divided into two categories, atypical and typical PKAN. Typical PKAN patients usually become symptomatic with gait and postural abnormalities around the age of 3–4 [29, 31]. Their mutational spectrum tends to show variations in *PANK2* that lead to protein truncation more often than mutations in atypical, late-onset PKAN cases which tend to be amino acid changes without consequent truncation effects [29]. Typical PKAN patients present with a more rapid but nonlinear progression to a full clinical spectrum of severe (in its early manifestation predominantly oromandibular and nonaxial) dystonia [29, 32], spasticity and hyperreflexia, parkinsonism, chorea, impaired saccadic pursuits as well as decelerated and hypometric vertical saccades, mental decline, and behavioral abnormalities [29, 33]. Pigmentary retinopathy occurs in up to 40 % of typical PKAN cases, whereas optic atrophy is infrequent [29, 34]. Given the disease progression with rapid deterioration intertwined with phases of stability, the majority of patients are nonambulatory within at most 15 years into the disease [29].

Atypical PKAN cases tend to be significantly older when the first obvious symptoms appear (age of onset at 13.7 ± 5.9 years [range, 1–28] in atypical vs. 3.4 ± 3.0 years [range, 0.5–12] in typical cases as reported in the original paper by Hayflick et al., 2003) [29]. Their pyramidal and extrapyramidal manifestations are generally milder and progress less rapidly; however, most atypical PKAN patients eventually lose their ambulatory independency [29]. Furthermore, speech defects like dysarthria or palilalia as well as psychiatric features like cognitive decline seem to be more prevalent in atypical cases [29].

In terms of radiographic findings, the eye-of-the-tiger sign, a T_2-weighted hypointense signal in the globus pallidus (GP) with a central region of hyperintensity, has lost its previously acclaimed pathognomonic status for *PANK2* [29, 35]. Patients with other genetic forms of NBIA or with a different neurodegenerative disease have been found to hold this sign [8, 36] as well as *PANK2*-positive patients lacking it [37]. The eye-of-the-tiger sign can even be present in individuals without any clinical symptoms [38]. Nonetheless it remains an important flag in clinical diagnostics pointing towards the group of NBIA disorders.

The human gene which is associated with this condition is *PANK2*. *PANK2* finds itself on chromosome 20, p13 [39]. It encodes the only human protein from the pantothenate kinase family that is thought to be expressed in mitochondria and therefore seems to be responsible for the intramitochondrial de novo synthesis of coenzyme A [39]. Pantothenate kinase is the key regulatory enzyme in coenzyme A synthesis and catalyzes the first step from pantothenate/vitamin B to 4'phosphopantothenate in this universally important pathway. Given its role in fatty acid metabolism, amino acid synthesis, and Krebs cycle, CoA is vital for the basic key metabolism of the cell [40].

PKAN is inherited in autosomal recessive manner. Its mutational spectrum includes mostly missense and nonsense mutations, which – depending on the location of the mutation and the corresponding conservation throughout species – result in reduced or no activity of pantothenate kinase in mitochondria. Additionally, deletions up to 6 kb, whole exon deletions, and splice site mutations and duplications have been observed, and all 7 exons of the gene can be affected [41]. A screening study of 2006 enrolled 72 patients with a clinical diagnosis of NBIA and could identify both mutated *PANK2* alleles in 48 patients. Thirty-three different mutations – mostly missense and nonsense – were reported; deletions of the gene were found in around 4 % of the mutated *PANK2* alleles [41]. The most frequent mutations in their study were c.1583C>T/p.Thr528Met ($n=11$), c.573delC/p.S191RfsX13 ($n=10$), and c.1561G>A/p.Gly521Arg ($n=10$). Over the years, authors used different transcripts to refer to the same common mutations in *PANK2*, while in effect c.1561G>A is found to be equal to c.1231G>A and c.1583C>T to c.1253C>T. In order to avoid confusion, we will only refer to the amino acid change in the following although even a certain amount of different annotations can be found throughout the literature. With increasing evidence, p.Gly521Arg (allele frequency ~ 25 %), p.Thr528Met (~8 %), and p.Arg451Ter (~3 %) are found to be the most common pathogenic variants [42, 43], while the residual spectrum of *PANK2* mutations includes mainly private mutations [29]. Two thirds of PKAN patients are compound heterozygotes [43]. As per example, one of the most common point mutations, leading to amino acid change p.Gly521Arg, has been shown to result in reduced production of the mature isoform of the *PANK2* enzyme [40]. Regarding the molecular pathology of PKAN, it has therefore been suggested that mutations in *PANK2* lead to reduced *PANK2* protein levels, impaired catalytic activity of *PANK2,* and consecutively altered neuronal mitochondrial lipid formation and metabolism [40]. However, it has to be noted that not all disease-associated point mutations result in significantly reduced catalytic activity of the enzyme [40]. The final transformation into clinical symptoms still remains equally elusive, and few attempts have been made to combine the mutational location and corresponding clinical features: As one example, Hartig et al. introduced an activity score to take into account the severity of the identified mutations and the predicted rest activity of the enzyme. They found the activity score of the mutations to be correlated with the age of onset of the disease, but not the loss of ambulation in their *PANK2*-positive cases [41]. In a different attempt, a correlation between the location of missense mutations and their biochemical properties with the disease features found mutations located in the dimer interface, the ATP binding site, and the interior of the protein to negatively impact the enzyme activity and to be mostly associated with classic, young-onset, and rapidly progressing disease. Mutations located on the surface that lead to slight instability, but seemed to preserve most of the enzyme' s catalytic activity, were associated with milder symptom presentation of PKAN [44]. Even though genotype-phenotype correlations in PKAN remain controversial and difficult, it is these arduous and small advances in trying to correlate the specific location of a mutation with functional and phenotypical properties that will shed further light on the gap between the genetic underlying causes and their transformation into clinical manifestations and will ultimately facilitate genetic counseling. However, one important restriction in our field of extremely rare conditions will always be the inherently small amount of cases available.

Despite the remaining gaps, as of current state of knowledge, some conclusions can be retained: As shown in the original work by Hayflick and colleagues, patients homozygous for the common p.Gly521Arg amino acid change have classic disease [29]. Furthermore, two null mutations seem to result in rapidly progressive, early-onset PKAN, while missense mutations with diminished but preserved enzyme function are likely to lead to atypical PKAN with later onset and slower progression. In our own clinical experience, we have now seen several compound heterozygous cases that seem to lead to atypical PKAN: Late disease onset in these cases goes along with rather preserved cognition, slow progression, and longer lifespan.

Neuropathologically, PKAN is part of the neuroaxonal dystrophy spectrum with two main classes of spheroids observed: large, granular bodies representing degenerating neurons and smaller eosinophilic spheroid-like structures indicative of dystrophic neurites [7]. Prior to gene identification, numerous cases of heterogeneous etiology under the former umbrella term "Hallervorden-Spatz syndrome" have been reported to show Lewy body pathology [13, 45–47]. These have been genetically unconfirmed cases which renders the interpretation of this histopathological finding uncertain and less trustworthy as retrospectively these cases are most likely to be *PANK2*-negative cases with possibly heterogeneous but finally undetermined underlying genetic defects. However, a recent neuropathological investigation strictly including only *PANK2*-positive patients observed no alpha-synuclein positivity, but some tau-positive inclusions, and concluded that PKAN is not a synucleinopathy [16] which neuropathologically distinguishes it from other NBIA disorders (PLAN, MPAN) where alpha-synuclein accumulation can occur.

Furthermore, the disease has been shown to be allelic to HARP syndrome, depicting hypoprebetalipoproteinemia, acanthocytosis, retinitis pigmentosa, and pallidal degeneration [48] which is now likewise considered to be part of the PKAN- continuum. PKAN is the only NBIA disorder where iron-mediating medical treatment has systematically been tested, and while treatment with the iron chelator deferiprone leads to a median reduction of 30 % of pallidal iron content, clinical benefits unfortunately remained nonsignificant in the initial report [49], while the recent four-year follow-up report has shown clinical stabilization upon treatment in 5/6 patients [50]. Furthermore, it is the only NBIA subgroup where preliminary data about the use of deep brain stimulation (DBS) of globus pallidus internus bilaterally in the treatment of dystonia are available [51, 52] showing that it may produce clinical benefit for the postoperational time observed but does not stop the ongoing neuronal degeneration.

PLA2G6-Associated Neurodegeneration (PLAN)

PLA2G6-associated neurodegeneration (PLAN) accounts for approximately 20 % and thereby for the largest proportion of NBIA disorders after PKAN [53]. Three main phenotypes have been described within the spectrum of *PLA2G6*-associated disease that is a striking example of allelic heterogeneity: classic infantile neuroaxonal dystrophy (INAD) [54], childhood-onset atypical neuroaxonal dystrophy (NAD) [14, 55], and adult-onset dystonia-parkinsonism [5]. Their unifying features are progressive cognitive decline and rapid deterioration of motor skills, but the three syndromes can be distinguished via the following:

INAD is attended by a disease onset between 6 and 36 months and usually manifests with initial hypotonia, developmental regression, progressive psychomotor delay, cerebellar features, bulbar dysfunction, and progressive spastic tetraparesis [55–58]. MRI findings include cerebellar atrophy, and electromyography typically shows denervation atrophy [59, 60]. Optic atrophy, fast rhythms on electroencephalogram (EEG), and seizures may be present. Prior to gene identification, the definitive diagnosis was confirmed on sural biopsy, depicting typical dystrophic axons in the peripheral nerves [57]. Most INAD patients die within the first decade of their life; isolated evidence suggests some surviving up to their early twenties [42].

Atypical NAD is less common than INAD and usually manifests between the first and eighth year of life, while a delayed onset in the late twenties is possible [58]. The disease course is less aggressive with a slower progression rate. Prominent symptoms are ataxia, spastic tetraparesis, dystonia, speech delay, and behavioral abnormalities ranging from impulsivity, poor attention span, and emotional lability to autistic behavior [14, 55]. Seizures, optic atrophy, and nystagmus seem to occur in NAD as frequently as in INAD, while fast rhythms, truncal hypotonia, and strabism are predominantly part of INAD [14].

The third phenotype, *PLA2G6*-related adult-onset dystonia-parkinsonism, is characterized by a later (second to third decade), subacute onset of dystonia-parkinsonism with rapid decline and initial dramatic response to levodopa. Pyramidal involvement, eye movement abnormalities, dystonia, dysarthria, psychiatric features, cognitive decline, and gait abnormalities were further common findings. Brain iron deposits were absent on MR imaging of these patients, whereas cerebral and cerebellar atrophy was prominent [5].

Phospholipase A2-associated neurodegeneration is inherited in autosomal recessive manner and caused by mutations in the widespread expressed gene *PLA2G6* [61]. *PLA2G6* is located on chromosome 22q and comprises 17 exons which underlie alternative splicing and result in the production of different isoforms [61]. The gene was discovered in 2006 following a linkage approach in families with INAD and NBIA [54] and was subsequently found to be mutated in the related Karak syndrome [62] which is now recognized to be part of atypical NAD. Prior to this discovery, the diagnosis was solely to be made clinically or histopathologically, and confirming the diagnosis via molecular genetic testing has since proven useful to reduce invasive tissue biopsies and alleviate genetic counseling.

In the initial study, the majority of 44 identified unique mutations were homozygous missense mutations [33], followed by frameshift-inducing deletions [5], nonsense mutations [3], deletions without subsequent frameshift [1], a splice site mutation, and a large deletion. Most mutations are private mutations. This frequency spectrum has since been reproduced in a slightly larger cohort [14]. So far, homozygous null mutations were only found in patients with INAD and not in individuals of the broader clinical category with iron dyshomeostasis without axonal spheroids [54] suggesting that mutations resulting in absent protein seem to be associated with severe phenotypes. As in *PANK2*, compound heterozygous missense mutations suggestive of remaining protein function correlate with the atypical, milder NAD phenotype [14].

The 85 kDa calcium-independent group 6 phospholipase A2 (iPLA$_2$-VI) is the encoded protein which plays an important role in the maintenance of cell membrane homeostasis, regulation of apoptosis, leukotriene and prostaglandin synthesis, catalysis of glycerophospholipid hydrolysis, and phospholipid remodeling [5, 14, 42, 53, 61, 63, 64]. Multiple isoforms are encoded by the *PLA2G6* transcript variants, whereof two are enzymatically active [61]. A subset of the reported mutations in the literature was found to alter the shorter enzymatically inactive isoforms and when incorporated into the tetramer iPLA$_2$-VI acts as dominant-negative inhibitors [61, 63]. Therefore, defects in iPLA$_2$-VI result in impaired phospholipid remodeling which is an essential component of physiological membrane repair and homeostasis [65]. Additionally, iPLA$_2$-VI can initiate apoptosis when exposed to oxidative stress [66], and deficiency in these vital cell protection and repair mechanisms results in neuronal damage and degeneration.

Histopathologically, the hallmark finding in PLAN is the presence of neuroaxonal spheroids which is thought to represent the degeneration of the inner mitochondrial membrane [67, 68]. This neuroaxonal degeneration with distended axons (spheroid bodies) is mainly present in the CNS but has been reported in peripheral nerves as well [57]. Furthermore, Lewy body pathology alongside tau-positive inclusions has been observed [69]. A second common finding is progressive brain iron deposition that can be detected neuropathologically as well as neuroradiologically with some time into the disease. Typical iron deposits in the globus pallidus can be missing in the initial radiographic brain imaging of INAD cases but usually develop within a certain course of the disease [54, 59]. Further common neuroradiographic features in PLAN are cerebellar hypoplasia or atrophy and T2-weighted high signal in the cerebellum, hypoplastic optic tracts/chiasm, and an elongated, vertically orientated splenium [59].

Mitochondrial Membrane Protein-Associated Neurodegeneration (MPAN)

Mitochondrial membrane protein-associated neurodegeneration (MPAN), also known as neurodegeneration associated with *C19orf12* mutations, accounts for 6–10 % of NBIA disorders and is the third most prevalent group after PKAN and PLAN [53, 70, 71]. Disease onset usually is in childhood to early adulthood. Common features are speech and gait difficulties, cognitive decline resulting in dementia, spasticity, dysarthria, optic atrophy, dystonia, parkinsonism, psychiatric features, and motor neuronopathy with early signs of upper motor neuron dysfunction, followed by affection of the second motor neuron later. Its natural history is slowly progressive; survival into adulthood is not uncommon. MPAN is more than other NBIA disorders associated with rapid progressive cognitive decline [53, 70, 71].

Neuroimaging shows iron accumulation in the globus pallidus and substantia nigra (SN) as well as cortical and cerebellar atrophy. Hyperintense streaking of the medial medullary lamina between globus pallidus internus and externus on

T_2-weighted images can be additionally present and is sometimes mistaken for an eye-of-the-tiger sign [71].

MPAN is caused by mutations in the orphan gene *C19orf12* and is inherited in autosomal recessive fashion. Homozygosity mapping followed by candidate gene sequencing identified the common founder mutation in *C19orf12* NM_001031726.3:c.204_214del11/NP_001026896.2:p.Gly69ArgfsTer10 in a Polish family in 2009 [70]. Subsequent screening in a Polish cohort of additional 23 index patients with the above described phenotype and negative for mutations in *PANK2*, *PLA2G6*, *FTL*, and *CP* revealed homozygous mutations in *C19orf12* in 18 of them. 12 carried the homozygous founder mutation which is thought to have arisen in a common founder at least 50–100 generations ago. Three remaining cases carried the deletion in combination with different missense mutations (p.Gly65Glu, p.Gly53Arg, and p.Thr11Met) in the compound heterozygous state. One remaining case carried two missense mutations, p.Gly69Arg and p.Lys142Glu, and two cases with homozygous missense mutations (p.Tyr11Met and p.Gly69Arg) were identified.

One additional compound heterozygous missense mutation (p.Gly69Arg and p.Lys142Glu) in *C19orf12* was identified in a patient with a late-onset (49 years) predominantly parkinsonian phenotype and in one young Polish patient with a mild impairment of fine motor skills and is therefore thought to result in milder phenotypes. A follow-up screening study on a larger and ethnically more diverse cohort of 161 idiopathic NBIA cases was published in 2013. It identified two mutated alleles in 23 cases and established MPAN as the third most common subform of NBIA to date. In addition to the common founder mutation, a variety of different, mostly "private" mutations (nonsense, frameshift, and missense) were identified throughout *C19orf12*. There was no evidence for large deletions and duplications. However, the occurrence of a single heterozygous mutant allele in three cases suggests the presence of occult mutations in intronic and regulatory sequences [71]. Furthermore, in their study, one single-mutation case had a family history compatible with autosomal dominant inheritance backed up by histological findings in the deceased father of the family. The identified single unique frameshift mutation induces a series of 32 amino acid substitutions and ultimately results in a premature stop codon 2 amino acids away from the physiological termination. Therefore, the authors discuss the possibility of this aberrant product escaping physiological nonsense-mediated mRNA decay and thereby presumably exerting dominant-negative effects on the normal protein. However, further studies are awaited to elucidate the pathogenesis of this single mutation and finally clarify the possibility of additional autosomal dominant inheritance in *C19orf12* [71].

Most evidence in *C19orf12* pathogenesis has been collected regarding the common founder mutation NM_001031726.3:c.204_214del11/NP_001026896.2:p.Gly69ArgfsTer10. This homozygous 11-bp deletion results in a frameshift that introduces a premature stop codon and is predicted to cause early truncation of the protein. Even though the deletion did not alter *C19orf12*-RNA levels in blood, the protein was undetectable with immunoblot analysis in patients' fibroblasts [70]. The missense mutation p.Lys142Glu changes a highly conserved positive lysine to a negatively charged glutamate. Three different missense mutations p.Gly53Arg, p.Gly65Glu, and p. Gly69Arg replace highly conserved glycines in the transmembrane region of *C19orf12* with a charged amino acid and therefore are likely to alter its function.

The exact gene function of *C19orf12* is unknown, but functional expression analyses suggest its mitochondrial location [70]. Analysis of respiratory chain complexes and mitochondrial morphology in fibroblasts of *C19orf12*-positive patients could not detect any significant abnormalities. However, analysis of *C19orf12-coregulated* genes in whole blood interestingly revealed strongest coregulation with genes involved in valine, leucine, and isoleucine degradation as well as fatty acid biogenesis. These processes are related to coenzyme A metabolism in mitochondria and therefore link MPAN to previous NBIA disorders with impairment in CoA pathways and lipid homeostasis (*PKAN*, *PLAN*, *CoPAN* (see later)).

Postmortem brain histopathology in two cases showed neuronal loss, iron deposits in the globus pallidus and substantia nigra, Lewy bodies, Lewy neurites in the globus pallidus, axonal spheroids, neurofibrillatory tangles, and tau-positive inclusions. The pyramidal tracts of the spinal cord and optic nerve displayed severe loss of myelin in one of them [70, 71].

Beta-Propeller Protein-Associated Neurodegeneration (BPAN, Formerly SENDA Syndrome)

Beta-propeller protein-associated neurodegeneration (BPAN) is also formerly known as static encephalopathy of childhood with neurodegeneration in adulthood.

(SENDA syndrome) accounts for about 1–2 % of NBIA disorders based on its prevalence in the International Registry for NBIA and Related Disorders from the Hayflick laboratory [53] and ~7 % according to a recent literature review [72].

Affected cases show a distinct phenotype of psychomotor developmental delay (mental retardation and early-onset spasticity of the lower limbs) in early childhood which remains fairly stable until a sudden onset and rapidly progressive complex of symptoms including dystonia, parkinsonism, and spasticity occurs in adulthood. Eye movement disorder, sleep disturbances, dysautonomia, seizures, and frontal release signs can additionally be present, and parkinsonian features usually show good response to L-dopa even though early motor fluctuations and dyskinesias often develop [1, 73]. Brain MRI shows a specific substantia nigra hyperintensity with central hypointensity on T1, iron accumulation in the globus pallidus and SN, and mild cerebellar atrophy along with white matter changes [74]. Preliminary brain pathology showed widespread tangles and threads in a single case (J. Holton, personal communication, 2014), and more BPAN patients will need to be autopsied to complement these observations.

Only recently, exome sequencing identified the underlying previously unknown genetic cause of this disease: De novo mutations in the beta-propeller scaffold protein *WDR45* at chromosome Xp11.23 were reported in affected SENDA cases establishing BPAN as the first x-linked dominant NBIA disorder [27]. All reported variants had unique occurrence in the index patient of the sequenced families suggesting de novo events, and loss-of-function mutations account for the majority of so far reported variants, followed by missense mutations in highly conserved residues [27, 73]. The majority of reported *WDR45*-positive cases are females [73, 75], while phenotypes of affected males do not substantially differ from females [27] which might be due to somatic mosaicism in the few surviving males and somatic and/or germline mutations and skewed X-chromosome inactivation in females.

WDR45 encodes WD repeat domain 45, one of the mammalian homologues of the autophagy-related gene *Atg18* in yeast that is thought to be a human core autophagy gene important in the early autophagy pathway [75–77]. In a recent experiment, *WDR45*-positive patient-derived lymphoblastoid cell lines showed accumulation of aberrant early autophagic bodies and decreased autophagic activity [75]. Together with the original findings [27], this provides further evidence for a strong connection between neurodegeneration and genetically defective autophagy.

Fatty Acid Hydroxylase-Associated Neurodegeneration (FAHN)

Fatty acid hydroxylase-associated neurodegeneration (FAHN) is another rare form of neurodegeneration with brain iron accumulation. It includes dysmyelinating leukodystrophy and spastic paraparesis with or without dystonia/spastic paraplegia 35 [78, 79], which had been recognized as distinct clinical entities previously but have now been included into the spectrum of FAHN [80, 81]. Clinically, FAHN is characterized by a pyramidal-extrapyramidal movement disorder with predominant gait difficulties due to severe spasticity and ataxic and dystonic features alongside to progressive intellectual impairment and the likely occurrence of optic atrophy, oculomotor abnormalities, and seizures. Usually, the disease manifests itself in childhood, but at the latest in the first or second decade of life. Typical neuroimaging features include bilateral GP hypointensity on T_2-weighted images, white matter lesions, mild cortical and pronounced pontocerebellar atrophy, and a thin corpus callosum [82]. Thin corpus callosum is not a common feature in the remaining NBIA disorders and should direct genetic testing to mutations in *FA2H*. However, it can be observed more frequently in other complex hereditary spastic paraplegias, mostly SPG11 and SPG15 [83, 84].

To date, less than 30 patients from different ethnic backgrounds are reported [78–80, 82, 85–87]. Reliable data on prevalence are still missing. Characteristics of the phenotype as well as the natural history of the disease can therefore only be reported with limited certainty and need to await further confirmation with more cases arising [87].

Neuropathological data from postmortem brain analysis have not yet been reported in this disorder. Sural nerve biopsy of one *FA2H*-positive case revealed a decrease of myelinated nerve fibers with intact myelin compaction and a normal amount of nonmyelinated fibers and normal ratio of large to small fibers [79]. Available muscle biopsy in another case from Dick et al. showed denervation and reinnervation without evidence of mitochondrial disease [78]. However, in another reported case, biopsies of the skin, muscle, and sural nerve were found to be normal [86], and although not mandatory for diagnosis, bone marrow biopsy in *FA2H*-positive patients may show accumulation of granular histiocytes. In animal models of *FA2H*, demyelination and profound axonal loss in the CNS as well as cerebellar abnormalities have been observed after 12 months, while at that timepoint peripheral nerves were principally normal in function and structure and only exhibited later-onset peripheral demyelinating and axonal neuropathy [88].

Fatty acid hydroxylase-associated neurodegeneration is inherited in autosomal recessive manner and is caused by mutations in the gene *FA2H* on chromosome 16q23.1. Human *FA2H* has seven exons and encodes the fatty acid 2 hydroxylase which alpha-hydroxylates incipient fatty acids enzymatically. The hydroxylation is required for the fatty acids in order to be incorporated into subsequent lipids that make up cell membranes and form myelin structures. All reported sequence variants in *FA2H* to date are "private" mutations, and it is thought that they exert their effect through a loss-of-function mechanism. Identified mutations lead to premature termination of the protein, and reduced protein levels of *FA2H* have been detected in D6P2T cells transfected with pcDNA-hFA2H R154C [82]. However, due to its rare occurrence, the functional implications so far remain poorly studied and understood.

Kufor-Rakeb Disease (*ATP13A2* Mutations/PARK9)

Kufor-Rakeb disease was originally described in a family with consanguineous background from Kufor-Rakeb, a small village in Jordan in 1994 [89]. The original paper reported juvenile-onset severe parkinsonian features in combination with pyramidal symptoms, dementia, and supranuclear upgaze paresis. Levodopa therapy usually improves the extrapyramidal dysfunction, while levodopa-induced dyskinesias are reported to develop early [90, 91]. MRI findings comprised severe atrophy of the globus pallidus and the pyramids and more generalized brain atrophy in later course of the disease. Later papers describe facial-faucial-finger myoclonus, visual hallucinations, autonomic dysfunction, slowing of saccadic pursuit and horizontal and vertical saccades, and oculogyric dystonic spasms in addition to the juvenile-onset parkinsonism, pyramidal signs, dementia, and supranuclear gaze palsy [90–93] and initially categorized Kufor-Rakeb disease as Parkinson's disease 9/*PARK9*. It was another 12 years from the original report in 1994 until the underlying genetic defect, a compound heterozygous loss-of-function mutation (c.3057delC/c.1306+5G>A) in a previously uncharacterized neuronal P-type ATPase gene, *ATP13A2*, was identified in a large nonconsanguineous Chilean sibship in 2006. Subsequent mutation screening in the original Jordanian family revealed a homozygous 22 bp duplication (c.1632_1653dup22) in all affected individuals [28]. Reports on the incidence of brain iron accumulation in the putamen and caudate [92, 94] in a proportion of *ATP13A2*-positive patients led to the inclusion of this disease entity into the NBIA spectrum [94]. It has been hypothesized that occurrence of iron might be associated exclusively with more severe mutations or may only develop later in the disease course [95].

Kufor-Rakeb disease is inherited in autosomal recessive manner and has been attributed to mutations in the *ATP13A2* gene on chromosome 1p. Affected patients predominantly carry homozygous mutations [28, 90, 94, 96, 97], but compound heterozygous cases have been reported and mutations seem to occur in various ethnical regions [28, 92, 98]. Human *ATP13A2* protein is a member of the lysosomal P5 subfamily of transport ATPases and contains 10 transmembrane domains [99]. The 1,180 amino acid protein encoded by 29 exons is expressed in dopaminergic neurons of the substantia nigra as well as in pyramidal cortex neurons [100]. Mutations in *ATP13A2* have been associated with mislocalization of the mutant *ATP13A2*, subsequent ER stress, modifications in the proteasomal pathways, and premature degradation of aberrant *ATP13A2* by the proteasomal but not the lysosomal pathways [98]. Further functional studies revealed the importance of *ATP13A2* for mitochondrial maintenance and renewal when *ATP13A2*-deficient cells showed impairments in autophagy, increased mitochondrial mass, affected mitochondrial renewal, and increased ROS production [101]. *ATP13A2*-positive patient's fibroblasts showed deficient mitochondrial clearance, increased oxygen consumption rates, increased fragmentation of the mitochondrial network, and increased occurrence of mitochondrial DNA lesions [102].

Up to now, no definitive and detailed brain pathology is available in *ATP13A2*-positive Kufor-Rakeb disease patients. However, *ATP13A2* mutations were identified retrospectively in a family with juvenile neuronal ceroid lipofuscinosis (NCL) displaying progressive spinocerebellar ataxia, intellectual decline, bulbar syndrome, and pyramidal and extrapyramidal syndrome where postmortem brain examination by that time showed widespread neuronal and glial lipofuscinosis sparing the white matter along with whorled lamellar inclusions in electron microscopy [103]. Furthermore, sural nerve biopsy in *ATP13A2*-positive cases revealed acute axonal degeneration with an accompanying mild chronic inflammation response with endoneurial and perineurial T cells. Abundant cytoplasmic inclusion bodies were seen within Schwann cells and epi- and perineurial cells (not within axons), and electron microscopy suggested their resemblance to irregular primary lysosomes [104].

Hereditary Ferritinopathy (*FTL*)

Hereditary ferritinopathy (*FTL*), or neuroferritinopathy, typically presents with extrapyramidal features comprising dystonia, oromandibular dyskinesias, blepharospasm, and chorea and is often thought to be phenotypically similar to neuroacanthocytosis or Morbus Huntington [25, 105]. Less frequent symptoms include parkinsonism, dysarthria, psychiatric features (depression, psychosis, cognitive decline), tremor, and cerebellar symptoms [25, 105]. Reported cases seem to cluster in Cumbria, Northern England, with the first and most common identified mutation c.460InsA in exon 4 of *FTL1*, but affected patients with at least seven different mutations from India, France, Japan, and elsewhere in the world have been reported in the meantime [22, 105, 106]. Adult age of onset is common, and MRI findings include iron accumulation in the caudate, GP, putamen, SN, and red nuclei alongside to cystic necrosis in the basal ganglia and bilateral pallidum. Interestingly, hypointense signal changes predated onset of symptoms, and the burden of T2* abnormalities increased with age [8, 107]. Radiological findings alongside with decreased ferritin levels can give important diagnostic hints and should lead to genetic testing of *FTL1* in order to identify this progressive disorder ideally before onset of neurological symptoms. Neuropathology revealed tau- and ubiquitin-positive neuroaxonal spheroids and neurofilaments as well as ferritin-positive inclusions in the cerebellum, the posterior putamen, and other iron-rich areas [108, 109].

Hereditary ferritinopathy is caused by mutations in ferritin light chain gene (*FTL1*) and is inherited in autosomal dominant manner. Its most common mutation, c.460InsA, leads to an extension of the peptide chain which alters its important ferritin dodecahedron structure and ultimately causes accumulation of ferritin and iron predominantly in central neurons that trigger oxidative stress, neuroinflammation, and neurodegeneration [22, 25, 109, 110].

Aceruloplasminemia (ACP)

Aceruloplasminemia is characterized by adult-onset (mean, 51; range, 16–71 years) movement disorder consisting of cerebellar ataxia and craniofacial dyskinesia plus predominant cognitive impairment, dysarthria, and retinal degeneration [21]. However, microcytic anemia and diabetes mellitus often predate neurologic symptoms by one or two decades and can be an important hint in diagnostics [111]. Its prevalence is estimated to be 1:2,000,000 in Japan where most of to date reported cases come from [112]. The disease is inherited in autosomal recessive manner and caused by loss-of-function mutations in the ceruloplasmin (*CP*) gene located on the long arm of chromosome 3. More than 40 different homozygous mutations (nonsense, missense, frameshift, as well as small deletions and insertions) are reported alongside few heterozygous cases with generally milder and more diverse phenotype ranging from chorea and athetosis to cerebellar signs and tremor [21]. The homozygous mutation carriers display characteristic imaging features on T2-weighted MRI with marked hypointensity of the thalami, the nuclei of the basal ganglia and the dentate, and the cerebral and cerebellar cortices [21]. Abundant iron deposits within mainly astrocytes and to a lesser extent within neurons in the basal ganglia, thalamus, and cerebellum and to a trivial amount in the frontal cortex mirror the condition neuropathologically [113, 114]. Astrocytic deformation with included globular structures that are proportional to the degree of iron deposition and react positively to anti-ubiquitin antibody and to the lipid peroxidation marker anti-4-hydroxynonenal antibody is a characteristic feature in aceruloplasminemia brains. There is no positivity to anti-α-synuclein antibodies.

Diagnostically, due to homozygous mutations in *CP*, ceruloplasmin is undetectable in blood serum, ferritin levels are elevated, and copper and iron are low [21].

The encoded protein ceruloplasmin, the most important carrier of copper in the human blood system, is an alpha-2-glycoprotein incorporating a ferroxidase activity that is crucial to iron mobilization [115]. Loss of this ferroxidase function leads to excessive iron accumulation within the pancreas, liver, and cerebral tissue with the main pathomechanism in the CNS being lipid peroxidation in astrocytes. Iron deposition is a trigger of free radical generation which consecutively causes oxidative damage to the vulnerable cells and leads to the pathology in the liver, pancreas, hematological system, and neuronal tissue [116–118].

COASY protein-associated neurodegeneration (*CoPAN*)

Recently, Dusi et al. identified recessive missense mutations in the human gene for coenzyme A synthase (*COASY*) in two unrelated individuals with previously idiopathic NBIA which led to the inclusion of *COASY* protein-associated neurodegeneration (CoPAN) into the spectrum of NBIA disorders [119]. CoPAN is inherited in autosomal recessive fashion with the human gene comprising 9 exons and being located on the long arm of chromosome 17. In a healthy organism, its encoded enzyme CoA synthase facilitates the coupling of ATP and phosphopantetheine to generate dephospho-CoA which is then enzymatically phosphorylated again by the bifunctional CoA synthase to finally generate CoA. Mutations in the coenzyme A synthase have been demonstrated to lead to alterations in RNA and protein expression and coenzyme A levels in fibroblasts from the affected patients as well as in a yeast model and are thought to be inherited in autosomal recessive fashion [119]. So far, more COASY-positive cases are awaited to further assess its prevalence and typical clinical presentation. Regarding its pathogenesis, CoPAN is strongly connected to PKAN, as both disorders are linked to coenzyme A – a vital key player in the cell's maintenance and regulation.

Brain Iron in Other Neurodegenerative Diseases

Additionally, brain iron accumulation with divergence regarding loci of highest iron content can also occur in different neurological disorders which bring back the unresolved question of iron accumulation as an accompanying epiphenomenon/result of neuroinflammation/neurodegeneration or of iron as the causal and incipient trigger of the neuronal loss observed in these diseases. Brain iron accumulation and dysregulation have been observed inter alia in multiple sclerosis [120]; Woodhouse-Sakati syndrome [121, 122]; GM1 gangliosidosis [123, 124]; alpha-mannosidosis [125]; Huntington' s disease [126]; frontotemporal dementia-amyotrophic lateral sclerosis complex [127]; RLS associated with hemochromatosis [128]; fucosidosis [129];

mucolipidosis type 4 [130]; superficial siderosis [131, 132]; Friedreich's ataxia [133]; atypical Parkinson syndromes like multiple system atrophy, cortical-basal ganglionic degeneration, and progressive supranuclear palsy; and classical Parkinson' s disease – even though still under some controversy [134–138]. Of these disorders, only Woodhouse-Sakati syndrome, due to mutations in *DCAF17*, is included into the NBIA disorder spectrum in some literature. However, it is beyond the scope of this chapter to review those, and interested readers must be relegated to the seminal review literature at this point (e.g., [139]).

Idiopathic NBIA

To date, there is still a rather large proportion of NBIA cases that is classified as idiopathic, meaning without detected genetic origin [71]. Dissecting their family history carefully, collecting samples from related individuals, and a combination of genetic techniques like linkage analysis, homozygosity mapping, and whole exome or whole genome sequencing will foster the ongoing excitement in the gene hunt and elucidate phenotype-genotype clarification in neurodegeneration with brain iron accumulation disorders. Collection of the idiopathic cases in international consortia and subsequent screening of those once a new gene has been identified will further reduce idiopathic NBIA in number and sharpen our understanding of this clinical spectrum. The advent of whole genome sequencing may introduce novel intronic variants associated with the disease that are linked to alternative splicing, nonsense-mediated mRNA decay, and altered transcription of disease-relevant proteins which may feed into the known or point to yet unknown novel therapeutically targetable pathways and may account for additional parts of the idiopathic cases. NBIA or pallidopyramidal syndromes are – despite their scarcity – an exciting and expanding field of study and may-due to their overlap in pathophysiology and clinical phenotypes with common diseases like PD and Alzheimer's-pave the avenue in understanding common pathways in clinical neurodegeneration.

Therapeutical Approaches: Which Pathways to Target and How?

To date, therapeutics in NBIA remain exclusively symptomatic. They may bring relief and are therefore important, but they do not target the origin of the disease and are incapable of stopping the neurodegenerative process. The development of specific, causal, and successful therapeutic agents in the future will therefore heavily depend upon our full understanding of the implicated pathways in this disease. Common pathways in NBIA include iron aggregation, mitochondrial deficiency, and lysosome and ceramide metabolism (for an overview of the different genes associated with NBIA to date and their role in the different pathways, see Fig. 13.2).

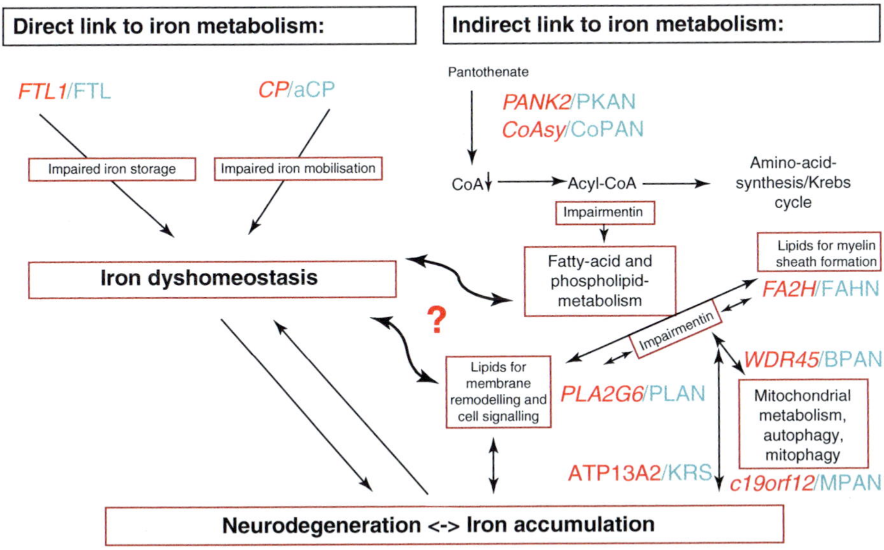

Fig. 13.2 NBIA genes and their suspected settlement within the different and interacting disease-associated pathways directly and indirectly linked to iron accumulation

Primarily the lysosomal function seems to be a promising candidate that needs closer investigation as it is the main metabolizer of ceramides which are crucial for many cellular processes [140] and seems to be involved in tauopathies equally as in Lewy body formation [82, 141] bonding NBIA closer to more common neurodegenerative diseases like atypical and typical Parkinson syndromes and potentially Alzheimer's dementia.

How induced Pluripotent Stem-Cell (iPSC) Technology Could Help to Foster Our Understanding of NBIA

So far, the lack of human neuronal cell models that faithfully recapitulate disease phenotypes in vitro has been one of the major hurdles in our efforts to study the mechanisms of NBIA disorders effectively. However, the recent discovery and rapid spread of induced pluripotent stem-cell technology may yield new important insights into NBIA pathophysiology within the upcoming years. This fascinating breakthrough technique enables us to model PKAN and other NBIA disorders with a defined genetic mutation in vitro via the pathophysiologic study of iPSC-derived neurons that carry the exact genetic information as our patients. Briefly, this technique involves collecting fibroblasts from genetically confirmed NBIA patients via skin biopsy and consecutive laboratory reprogrammation into induced pluripotent stem cell state, e.g. via episomal gene delivery [142]. Subsequently, neural induction is initiated via treatment with dual SMAD inhibitors [143] followed by exposition to default neural inductive conditions in the presence of retinoids to produce cortical or other region-specific neurons [144] derived from the patient' s original skin cells and ready for experimental readout. Thereby, extensive characterization of the iPSC-derived neurons carrying the genetic defect inclusive high-throughput screening for possible therapeutic rescues becomes possible. The results may give us a better idea of mechanisms and triggers of iron accumulation, transport deregulation, mitochondrial fitness including ATP generation, mitochondrial membrane potential, generation of reactive oxygen species, as well as generation of tau and acetyl-CoA protein and RNA expression in *PANK2* NBIA neurons.

These studies will lead to better understanding of disease mechanisms and ultimately could help with disease management.

Note on variant classification: Variants listed in the text have been provided by the author(s) of the respective studies and have been taken without adaptation or independent verification.

References

1. Gregory A, Hayflick SJ. Genetics of neurodegeneration with brain iron accumulation. Curr Neurol Neurosci Rep. 2011;11(3):254–61.
2. Schneider SA, Bhatia KP. Syndromes of neurodegeneration with brain iron accumulation. Semin Pediatr Neurol. 2012;19(2):57–66.
3. Aggarwal A, Schneider SA, Houlden H, Silverdale M, Paudel R, Paisan-Ruiz C, et al. Indian-subcontinent NBIA: unusual phenotypes, novel PANK2 mutations, and undetermined genetic forms. Mov Disord. 2010;25(10):1424–31.
4. Hayflick SJ, Hartman M, Coryell J, Gitschier J, Rowley H. Brain MRI in neurodegeneration with brain iron accumulation with and without PANK2 mutations. AJNR Am J Neuroradiol. 2006;27(6):1230–3.
5. Paisan-Ruiz C, Bhatia KP, Li A, Hernandez D, Davis M, Wood NW, et al. Characterization of PLA2G6 as a locus for dystonia-parkinsonism. Ann Neurol. 2009;65(1):19–23.
6. Yoshino H, Tomiyama H, Tachibana N, Ogaki K, Li Y, Funayama M, et al. Phenotypic spectrum of patients with PLA2G6 mutation and PARK14-linked parkinsonism. Neurology. 2010;75(15):1356–61.
7. Kruer MC, Hiken M, Gregory A, Malandrini A, Clark D, Hogarth P, et al. Novel histopathologic findings in molecularly-confirmed pantothenate kinase-associated neurodegeneration. Brain. 2011;134(Pt 4):947–58.
8. McNeill A, Birchall D, Hayflick SJ, Gregory A, Schenk JF, Zimmerman EA, et al. T2* and FSE MRI distinguishes four subtypes of neurodegeneration with brain iron accumulation. Neurology. 2008;70(18):1614–9.
9. Stamelou M, Lai SC, Aggarwal A, Schneider SA, Houlden H, Yeh TH, et al. Dystonic opisthotonus: a "red flag" for neurodegeneration with brain iron accumulation syndromes? Mov Disord. 2013;28(10):1325–9.
10. Kruer MC, Boddaert N. Neurodegeneration with brain iron accumulation: a diagnostic algorithm. Semin Pediatr Neurol. 2012;19(2):67–74.
11. Defendini R, Markesbery WR, Mastri AR, Duffy PE. Hallervorden-Spatz disease and infantile neuroaxonal dystrophy. Ultrastructural observations, anatomical pathology and nosology. J Neurol Sci. 1973;20(1):7–23.
12. Savoiardo M, Halliday WC, Nardocci N, Strada L, D'Incerti L, Angelini L, et al. Hallervorden-Spatz disease: MR and pathologic findings. AJNR Am J Neuroradiol. 1993;14(1):155–62.

13. Wakabayashi K, Yoshimoto M, Fukushima T, Koide R, Horikawa Y, Morita T, et al. Widespread occurrence of alpha-synuclein/NACP-immunoreactive neuronal inclusions in juvenile and adult-onset Hallervorden-Spatz disease with Lewy bodies. Neuropathol Appl Neurobiol. 1999;25(5):363–8.
14. Gregory A, Westaway SK, Holm IE, Kotzbauer PT, Hogarth P, Sonek S, et al. Neurodegeneration associated with genetic defects in phospholipase A(2). Neurology. 2008;71(18):1402–9.
15. Haraguchi T, Terada S, Ishizu H, Yokota O, Yoshida H, Takeda N, et al. Coexistence of TDP-43 and tau pathology in neurodegeneration with brain iron accumulation type 1 (NBIA-1, formerly Hallervorden-Spatz syndrome). Neuropathol Off J Jpn Soc Neuropathol. 2011;31(5):531–9.
16. Li A, Paudel R, Johnson R, Courtney R, Lees AJ, Holton JL, et al. Pantothenate kinase-associated neurodegeneration is not a synucleinopathy. Neuropathol Appl Neurobiol. 2012;39(2):121–131.
17. Eidelberg D, Sotrel A, Joachim C, Selkoe D, Forman A, Pendlebury WW, et al. Adult onset Hallervorden-Spatz disease with neurofibrillary pathology. A discrete clinicopathological entity. Brain. 1987;110(Pt 4):993–1013.
18. Hartmann HA, White SK, Levine RL. Neuroaxonal dystrophy with neuromelanin deposition, neurofibrillary tangles, and neuronal loss. Light- and electron-microscopic changes in a 45-year-old woman with progressive psychomotor deterioration. Acta Neuropathol. 1983; 61(3–4):169–72.
19. Keogh MJ, Chinnery PF. Current concepts and controversies in neurodegeneration with brain iron accumulation. Semin Pediatr Neurol. 2012;19(2):51–6.
20. Miyajima H, Nishimura Y, Mizoguchi K, Sakamoto M, Shimizu T, Honda N. Familial apoceruloplasmin deficiency associated with blepharospasm and retinal degeneration. Neurology. 1987;37(5):761–7.
21. McNeill A, Pandolfo M, Kuhn J, Shang H, Miyajima H. The neurological presentation of ceruloplasmin gene mutations. Eur Neurol. 2008;60(4):200–5.
22. Curtis AR, Fey C, Morris CM, Bindoff LA, Ince PG, Chinnery PF, et al. Mutation in the gene encoding ferritin light polypeptide causes dominant adult-onset basal ganglia disease. Nat Genet. 2001;28(4):350–4.
23. Ohta E, Nagasaka T, Shindo K, Toma S, Nagasaka K, Ohta K, et al. Neuroferritinopathy in a Japanese family with a duplication in the ferritin light chain gene. Neurology. 2008;70 (16 Pt 2):1493–4.
24. Ory-Magne F, Brefel-Courbon C, Payoux P, Debruxelles S, Sibon I, Goizet C, et al. Clinical phenotype and neuroimaging findings in a French family with hereditary ferritinopathy (FTL498-499InsTC). Mov Disord. 2009;24(11):1676–83.
25. Vidal R, Ghetti B, Takao M, Brefel-Courbon C, Uro-Coste E, Glazier BS, et al. Intracellular ferritin accumulation in neural and extraneural tissue characterizes a neurodegenerative disease associated with a mutation in the ferritin light polypeptide gene. J Neuropathol Exp Neurol. 2004;63(4):363–80.
26. Khateeb S, Flusser H, Ofir R, Shelef I, Narkis G, Vardi G, et al. PLA2G6 mutation underlies infantile neuroaxonal dystrophy. Am J Hum Genet. 2006;79(5):942–8.
27. Haack TB, Hogarth P, Kruer MC, Gregory A, Wieland T, Schwarzmayr T, et al. Exome sequencing reveals de novo WDR45 mutations causing a phenotypically distinct, X-linked dominant form of NBIA. Am J Hum Genet. 2012;91(6):1144–9.
28. Ramirez A, Heimbach A, Grundemann J, Stiller B, Hampshire D, Cid LP, et al. Hereditary parkinsonism with dementia is caused by mutations in ATP13A2, encoding a lysosomal type 5 P-type ATPase. Nat Genet. 2006;38(10):1184–91.
29. Hayflick SJ, Westaway SK, Levinson B, Zhou B, Johnson MA, Ching KH, et al. Genetic, clinical, and radiographic delineation of Hallervorden-Spatz syndrome. N Engl J Med. 2003; 348(1):33–40.
30. Zeidman LA, Pandey DK. Declining use of the Hallervorden-Spatz disease eponym in the last two decades. J Child Neurol. 2012;27(10):1310–5.
31. Hayflick SJ. Neurodegeneration with brain iron accumulation: from genes to pathogenesis. Semin Pediatr Neurol. 2006;13(3):182–5.

32. Schneider SA, Aggarwal A, Bhatt M, Dupont E, Tisch S, Limousin P, et al. Severe tongue protrusion dystonia: clinical syndromes and possible treatment. Neurology. 2006;67(6):940–3.
33. Marelli C, Piacentini S, Garavaglia B, Girotti F, Albanese A. Clinical and neuropsychological correlates in two brothers with pantothenate kinase-associated neurodegeneration. Mov Disord. 2005;20(2):208–12.
34. Egan RA, Weleber RG, Hogarth P, Gregory A, Coryell J, Westaway SK, et al. Neuro-ophthalmologic and electroretinographic findings in pantothenate kinase-associated neurodegeneration (formerly Hallervorden-Spatz syndrome). Am J Ophthalmol. 2005;140(2):267–74.
35. Chang CL, Lin CM. Eye-of-the-tiger sign is not pathognomonic of pantothenate kinase-associated neurodegeneration in adult cases. Brain Behavior. 2011;1(1):55–6.
36. Strecker K, Hesse S, Wegner F, Sabri O, Schwarz J, Schneider JP. Eye of the tiger sign in multiple system atrophy. Eur J Neurol. 2007;14(11):e1–2.
37. Delgado RF, Sanchez PR, Speckter H, Then EP, Jimenez R, Oviedo J, et al. Missense PANK2 mutation without "eye of the tiger" sign: MR findings in a large group of patients with pantothenate kinase-associated neurodegeneration (PKAN). J Magn Reson Imaging JMRI. 2012;35(4):788–94.
38. van den Bogaard SJ, Kruit MC, Dumas EM, Roos RA. Eye-of-the-tiger-sign in a 48 year healthy adult. J Neurol Sci. 2014;336(1–2):254–6.
39. Hortnagel K, Prokisch H, Meitinger T. An isoform of hPANK2, deficient in pantothenate kinase-associated neurodegeneration, localizes to mitochondria. Hum Mol Genet. 2003;12(3):321–7.
40. Kotzbauer PT, Truax AC, Trojanowski JQ, Lee VM. Altered neuronal mitochondrial coenzyme A synthesis in neurodegeneration with brain iron accumulation caused by abnormal processing, stability, and catalytic activity of mutant pantothenate kinase 2. J Neurosci. 2005;25(3):689–98.
41. Hartig MB, Hortnagel K, Garavaglia B, Zorzi G, Kmiec T, Klopstock T, et al. Genotypic and phenotypic spectrum of PANK2 mutations in patients with neurodegeneration with brain iron accumulation. Ann Neurol. 2006;59(2):248–56.
42. Gregory A, Polster BJ, Hayflick SJ. Clinical and genetic delineation of neurodegeneration with brain iron accumulation. J Med Genet. 2009;46(2):73–80.
43. Gregory A, Hayflick SJ. Pantothenate kinase-associated neurodegeneration. In: Pagon RA, Adam MP, Ardinger HH, Bird TD, Dolan CR, Fong CT, et al., editors. GeneReviews(R). Seattle, WA: University of Washington; 1993.
44. Hong BS, Senisterra G, Rabeh WM, Vedadi M, Leonardi R, Zhang YM, et al. Crystal structures of human pantothenate kinases. Insights into allosteric regulation and mutations linked to a neurodegeneration disorder. J Biol Chem. 2007;282(38):27984–93.
45. Saito Y, Kawai M, Inoue K, Sasaki R, Arai H, Nanba E, et al. Widespread expression of alpha-synuclein and tau immunoreactivity in Hallervorden-Spatz syndrome with protracted clinical course. J Neurol Sci. 2000;177(1):48–59.
46. Neumann M, Adler S, Schluter O, Kremmer E, Benecke R, Kretzschmar HA. Alpha-synuclein accumulation in a case of neurodegeneration with brain iron accumulation type 1 (NBIA-1, formerly Hallervorden-Spatz syndrome) with widespread cortical and brainstem-type Lewy bodies. Acta Neuropathol. 2000;100(5):568–74.
47. Galvin JE, Giasson B, Hurtig HI, Lee VM, Trojanowski JQ. Neurodegeneration with brain iron accumulation, type 1 is characterized by alpha-, beta-, and gamma-synuclein neuropathology. Am J Pathol. 2000;157(2):361–8.
48. Houlden H, Lincoln S, Farrer M, Cleland PG, Hardy J, Orrell RW. Compound heterozygous PANK2 mutations confirm HARP and Hallervorden-Spatz syndromes are allelic. Neurology. 2003;61(10):1423–6.
49. Zorzi G, Zibordi F, Chiapparini L, Bertini E, Russo L, Piga A, et al. Iron-related MRI images in patients with pantothenate kinase-associated neurodegeneration (PKAN) treated with deferiprone: results of a phase II pilot trial. Mov Disord. 2011;26(9):1756–9.
50. Cossu G, Abbruzzese G, Matta G, Murgia D, Melis M, Ricchi V, et al. Efficacy and safety of deferiprone for the treatment of pantothenate kinase-associated neurodegeneration (PKAN)

and neurodegeneration with brain iron accumulation (NBIA): results from a four years follow-up. Parkinsonism Relat Disord. 2014;20(6):651–4.
51. Timmermann L, Pauls KA, Wieland K, Jech R, Kurlemann G, Sharma N, et al. Dystonia in neurodegeneration with brain iron accumulation: outcome of bilateral pallidal stimulation. Brain. 2010;133(Pt 3):701–12.
52. Mikati MA, Yehya A, Darwish H, Karam P, Comair Y. Deep brain stimulation as a mode of treatment of early onset pantothenate kinase-associated neurodegeneration. Eur J Paediatr Neurol EJPN Off J Eur Paediatr Neurol Soc. 2009;13(1):61–4.
53. Gregory A, Hayflick S. Neurodegeneration with brain iron accumulation disorders overview. In: Pagon RA, Adam MP, Ardinger HH, Bird TD, Dolan CR, Fong CT, et al., editors. GeneReviews(R). Seattle, WA: University of Washington; 1993.
54. Morgan NV, Westaway SK, Morton JE, Gregory A, Gissen P, Sonek S, et al. PLA2G6, encoding a phospholipase A2, is mutated in neurodegenerative disorders with high brain iron. Nat Genet. 2006;38(7):752–4.
55. Kurian MA, Morgan NV, MacPherson L, Foster K, Peake D, Gupta R, et al. Phenotypic spectrum of neurodegeneration associated with mutations in the PLA2G6 gene (PLAN). Neurology. 2008;70(18):1623–9.
56. Aicardi J, Castelein P. Infantile neuroaxonal dystrophy. Brain. 1979;102(4):727–48.
57. Nardocci N, Zorzi G, Farina L, Binelli S, Scaioli W, Ciano C, et al. Infantile neuroaxonal dystrophy: clinical spectrum and diagnostic criteria. Neurology. 1999;52(7):1472–8.
58. Gregory A, Kurian MA, Maher ER, Hogarth P, Hayflick SJ. PLA2G6-associated neurodegeneration. In: Pagon RA, Adam MP, Ardinger HH, Bird TD, Dolan CR, Fong CT, et al., editors. GeneReviews(R). Seattle, WA: University of Washington; 1993.
59. Illingworth MA, Meyer E, Chong WK, Manzur AY, Carr LJ, Younis R, et al. PLA2G6-associated neurodegeneration (PLAN): further expansion of the clinical, radiological and mutation spectrum associated with infantile and atypical childhood-onset disease. Mol Genet Metab. 2014;114(2):183–9.
60. Kurian MA, McNeill A, Lin JP, Maher ER. Childhood disorders of neurodegeneration with brain iron accumulation (NBIA). Dev Med Child Neurol. 2011;53(5):394–404.
61. Larsson PK, Claesson HE, Kennedy BP. Multiple splice variants of the human calcium-independent phospholipase A2 and their effect on enzyme activity. J Biol Chem. 1998;273(1):207–14.
62. Mubaidin A, Roberts E, Hampshire D, Dehyyat M, Shurbaji A, Mubaidien M, et al. Karak syndrome: a novel degenerative disorder of the basal ganglia and cerebellum. J Med Genet. 2003;40(7):543–6.
63. Balsinde J, Balboa MA. Cellular regulation and proposed biological functions of group VIA calcium-independent phospholipase A2 in activated cells. Cell Signal. 2005;17(9):1052–62.
64. Strokin M, Seburn KL, Cox GA, Martens KA, Reiser G. Severe disturbance in the Ca2+ signaling in astrocytes from mouse models of human infantile neuroaxonal dystrophy with mutated Pla2g6. Hum Mol Genet. 2012;21(12):2807–14.
65. Lands WE. Metabolism of glycerolipids. 2. The enzymatic acylation of lysolecithin. J Biol Chem. 1960;235:2233–7.
66. Perez R, Melero R, Balboa MA, Balsinde J. Role of group VIA calcium-independent phospholipase A2 in arachidonic acid release, phospholipid fatty acid incorporation, and apoptosis in U937 cells responding to hydrogen peroxide. J Biol Chem. 2004;279(39):40385–91.
67. Shinzawa K, Sumi H, Ikawa M, Matsuoka Y, Okabe M, Sakoda S, et al. Neuroaxonal dystrophy caused by group VIA phospholipase A2 deficiency in mice: a model of human neurodegenerative disease. J Neurosci. 2008;28(9):2212–20.
68. Malik I, Turk J, Mancuso DJ, Montier L, Wohltmann M, Wozniak DF, et al. Disrupted membrane homeostasis and accumulation of ubiquitinated proteins in a mouse model of infantile neuroaxonal dystrophy caused by PLA2G6 mutations. Am J Pathol. 2008;172(2):406–16.
69. Paisan-Ruiz C, Li A, Schneider SA, Holton JL, Johnson R, Kidd D, et al. Widespread Lewy body and tau accumulation in childhood and adult onset dystonia-parkinsonism cases with PLA2G6 mutations. Neurobiol Aging. 2012;33(4):814–23.

70. Hartig MB, Iuso A, Haack T, Kmiec T, Jurkiewicz E, Heim K, et al. Absence of an orphan mitochondrial protein, c19orf12, causes a distinct clinical subtype of neurodegeneration with brain iron accumulation. Am J Hum Genet. 2011;89(4):543–50.
71. Hogarth P, Gregory A, Kruer MC, Sanford L, Wagoner W, Natowicz MR, et al. New NBIA subtype: genetic, clinical, pathologic, and radiographic features of MPAN. Neurology. 2013;80(3):268–75.
72. Hogarth P. Neurodegeneration with brain iron accumulation: diagnosis and management. Journal of Movement Disorders, 2015;8(1):1–13. doi:10.14802/jmd.14034.
73. Hayflick SJ, Kruer MC, Gregory A, Haack TB, Kurian MA, Houlden HH, et al. Beta-propeller protein-associated neurodegeneration: a new X-linked dominant disorder with brain iron accumulation. Brain. 2013;136(Pt 6):1708–17.
74. Kruer MC, Boddaert N, Schneider SA, Houlden H, Bhatia KP, Gregory A, et al. Neuroimaging features of neurodegeneration with brain iron accumulation. AJNR Am J Neuroradiol. 2012;33(3):407–14.
75. Saitsu H, Nishimura T, Muramatsu K, Kodera H, Kumada S, Sugai K, et al. De novo mutations in the autophagy gene WDR45 cause static encephalopathy of childhood with neurodegeneration in adulthood. Nat Genet. 2013;45(4):445–9, 449e1.
76. Lu Q, Yang P, Huang X, Hu W, Guo B, Wu F, et al. The WD40 repeat PtdIns(3)P-binding protein EPG-6 regulates progression of omegasomes to autophagosomes. Dev Cell. 2011; 21(2):343–57.
77. Nakatogawa H, Suzuki K, Kamada Y, Ohsumi Y. Dynamics and diversity in autophagy mechanisms: lessons from yeast. Nat Rev Mol Cell Biol. 2009;10(7):458–67.
78. Dick KJ, Eckhardt M, Paisan-Ruiz C, Alshehhi AA, Proukakis C, Sibtain NA, et al. Mutation of FA2H underlies a complicated form of hereditary spastic paraplegia (SPG35). Hum Mutat. 2010;31(4):E1251–60.
79. Edvardson S, Hama H, Shaag A, Gomori JM, Berger I, Soffer D, et al. Mutations in the fatty acid 2-hydroxylase gene are associated with leukodystrophy with spastic paraparesis and dystonia. Am J Hum Genet. 2008;83(5):643–8.
80. Garone C, Pippucci T, Cordelli DM, Zuntini R, Castegnaro G, Marconi C, et al. FA2H-related disorders: a novel c.270+3A>T splice-site mutation leads to a complex neurodegenerative phenotype. Dev Med Child Neurol. 2011;53(10):958–61.
81. Schneider SA, Bhatia KP. Three faces of the same gene: FA2H links neurodegeneration with brain iron accumulation, leukodystrophies, and hereditary spastic paraplegias. Ann Neurol. 2010;68(5):575–7.
82. Kruer MC, Paisan-Ruiz C, Boddaert N, Yoon MY, Hama H, Gregory A, et al. Defective FA2H leads to a novel form of neurodegeneration with brain iron accumulation (NBIA). Ann Neurol. 2010;68(5):611–8.
83. Stevanin G, Azzedine H, Denora P, Boukhris A, Tazir M, Lossos A, et al. Mutations in SPG11 are frequent in autosomal recessive spastic paraplegia with thin corpus callosum, cognitive decline and lower motor neuron degeneration. Brain. 2008;131(Pt 3):772–84.
84. Schule R, Schols L. Genetics of hereditary spastic paraplegias. Semin Neurol. 2011;31(5): 484–93.
85. Liao X, Luo Y, Zhan Z, Du J, Hu Z, Wang J, et al. SPG35 contributes to the second common subtype of AR-HSP in China: frequency analysis and functional characterization of FA2H gene mutations. Clin Genet. 2015;87(1):85–9.
86. Pierson TM, Simeonov DR, Sincan M, Adams DA, Markello T, Golas G, et al. Exome sequencing and SNP analysis detect novel compound heterozygosity in fatty acid hydroxylase-associated neurodegeneration. Eur J Hum Genet. 2012;20(4):476–9.
87. Kruer MC, Gregory A, Hayflick SJ. Fatty Acid hydroxylase-associated neurodegeneration. In: Pagon RA, Adam MP, Ardinger HH, Bird TD, Dolan CR, Fong CT, et al., editors. GeneReviews(R). Seattle, WA: University of Washington; 1993.
88. Potter KA, Kern MJ, Fullbright G, Bielawski J, Scherer SS, Yum SW, et al. Central nervous system dysfunction in a mouse model of FA2H deficiency. Glia. 2011;59(7):1009–21.

89. Najim al-Din AS, Wriekat A, Mubaidin A, Dasouki M, Hiari M. Pallido-pyramidal degeneration, supranuclear upgaze paresis and dementia: Kufor-Rakeb syndrome. Acta Neurol Scand. 1994;89(5):347–52.
90. Di Fonzo A, Chien HF, Socal M, Giraudo S, Tassorelli C, Iliceto G, et al. ATP13A2 missense mutations in juvenile parkinsonism and young onset Parkinson disease. Neurology. 2007;68(19):1557–62.
91. Williams DR, Hadeed A, Al-Din AS, Wreikat AL, Lees AJ. Kufor Rakeb disease: autosomal recessive, levodopa-responsive parkinsonism with pyramidal degeneration, supranuclear gaze palsy, and dementia. Mov Disord. 2005;20(10):1264–71.
92. Behrens MI, Bruggemann N, Chana P, Venegas P, Kagi M, Parrao T, et al. Clinical spectrum of Kufor-Rakeb syndrome in the Chilean kindred with ATP13A2 mutations. Mov Disord. 2010;25(12):1929–37.
93. Machner B, Sprenger A, Behrens MI, Ramirez A, Bruggemann N, Klein C, et al. Eye movement disorders in ATP13A2 mutation carriers (PARK9). Mov Disord. 2010; 25(15):2687–9.
94. Schneider SA, Paisan-Ruiz C, Quinn NP, Lees AJ, Houlden H, Hardy J, et al. ATP13A2 mutations (PARK9) cause neurodegeneration with brain iron accumulation. Mov Disord. 2010;25(8):979–84.
95. Chien HF, Bonifati V, Barbosa ER. ATP13A2-related neurodegeneration (PARK9) without evidence of brain iron accumulation. Mov Disord. 2011;26(7):1364–5.
96. Crosiers D, Ceulemans B, Meeus B, Nuytemans K, Pals P, Van Broeckhoven C, et al. Juvenile dystonia-parkinsonism and dementia caused by a novel ATP13A2 frameshift mutation. Parkinsonism Relat Disord. 2011;17(2):135–8.
97. Santoro L, Breedveld GJ, Manganelli F, Iodice R, Pisciotta C, Nolano M, et al. Novel ATP13A2 (PARK9) homozygous mutation in a family with marked phenotype variability. Neurogenetics. 2011;12(1):33–9.
98. Park JS, Mehta P, Cooper AA, Veivers D, Heimbach A, Stiller B, et al. Pathogenic effects of novel mutations in the P-type ATPase ATP13A2 (PARK9) causing Kufor-Rakeb syndrome, a form of early-onset parkinsonism. Hum Mutat. 2011;32(8):956–64.
99. Schultheis PJ, Hagen TT, O'Toole KK, Tachibana A, Burke CR, McGill DL, et al. Characterization of the P5 subfamily of P-type transport ATPases in mice. Biochem Biophys Res Commun. 2004;323(3):731–8.
100. Ramonet D, Podhajska A, Stafa K, Sonnay S, Trancikova A, Tsika E, et al. PARK9-associated ATP13A2 localizes to intracellular acidic vesicles and regulates cation homeostasis and neuronal integrity. Hum Mol Genet. 2012;21(8):1725–43.
101. Gusdon AM, Zhu J, Van Houten B, Chu CT. ATP13A2 regulates mitochondrial bioenergetics through macroautophagy. Neurobiol Dis. 2012;45(3):962–72.
102. Grunewald A, Arns B, Seibler P, Rakovic A, Munchau A, Ramirez A, et al. ATP13A2 mutations impair mitochondrial function in fibroblasts from patients with Kufor-Rakeb syndrome. Neurobiol Aging. 2012;33(8):1843.e1–7.
103. Bras J, Verloes A, Schneider SA, Mole SE, Guerreiro RJ. Mutation of the parkinsonism gene ATP13A2 causes neuronal ceroid-lipofuscinosis. Hum Mol Genet. 2012;21(12):2646–50.
104. Paisan-Ruiz C, Guevara R, Federoff M, Hanagasi H, Sina F, Elahi E, et al. Early-onset L-dopa-responsive parkinsonism with pyramidal signs due to ATP13A2, PLA2G6, FBXO7 and spatacsin mutations. Mov Disord. 2010;25(12):1791–800.
105. Chinnery PF, Crompton DE, Birchall D, Jackson MJ, Coulthard A, Lombes A, et al. Clinical features and natural history of neuroferritinopathy caused by the FTL1 460InsA mutation. Brain. 2007;130(Pt 1):110–9.
106. McNeill A, Chinnery PF. Neuroferritinopathy: update on clinical features and pathogenesis. Curr Drug Targets. 2012;13(9):1200–3.
107. Keogh MJ, Jonas P, Coulthard A, Chinnery PF, Burn J. Neuroferritinopathy: a new inborn error of iron metabolism. Neurogenetics. 2012;13(1):93–6.

108. Hautot D, Pankhurst QA, Morris CM, Curtis A, Burn J, Dobson J. Preliminary observation of elevated levels of nanocrystalline iron oxide in the basal ganglia of neuroferritinopathy patients. Biochim Biophys Acta. 2007;1772(1):21–5.
109. Mancuso M, Davidzon G, Kurlan RM, Tawil R, Bonilla E, Di Mauro S, et al. Hereditary ferritinopathy: a novel mutation, its cellular pathology, and pathogenetic insights. J Neuropathol Exp Neurol. 2005;64(4):280–94.
110. Maciel P, Cruz VT, Constante M, Iniesta I, Costa MC, Gallati S, et al. Neuroferritinopathy: missense mutation in FTL causing early-onset bilateral pallidal involvement. Neurology. 2005;65(4):603–5.
111. Ogimoto M, Anzai K, Takenoshita H, Kogawa K, Akehi Y, Yoshida R, et al. Criteria for early identification of aceruloplasminemia. Intern Med. 2011;50(13):1415–8.
112. Miyajima H, Takahashi Y, Kono S. Aceruloplasminemia, an inherited disorder of iron metabolism. Biometals. 2003;16(1):205–13.
113. Kono S, Miyajima H. Molecular and pathological basis of aceruloplasminemia. Biol Res. 2006;39(1):15–23.
114. Miyajima H. Aceruloplasminemia, an iron metabolic disorder. Neuropathol Off J Jpn Soc Neuropathol. 2003;23(4):345–50.
115. Hellman NE, Gitlin JD. Ceruloplasmin metabolism and function. Annu Rev Nutr. 2002; 22:439–58.
116. Gonzalez-Cuyar LF, Perry G, Miyajima H, Atwood CS, Riveros-Angel M, Lyons PF, et al. Redox active iron accumulation in aceruloplasminemia. Neuropathol Off J Jpn Soc Neuropathol. 2008;28(5):466–71.
117. Oide T, Yoshida K, Kaneko K, Ohta M, Arima K. Iron overload and antioxidative role of perivascular astrocytes in aceruloplasminemia. Neuropathol Appl Neurobiol. 2006;32(2):170–6.
118. Yoshida K, Kaneko K, Miyajima H, Tokuda T, Nakamura A, Kato M, et al. Increased lipid peroxidation in the brains of aceruloplasminemia patients. J Neurol Sci. 2000;175(2):91–5.
119. Dusi S, Valletta L, Haack TB, Tsuchiya Y, Venco P, Pasqualato S, et al. Exome sequence reveals mutations in CoA synthase as a cause of neurodegeneration with brain iron accumulation. Am J Hum Genet. 2014;94(1):11–22.
120. Burgetova A, Seidl Z, Krasensky J, Horakova D, Vaneckova M. Multiple sclerosis and the accumulation of iron in the Basal Ganglia: quantitative assessment of brain iron using MRI t(2) relaxometry. Eur Neurol. 2010;63(3):136–43.
121. Al-Semari A, Bohlega S. Autosomal-recessive syndrome with alopecia, hypogonadism, progressive extra-pyramidal disorder, white matter disease, sensory neural deafness, diabetes mellitus, and low IGF1. Am J Med Genet A. 2007;143(2):149–60.
122. Alazami AM, Al-Saif A, Al-Semari A, Bohlega S, Zlitni S, Alzahrani F, et al. Mutations in C2orf37, encoding a nucleolar protein, cause hypogonadism, alopecia, diabetes mellitus, mental retardation, and extrapyramidal syndrome. Am J Hum Genet. 2008;83(6):684–91.
123. Muthane U, Chickabasaviah Y, Kaneski C, Shankar SK, Narayanappa G, Christopher R, et al. Clinical features of adult GM1 gangliosidosis: report of three Indian patients and review of 40 cases. Mov Disord. 2004;19(11):1334–41.
124. Tanaka R, Momoi T, Yoshida A, Okumura M, Yamakura S, Takasaki Y, et al. Type 3 GM1 gangliosidosis: clinical and neuroradiological findings in an 11-year-old girl. J Neurol. 1995;242(5):299–303.
125. Zoons E, de Koning TJ, Abeling NG, Tijssen MA. Neurodegeneration with brain iron accumulation on MRI: an adult case of alpha-mannosidosis. JIMD Rep. 2012;4:99–102.
126. Bartzokis G, Cummings J, Perlman S, Hance DB, Mintz J. Increased basal ganglia iron levels in Huntington disease. Arch Neurol. 1999;56(5):569–74.
127. Santillo AF, Skoglund L, Lindau M, Eeg-Olofsson KE, Tovi M, Engler H, et al. Frontotemporal dementia-amyotrophic lateral sclerosis complex is simulated by neurodegeneration with brain iron accumulation. Alzheimer Dis Assoc Disord. 2009;23(3):298–300.
128. Haba-Rubio J, Staner L, Petiau C, Erb G, Schunck T, Macher JP. Restless legs syndrome and low brain iron levels in patients with haemochromatosis. J Neurol Neurosurg Psychiatry. 2005;76(7):1009–10.

129. Gautschi M, Merlini L, Calza AM, Hayflick S, Nuoffer JM, Fluss J. Late diagnosis of fucosidosis in a child with progressive fixed dystonia, bilateral pallidal lesions and red spots on the skin. Eur J Paediatr Neurol EJPN Off J Eur Paediatr Neurol Soc. 2014;18(4):516–9.
130. Altarescu G, Sun M, Moore DF, Smith JA, Wiggs EA, Solomon BI, et al. The neurogenetics of mucolipidosis type IV. Neurology. 2002;59(3):306–13.
131. Levy M, Turtzo C, Llinas RH. Superficial siderosis: a case report and review of the literature. Nat Clin Pract Neurol. 2007;3(1):54–8; quiz 9.
132. Spengos K, Koutsis G, Tsivgoulis G, Panas M, Vemmos K, Vassilopoulos D. Superficial siderosis of the CNS. Case report and literature review. Nervenarzt. 2004;75(5):492–5.
133. Waldvogel D, van Gelderen P, Hallett M. Increased iron in the dentate nucleus of patients with Friedrich's ataxia. Ann Neurol. 1999;46(1):123–5.
134. Visanji NP, Collingwood JF, Finnegan ME, Tandon A, House E, Hazrati LN. Iron deficiency in parkinsonism: region-specific iron dysregulation in Parkinson's disease and multiple system atrophy. J Parkinsons Dis. 2013;3(4):523–37.
135. Berg D, Hochstrasser H. Iron metabolism in Parkinsonian syndromes. Mov Disord. 2006;21(9):1299–310.
136. Wang Y, Butros SR, Shuai X, Dai Y, Chen C, Liu M, et al. Different iron-deposition patterns of multiple system atrophy with predominant parkinsonism and idiopathetic Parkinson diseases demonstrated by phase-corrected susceptibility-weighted imaging. AJNR Am J Neuroradiol. 2012;33(2):266–73.
137. Davie CA, Barker GJ, Machado C, Miller DH, Lees AJ. Proton magnetic resonance spectroscopy in Steele-Richardson-Olszewski syndrome. Mov Disord. 1997;12(5):767–71.
138. Molinuevo JL, Munoz E, Valldeoriola F, Tolosa E. The eye of the tiger sign in cortical-basal ganglionic degeneration. Mov Disord. 1999;14(1):169–71.
139. Dusek P, Jankovic J, Le W. Iron dysregulation in movement disorders. Neurobiol Dis. 2012;46(1):1–18.
140. Ogretmen B, Hannun YA. Biologically active sphingolipids in cancer pathogenesis and treatment. Nat Rev Cancer. 2004;4(8):604–16.
141. Bras J, Singleton A, Cookson MR, Hardy J. Emerging pathways in genetic Parkinson's disease: Potential role of ceramide metabolism in Lewy body disease. FEBS J. 2008;275(23):5767–73.
142. Okita K, Matsumura Y, Sato Y, Okada A, Morizane A, Okamoto S, et al. A more efficient method to generate integration-free human iPS cells. Nat Methods. 2011;8(5):409–12.
143. Chambers SM, Fasano CA, Papapetrou EP, Tomishima M, Sadelain M, Studer L. Highly efficient neural conversion of human ES and iPS cells by dual inhibition of SMAD signaling. Nat Biotechnol. 2009;27(3):275–80.
144. Shi Y, Kirwan P, Livesey FJ. Directed differentiation of human pluripotent stem cells to cerebral cortex neurons and neural networks. Nat Protoc. 2012;7(10):1836–46.

Chapter 14
Genetics of Metal Disorders (Excluding NBIA)

Petr Dusek and Daniela Zahorakova

Abstract In this chapter, we describe genetic movement disorders arising from endogenous dysregulation of calcium, copper, and manganese homeostasis. In general, dysregulation of metal homeostasis may lead to regional brain metal accumulation, systemic metal accumulation affecting the whole brain and other organs, or brain metal deficiency.

Primary familial brain calcification leading to regional brain calcium deposits is caused by mutations in inorganic phosphate transporter 2 (PiT2), platelet-derived growth factor (PDGFβ), or platelet-derived growth factor receptor-β (PDGFRβ). Mutations in these three genes explain 50 % of cases and further causative genes are likely involved.

Systemic accumulation of copper is the hallmark of Wilson disease and MEDNIK syndrome caused by mutations in *ATP7B* and *AP1S1* genes, respectively. Menkes disease, caused by mutations in *ATP7A*, is an example of disorder of systemic copper deficiency.

Systemic accumulation of manganese has been described in manganese transporter deficiency caused by *SLC30A10* mutations. The brain and liver are the most affected organs in these systemic disorders. Kufor-Rakeb syndrome, caused by mutations in *ATP13A2*, is likely also related to manganese toxicity.

Keywords Wilson disease • Menkes disease • Fahr's disease • Copper • Manganese • Calcium

P. Dusek, MD, PhD (✉)
Department of Neurology and Center of Clinical Neuroscience, Charles University, Prague, Czech Republic

1st Faculty of Medicine, General University Hospital, Prague 2, 12000, Czech Republic
e-mail: pdusek@gmail.com

D. Zahorakova, RNDr, PhD
First Faculty of Medicine, Charles University, Prague 2, 12000, Czech Republic

Department of Pediatrics and Adolescent Medicine, General University Hospital, Prague 2, 121 00, Czech Republic

S.A. Schneider, J.M.T. Brás (eds.), *Movement Disorder Genetics*,
DOI 10.1007/978-3-319-17223-1_14

Abbreviations

AP1S1	Adaptor-related protein complex 1, subunit σ1A
AT1	Acetyl-CoA transporter
ATOX1	Antioxidant 1 copper chaperone
ATP	Adenosine triphosphate
ATP7A	ATPase, Cu2+ transporting, alpha polypeptide
ATP7B	ATPase, Cu2+ transporting, beta polypeptide
BBB	Blood-brain barrier
BCB	Blood-cerebrospinal fluid barrier
BG	Basal ganglia
Ca	Calcium
CCS	Copper chaperone for superoxide dismutase 1
Cd	Cadmium
COMMD1	Copper metabolism (Murr1) domain-containing 1 protein
COX17	Cytochrome c oxidase copper chaperone
CP	Ceruloplasmin
CSF	Cerebrospinal fluid
CT	Computerized tomography
Cu	Copper
DHPG	Dihydroxyphenylglycol
DMT1	Divalent metal transporter 1
DOPAC	Dihydroxyphenylacetic acid
ER	Endoplasmic reticulum
Fe	Iron
FPN1	Ferroportin 1
GHS	Glutathione
GP	Globus pallidus
hCTR	Human copper transporter protein
HEPH	Hephaestin
ITPR	Inositol 1,4,5-trisphosphate receptor
K-F ring	Kayser-Fleischer ring
MBD	Metal-binding domain
MCT1	Monocarboxylic acid transporter
MD	Menkes disease
Mn	Manganese
MRI	Magnetic resonance imaging
NBIA	Neurodegeneration with brain iron accumulation
Ni	Nickel
NMDA	N-methyl D-aspartate
OHS	Occipital horn syndrome
P2RX1	Purinergic receptor type P2X1
Pb	Lead
PD	Parkinson's disease

PDGF-B	Platelet-derived growth factor-β
PDGFRβ	Platelet-derived growth factor receptor-β
PFBC	Primary familial brain calcification
PiT1	Phosphate transporter 1
PiT2	Phosphate transporter 2
RYR	Ryanodine receptor
SCA	Spinocerebellar ataxia
SERCA	Sarcoplasmic/endoplasmic reticulum calcium ATPase
SLC	Solute carrier family
SLC30A10	Solute carrier family 30, member 10
T1w	T1-weighted image
T2w	T2-weighted image
TD	Transmembrane domain
TFRC	Transferrin receptor
TGN	Trans-Golgi network
TRPM7	TRP, subfamily M, member 7
TRPs	Transient receptor potential cation channels
WD	Wilson disease
ZDHHC17	Zinc finger DHHC domain-containing protein 17
Zn	Zinc

Introduction

Trace elements including iron (Fe), copper (Cu), manganese (Mn), and calcium (Ca), which are essential constituents necessary for cellular homeostasis, become toxic when present in excess quantities. Tight regulation of metal uptake and efflux is therefore necessary for sufficient synthesis of metalloproteins on one side and prevention of excessive oxidative stress on the other side. In this chapter, we describe genetic movement disorders arising from endogenous dysregulation of metal homeostasis. In general, there are three subgroups of brain metal dysregulation disorders: (1) regional brain metal accumulation, mostly in globus pallidus (GP), which is susceptible to accumulation of divalent metal ions, (2) metal accumulation affecting the whole brain as a manifestation of systemic metal accumulation, and (3) brain metal deficiency.

Metabolism of Metals

Transport systems involved in cellular metal homeostasis are redundant, but individual transport proteins may have different importance for transporting particular metal, and their dysfunction may thus lead to dyshomeostasis of various severities.

Transport proteins can be specific for particular metal species or may be capable of transporting more species leading to interdependencies in the metabolism of various metals. There are several protein families involved in regulating metal homeostasis: (1) solute carrier (SLC) family includes transmembrane proteins that are either facilitative transporters shifting metals along their electrochemical gradient or secondary active transporters using electrochemical gradient of another substance for symport or antiport, (2) P-type ATPases are transmembrane proteins using energy from adenosine triphosphate (ATP) hydrolysis for primary active transport of metals against their electrochemical gradient, and (3) chaperons assist in metal storage, trafficking, and delivery to the sites of metalloprotein synthesis. Metals can be also transported across the cellular membrane via ion channels, receptor-mediated endocytosis, and possibly also by exocytosis. Proteins involved in cellular import, export, trafficking, and storage of Cu, Ca, and Mn are summarized in Table 14.1 [1–5].

Calcium

Regulation of cellular Ca metabolism is different compared to other metals because Ca2+ is a ubiquitous ion involved in a wide spectrum of physiological functions, including signal transduction, muscle contraction, secretion of hormones and neurotransmitters, regulation of gene expression, apoptosis, mitochondrial oxidative phosphorylation, and autophagy [6].

Cellular Ca2+ entry is mediated by voltage-operated channels, receptor-operated channels, and store-operated channels. There are several types of voltage-operated Ca2+ channels to carry out specific functions. The L-type channel is responsible for mediating muscle contraction and transduction of signal from proximal neuronal dendrites, while the N-type and the P/Q-type trigger release of neurotransmitters at synaptic endings [7]. It has been suggested that the L-type Ca2+ channels may be an alternative route for cellular Fe and Mn uptake suggesting interdependencies between Ca, Mn, and Fe pathways [8, 9]. N-methyl D-aspartate (NMDA) glutamate ionotropic receptor is responsible for receptor-mediated cellular Ca2+ influx [5]. Store-operated channels are responsible for capacitative Ca2+ entry, which occurs when endoplasmic reticulum (ER) Ca2+ stores are depleted. This group includes calcium release-activated calcium channel proteins 1–3 encoded by *ORAI1–3* genes and a family of transient receptor potential cation channels (TRPs) that consists of three subfamilies A, C, and M [10].

Calcium efflux from the cell is conducted via plasma membrane Ca2+-transporting ATPases (ATP2B1–4) [11] and via Na+/Ca2+ exchangers (SLC8A1–3) [5]. Within the cell, Ca2+ concentration is low in the cytoplasm, while high quantities of Ca2+ are stored in ER as well as in trans-Golgi network (TGN) and lysosomes. The major Ca2+ storage organelle of the cell is the ER, and Ca2+ accumulation in its lumen is mediated by the sarcoplasmic/endoplasmic reticulum calcium ATPases 1–3 (SERCA 1–3 aka ATP2A3) [5]. Within the ER lumen, Ca2+ is bound to a variety of chaperone proteins [6] maintaining its concentration gradient

Table 14.1 Major proteins involved in metal homeostasis

Gene/protein symbol	Protein name	Synonym	Major substrate	Other substrates	Comments
Cellular import					
CACNA1[a]	Calcium channel, voltage dependent		Ca2+	Mn2+, Fe2+	N, L, R, T, and P/Q types (many subunits)
GRIN	Glutamate receptor, ionotropic, N-methyl D-aspartate	GluN	Ca2+		Subunits 1, 2A, 2B, 2C, 2D, 3A, 3B
ORAI1–3	Calcium release-activated calcium channel protein 1–3	CRACM	Ca2+	Mn2+?	
P2RX1	Purinergic receptor type P2X1		Ca2+	Mn2+?	
SLC11A2[b]	Solute carrier family 11 member 2	Divalent metal transporter 1 (DMT1)	Fe2+	Mn2+, Cd2+, Ni2+, Zn2+, Co2+, Pb2+, Cu1+	
SLC16A1	Solute carrier family 16, member 1	Monocarboxylic acid transporter 1/ MCT1	citrate	Mn-citrate	
SLC31A1	Solute carrier family 31 member 1	Human copper transport protein 1 (hCTR1)	Cu1+	Cisplatin, carboplatin, oxaliplatin	Homolog SLC31A2/hCTR2
SLC39A14	Solute carrier family 39 member 14	ZIP 14	Mn2+	Fe2+, Zn2+, Cd2+, Cu1+?	
SLC39A8	Solute carrier family 39 member 8	ZIP 8	Mn2+	Fe2+, Zn2+, Cd2+	
TFRC	Transferrin receptor	CD71, p90	Fe3+	Mn3+	
TRPM	Transient receptor potential cation channels		Ca2+	Mn2+?	Subfamilies A, M, C

(continued)

Table 14.1 (continued)

Gene/protein symbol	Protein name	Synonym	Major substrate	Other substrates	Comments
ZDHHC17	Zinc finger DHHC domain-containing protein 17		Ca2+	Mg2+, Mn2+?	
Cellular export					
AP1S1[a]	Adaptor-related protein complex 1, σ1 subunit	Sigma1A-adaptin			Regulates trafficking of ATP7A and ATP7B
ATP2B1–4[a]	ATPase, Ca++ transporting, plasma membrane 1–4	Plasma membrane calcium-transporting ATPase 1–4/PMCA 1–4	Ca2+		
ATP7A[a]	ATPase, Cu++ transporting, alpha polypeptide		Cu1+		Also cellular Cu trafficking
ATP7B[a]	ATPase, Cu++ transporting, beta polypeptide		Cu1+		Also cellular Cu trafficking
COMMD1[b]	Copper metabolism (Murr1) domain-containing 1	MURR1			Regulates degradation of ATP7A and ATP7B
CP[a]	Ceruloplasmin		Fe2+	Mn2+	Ferroxidase
HEPH	Hephaestin		Fe2+	Mn2+	Ferroxidase, CP homolog
SLC30A10[a]	Solute carrier family 30 member 10	Manganese transporter	Mn2+		Also cellular Mn trafficking (sequestering into TGN)
SLC40A1	Solute carrier family 40 member 1	Ferroportin (FPN1)	Fe2+	Mn2+?	
SLC8A1–3	Solute carrier family 8 (sodium/calcium exchanger), member 1–3	Na+/Ca2+ exchanger	Ca2+		

Cellular trafficking					
ATOX1	Antioxidant 1 copper chaperone	HAH1	Cu2+		
ATP13A2[a]	ATPase type 13A member 2	PARK9	Mn2+?	Zn2+?	Sequestering into lysosomes
ATP2A1–3	ATPase, Ca++ transporting	Sarcoplasmic/endoplasmic reticulum calcium ATPase 1–3/ SERCA1–3	Ca2+		Sequestering into ER
ATP2C1, 2	ATPase type 2C member 1, 2	secretory pathway Ca2+/Mn2+ ATPases/ SPCA1,2	Ca2+, Mn2+		Sequestering into TGN
CCS	Copper chaperone for superoxide dismutase 1		Cu2+		
COX17	COX17 cytochrome c oxidase copper chaperone		Cu2+		
ITPR1–3[a]	Inositol 1,4,5-trisphosphate receptor, type 1–3		Ca2+		Release from ER
RYR1–3	Ryanodine receptors 1–3		Ca2+		Release from ER

ER endoplasmic reticulum, *TGN* trans-Golgi network
[a]Monogenic cause of neurological disorder
[b]Polymorphism related to risk of neurological disorder

that allows for a rapid release of Ca2+ to cytoplasm upon opening of receptor-operated Ca2+ release channels residing in the ER membrane, namely, inositol 1,4,5-trisphosphate receptors, type 1–3 (ITPR1–3) [12, 13], and ryanodine receptors 1–3 (RYR1–3) [14]. Transport of Ca2+ to the TGN is mediated by the secretory pathway Ca2+/Mn2+ ATPases 1 and 2 (SPCA1,2 aka ATP2C1,2) that are also capable of transporting Mn [15].

None of the genes involved in the Ca2+ pathway have been described as a cause of the primary familial brain calcification syndrome, but mutations in several genes encoding proteins from the Ca2+ pathway were identified as causes of spinocerebellar ataxias (SCA). Mutations in *ITPR1* cause SCA15/16, mutations in *CACNA1A* cause SCA6 aka episodic ataxia type 2 [16], and mutations in *ATP2B3* cause X-linked SCAX1 [17].

Copper

Human copper transporter protein 1 (hCTR1 aka SLC31A1) is the most important transporter mediating and regulating Cu uptake in the vast majority of tissues, while the role of its homolog, hCTR2, remains unknown [18]. There is probably a minor role of divalent metal transporter 1 (DMT1 aka SLC11A2) in Cu transport across the blood-brain barrier (BBB) and the blood-cerebrospinal fluid barrier (BCB) [19]. Two P-type ATPases, ATPase, Cu2+ transporting, alpha polypeptide (ATP7A) [20] and ATPase, Cu2+ transporting, beta polypeptide (ATP7B) [21, 22] have a dual role in the Cu metabolism. They facilitate Cu transport from the cytoplasm to the TGN where it is provided for incorporation into cuproenzymes, namely, ceruloplasmin, hephaestin, lysyl oxidase, dopamine-β-hydroxylase, peptidyl-α-amidating monooxygenase, and tyrosinase [23]. Under the condition of excess Cu levels, they translocate to plasma membrane or vesicular compartment near the plasma membrane to facilitate Cu efflux. Protein copper metabolism (Murr1) domain-containing 1 (COMMD1) is also involved in Cu efflux by regulating degradation of the ATP7B [24]. At the BBB, the ATP7A is involved in brain Cu uptake because it facilitates efflux from endothelial cells. There are three main intracellular Cu chaperones, namely, antioxidant 1 copper chaperone (ATOX1) shuttling Cu to the secretory pathway represented by ATP7A and ATP7B [25], COX17 cytochrome c oxidase copper chaperone facilitating assembly of mitochondrial cytochrome c oxidase, and copper chaperone for superoxide dismutase 1 (CCS) [26, 27].

Intracellular Cu storage and exchangeable pool are maintained by metallothioneins and glutathione (GSH), proteins that form stable complexes with Cu [28]. Family of metallothioneins, encoded by a cluster of genes on the chromosome 16, is a group of cytoplasmic proteins binding free Cu, zinc (Zn), and other metals in order to protect cells from their toxic effects [29, 30]. The GSH is not only involved in sequestering intracellular Cu but seems to be also involved in posttranslational regulation of ATP7A and ATP7B activity [31]. Adaptor-related protein complex 1, subunit σ1A (AP1S1), also regulates intracellular trafficking of ATP7A and ATP7B, and its dysfunction leads to a severe phenotype [32, 33]. Interactions between Fe, Mn, and Cu metabolism have been reported. Mn exposure and Fe deficiency both lead to increase of brain Cu concentration probably due to upregulation of hCTR1 and DMT1, respectively [19, 34].

Mutations in genes encoding ATP7A, ATP7B, and AP1S1 give rise to neurological disorders. Polymorphism c.492T>C in *COMMD1* gene was associated with age of onset in Wilson disease [35], but it was not confirmed in subsequent studies.

Manganese

Many transport systems are involved in cellular Mn uptake as well as in its transport across the BBB and BCB [1, 9, 36]. These include uptake via transferrin receptor (TFRC) and DMT1, proteins that are also involved in Fe uptake [37]. DMT1 has a broad substrate specificity for various divalent cations besides Fe and Mn including cadmium (Cd), nickel (Ni), cobalt (Co), and lead (Pb) [38]. Fe deficiency leads to TFRC and DMT1 upregulation, and since Mn shares this transport pathway [39, 40], it has been suggested that Fe deficit increases brain influx of Mn via this mechanism [41–44]. There is however controversy to what extent the DMT1 is involved in Mn transport under physiological conditions [9, 45].

Other ways for Mn cellular uptake are shared with Ca2+ underlining the close relationship of transport pathways of these two elements [46]. All of the cellular Ca2+ uptake channels, that is, NMDA glutamate ionotropic receptor [47], L-type voltage-operated Ca2+ channels, and store-operated Ca2+ channels, specifically TRP, subfamily M, member 7 (TRPM7), were suggested to transport also Mn ions [48, 49]. Hypothetically, Mn may share another transport mechanism with Ca2+ through purinergic receptor type P2X1 (P2RX1) [50] and with other divalent metals through zinc finger DHHC domain-containing protein 17 (ZDHHC17) [51]. Through these interdependencies, low Ca2+ concentration supposedly increases the Mn uptake [48]. Independent on the Ca2+ channels, two members of the SLC39 family, ZIP-8 (SLC39A8) [52] and ZIP-14 (SLC39A14) [53], may be also involved in Mn uptake using the HCO3- gradient across the plasma membrane for symport. The SLC39 family includes multisubstrate divalent cation transporters that may regulate also Fe, Zn, and Cd transport. Contributions of the abovementioned pathways to in vivo Mn uptake into brain cells in humans are not clear, but it was suggested that Mn enters the brain predominantly through the BCB as Mn-citrate species using various organic acid transporters, such as monocarboxylic acid transporter 1 (MCT1 aka SLC16A1), using the gradient of H+ for cotransport [54–56].

Two types of carriers are known to be involved in sequestering cytosolic Mn into TGN: (1) Ca2+/Mn2+ (P-type) ATPases of the secretory pathway, ATP2C1 and ATP2C2 [57–59], and (2) manganese transporter SLC30A10 [60, 61]. Another P5-type cation transporting ATPase, ATP13A2, is likely involved in sequestration of Mn into lysosomes [62]. SLC30A10 is involved in cellular Mn efflux since its dysfunction causes a profound Mn accumulation, but the mechanism is unclear. No other cellular exporter specific for Mn is known and Mn export may share the efflux pathway with Fe supposedly using ferroportin 1 (FPN1 aka SLC40A1) complex associated with ferroxidases, ceruloplasmin (CP), and hephaestin (HEPH) [63].

Neurological symptoms were described in genetic disorders caused by deficits of two of the abovementioned transporters, ATP13A2 and SLC30A10, respectively. Furthermore, DMT1 haplotype (C alleles of 1254C/T and IVS4 + 44C/A) has been identified as a risk factor for Parkinson disease (PD) in one study with odds ratio 1.72 in Chinese population [64].

Disorders of Copper Metabolism

Wilson Disease

Initially, Wilson disease (WD) was not regarded as a hereditary disorder. Its genetic origin with autosomal recessive inheritance was reported several decades after the Wilson's first description of the disease [65]. In 1993, the causative gene *ATP7B* (OMIM 606882) was identified and cloned [21, 22]. *ATP7B* is a large gene spanning approximately 80 kb of genomic DNA on chromosome 13 (13q14). The gene consists of 21 exons, which encode a 1,465-amino acid protein, ATP7B.

ATP7B protein is a member of the P-type ATPase family of membrane proteins that pump ions and lipids across the cellular membranes and the key regulator of cellular Cu metabolism in human [66]. The protein contains several highly conserved functional domains: six metal-binding domains (MBDs), each with a metal-binding motif GMxCxxC; eight hydrophobic transmembrane domains (TMs) that form a path through cell membranes for Cu translocation; the phosphatase domain (A-domain); the phosphorylation domain (P-domain); and the ATP-binding domain (N-domain). Expression of ATP7B is predominant in the liver. Lower expression levels are detected in the brain, heart, lungs, kidney, and placenta [21, 22]. ATP7B has a dual function in cells. Biosynthetic role is represented by Cu delivery for incorporation into copper-dependent enzymes such as CP [67], and homeostatic role is fulfilled by removal of excess Cu from cells [68]. Symptoms of WD are consequences of (1) impaired Cu excretion from the liver to bile resulting in its accumulation in the liver and (2) dysfunctional incorporation of Cu into CP leading to hypoceruloplasminemia. When the capacity of the liver to store Cu is exceeded, free Cu is released into the bloodstream and deposited in various organs, predominantly the brain, cornea, and kidneys.

More than 700 mutations have been reported in *ATP7B* gene (HGMD Professional 2014.2) and most patients are compound-heterozygous. The mutations are scattered throughout the gene and are mostly missense (Table 14.2). They affect protein stability, intracellular localization, various activities depending on afflicted domain (catalytic, transport, phosphorylation), as well as protein expression levels.

Pathogenic mutations are found in up to 98 % of WD patients [69, 70], but most studies report lower detection rate, approximately 70–85 %. Failure to identify two *ATP7B* mutations in a given patient should not exclude the diagnosis of WD. Allele

Table 14.2 Spectrum and frequency of *ATP7B* mutations (HGMD Professional 2014.2)

Mutation type	Number of mutations	Frequency (%)
Missense	424	55
Nonsense	63	8
Splicing	64	8
Regulatory	12	2
Small deletions	131	17
Small insertions	55	7
Small indels	8	1
Gross deletions	12	2
Complex rearrangements	1	0.1
Total	*770*	*100*

frequency of most mutations is very low. Only several mutations occur with a high frequency in certain populations due to a founder effect. For instance, p.His1069Gln is the most common *ATP7B* mutation in Europe, accounting for 30–70 % of all detected mutations [71–74]. Mutation p.Arg778Leu is the most common one among Chinese and Taiwanese WD patients (20–40 %) [75–78]. In Sardinian WD patients, mutation c.-441_-427del predominates with frequency 60.5 % of detected mutations [79], and in Saudi Arabia, p.Gln1399Argfs*6 mutation is the most common one [80, 81]. In Indian patients, mutation p.Cys271* is observed with the highest frequency (20–24 %) [69, 82]. Identification of population-specific prevalent mutations facilitates genetic testing in given populations, but the analysis of the entire coding region of *ATP7B* as well as the copy number analysis (to detect deletions of one or more exons) may still be desirable.

The most commonly reported numbers are 1:30,000 for worldwide WD prevalence and 1 % for population frequency of heterozygous mutation carriers [83]. Recent data from the United Kingdom however suggest that WD may be considerably more common with the prevalence of 1:7,000 and carrier frequency of 2.2–5 % [70].

The typical age of onset is between 5 and 35 years, but approximately 4 % of patients become symptomatic in the fifth decade or later [84]. The most common manifestations of WD are hepatic (50 %) and neuropsychiatric (50 %), but more than 60 % of neuropsychiatric patients have liver cirrhosis at the time of diagnosis [72]. The hepatic manifestation of WD occurs almost 10 years earlier than neurological symptoms with the mean age of onset 15 years [85]. The hepatic presentation of WD can be divided into several forms: asymptomatic elevation of liver enzymes, acute hepatitis mimicking viral hepatitis with jaundice, acute liver failure usually accompanied by hemolytic anemia, and chronic hepatitis with liver cirrhosis [83].

The mean age of onset in neurologically presenting patients is 20 years [85]; however, the earliest onset of neurological symptoms was 6 years and the latest was 72 years [83]. The neurological presentation is divided into four phenotypes with a significant overlap: parkinsonism, tremors, ataxia, and dystonia [83]. Tremor, occurring in almost 80 % of patients with the neurological manifestation, is the most frequent neurological symptom [86]. Classically, high-amplitude low-frequency coarse proximal "wing-beating" tremor has been described, but WD patients can manifest with any type and combination of tremors, resting, intentional, and/or postural. Dysarthria occurs in more than 70 % of WD patients and most frequently is of mixed type with varying spastic, cerebellar, hypokinetic, and dystonic components [87]. Parkinsonism, commonly manifesting as symmetric akinesia and rigidity, hypomimia, dysarthria, and drooling, occurs in almost 40 % of patients with neurological presentation. Parkinsonism can be also the manifestation of hepatic encephalopathy in severe cirrhosis. Dystonic phenotype, occurring in 10–30 % of cases, is usually most severe and resistant to treatment [86]. Dystonia can be focal, commonly in the orofacial region causing the typical facies with "vacuous smile" or in the hand region, but can be also segmental or generalized in some patients. Other movement disorders like chorea, balism, myoclonus as well as pyramidal signs and autonomic system impairment are less frequent.

Psychiatric symptoms affect more than 60 % of patients during the disease progression and can be the initial presentation in 20–40 % of patients [88–90]. The most common psychiatric symptoms include mood disorders, anxiety, and personality changes such as irritability, aggressiveness, and disinhibition, while psychotic symptoms occur less frequently. Cognitive disorders in patients with neuropsychiatric presentation are common but variable and rarely lead to dementia [91]. The most severely affected cognitive domain is executive functions, particularly attention [92].

Ophthalmologic manifestations include the Kayser-Fleischer ring (K-F ring) and sunflower cataract caused by copper deposition in the corneal Descemet's membrane and anterior lens capsule, respectively. The K-F ring is detectable in 80–95 % of patients with neurological presentation as golden brownish coloration seen at the periphery of the cornea [93], while sunflower cataract is less common. Other manifestations of WD include hematologic changes (thrombocytopenia, leukopenia, hemolytic anemia), bone and joint involvement (pain, osteoporosis, spontaneous fractures), and renal involvement (hypercalciuria, hyperphosphaturia, nephrocalcinosis).

Genotype-phenotype correlation in WD is challenging due to the great clinical variability and high prevalence of patients carrying two different mutations. The correlation studies are hampered by a paucity of heterozygotes with the same *ATP7B* genotype as well as homozygotes for less frequent mutations. However, some associations have been proposed. The mutation p.His1069Gln tends to cause later-onset (the second to the third decade) and neurological phenotype, while the mutations p. Cys271* and p.E122fs, common in Indian population, more often lead to earlier-onset (the first to the second decade) and more severe phenotype [69, 94–96].

Age of onset and clinical presentations often vary even among the patients carrying the same *ATP7B* mutation or the patients with different mutations leading to a similar protein defect. Heterogeneity of clinical phenotype proposed the speculations that there might be other loci modulating the basic WD phenotype. The most perspective candidates are genes encoding other members of copper homeostasis pathway, such as *ATOX1* and *COMMD1*. However, the results of association studies have been so far inconclusive [35, 97–99], suggesting that these genes do not play a major role as modifying factors in WD. The factors and mechanism underlining the clinical variability are probably more complex since even monozygotic twins can manifest different features and severity of WD [100, 101].

Timely diagnosis is important since early treatment with chelation drugs such as d-penicillamine or trientine or zinc supplementation may improve symptoms and prevent irreversible liver and brain damage [102]. WD diagnosis is based mainly on findings of abnormal Cu metabolism, that is, serum CP level, serum Cu level, 24-h urinary Cu excretion, and Cu concentration in liver biopsy. The serum CP level is decreased to <0.2 g/L in almost 95 % of WD patients. The total serum Cu level in WD patients is usually decreased since it mostly represents the Cu bound to CP. Free, non-ceruloplasmin-bound Cu calculated manually as difference between total and CP bound serum Cu is more relevant for the WD diagnosis; it is typically increased to >1.6 μmol/L in non-treated WD patients. Daily urinary copper excretion >1.6 μmol/24 h is the best single test for WD diagnosis with sensitivity and specificity both above 90 %. Hepatic parenchymal copper content in liver biopsy elevated to >250 μg/g of dry weight is highly suggestive of WD, while values <50 μg/g virtually exclude WD [102]. Typical magnetic resonance imaging (MRI) findings include symmetrical hyperintensity in T2-weighted (T2w) images in basal ganglia (BG) and brainstem along with generalized atrophy. Supposedly pathognomonic MRI findings including "the face of the giant panda" and the "bright claustrum" are present in less than 14 % of WD patients. Altogether, MRI abnormalities occur in almost 90–100 % of neuropsychiatric, 40–75 % of hepatic, and 20–30 % of asymptomatic patients [103, 104]. Genetic testing confirms the WD diagnosis but is not necessary for diagnosis in typical cases. It is particularly helpful in patients with inconclusive biochemical findings and in asymptomatic WD patients, mostly relatives of WD cases, who may not manifest typical biochemical abnormalities. A scoring system for the WD diagnosis includes results of all the abovementioned methods (Table 14.3). The resulting Ferenci aka Leipzig score is the gold standard for WD diagnosis and is currently recommended in the guidelines for WD diagnosis and treatment [105].

Menkes Disease and Other ATP7A-Related Diseases

The *ATP7A* gene (OMIM 300011) is located on chromosome X (Xq21.1), spans about 140 kb of genomic region, and is organized in 23 exons (the first exon in non-coding). The gene also shows a considerable similarity to exonic structure of the *ATP7B* gene, especially in the 3′ two-thirds, suggesting both genes have a common evolutionary ancestor [106, 107]. The gene product is a transmembrane copper-transporting P-type ATPase, ATP7A [108–110], which is 1,500 amino acids long. The protein shares about 60 % of sequence identity with the ATP7B protein. The N-terminus of the ATP7A protein includes six homologous metal-binding domains (MBDs), each containing a copper-binding motif GMxCxxC [111]. Eight transmembrane domains (TMs) anchor the protein to a membrane and form a channel for Cu translocation. Other domains include the phosphatase domain (A-domain), the

Table 14.3 Ferenci score – scoring system for the diagnosis of Wilson's disease

Finding		Points
K-F rings	Absent	0
	Present	2
Neuropsychiatric symptoms suggestive of WD (or typical brain MRI)	Absent	0
	Present	2
Coombs-negative hemolytic anemia or free Cu in plasma >1.6 μmol/L	Absent	0
	Present	1
24-h urinary copper excretion (in the absence of acute hepatitis)	Normal	0
	1–2× ULN (1–2 μmol/24 h)	1
	>2× ULN (>2 μmol/24 h)	2
	>5× ULN after D-penicillamine challenge	2
Liver copper quantitative	Normal (<50 μg/g)	−1
	<5× ULN (50–250 μg/g)	1
	>5× ULN (>250 μg/g)	2
Rhodanine-positive hepatocytes (only if quantitative Cu measurement is not available)	Absent	0
	Present	1
Serum ceruloplasmin	Normal	0
	0.1–0.2 g/L	1
	<0.1 g/L	2
Mutation analysis	Disease-causing mutations on both chromosomes	4
	Disease-causing mutation on one chromosome	1
	No mutation detected	0

Assessment of the WD diagnosis score:
≥4 points: diagnosis of WD highly likely
2–3 points: diagnosis of WD probable, more investigations needed
0–1 points: diagnosis of WD unlikely
MRI magnetic resonance imaging, *ULN* upper limit of normal

phosphorylation domain (P-domain), and the ATP-binding domain (N-domain), and they mediate the catalytic activity of ATP7A. Besides the structure, both proteins are also highly related in function. Unlike ATP7B, expression of ATP7A is ubiquitous, with a low level in liver, suggesting its housekeeping role [108, 110]. The protein has two main functions: (1) the biosynthetic function, which involves transporting Cu to cuproenzymes at the secretory pathway, and (2) the homeostatic function of exporting of excess Cu from cells and transporting Cu across the gut mucosal wall and the BBB [112]. ATP7A is required during neuronal development probably due to its important role in synaptogenesis [113]. Apart from that, it has a role in NMDA glutamatergic signaling in hippocampal neurons [114]. Clinical symptoms in *ATP7A* mutations result from generalized hypocupremia and subsequent dysfunction of cuproenzymes. Relative Cu accumulation occurs in enterocytes,

Table 14.4 Spectrum and frequency of *ATP7A* mutations (HGMD Professional 2014.2.)

Mutation type	Number of mutations	Frequency (%)
Missense	65	20.3
Nonsense	37	11.6
Splicing	67	21
Small deletions	48	15
Small insertions	17	5.3
Small indels	1	0.3
Gross deletions	54	17
Gross insertions/duplications	23	7.2
Complex rearrangements[a]	7	2.2
Total	*319*	*100*

[a]The number of complex rearrangements according to review by Tumer [115]

endothelia of the BBB, and kidney epithelia because its influx into barrier cells is intact, while its efflux is blocked due to ATP7A dysfunction [23].

Mutations in the *ATP7A* gene are inherited in X-linked recessive manner; therefore, affected patients are almost exclusively males, while heterozygous females are mostly asymptomatic carriers. To date above 300 different *ATP7A* mutations have been reported, and they range from single nucleotide changes to gross deletions or duplications [115] (HGMD Professional 2014.2). The most common mutation types, accounting for almost two-thirds of all mutations, are missense mutations, splice-site mutations, and gross deletions ranging from one to several exons (Table 14.4). The mutations are usually unique to each affected family, and the most recurrent mutation is c.2179G>A (p.Gly727Arg) with the estimated frequency of 2.7 %. The donor splice site of intron 8 also seems to be a mutation hot spot of *ATP7A*, since nine different mutations occur in this location. Interestingly, no missense mutations were observed in exons 2–7, which encode MBDs of ATP7A, suggesting that variations in these regions are more acceptable regarding the normal protein function [115].

The mutations may affect various features and functions of normal ATP7A, such as protein stability, intracellular localization, trafficking, Cu transport, and catalytic activity as reviewed by Tumer [115]. Incidentally, splice-site mutations do not necessarily lead to a complete disruption of splicing, but a small amount of normal transcript and subsequently normal protein can be produced [116–118].

Mutations in the *ATP7A* gene are associated with three clinical entities: Menkes disease (MD) (OMIM 309400), occipital horn syndrome (OHS) (OMIM 304150), and X-linked distal motor neuropathy (OMIM 300489) [119].

The estimated incidence of MD ranges between 1:40,000 and 1:360,000 live births [120]. MD clinically manifests as infantile-onset cerebral and cerebellar neurodegeneration, failure to thrive, coarse hair (kinky hair or pili torti), and connective tissue abnormalities. Affected infants may present with prolonged jaundice, hypothermia, hypoglycemia, and feeding difficulties in the early neonatal period. They develop often intractable epileptic seizures, hypotonia, vomiting, diarrhea, and developmental regression in the 2nd or 3rd month of life and usually die within first 3 years of life [121, 122]. Approximately 6 % of patients manifest slightly milder MD phenotype [120]. Biochemical findings include low Cu and CP levels and increased ratio of dopamine metabolite dihydroxyphenylacetic acid (DOPAC) and the norepinephrine metabolite dihydroxyphenylglycol (DHPG) in the blood and cerebrospinal fluid (CSF) [123, 124]. Connective tissue disorders manifest as loose skin (cutis laxa) particularly in the neck and axillar regions, arterial aneurysms, fragile bones, and other structural bone abnormalities particularly in the rib cage (pectus excavatum). Brain MRI abnormalities become evident several months after birth and include diffuse atrophy, ventriculomegaly, tortuosity of cerebral blood vessels, delayed myelination, signal abnormalities in BG, and high incidence of subdural hematomas [125, 126]. Subcutaneous Cu replacement in the first 2 postnatal weeks improves survival and may even normalize developmental outcomes in some patients with residual ATP7A activity [127–131]. During the critical period for treatment, MD cannot be diagnosed clinically, and biochemical or genetic screening of newborns at risk is necessary.

OHS has a milder clinical presentation with a usual symptoms onset between 3 and 10 years and less severe neurological deficit including slight muscle weakness, clumsiness, dysautonomia (orthostatic hypotension, chronic diarrhea, and heart conduction disorders), and variably subnormal cognitive function. The name refers to the wedge-shaped calcifications that form bilaterally within the occipital attachments of trapezius and sternocleidomastoid muscles [122]. Connective tissue abnormalities in OHS are similar to MD, but since these patients survive longer, various bone and joint deformities become apparent during development. Bladder diverticula lead to chronic urinary infections. Biochemical findings include low to normal levels of Cu and CP in the blood and abnormal plasma and CSF catecholamine levels. Life expectancy is variable and some patients may survive until the sixth decade [122, 132]. It has been estimated that approximately 3 % of *ATP7A* mutations manifest as OHS [120].

ATP7A-related distal motor neuropathy is the mildest phenotype manifesting as a monosymptomatic progressive peripheral neuropathy that has been classified within the group of distal hereditary motor neuropathies. It presents between 10 and 35 years of age in majority of patients. No overt Cu metabolic abnormalities can be detected in this phenotype [133, 134].

No obvious correlation between *ATP7A* mutations and the clinical severity of MD has been described, but in general, the severe classic form of MD with early death is caused mostly by nonsense mutations, early truncating mutations, and gross deletions. Patients with the mild form of MD and OHS often carry late truncating mutations [135, 136], mutations leading to synthesis of partially functional protein or reduced amount of normal protein [116–118, 137]. Skipping of exons with mutations has also been observed in mildly affected patients [138, 139]. Several missense mutations causing amino acids substitutions within or near TMs are associated with the distal motor neuropathy phenotype [133, 134]. These mutations supposedly do not affect Cu-transporting function but rather cause aberrant intracellular

Table 14.5 Mutations in the *SLC33A1* gene in patients with Huppke-Brendel syndrome [149]

cDNA	Protein
c.328G>C	p.Ala110Pro
c.614dupT	p.Leu205Phefs*31
c.1098C>G	p.Tyr366*
c.1267-1G>A	–
c.1474_1482+9del18	–

The nucleotide numbering is based on the GenBank reference sequence NM_004733.3

localization of ATP7A [140]. Nevertheless, the phenotypic variability is often observed even in the family members with the same *ATP7A* mutation illustrating that other factors, genetic and non-genetic, may underlie phenotypic variability of *ATP7A*-related diseases [141–143].

A few females with the phenotype of MD have been identified, most of them carrying chromosomal aberrations, especially an X-autosome translocations, which disrupt the *ATP7A* gene [144–147]. The classical severe phenotype observed in some cases may be attributed to a preferential inactivation of the normal X chromosome, but clinical features of female MD patients are usually milder with much longer life expectancy than in males [148].

Other Inborn Errors of Copper Metabolism

Huppke-Brendel Syndrome

Huppke-Brendel syndrome (OMIM 614482 as CCHLND) is a severe autosomal recessive disorder leading to death in early childhood. It is characterized by congenital cataracts, hearing loss, severe developmental delay, nystagmus, and epileptic seizures associated with low total serum Cu and CP [149, 150]. MRI pathology includes cerebellar hypoplasia, cortical atrophy, and hypomyelination. Genetic basis of the disease was revealed by the linkage analysis and sequencing of candidate region (3q25) in four patients from three consanguineous families. All four patients carried homozygous mutations, and one additional patient from a nonconsanguineous family carried two heterozygous mutations in the *SLC33A1* gene (OMIM 603690) (Table 14.5) [149]. The gene codes for the acetyl-CoA transporter (AT-1), a transmembrane protein transporting acetyl-CoA into the lumen of the ER [151]. The precise mechanism by which defective or absent AT-1 causes the reduction of Cu and CP levels is not clear, yet. A proposed explanation is that non-functional AT-1 impairs transient acetylation of CP, which is normally required for its proper function. Low plasma CP is the cause of low plasmatic Cu levels. Thus, Huppke-Brendel syndrome, along with WD, MD, and aceruloplasminemia, belongs to the differential diagnosis of hypoceruloplasminemia [149].

Table 14.6 Mutations in the *AP1S1* gene (HGMD Professional 2014.2)

cDNA	Protein	Reference
c.183-2A>G	–	[153]
c.364dupG	p.Asp322Glyfs*17	[32]

The nucleotide numbering is based on the GenBank reference sequence NM_001283.3

MEDNIK Syndrome

MEDNIK syndrome, the abbreviation for mental retardation, enteropathy, deafness, peripheral neuropathy, ichthyosis, and keratoderma (OMIM 609313), is a rare, severe, autosomal recessive, multisystem disorder. It was first described, under the name of erythrokeratodermia variabilis-3, in a relatively isolated population in Quebec [152] and the causative gene, *AP1S1* (OMIM 603531), was identified on chromosome 7 (7q22.1) [153]. It encodes the ubiquitously expressed small subunit σ1A of adaptor protein complex AP-1, which has been shown to regulate intracellular trafficking of copper pumps ATP7A and ATP7B and hence affect the Cu transport in cells. Patients manifest symptoms similar to WD (hepatopathy, low plasma CP and total Cu, high free Cu) and MD (mental retardation, connective tissue disorders). Brain MRI shows cerebral atrophy and mild signal changes in BG. To date, two *AP1S1* mutations, both homozygous, have been observed in five French-Canadian patients from the original Quebec cohort and in one Italian patient, respectively (Table 14.6) [32, 154].

Disorders of Manganese Metabolism

SLC30A10 Mutations

Several acquired causes of hypermanganesemia have been described, but the first inherited inborn error of Mn metabolism was identified only recently. This autosomal recessive disorder, which is caused by mutations in the *SLC30A10* gene (OMIM 611146), is characterized by hypermanganesemia with dystonia, polycythemia, and cirrhosis (OMIM 613280) [60, 61]. The gene is located on chromosome 1 (1q41) and codes for a SLC family 30, member 10. SLC30A10 is highly expressed in liver and brain and, due to the sequence homology with other members of the same family, was initially presumed to be a Zn transporter [155]. However, recent studies confirm that it plays a key role in Mn transport and cell protection from Mn toxicity [61]. *SLC30A10* mutations are predicted to give rise to a truncated protein or affect its normal function due to the disruption of a highly conserved area or functional domain. Nevertheless, no apparent genotype-phenotype correlation could be outlined since only 12 homozygous *SLC30A10* mutations in 20 patients have been reported so far (Table 14.7) [60, 61].

Clinical symptoms include a childhood-onset chronic liver disease and a movement disorder. Neurological symptoms typically develop in the first decade and

Table 14.7 Mutations in the *SLC30A10* gene (HGMD Professional 2014.2)

cDNA	Protein	Reference
g.218,057,426_218,158,564del[a]	–	[61]
c.266T>C	p.Leu89Pro	[61]
c.292_402del	p.Val98_Phe134del	[61]
c.314_322del	p.Ala105_Pro107del	[61]
c.507delG	p.Pro170Leufs*22	[60]
c.585delG	p.Thr196Profs*17	[61]
c.765_767delGGT	p.Val256del	[61]
c.922C>T	p.Gln308*	[61]
c.1046T>C	p.Leu349Pro	[61]
c.1235delA	p.Gln412Argfs*26	[60]

The nucleotide numbering (except the gross deletion) is based on the GenBank reference sequence NM_018713.2

[a]Deletion of approximately 101 kb including exons 1–2

manifest as dystonia with a characteristic high-stepping (cock-walk) gait variably accompanied by dysarthria, spastic paraparesis, parkinsonism, psychiatric symptoms, and motor neuropathy [61]. Rare cases with adult-onset parkinsonism were also reported [60]. Severity of liver involvement is highly variable, ranging from mildly elevated liver transaminases to liver failure due to cirrhosis.

MRI is specific for Mn deposits showing typical hyperintensities predominantly in GP, extending also to striatum, cerebellum, pituitary, and white matter in T1w images, while only mild GP hypointensities are seen in T2w images. In an autopsy case, 16-fold increase of Mn concentration was documented in BG along with neuronal loss, reactive astrocytosis, activated microglia, myelin loss, spongiosis, and rare axonal spheroids, predominantly in GP [156]. Neuropathological findings are similar to those found in neurodegeneration with brain iron accumulation (NBIA) and WD [157, 158] suggesting that mechanisms of brain damage may be similar for various metal species. Increased Mn levels can be detected in blood, urine, and liver biopsy. Other laboratory findings are polycythemia, low plasma ferritin, and Fe levels [61]. This disorder is treatable; clinical improvement can be achieved by Fe supplementation and chelation treatment with disodium calcium edetate [159, 160].

ATP13A2 Mutations

Mutations in the *ATP13A2* gene (*PARK9*, OMIM 610513) have been identified in patients with Kufor-Rakeb syndrome (OMIM 606693), a rare autosomal recessive form of juvenile-onset parkinsonism [161]. The gene was mapped to chromosome 1 (1p36.13) and encodes a lysosomal P5-type ATPase. The protein is involved in protection from Mn-induced cell death [62, 162], Zn homeostasis, and accumulation of α-synuclein [163–165], all of which are also implicated in the pathogenesis

Table 14.8 Mutations in the *ATP13A2* gene (HGMD Professional 2014.2)

cDNA	Protein	Reference	Phenotype
c.35C>T	p.Thr12Met	[166]	EOPD
c.546C>A	p.Phe182Leu	[167]	KRS
c.746C>T	p.Ala249Val	[168]	EOPD
c.844A>T	p.Ser282Cys	[168]	EOPD
c.1101_1102dupGA	p.Thr367Argfs*29	[169]	KRS
c.1108_1120del13	p.Arg370Serfs*22	[170]	EOPD
c.1306+5G>A	–	[161]	KRS
c.1346G>A	p.Arg449Gln	[168]	EOPD
c.1510G>C	p.Gly504Arg	[166]	KRS
c.1550C>T	p.Thr517Ile	[171]	KRS
c.1597G>A	p.Gly533Arg	[166]	EOPD
c.1632_1653dup22	p.Leu552Profs*238	[161]	KRS
c.2473delCinsAA	p.Leu825Asnfs*32	[172]	KRS
c.2543G>A	p.Gly848Asp	[173]	HSP with parkinsonism
c.2552_2553delTT	p.Phe851Cysfs*6	[174]	KRS
c.2561T>G	p.Met854Arg	[175]	NCL
c.2629G>A	p.Gly877Arg	[176]	KRS
c.2762C>T	p.Gln858*	[177]	KRS
c.2939G>A	p.Arg980His	[168]	EOPD
c.3057delC	p.Tyr1020Thrfs*3	[161]	KRS
c.3176T>G	p.Leu1059Arg	[178]	KRS
c.3253delC	p.Leu1085Trpfs*1088	[178]	KRS
Deletion of exon 2	–	[179]	KRS

The nucleotide numbering is based on the GenBank reference sequence NM_022089.2
EOPD early-onset Parkinson's disease, *KRS* Kufor-Rakeb syndrome, *NCL* neuronal ceroid lipofuscinosis, *HSP* hereditary spastic paraparesis

of PD. To date, 23 homozygous or compound-heterozygous mutations have been identified in *ATP13A2* (Table 14.8), and they lead to mRNA degradation, protein misfolding, truncation, and/or degradation [178, 180, 181].

Although there is no direct evidence of Mn metabolism dysregulation in human patients, in vitro and animal data suggest that ATP13A2 protein is a Mn transporter protecting cells from excess Mn toxicity and that its dysfunction leads to cellular Mn accumulation [62, 182]. Brain MRI shows diffuse moderate generalized atrophy in majority and paramagnetic deposits in caudate and putamen in some patients [169, 183]. These paramagnetic deposits presenting as hypointensities in T2w images accompanied by normal intensity in T1w images are suggestive of Fe rather than Mn deposits. The only autopsy case showed lysosomal accumulation of the pigment lipofuscin, suggesting that Kufor-Rakeb syndrome may belong to the neuronal ceroid lipofuscinoses group [175].

Kufor-Rakeb syndrome was originally described in a consanguineous Jordanian family from the village of Kufor-Rakeb [184]. The associated gene was later identified in a large Chilean sibship [161], and since then, other cases have been identified worldwide [185]. The clinical phenotype comprises juvenile parkinsonism accompanied by ocular symptoms including slowed vertical and horizontal saccades and supranuclear upgaze palsy and psychiatric symptoms including early cognitive decline and visual hallucinations. Oculogyric spasms, facial-faucial finger mini-myoclonus, autonomic dysfunction, and pyramidal tract signs may be present in some patients. Response to levodopa is good in the initial stage, but severe dyskinesias tend to develop early [176, 183]. In some patients, ataxia, dysarthria, and myoclonus may dominate rather than parkinsonism [172].

Several reports suggested that heterozygous missense *ATP13A2* mutations may be etiologically related to early-onset PD without other symptoms described in Kufor-Rakeb syndrome [166, 168, 170].

ATP13A2 has also been shown to be a possible modifier gene of Mn neurotoxicity. Carriers of *ATP13A2* rs4920608 CT and CC and rs2871776 GG and GA genotypes with long-term environmental Mn exposure suffer from significantly impaired motor coordination in their old age compared to rs4920608 TT and rs2871776 AA genotypes [186].

Genetics of Primary Familial Brain Calcification

Primary familial brain calcification (PFBC), formerly referred to as Fahr's disease or idiopathic BG calcifications, is a disorder characterized by extensive calcifications in GP and other locations including BG, thalamus, cerebellum, brainstem, capsula interna, cerebral cortex, and subcortical white matter. PFBC is a genetically heterogeneous disease transmitted in an autosomal dominant manner. Initially, linkage and haplotype analyses revealed at least three PFBC-associated loci: *IBGC1* on 14q13 [187], *IBGC2* on 2q37 [188], and *IBGC3* on 8q21.1-q11.23 [189], but these candidates were excluded in different families, thus highlighting the genetic heterogeneity of the disease. The first causative genes were only discovered in the past 2 years: *SLC20A2* [190], *PDGFRB* [191], and *PDGFB* [192]. The proportion of sporadic cases caused by de novo mutations is yet to be determined, but these cases seem to be rather rare.

The phenotypic spectrum of PFBC of different genetic background and of patients with brain calcifications caused by secondary causes is similar and comprises movement disorders including parkinsonism, postural tremor, chorea, focal or generalized dystonia, and ataxia, accompanied by dysarthria, pyramidal signs, cognitive decline, seizures, headaches, and psychiatric symptoms [193, 194]. A phenotype resembling paroxysmal kinesigenic dyskinesia has been also reported [195]. Psychiatric symptoms including mood disorders and psychosis are common, affecting 50–83 % of patients, and they may be also the presenting symptom [193]. Age of symptoms onset is highly variable, ranging from the first to the seventh decade, but some subjects with profound calcium deposits may be asymptomatic [196]. Computerized tomography (CT) is the most helpful neuroimaging method depicting calcifications as hyperdense areas. MRI is less reliable since calcifications may be depicted as hypo-, iso-, or hyperintense areas. The most common presentations however are hypointensities in T2w images. White matter hyperintensities of presumed vascular origin are also a frequent MRI finding [191]. In differential diagnosis of PFBC, it is important to exclude secondary causes, namely, endocrine disorders such as hypoparathyroidism, pseudohypoparathyroidism, or autoimmune polyglandular syndrome [197]. Calcifications limited to GP found incidentally in elderly subjects are prevalent (5.5–20 %) but likely of no clinical significance [198–200].

Pathophysiologically, in primary and secondary causes of brain calcifications, Ca deposits generally appear to initially develop within the vessel wall and in the perivascular space in GP. This points to endothelial and smooth muscle cells of GP vessels to be the most susceptible to build calcium deposits in response to various metabolic triggers [201]. Involvement of PDGFB pathway, which plays a significant role in the angiogenesis and mesenchymal cells differentiation, in the etiology of the PFBC further stresses the crucial role of vessel wall in the pathophysiology of brain calcifications. It has been suggested that Ca deposits are secondary unspecific consequence of brain tissue damage [197]. It has been also hypothesized that Ca aggregates may have protective effect against toxic effects of excess free Ca2+, and they are thus part of the compensatory mechanisms for excitotoxic neuronal damage [202, 203]. Abnormal transport of inorganic phosphate, as documented in the *SLC20A2* mutation, could increase the hydroxyapatite aggregates formation and may thus be another pathway contributing to Ca deposits.

SLC20A2 Mutations

SLC20A2 gene (OMIM 158378) is located on chromosome 8 (8p12) and encodes a type III sodium-dependent phosphate transporter 2 (PiT2). Its expression occurs in a wide variety of tissues and points to its housekeeping role in cellular phosphate uptake and homeostasis [204–207]. Over 30 pathogenic mutations, mostly missense and nonsense, have been reported in various ethnicities as listed in HGMD Professional 2014.2 database, and according to several records, they account for 20–50 % of familial PFBC cases (Table 14.9) [101, 190, 194, 199, 208]. Analysis of several PiT2 mutants and mRNA expression profiles proposes the haploinsufficiency as an underlying mechanism in PFBC pathology. Deficient phosphate transport capacity of PiT2 subsequently affects phosphate-dependent processes in the cells, including calcification [65, 209]. Genotype-phenotype correlation studies did not reveal any apparent association, but only a limited number of cases with the same mutation could have been analyzed so far. In *SLC20A2* mutation carriers, clinical onset appeared to be later and the extent of calcifications on CT larger compared to *PDGFRB*-related PFBC [193].

Interestingly, *SLC20A1* gene, which codes for the phosphate transporter 1 (PiT1), has also been screened in PFBC patients. Up to now, the search has not yielded any

Table 14.9 Spectrum and frequency of *SLC20A2* mutations (HGMD Professional 2014.2)

Mutation type	Number of mutations	Frequency (%)
Missense	19	47.5
Nonsense	6	15
Splicing	5	12.5
Small deletions	9	22.5
Gross deletions	1	2.5
Total	*40*	*100*

Table 14.10 Mutations in the *PDGFRB* gene

cDNA	Protein	Reference
c.1973T>C	p.Leu658Pro	[191]
c.2083C>T	p.Arg695Cys	[215]
c.2959C>T	p.Arg987Trp	[191]
c.3212A>T	p.Glu1071Val	[193]

The nucleotide numbering is based on the GenBank reference sequence NM_002609.3

positive result suggesting that these mutations might be too deleterious for embryonic survival or normal development [197] as demonstrated in transgenic mice [210, 211].

PDGFRB Mutations

The second PFBC-associated gene is *PDGFRB* (OMIM 173410) located on chromosome 5 (5q32). Its product is the platelet-derived growth factor receptor-β (PDGFRβ), a cell-surface tyrosine kinase receptor, which plays an essential role in various signaling pathways involved in the regulation of cell proliferation, differentiation, survival, and migration [212]. *PDGFRB* is expressed in various tissues including the human brain, particularly in BG and cerebellar dentate nucleus [213, 214]. Four mutations, all missense, have been reported in *PDGFRB*, one of them in a patient with BG calcification of unknown etiology (Table 14.10) [191, 193, 215]. Functional characterization of known mutations suggests that in addition to protein stability, mutations in tyrosine kinase domain may differently affect receptor activation and the activation of its downstream effectors [215]. Nicolas et al. proposed two pathophysiologic hypotheses explaining the calcification in PFBD due to mutations in the *PDGFRB*. According to the first one, the integrity of the BBB is compromised, which secondarily induces vascular and perivascular calcium depositions. The second hypothesis proposes that the mutations lead to overactivation of the receptor thus impacting the PDGF-PiT1 pathway and directly induce vascular calcification [191]. Analysis of the clinical phenotype of PFBC patients has revealed that *SLC20A2* mutation carriers tend to suffer from more severe calcification with different pattern than *PDGFRB* mutation carriers, but more unrelated patients with *PDGFRB* mutations should be examined to confirm these findings [193].

Table 14.11 Mutations in the *PDGFB* gene

cDNA	Protein	Reference
c.3G>A	p.Met1Ile	[192]
c.26T>G	p.Leu9Arg	[192]
c.356T>C	p.Leu119Pro	[192]
c.433C>T	p.Gln145*	[192]
c.439C>T	p.Gln147*	[220]
c.445C>T	p.Arg149*	[192]
c.726G>C	p.*242Tyr	[192]
g.39629767_39622528del[a]	–	[221]

The nucleotide numbering is based on the GenBank reference sequence NM_002608.2
[a]Gross deletion including exons 3–5

PDGFB Mutations

Very recently, mutations in *PDGFB* gene (OMIM 190040) were identified in six families with PFBC [192]. The gene is located on chromosome 22 (22q13.1) and codes for the platelet-derived growth factor-β (PDGF-B), the main ligand of PDGFRβ. PDGF-B serves as a proliferation, growth, and motility factor in many tissues, and with its receptor, it is involved in multiple processes, such as the BBB maintenance, angiogenesis, and pericyte survival [216–219]. The position of *PDGFB* among the causative genes associated with PFBC has recently been supported by additional reports: a confirmed de novo mutation in a sporadic patient with BG calcification and laryngeal dystonia [220] and a partial intragenic deletion in a patient with brain calcification and leukoencephalopathy (Table 14.11) [221].

Mutations in the *PDGFRB* and *PDGFB* genes accentuate the significant role of the PDGFRβ/PDGF-B signaling pathway in the development of brain calcifications, although the precise mechanisms remain unclear.

Other Candidate Genes in PFBC

The number and spectrum of mutations in *SLC20A2*, *PDGFRB*, and *PDGFB* will certainly grow in the future as more affected patients will undergo the genetic testing. Nevertheless, efforts to identify further PFBC-linked genes should be pursued, since about 50 % of tested families do not carry a pathogenic mutation in neither of already known causative genes. Identification of other causative genes and characterization of mutations in already known genes are crucial for understanding the pathogenic mechanisms leading to various clinical expressions of PFBC and might also shed more light in the molecular background of other clinical conditions with similar neuropathological features.

Conclusion

Genetic disorders affecting brain metal homeostasis are rare but important from the therapeutic perspective. In disorders with increased systemic metal deposits, such as WD and Mn transporter deficiency, metal accumulation advances insidiously and may be asymptomatic for a long time. When the diagnosis is not made early enough, profound metal accumulation and irreversible brain damage are done before chelation therapy is initiated. In disorders with brain metal insufficiency such as MD, there is a very short therapeutic window to initiate replacement therapy to prevent irreversible consequences. Genetic testing plays an important role in early and presymptomatic diagnosis of these disorders. Currently, there is no effective treatment for the PFBC, but understanding their pathophysiological pathway may bring important information regarding cerebral response to damage.

Acknowledgements This work was supported by the research grants PRVOUKP26/LF1/4, UNCE 204011/12, and RVO-VFN64165/2012.

References

1. Zheng W, Monnot AD. Regulation of brain iron and copper homeostasis by brain barrier systems: implication in neurodegenerative diseases. Pharmacol Ther. 2012;133(2):177–88. PubMed PMID: 22115751. Pubmed Central PMCID: 3268876. Epub 2011/11/26. eng.
2. Tuschl K, Mills PB, Clayton PT. Manganese and the brain. Int Rev Neurobiol. 2013;110:277–312. PubMed PMID: 24209443.
3. Madsen E, Gitlin JD. Copper and iron disorders of the brain. Annu Rev Neurosci. 2007;30:317–37. PubMed PMID: 17367269. Epub 2007/03/21. eng.
4. Scheiber IF, Mercer JF, Dringen R. Metabolism and functions of copper in brain. Prog Neurobiol. 2014;116:33–57. PubMed PMID: 24440710.
5. Berridge MJ, Lipp P, Bootman MD. The versatility and universality of calcium signalling. Nat Rev Mol Cell Biol. 2000;1(1):11–21. PubMed PMID: 11413485.
6. Kaufman RJ, Malhotra JD. Calcium trafficking integrates endoplasmic reticulum function with mitochondrial bioenergetics. Biochim Biophys Acta. 2014;1843(10):2233–9. PubMed PMID: 24690484.
7. Catterall WA, Perez-Reyes E, Snutch TP, Striessnig J. International Union of Pharmacology. XLVIII. Nomenclature and structure-function relationships of voltage-gated calcium channels. Pharmacol Rev. 2005;57(4):411–25. PubMed PMID: 16382099.
8. Gaasch JA, Geldenhuys WJ, Lockman PR, Allen DD, Van der Schyf CJ. Voltage-gated calcium channels provide an alternate route for iron uptake in neuronal cell cultures. Neurochem Res. 2007;32(10):1686–93. PubMed PMID: 17404834.
9. Yokel RA. Manganese flux across the blood-brain barrier. Neuromolecular Med. 2009;11(4):297–310. PubMed PMID: 19902387.
10. Smyth JT, Hwang SY, Tomita T, DeHaven WI, Mercer JC, Putney JW. Activation and regulation of store-operated calcium entry. J Cell Mol Med. 2010;14(10):2337–49. PubMed PMID: 20807283. Pubmed Central PMCID: 3074973.
11. Olson S, Wang MG, Carafoli E, Strehler EE, McBride OW. Localization of two genes encoding plasma membrane Ca2(+)-transporting ATPases to human chromosomes 1q25-32 and 12q21-23. Genomics. 1991;9(4):629–41. PubMed PMID: 1674727.

12. Nucifora Jr FC, Li SH, Danoff S, Ullrich A, Ross CA. Molecular cloning of a cDNA for the human inositol 1,4,5-trisphosphate receptor type 1, and the identification of a third alternatively spliced variant. Brain Res Mol Brain Res. 1995;32(2):291–6. PubMed PMID: 7500840.
13. Yamamoto-Hino M, Sugiyama T, Hikichi K, Mattei MG, Hasegawa K, Sekine S, et al. Cloning and characterization of human type 2 and type 3 inositol 1,4,5-trisphosphate receptors. Receptors Channels. 1994;2(1):9–22. PubMed PMID: 8081734.
14. Sorrentino V, Giannini G, Malzac P, Mattei MG. Localization of a novel ryanodine receptor gene (RYR3) to human chromosome 15q14-q15 by in situ hybridization. Genomics. 1993;18(1):163–5. PubMed PMID: 8276408.
15. Hu Z, Bonifas JM, Beech J, Bench G, Shigihara T, Ogawa H, et al. Mutations in ATP2C1, encoding a calcium pump, cause Hailey-Hailey disease. Nat Genet. 2000;24(1):61–5. PubMed PMID: 10615129.
16. Schorge S, van de Leemput J, Singleton A, Houlden H, Hardy J. Human ataxias: a genetic dissection of inositol triphosphate receptor (ITPR1)-dependent signaling. Trends Neurosci. 2010;33(5):211–9. PubMed PMID: 20226542.
17. Bertini E, des Portes V, Zanni G, Santorelli F, Dionisi-Vici C, Vicari S, et al. X-linked congenital ataxia: a clinical and genetic study. Am J Med Genet. 2000;92(1):53–6. PubMed PMID: 10797423.
18. Zhou B, Gitschier J. hCTR1: a human gene for copper uptake identified by complementation in yeast. Proc Natl Acad Sci U S A. 1997;94(14):7481–6. PubMed PMID: 9207117. Pubmed Central PMCID: 23847.
19. Zheng G, Chen J, Zheng W. Relative contribution of CTR1 and DMT1 in copper transport by the blood-CSF barrier: implication in manganese-induced neurotoxicity. Toxicol Appl Pharmacol. 2012;260(3):285–93. PubMed PMID: 22465424. Pubmed Central PMCID: 3336026.
20. Tumer Z, Moller LB, Horn N. Mutation spectrum of ATP7A, the gene defective in Menkes disease. Adv Exp Med Biol. 1999;448:83–95. PubMed PMID: 10079817.
21. Tanzi RE, Petrukhin K, Chernov I, Pellequer JL, Wasco W, Ross B, et al. The Wilson disease gene is a copper transporting ATPase with homology to the Menkes disease gene. Nat Genet. 1993;5(4):344–50. PubMed PMID: 8298641. Epub 1993/12/01. eng.
22. Bull PC, Thomas GR, Rommens JM, Forbes JR, Cox DW. The Wilson disease gene is a putative copper transporting P-type ATPase similar to the Menkes gene. Nat Genet. 1993;5(4):327–37. PubMed PMID: 8298639. Epub 1993/12/01. eng.
23. Telianidis J, Hung YH, Materia S, Fontaine SL. Role of the P-Type ATPases, ATP7A and ATP7B in brain copper homeostasis. Front Aging Neurosci. 2013;5:44. PubMed PMID: 23986700. Pubmed Central PMCID: 3750203.
24. van De Sluis B, Rothuizen J, Pearson PL, van Oost BA, Wijmenga C. Identification of a new copper metabolism gene by positional cloning in a purebred dog population. Hum Mol Genet. 2002;11(2):165–73. PubMed PMID: 11809725.
25. Klomp LW, Lin SJ, Yuan DS, Klausner RD, Culotta VC, Gitlin JD. Identification and functional expression of HAH1, a novel human gene involved in copper homeostasis. J Biol Chem. 1997;272(14):9221–6. PubMed PMID: 9083055.
26. Kristinsson J, Snaedal J, Torsdottir G, Johannesson T. Ceruloplasmin and iron in Alzheimer's disease and Parkinson's disease: a synopsis of recent studies. Neuropsychiatr Dis Treat. 2012;8:515–21. PubMed PMID: 23144563. Pubmed Central PMCID: 3493298.
27. Cobine PA, Pierrel F, Winge DR. Copper trafficking to the mitochondrion and assembly of copper metalloenzymes. Biochim Biophys Acta. 2006;1763(7):759–72. PubMed PMID: 16631971.
28. Freedman JH, Ciriolo MR, Peisach J. The role of glutathione in copper metabolism and toxicity. J Biol Chem. 1989;264(10):5598–605. PubMed PMID: 2564391. Epub 1989/04/05. eng.
29. West AK, Stallings R, Hildebrand CE, Chiu R, Karin M, Richards RI. Human metallothionein genes: structure of the functional locus at 16q13. Genomics. 1990;8(3):513–8. PubMed PMID: 2286373.
30. Karin M, Eddy RL, Henry WM, Haley LL, Byers MG, Shows TB. Human metallothionein genes are clustered on chromosome 16. Proc Natl Acad Sci U S A. 1984;81(17):5494–8. PubMed PMID: 6089206. Pubmed Central PMCID: 391732.

31. Singleton WC, McInnes KT, Cater MA, Winnall WR, McKirdy R, Yu Y, et al. Role of glutaredoxin1 and glutathione in regulating the activity of the copper-transporting P-type ATPases, ATP7A and ATP7B. J Biol Chem. 2010;285(35):27111–21. PubMed PMID: 20566629. Pubmed Central PMCID: 2930710. Epub 2010/06/23. eng.
32. Martinelli D, Travaglini L, Drouin CA, Ceballos-Picot I, Rizza T, Bertini E, et al. MEDNIK syndrome: a novel defect of copper metabolism treatable by zinc acetate therapy. Brain. 2013;136(Pt 3):872–81. PubMed PMID: 23423674.
33. Holloway ZG, Velayos-Baeza A, Howell GJ, Levecque C, Ponnambalam S, Sztul E, et al. Trafficking of the Menkes copper transporter ATP7A is regulated by clathrin-, AP-2-, AP-1-, and Rab22-dependent steps. Mol Biol Cell. 2013;24(11):1735–48, S1–8. PubMed PMID: 23596324. Pubmed Central PMCID: 3667726.
34. Monnot AD, Zheng G, Zheng W. Mechanism of copper transport at the blood-cerebrospinal fluid barrier: influence of iron deficiency in an in vitro model. Exp Biol Med (Maywood). 2012;237(3):327–33. PubMed PMID: 22442359. Pubmed Central PMCID: 3982225.
35. Stuehler B, Reichert J, Stremmel W, Schaefer M. Analysis of the human homologue of the canine copper toxicosis gene MURR1 in Wilson disease patients. J Mol Med. 2004;82(9):629–34. PubMed PMID: 15205742. Epub 2004/06/19. eng.
36. Zheng W, Aschner M, Ghersi-Egea JF. Brain barrier systems: a new frontier in metal neurotoxicological research. Toxicol Appl Pharmacol. 2003;192(1):1–11. PubMed PMID: 14554098. Pubmed Central PMCID: 3982148.
37. Gunter TE, Gerstner B, Gunter KK, Malecki J, Gelein R, Valentine WM, et al. Manganese transport via the transferrin mechanism. Neurotoxicology. 2013;34:118–27. PubMed PMID: 23146871. Pubmed Central PMCID: 3576891.
38. Gunshin H, Mackenzie B, Berger UV, Gunshin Y, Romero MF, Boron WF, et al. Cloning and characterization of a mammalian proton-coupled metal-ion transporter. Nature. 1997;388(6641):482–8. PubMed PMID: 9242408. Epub 1997/07/31. eng.
39. Aschner M, Gannon M. Manganese (Mn) transport across the rat blood-brain barrier: saturable and transferrin-dependent transport mechanisms. Brain Res Bull. 1994;33(3):345–9. PubMed PMID: 8293318.
40. Fitsanakis VA, Zhang N, Garcia S, Aschner M. Manganese (Mn) and iron (Fe): interdependency of transport and regulation. Neurotox Res. 2010;18(2):124–31. PubMed PMID: 19921534.
41. Mena I, Horiuchi K, Burke K, Cotzias GC. Chronic manganese poisoning. Individual susceptibility and absorption of iron. Neurology. 1969;19(10):1000–6. PubMed PMID: 5387706.
42. Erikson KM, Syversen T, Steinnes E, Aschner M. Globus pallidus: a target brain region for divalent metal accumulation associated with dietary iron deficiency. J Nutr Biochem. 2004;15(6):335–41. PubMed PMID: 15157939. Epub 2004/05/26. eng.
43. Erikson KM, Syversen T, Aschner JL, Aschner M. Interactions between excessive manganese exposures and dietary iron-deficiency in neurodegeneration. Environ Toxicol Pharmacol. 2005;19(3):415–21. PubMed PMID: 21783506. Epub 2005/05/01.
44. Wang X, Li GJ, Zheng W. Upregulation of DMT1 expression in choroidal epithelia of the blood-CSF barrier following manganese exposure in vitro. Brain Res. 2006;1097(1):1–10. PubMed PMID: 16729984. Pubmed Central PMCID: 3980874. Epub 2006/05/30. eng.
45. Crossgrove JS, Yokel RA. Manganese distribution across the blood-brain barrier III. The divalent metal transporter-1 is not the major mechanism mediating brain manganese uptake. Neurotoxicology. 2004;25(3):451–60. PubMed PMID: 15019308.
46. Gavin CE, Gunter KK, Gunter TE. Manganese and calcium transport in mitochondria: implications for manganese toxicity. Neurotoxicology. 1999;20(2–3):445–53. PubMed PMID: 10385903.
47. Kannurpatti SS, Joshi PG, Joshi NB. Calcium sequestering ability of mitochondria modulates influx of calcium through glutamate receptor channel. Neurochem Res. 2000;25(12): 1527–36. PubMed PMID: 11152381.
48. Crossgrove JS, Yokel RA. Manganese distribution across the blood-brain barrier. IV. Evidence for brain influx through store-operated calcium channels. Neurotoxicology. 2005;26(3): 297–307. PubMed PMID: 15935202.

49. Riccio A, Mattei C, Kelsell RE, Medhurst AD, Calver AR, Randall AD, et al. Cloning and functional expression of human short TRP7, a candidate protein for store-operated Ca2+ influx. J Biol Chem. 2002;277(14):12302–9. PubMed PMID: 11805119.
50. Wang X, Kim SU, van Breemen C, McLarnon JG. Activation of purinergic P2X receptors inhibits P2Y-mediated Ca2+ influx in human microglia. Cell Calcium. 2000;27(4):205–12. PubMed PMID: 10858666.
51. Goytain A, Hines RM, Quamme GA. Huntingtin-interacting proteins, HIP14 and HIP14L, mediate dual functions, palmitoyl acyltransferase and Mg2+ transport. J Biol Chem. 2008;283(48):33365–74. PubMed PMID: 18794299. Pubmed Central PMCID: 2662264.
52. He L, Girijashanker K, Dalton TP, Reed J, Li H, Soleimani M, et al. ZIP8, member of the solute-carrier-39 (SLC39) metal-transporter family: characterization of transporter properties. Mol Pharmacol. 2006;70(1):171–80. PubMed PMID: 16638970.
53. Pinilla-Tenas JJ, Sparkman BK, Shawki A, Illing AC, Mitchell CJ, Zhao N, et al. Zip14 is a complex broad-scope metal-ion transporter whose functional properties support roles in the cellular uptake of zinc and nontransferrin-bound iron. Am J Physiol Cell Physiol. 2011;301(4):C862–71. PubMed PMID: 21653899. Pubmed Central PMCID: 3191563.
54. Yokel RA, Crossgrove JS. Manganese toxicokinetics at the blood-brain barrier. Res Rep Health Eff Inst. 2004;(119):7–58; discussion 59–73. PubMed PMID: 15043400.
55. Michalke B, Berthele A, Mistriotis P, Ochsenkuhn-Petropoulou M, Halbach S. Manganese species from human serum, cerebrospinal fluid analyzed by size exclusion chromatography-, capillary electrophoresis coupled to inductively coupled plasma mass spectrometry. J Trace Elem Med Biol. 2007;21 Suppl 1:4–9. PubMed PMID: 18039486.
56. Michalke B, Lucio M, Berthele A, Kanawati B. Manganese speciation in paired serum and CSF samples using SEC-DRC-ICP-MS and CE-ICP-DRC-MS. Anal Bioanal Chem. 2013;405(7):2301–9. PubMed PMID: 23325402.
57. Mukhopadhyay S, Linstedt AD. Identification of a gain-of-function mutation in a Golgi P-type ATPase that enhances Mn2+ efflux and protects against toxicity. Proc Natl Acad Sci U S A. 2011;108(2):858–63. PubMed PMID: 21187401. Pubmed Central PMCID: 3021037.
58. Ton VK, Mandal D, Vahadji C, Rao R. Functional expression in yeast of the human secretory pathway Ca(2+), Mn(2+)-ATPase defective in Hailey-Hailey disease. J Biol Chem. 2002;277(8):6422–7. PubMed PMID: 11741891.
59. Sepulveda MR, Wuytack F, Mata AM. High levels of Mn(2)(+) inhibit secretory pathway Ca(2)(+)/Mn(2)(+)-ATPase (SPCA) activity and cause Golgi fragmentation in neurons and glia. J Neurochem. 2012;123(5):824–36. PubMed PMID: 22845487.
60. Quadri M, Federico A, Zhao T, Breedveld GJ, Battisti C, Delnooz C, et al. Mutations in SLC30A10 cause parkinsonism and dystonia with hypermanganesemia, polycythemia, and chronic liver disease. Am J Hum Genet. 2012;90(3):467–77. PubMed PMID: 22341971. Pubmed Central PMCID: 3309204. English.
61. Tuschl K, Clayton PT, Gospe Jr SM, Gulab S, Ibrahim S, Singhi P, et al. Syndrome of hepatic cirrhosis, dystonia, polycythemia, and hypermanganesemia caused by mutations in SLC30A10, a manganese transporter in man. Am J Hum Genet. 2012;90(3):457–66. PubMed PMID: 22341972. Pubmed Central PMCID: 3309187.
62. Tan J, Zhang T, Jiang L, Chi J, Hu D, Pan Q, et al. Regulation of intracellular manganese homeostasis by Kufor-Rakeb syndrome-associated ATP13A2 protein. J Biol Chem. 2011;286(34):29654–62. PubMed PMID: 21724849. Pubmed Central PMCID: 3191006. Epub 2011/07/05. Eng.
63. Yin Z, Jiang H, Lee ES, Ni M, Erikson KM, Milatovic D, et al. Ferroportin is a manganese-responsive protein that decreases manganese cytotoxicity and accumulation. J Neurochem. 2010;112(5):1190–8. PubMed PMID: 20002294. Pubmed Central PMCID: 2819584.
64. He Q, Du T, Yu X, Xie A, Song N, Kang Q, et al. DMT1 polymorphism and risk of Parkinson's disease. Neurosci Lett. 2011;501(3):128–31. PubMed PMID: 21777657. Epub 2011/07/23. eng.
65. Bearn AG. Genetic and biochemical aspects of Wilson's disease. Am J Med. 1953;15(4): 442–9. PubMed PMID: 13092113. Epub 1953/10/01. eng.

66. Palmgren MG, Nissen P. P-type ATPases. Annu Rev Biophys. 2011;40:243–66. PubMed PMID: 21351879. Epub 2011/03/01. eng.
67. Terada K, Nakako T, Yang XL, Iida M, Aiba N, Minamiya Y, et al. Restoration of holoceruloplasmin synthesis in LEC rat after infusion of recombinant adenovirus bearing WND cDNA. J Biol Chem. 1998;273(3):1815–20. PubMed PMID: 9430732. Epub 1998/01/27. eng.
68. Terada K, Aiba N, Yang XL, Iida M, Nakai M, Miura N, et al. Biliary excretion of copper in LEC rat after introduction of copper transporting P-type ATPase, ATP7B. FEBS Lett. 1999;448(1):53–6. PubMed PMID: 10217409. Epub 1999/04/27. eng.
69. Aggarwal A, Chandhok G, Todorov T, Parekh S, Tilve S, Zibert A, et al. Wilson disease mutation pattern with genotype-phenotype correlations from Western India: confirmation of p.C271* as a common Indian mutation and identification of 14 novel mutations. Ann Hum Genet. 2013;77(4):299–307. PubMed PMID: 23551039. Epub 2013/04/05. Eng.
70. Coffey AJ, Durkie M, Hague S, McLay K, Emmerson J, Lo C, et al. A genetic study of Wilson's disease in the United Kingdom. Brain. 2013;136(Pt 5):1476–87. PubMed PMID: 23518715. Pubmed Central PMCID: 3634195.
71. Tomic A, Dobricic V, Novakovic I, Svetel M, Pekmezovic T, Kresojevic N, et al. Mutational analysis of ATP7B gene and the genotype-phenotype correlation in patients with Wilson's disease in Serbia. Vojnosanit Pregl Mil Med Pharm Rev. 2013;70(5):457–62. PubMed PMID: 23789284. English.
72. Bruha R, Marecek Z, Pospisilova L, Nevsimalova S, Vitek L, Martasek P, et al. Long-term follow-up of Wilson disease: natural history, treatment, mutations analysis and phenotypic correlation. Liver Int. 2011;31(1):83–91. PubMed PMID: 20958917. Epub 2010/10/21. eng.
73. Todorov T, Savov A, Jelev H, Panteleeva E, Konstantinova D, Krustev Z, et al. Spectrum of mutations in the Wilson disease gene (ATP7B) in the Bulgarian population. Clin Genet. 2005;68(5):474–6. PubMed PMID: 16207219. Epub 2005/10/07. eng.
74. Ferenci P. Regional distribution of mutations of the ATP7B gene in patients with Wilson disease: impact on genetic testing. Hum Genet. 2006;120(2):151–9. PubMed PMID: 16791614. Epub 2006/06/23. eng.
75. Li K, Zhang WM, Lin S, Wen L, Wang ZF, Xie D, et al. Mutational analysis of ATP7B in north Chinese patients with Wilson disease. J Hum Genet. 2013;58(2):67–72. PubMed PMID: 23235335.
76. Andreadou E, Anagnostouli M, Vasdekis V, Kararizou E, Rentzos M, Kontaxis T, et al. The impact of comorbidity and other clinical and sociodemographic factors on health-related quality of life in Greek patients with Parkinson's disease. Aging Ment Health. 2011;15(7):913–21. PubMed PMID: 21547746. Epub 2011/05/07. eng.
77. Wan L, Tsai CH, Tsai Y, Hsu CM, Lee CC, Tsai FJ. Mutation analysis of Taiwanese Wilson disease patients. Biochem Biophys Res Commun. 2006;345(2):734–8. PubMed PMID: 16696937. Epub 2006/05/16. eng.
78. Lin CW, Er TK, Tsai FJ, Liu TC, Shin PY, Chang JG. Development of a high-resolution melting method for the screening of Wilson disease-related ATP7B gene mutations. Clin Chim Acta. 2010;411(17–18):1223–31. PubMed PMID: 20465995. Epub 2010/05/15. eng.
79. Loudianos G, Dessi V, Lovicu M, Angius A, Figus A, Lilliu F, et al. Molecular characterization of wilson disease in the Sardinian population–evidence of a founder effect. Hum Mutat. 1999;14(4):294–303. PubMed PMID: 10502776. Epub 1999/09/30. eng.
80. Majumdar R, Al Jumah M, Fraser M. 4193delC, a common mutation causing Wilson's disease in Saudi Arabia: rapid molecular screening of patients and carriers. Mol Pathol. 2003;56(5):302–4. PubMed PMID: 14514926. Pubmed Central PMCID: 1187343. Epub 2003/09/30. eng.
81. Majumdar R, Al Jumah M, Al Rajeh S, Fraser M, Al Zaben A, Awada A, et al. A novel deletion mutation within the carboxyl terminus of the copper-transporting ATPase gene causes Wilson disease. J Neurol Sci. 2000;179(S 1–2):140–3. PubMed PMID: 11054498. Epub 2000/10/31. eng.
82. Mukherjee S, Dutta S, Majumdar S, Biswas T, Jaiswal P, Sengupta M, et al. Genetic defects in Indian Wilson disease patients and genotype-phenotype correlation. Parkinsonism Relat Disord. 2014;20(1):75–81. PubMed PMID: 24094725.

83. European Association for Study of Liver. EASL clinical practice guidelines: Wilson's disease. J Hepatol. 2012;56(3):671–85. PubMed PMID: 22340672. Epub 2012/02/22. eng.
84. Ferenci P, Czlonkowska A, Merle U, Ferenc S, Gromadzka G, Yurdaydin C, et al. Late-onset Wilson's disease. Gastroenterology. 2007;132(4):1294–8. PubMed PMID: 17433323. Epub 2007/04/17. eng.
85. Merle U, Schaefer M, Ferenci P, Stremmel W. Clinical presentation, diagnosis and long-term outcome of Wilson's disease: a cohort study. Gut. 2007;56(1):115–20. PubMed PMID: 16709660. Pubmed Central PMCID: 1856673. Epub 2006/05/20. eng.
86. Burke JF, Dayalu P, Nan B, Askari F, Brewer GJ, Lorincz MT. Prognostic significance of neurologic examination findings in Wilson disease. Parkinsonism Relat Disord. 2011;17(7):551–6. PubMed PMID: 21641265. Epub 2011/06/07. eng.
87. Lorincz MT. Neurologic Wilson's disease. Ann N Y Acad Sci. 2010;1184:173–87. PubMed PMID: 20146697. Epub 2010/02/12. eng.
88. Akil M, Schwartz JA, Dutchak D, Yuzbasiyan-Gurkan V, Brewer GJ. The psychiatric presentations of Wilson's disease. J Neuropsychiatry Clin Neurosci. 1991;3(4):377–82. PubMed PMID: 1821256. Epub 1991/01/01. eng.
89. Svetel M, Potrebic A, Pekmezovic T, Tomic A, Kresojevic N, Jesic R, et al. Neuropsychiatric aspects of treated Wilson's disease. Parkinsonism Relat Disord. 2009;15(10):772–5. PubMed PMID: 19559640. Epub 2009/06/30. eng.
90. Zimbrean PC, Schilsky ML. Psychiatric aspects of Wilson disease: a review. Gen Hosp Psychiatry. 2014;36(1):53–62. PubMed PMID: 24120023.
91. Seniow J, Bak T, Gajda J, Poniatowska R, Czlonkowska A. Cognitive functioning in neurologically symptomatic and asymptomatic forms of Wilson's disease. Mov Disord. 2002;17(5):1077–83. PubMed PMID: 12360563. Epub 2002/10/03. eng.
92. Iwanski S, Seniow J, Lesniak M, Litwin T, Czlonkowska A. Diverse attention deficits in patients with neurologically symptomatic and asymptomatic Wilson's disease. Neuropsychology. 2015;29(1):25–30. PubMed PMID: 24885450.
93. Cairns JE, Williams HP, Walshe JM. "Sunflower cataract" in Wilson's disease. Br Med J. 1969;3(5662):95–6. PubMed PMID: 5790274. Pubmed Central PMCID: 1983879. Epub 1969/07/12. eng.
94. Stapelbroek JM, Bollen CW, van Amstel JK, van Erpecum KJ, van Hattum J, van den Berg LH, et al. The H1069Q mutation in ATP7B is associated with late and neurologic presentation in Wilson disease: results of a meta-analysis. J Hepatol. 2004;41(5):758–63. PubMed PMID: 15519648. Epub 2004/11/03. eng.
95. Taly AB, Meenakshi-Sundaram S, Sinha S, Swamy HS, Arunodaya GR. Wilson disease: description of 282 patients evaluated over 3 decades. Medicine (Baltimore). 2007;86(2):112–21. PubMed PMID: 17435591. Epub 2007/04/17. eng.
96. Lee BH, Kim JH, Lee SY, Jin HY, Kim KJ, Lee JJ, et al. Distinct clinical courses according to presenting phenotypes and their correlations to ATP7B mutations in a large Wilson's disease cohort. Liver Int. 2011;31(6):831–9. PubMed PMID: 21645214. Epub 2011/06/08. eng.
97. de Bie P, van de Sluis B, Burstein E, van de Berghe PV, Muller P, Berger R, et al. Distinct Wilson's disease mutations in ATP7B are associated with enhanced binding to COMMD1 and reduced stability of ATP7B. Gastroenterology. 2007;133(4):1316–26. PubMed PMID: 17919502. Pubmed Central PMCID: 2857755. Epub 2007/10/09. eng.
98. Simon I, Schaefer M, Reichert J, Stremmel W. Analysis of the human Atox 1 homologue in Wilson patients. World J Gastroenterol. 2008;14(15):2383–7. PubMed PMID: 18416466. Pubmed Central PMCID: 2705094. Epub 2008/04/18. eng.
99. Bost M, Piguet-Lacroix G, Parant F, Wilson CM. Molecular analysis of Wilson patients: direct sequencing and MLPA analysis in the ATP7B gene and Atox1 and COMMD1 gene analysis. J Trace Elem Med Biol. 2012;26(2–3):97–101. PubMed PMID: 22677543. Epub 2012/06/09. eng.
100. Czlonkowska A, Gromadzka G, Chabik G. Monozygotic female twins discordant for phenotype of Wilson's disease. Mov Disord. 2009;24(7):1066–9. PubMed PMID: 19306278. Epub 2009/03/24. eng.

101. Kegley KM, Sellers MA, Ferber MJ, Johnson MW, Joelson DW, Shrestha R. Fulminant Wilson's disease requiring liver transplantation in one monozygotic twin despite identical genetic mutation. Am J Transplant. 2010;10(5):1325–9. PubMed PMID: 20346064. Epub 2010/03/30. eng.
102. Roberts EA, Schilsky ML, American Association for Study of Liver Diseases (AASLD). Diagnosis and treatment of Wilson disease: an update. Hepatology. 2008;47(6):2089–111. PubMed PMID: 18506894. Epub 2008/05/29. eng.
103. Sinha S, Taly AB, Prashanth LK, Ravishankar S, Arunodaya GR, Vasudev MK. Sequential MRI changes in Wilson's disease with de-coppering therapy: a study of 50 patients. Br J Radiol. 2007;80(957):744–9. PubMed PMID: 17709362. Epub 2007/08/22. eng.
104. Das M, Misra UK, Kalita J. A study of clinical, MRI and multimodality evoked potentials in neurologic Wilson disease. Eur J Neurol. 2007;14(5):498–504. PubMed PMID: 17437607. Epub 2007/04/18. eng.
105. Ferenci P, Caca K, Loudianos G, Mieli-Vergani G, Tanner S, Sternlieb I, et al. Diagnosis and phenotypic classification of Wilson disease. Liver Int. 2003;23(3):139–42. PubMed PMID: 12955875. Epub 2003/09/06. eng.
106. Tumer Z, Vural B, Tonnesen T, Chelly J, Monaco AP, Horn N. Characterization of the exon structure of the Menkes disease gene using vectorette PCR. Genomics. 1995;26(3):437–42. PubMed PMID: 7607665.
107. Dierick HA, Ambrosini L, Spencer J, Glover TW, Mercer JF. Molecular structure of the Menkes disease gene (ATP7A). Genomics. 1995;28(3):462–9. PubMed PMID: 7490081. Epub 1995/08/10. eng.
108. Chelly J, Tumer Z, Tonnesen T, Petterson A, Ishikawa-Brush Y, Tommerup N, et al. Isolation of a candidate gene for Menkes disease that encodes a potential heavy metal binding protein. Nat Genet. 1993;3(1):14–9. PubMed PMID: 8490646.
109. Mercer JF, Livingston J, Hall B, Paynter JA, Begy C, Chandrasekharappa S, et al. Isolation of a partial candidate gene for Menkes disease by positional cloning. Nat Genet. 1993;3(1):20–5. PubMed PMID: 8490647. Epub 1993/01/01. eng.
110. Vulpe C, Levinson B, Whitney S, Packman S, Gitschier J. Isolation of a candidate gene for Menkes disease and evidence that it encodes a copper-transporting ATPase. Nat Genet. 1993;3(1):7–13. PubMed PMID: 8490659.
111. Gitschier J, Moffat B, Reilly D, Wood WI, Fairbrother WJ. Solution structure of the fourth metal-binding domain from the Menkes copper-transporting ATPase. Nat Struct Biol. 1998;5(1):47–54 PubMed PMID: 9437429. Epub 1998/01/23. eng.
112. Lutsenko S, LeShane ES, Shinde U. Biochemical basis of regulation of human copper-transporting ATPases. Arch Biochem Biophys. 2007;463(2):134–48. PubMed PMID: 17562324. Pubmed Central PMCID: 2025638. Epub 2007/06/15. eng.
113. El Meskini R, Cline LB, Eipper BA, Ronnett GV. The developmentally regulated expression of Menkes protein ATP7A suggests a role in axon extension and synaptogenesis. Dev Neurosci. 2005;27(5):333–48. PubMed PMID: 16137991.
114. Schlief ML, Craig AM, Gitlin JD. NMDA receptor activation mediates copper homeostasis in hippocampal neurons. J Neurosci. 2005;25(1):239–46 PubMed PMID: 15634787.
115. Tumer Z. An overview and update of ATP7A mutations leading to Menkes disease and occipital horn syndrome. Hum Mutat. 2013;34(3):417–29. PubMed PMID: 23281160.
116. Moller LB, Tumer Z, Lund C, Petersen C, Cole T, Hanusch R, et al. Similar splice-site mutations of the ATP7A gene lead to different phenotypes: classical Menkes disease or occipital horn syndrome. Am J Hum Genet. 2000;66(4):1211–20. PubMed PMID: 10739752. Pubmed Central PMCID: 1288188.
117. Das S, Levinson B, Vulpe C, Whitney S, Gitschier J, Packman S. Similar splicing mutations of the Menkes/mottled copper-transporting ATPase gene in occipital horn syndrome and the blotchy mouse. Am J Hum Genet. 1995;56(3):570–6. PubMed PMID: 7887410. Pubmed Central PMCID: 1801180. Epub 1995/03/01. eng.
118. Levinson B, Gitschier J, Vulpe C, Whitney S, Yang S, Packman S. Are X-linked cutis laxa and Menkes disease allelic? Nat Genet. 1993;3(1):6. PubMed PMID: 8490656.

119. Kaler SG. ATP7A-related copper transport diseases-emerging concepts and future trends. Nat Rev Neurol. 2011;7((1):15–29. PubMed PMID: 21221114.
120. Moller LB, Mogensen M, Horn N. Molecular diagnosis of Menkes disease: genotype-phenotype correlation. Biochimie. 2009;91(10):1273–7. PubMed PMID: 19501626.
121. Verrotti A, Carelli A, Coppola G. Epilepsy in children with Menkes disease: a systematic review of literature. J Child Neurol. 2014;29(12):1757–64. PubMed PMID: 25038123.
122. Tumer Z, Moller LB. Menkes disease. Eur J Hum Genet. 2010;18(5):511–8. PubMed PMID: 19888294. Pubmed Central PMCID: 2987322.
123. Kaler SG, Goldstein DS, Holmes C, Salerno JA, Gahl WA. Plasma and cerebrospinal fluid neurochemical pattern in Menkes disease. Ann Neurol. 1993;33(2):171–5. PubMed PMID: 8434878.
124. Kaler SG, Holmes CS, Goldstein DS, Tang J, Godwin SC, Donsante A, et al. Neonatal diagnosis and treatment of Menkes disease. N Engl J Med. 2008;358(6):605–14. PubMed PMID: 18256395. Pubmed Central PMCID: 3477514.
125. Lee JS, Lim BC, Kim KJ, Hwang YS, Cheon JE, Kim IO, et al. Menkes disease in Korea: ATP7A mutation and epilepsy phenotype. Brain Dev. 2015;37(2):223–9. PubMed PMID: 24882692.
126. Bindu PS, Taly AB, Kothari S, Christopher R, Gayathri N, Sinha S, et al. Electro-clinical features and magnetic resonance imaging correlates in Menkes disease. Brain Dev. 2013;35(5):398–405. PubMed PMID: 22921468.
127. Tang J, Donsante A, Desai V, Patronas N, Kaler SG. Clinical outcomes in Menkes disease patients with a copper-responsive ATP7A mutation, G727R. Mol Genet Metab. 2008;95(3):174–81. PubMed PMID: 18752978. Pubmed Central PMCID: 2654537.
128. Kim BE, Smith K, Petris MJ. A copper treatable Menkes disease mutation associated with defective trafficking of a functional Menkes copper ATPase. J Med Genet. 2003;40(4):290–5. PubMed PMID: 12676902. Pubmed Central PMCID: 1735426.
129. Kaler SG, Das S, Levinson B, Goldstein DS, Holmes CS, Patronas NJ, et al. Successful early copper therapy in Menkes disease associated with a mutant transcript containing a small In-frame deletion. Biochem Mol Med. 1996;57(1):37–46. PubMed PMID: 8812725.
130. Sheela SR, Latha M, Liu P, Lem K, Kaler SG. Copper-replacement treatment for symptomatic Menkes disease: ethical considerations. Clin Genet. 2005;68(3):278–83. PubMed PMID: 16098018.
131. Kreuder J, Otten A, Fuder H, Tumer Z, Tonnesen T, Horn N, et al. Clinical and biochemical consequences of copper-histidine therapy in Menkes disease. Eur J Pediatr. 1993;152(10):828–32. PubMed PMID: 8223785.
132. Proud VK, Mussell HG, Kaler SG, Young DW, Percy AK. Distinctive Menkes disease variant with occipital horns: delineation of natural history and clinical phenotype. Am J Med Genet. 1996;65(1):44–51. PubMed PMID: 8914740.
133. Kennerson ML, Nicholson GA, Kaler SG, Kowalski B, Mercer JF, Tang J, et al. Missense mutations in the copper transporter gene ATP7A cause X-linked distal hereditary motor neuropathy. Am J Hum Genet. 2010;86(3):343–52. PubMed PMID: 20170900. Pubmed Central PMCID: 2833394.
134. Yi L, Donsante A, Kennerson ML, Mercer JF, Garbern JY, Kaler SG. Altered intracellular localization and valosin-containing protein (p97 VCP) interaction underlie ATP7A-related distal motor neuropathy. Hum Mol Genet. 2012;21(8):1794–807. PubMed PMID: 22210628. Pubmed Central PMCID: 3313796.
135. Tumer Z, Birk Moller L, Horn N. Screening of 383 unrelated patients affected with Menkes disease and finding of 57 gross deletions in ATP7A. Hum Mutat. 2003;22(6):457–64. PubMed PMID: 14635105.
136. Dagenais SL, Adam AN, Innis JW, Glover TW. A novel frameshift mutation in exon 23 of ATP7A (MNK) results in occipital horn syndrome and not in Menkes disease. Am J Hum Genet. 2001;69(2):420–7. PubMed PMID: 11431706. Pubmed Central PMCID: 1235313.
137. Moller LB, Bukrinsky JT, Molgaard A, Paulsen M, Lund C, Tumer Z, et al. Identification and analysis of 21 novel disease-causing amino acid substitutions in the conserved part of ATP7A. Hum Mutat. 2005;26(2):84–93. PubMed PMID: 15981243.

138. Das S, Levinson B, Whitney S, Vulpe C, Packman S, Gitschier J. Diverse mutations in patients with Menkes disease often lead to exon skipping. Am J Hum Genet. 1994;55(5):883–9. PubMed PMID: 7977350. Pubmed Central PMCID: 1918324. Epub 1994/11/01. eng.
139. Ronce N, Moizard MP, Robb L, Toutain A, Villard L, Moraine C. A C2055T transition in exon 8 of the ATP7A gene is associated with exon skipping in an occipital horn syndrome family. Am J Hum Genet. 1997;61(1):233–8. PubMed PMID: 9246006. Pubmed Central PMCID: 1715861. Epub 1997/07/01. eng.
140. Yi L, Kaler S. ATP7A trafficking and mechanisms underlying the distal motor neuropathy induced by mutations in ATP7A. Ann N Y Acad Sci. 2014;1314:49–54. PubMed PMID: 24754450. Pubmed Central PMCID: 4041065.
141. Vonk WI, de Bie P, Wichers CG, van den Berghe PV, van der Plaats R, Berger R, et al. The copper-transporting capacity of ATP7A mutants associated with Menkes disease is ameliorated by COMMD1 as a result of improved protein expression. Cell Mol Life Sci CMLS. 2012;69(1):149–63. PubMed PMID: 21667063. Pubmed Central PMCID: 3249196. Epub 2011/06/15. eng.
142. Borm B, Moller LB, Hausser I, Emeis M, Baerlocher K, Horn N, et al. Variable clinical expression of an identical mutation in the ATP7A gene for Menkes disease/occipital horn syndrome in three affected males in a single family. J Pediatr. 2004;145(1):119–21. PubMed PMID: 15238919.
143. Donsante A, Tang J, Godwin SC, Holmes CS, Goldstein DS, Bassuk A, et al. Differences in ATP7A gene expression underlie intrafamilial variability in Menkes disease/occipital horn syndrome. J Med Genet. 2007;44(8):492–7. PubMed PMID: 17496194. Pubmed Central PMCID: 2597922.
144. Beck J, Enders H, Schliephacke M, Buchwald-Saal M, Tumer Z. X;1 translocation in a female Menkes patient: characterization by fluorescence in situ hybridization. Clin Genet. 1994;46(4):295–8. PubMed PMID: 7834894.
145. Abusaad I, Mohammed SN, Ogilvie CM, Ritchie J, Pohl KR, Docherty Z. Clinical expression of Menkes disease in a girl with X;13 translocation. Am J Med Genet. 1999;87(4):354–9. PubMed PMID: 10588844. Epub 1999/12/10. eng.
146. Sirleto P, Surace C, Santos H, Bertini E, Tomaiuolo AC, Lombardo A, et al. Lyonization effects of the t(X;16) translocation on the phenotypic expression in a rare female with Menkes disease. Pediatr Res. 2009;65(3):347–51. PubMed PMID: 19092723. Epub 2008/12/19. eng.
147. Sugio Y, Kuwano A, Miyoshi O, Yamada K, Niikawa N, Tsukahara M. Translocation t(X;21)(q13.3; p11.1) in a girl with Menkes disease. Am J Med Genet. 1998;79(3):191–4. PubMed PMID: 9788559. Epub 1998/10/27. eng.
148. Moller LB, Lenartowicz M, Zabot MT, Josiane A, Burglen L, Bennett C, et al. Clinical expression of Menkes disease in females with normal karyotype. Orphanet J Rare Dis. 2012;7:6. PubMed PMID: 22264391. Pubmed Central PMCID: 3298521.
149. Huppke P, Brendel C, Kalscheuer V, Korenke GC, Marquardt I, Freisinger P, et al. Mutations in SLC33A1 cause a lethal autosomal-recessive disorder with congenital cataracts, hearing loss, and low serum copper and ceruloplasmin. Am J Hum Genet. 2012;90(1):61–8. PubMed PMID: 22243965. Pubmed Central PMCID: 3257879.
150. Horvath R, Freisinger P, Rubio R, Merl T, Bax R, Mayr JA, et al. Congenital cataract, muscular hypotonia, developmental delay and sensorineural hearing loss associated with a defect in copper metabolism. J Inherit Metab Dis. 2005;28(4):479–92. PubMed PMID: 15902551. Epub 2005/05/20. eng.
151. Kanamori A, Nakayama J, Fukuda MN, Stallcup WB, Sasaki K, Fukuda M, et al. Expression cloning and characterization of a cDNA encoding a novel membrane protein required for the formation of O-acetylated ganglioside: a putative acetyl-CoA transporter. Proc Natl Acad Sci U S A. 1997;94(7):2897–902. PubMed PMID: 9096318. Pubmed Central PMCID: 20294. Epub 1997/04/01. eng.
152. Saba TG, Montpetit A, Verner A, Rioux P, Hudson TJ, Drouin R, et al. An atypical form of erythrokeratodermia variabilis maps to chromosome 7q22. Hum Genet. 2005;116(3):167–71. PubMed PMID: 15668823. Epub 2005/01/26. eng.

153. Montpetit A, Cote S, Brustein E, Drouin CA, Lapointe L, Boudreau M, et al. Disruption of AP1S1, causing a novel neurocutaneous syndrome, perturbs development of the skin and spinal cord. PLoS Genet. 2008;4(12):e1000296. PubMed PMID: 19057675. Pubmed Central PMCID: 2585812. Epub 2008/12/06. eng.
154. Martinelli D, Dionisi-Vici C. AP1S1 defect causing MEDNIK syndrome: a new adaptinopathy associated with defective copper metabolism. Ann N Y Acad Sci. 2014;1314:55–63. PubMed PMID: 24754424. Epub 2014/04/24. eng.
155. Seve M, Chimienti F, Devergnas S, Favier A. In silico identification and expression of SLC30 family genes: an expressed sequence tag data mining strategy for the characterization of zinc transporters' tissue expression. BMC Genomics. 2004;5(1):32. PubMed PMID: 15154973. Pubmed Central PMCID: 428573. Epub 2004/05/25. eng.
156. Lechpammer M, Clegg MS, Muzar Z, Huebner PA, Jin LW, Gospe Jr SM. Pathology of inherited manganese transporter deficiency. Ann Neurol. 2014;75(4):608–12. PubMed PMID: 24599576.
157. Horoupian DS, Sternlieb I, Scheinberg IH. Neuropathological findings in penicillamine-treated patients with Wilson's disease. Clin Neuropathol. 1988;7(2):62–7. PubMed PMID: 3390974. Epub 1988/03/01. eng.
158. Kruer MC. The neuropathology of neurodegeneration with brain iron accumulation. Int Rev Neurobiol. 2013;110:165–94. PubMed PMID: 24209439.
159. Stamelou M, Tuschl K, Chong WK, Burroughs AK, Mills PB, Bhatia KP, et al. Dystonia with brain manganese accumulation resulting from SLC30A10 mutations: a new treatable disorder. Mov Disord. 2012;27(10):1317–22. PubMed PMID: 22926781. Pubmed Central PMCID: 3664426.
160. Di Toro Mammarella L, Mignarri A, Battisti C, Monti L, Bonifati V, Rasi F, et al. Two-year follow-up after chelating therapy in a patient with adult-onset parkinsonism and hypermanganesaemia due to SLC30A10 mutations. J Neurol. 2014;261(1):227–8. PubMed PMID: 24276520.
161. Ramirez A, Heimbach A, Grundemann J, Stiller B, Hampshire D, Cid LP, et al. Hereditary parkinsonism with dementia is caused by mutations in ATP13A2, encoding a lysosomal type 5 P-type ATPase. Nat Genet. 2006;38(10):1184–91. PubMed PMID: 16964263. Epub 2006/09/12. eng.
162. Schmidt K, Wolfe DM, Stiller B, Pearce DA. Cd2+, Mn2+, Ni2+ and Se2+ toxicity to Saccharomyces cerevisiae lacking YPK9p the orthologue of human ATP13A2. Biochem Biophys Res Commun. 2009;383(2):198–202. PubMed PMID: 19345671. Pubmed Central PMCID: 3906623. Epub 2009/04/07. eng.
163. Kong SM, Chan BK, Park JS, Hill KJ, Aitken JB, Cottle L, et al. Parkinson's disease-linked human PARK9/ATP13A2 maintains zinc homeostasis and promotes alpha-Synuclein externalization via exosomes. Hum Mol Genet. 2014;23(11):2816–33. PubMed PMID: 24603074.
164. Park JS, Koentjoro B, Veivers D, Mackay-Sim A, Sue CM. Parkinson's disease-associated human ATP13A2 (PARK9) deficiency causes zinc dyshomeostasis and mitochondrial dysfunction. Hum Mol Genet. 2014;23(11):2802–15. PubMed PMID: 24399444. Pubmed Central PMCID: 4014187.
165. Tsunemi T, Krainc D. Zn(2)(+) dyshomeostasis caused by loss of ATP13A2/PARK9 leads to lysosomal dysfunction and alpha-synuclein accumulation. Hum Mol Genet. 2014;23(11):2791–801. PubMed PMID: 24334770. Pubmed Central PMCID: 4014186.
166. Di Fonzo A, Chien HF, Socal M, Giraudo S, Tassorelli C, Iliceto G, et al. ATP13A2 missense mutations in juvenile parkinsonism and young onset Parkinson disease. Neurology. 2007;68(19):1557–62. PubMed PMID: 17485642. Epub 2007/05/09. eng.
167. Ning YP, Kanai K, Tomiyama H, Li Y, Funayama M, Yoshino H, et al. PARK9-linked parkinsonism in eastern Asia: mutation detection in ATP13A2 and clinical phenotype. Neurology. 2008;70(16 Pt 2):1491–3. PubMed PMID: 18413573. Epub 2008/04/17. eng.
168. Djarmati A, Hagenah J, Reetz K, Winkler S, Behrens MI, Pawlack H, et al. ATP13A2 variants in early-onset Parkinson's disease patients and controls. Mov Disord. 2009;24(14):2104–11. PubMed PMID: 19705361. Epub 2009/08/26. eng.

169. Schneider SA, Paisan-Ruiz C, Quinn NP, Lees AJ, Houlden H, Hardy J, et al. ATP13A2 mutations (PARK9) cause neurodegeneration with brain iron accumulation. Mov Disord. 2010;25(8):979–84. PubMed PMID: 20310007. Epub 2010/03/24. eng.
170. Fong CY, Rolfs A, Schwarzbraun T, Klein C, O'Callaghan FJ. Juvenile parkinsonism associated with heterozygous frameshift ATP13A2 gene mutation. Eur J Paediatr Neurol. 2011;15(3):271–5. PubMed PMID: 21316993. Epub 2011/02/15. Eng.
171. Usenovic M, Tresse E, Mazzulli JR, Taylor JP, Krainc D. Deficiency of ATP13A2 leads to lysosomal dysfunction, alpha-synuclein accumulation, and neurotoxicity. J Neurosci. 2012;32(12):4240–6. PubMed PMID: 22442086. Pubmed Central PMCID: 3462811. Epub 2012/03/24. eng.
172. Eiberg H, Hansen L, Korbo L, Nielsen IM, Svenstrup K, Bech S, et al. Novel mutation in ATP13A2 widens the spectrum of Kufor-Rakeb syndrome (PARK9). Clin Genet. 2012;82(3):256–63. PubMed PMID: 21696388.
173. Neveling K, Feenstra I, Gilissen C, Hoefsloot LH, Kamsteeg EJ, Mensenkamp AR, et al. A post-hoc comparison of the utility of sanger sequencing and exome sequencing for the diagnosis of heterogeneous diseases. Hum Mutat. 2013;34(12):1721–6. PubMed PMID: 24123792. Epub 2013/10/15. eng.
174. Crosiers D, Ceulemans B, Meeus B, Nuytemans K, Pals P, Van Broeckhoven C, et al. Juvenile dystonia-parkinsonism and dementia caused by a novel ATP13A2 frameshift mutation. Parkinsonism Relat Disord. 2011;17(2):135–8. PubMed PMID: 21094623. Epub 2010/11/26. eng.
175. Bras J, Verloes A, Schneider SA, Mole SE, Guerreiro RJ. Mutation of the parkinsonism gene ATP13A2 causes neuronal ceroid-lipofuscinosis. Hum Mol Genet. 2012;21(12):2646–50. PubMed PMID: 22388936. Pubmed Central PMCID: 3363329.
176. Santoro L, Breedveld GJ, Manganelli F, Iodice R, Pisciotta C, Nolano M, et al. Novel ATP13A2 (PARK9) homozygous mutation in a family with marked phenotype variability. Neurogenetics. 2011;12(1):33–9. PubMed PMID: 20853184. Pubmed Central PMCID: 3029807. Epub 2010/09/21. eng.
177. Malakouti-Nejad M, Shahidi GA, Rohani M, Shojaee SM, Hashemi M, Klotzle B, et al. Identification of p.Gln858* in ATP13A2 in two EOPD patients and presentation of their clinical features. Neurosci Lett. 2014;577C:106–11. PubMed PMID: 24949580. Epub 2014/06/21. Eng.
178. Park JS, Mehta P, Cooper AA, Veivers D, Heimbach A, Stiller B, et al. Pathogenic effects of novel mutations in the P-type ATPase ATP13A2 (PARK9) causing Kufor-Rakeb syndrome, a form of early-onset parkinsonism. Hum Mutat. 2011;32(8):956–64. PubMed PMID: 21542062. Epub 2011/05/05. eng.
179. Darvish H, Movafagh A, Omrani MD, Firouzabadi SG, Azargashb E, Jamshidi J, et al. Detection of copy number changes in genes associated with Parkinson's disease in Iranian patients. Neurosci Lett. 2013;551:75–8. PubMed PMID: 23880019. Epub 2013/07/25. eng.
180. Ugolino J, Fang S, Kubisch C, Monteiro MJ. Mutant Atp13a2 proteins involved in parkinsonism are degraded by ER-associated degradation and sensitize cells to ER-stress induced cell death. Hum Mol Genet. 2011;20(18):3565–77. PubMed PMID: 21665991. Pubmed Central PMCID: 3159557. Epub 2011/06/15. eng.
181. Podhajska A, Musso A, Trancikova A, Stafa K, Moser R, Sonnay S, et al. Common pathogenic effects of missense mutations in the P-type ATPase ATP13A2 (PARK9) associated with early-onset parkinsonism. PLoS One. 2012;7(6):e39942. PubMed PMID: 22768177. Pubmed Central PMCID: 3386943. Epub 2012/07/07. eng.
182. Gitler AD, Chesi A, Geddie ML, Strathearn KE, Hamamichi S, Hill KJ, et al. Alpha-synuclein is part of a diverse and highly conserved interaction network that includes PARK9 and manganese toxicity. Nat Genet. 2009;41(3):308–15. PubMed PMID: 19182805. Pubmed Central PMCID: 2683786. Epub 2009/02/03. eng.
183. Behrens MI, Bruggemann N, Chana P, Venegas P, Kagi M, Parrao T, et al. Clinical spectrum of Kufor-Rakeb syndrome in the Chilean kindred with ATP13A2 mutations. Mov Disord. 2010;25(12):1929–37. PubMed PMID: 20683840. Epub 2010/08/05. eng.

184. Najim al-Din AS, Wriekat A, Mubaidin A, Dasouki M, Hiari M. Pallido-pyramidal degeneration, supranuclear upgaze paresis and dementia: Kufor-Rakeb syndrome. Acta Neurol Scand. 1994;89(5):347–52. PubMed PMID: 8085432. Epub 1994/05/01. eng.
185. Schneider SA, Dusek P, Hardy J, Westenberger A, Jankovic J, Bhatia KP. Genetics and pathophysiology of neurodegeneration with brain iron accumulation (NBIA). Curr Neuropharmacol. 2013;11(1):59–79. PubMed PMID: 23814539. Pubmed Central PMCID: 3580793. English.
186. Rentschler G, Covolo L, Haddad AA, Lucchini RG, Zoni S, Broberg K. ATP13A2 (PARK9) polymorphisms influence the neurotoxic effects of manganese. Neurotoxicology. 2012;33(4):697–702. PubMed PMID: 22285144. Pubmed Central PMCID: 3997180.
187. Geschwind DH, Loginov M, Stern JM. Identification of a locus on chromosome 14q for idiopathic basal ganglia calcification (Fahr disease). Am J Hum Genet. 1999;65(3):764–72. PubMed PMID: 10441584. Pubmed Central PMCID: 1377984.
188. Volpato CB, De Grandi A, Buffone E, Facheris M, Gebert U, Schifferle G, et al. 2q37 as a susceptibility locus for idiopathic basal ganglia calcification (IBGC) in a large South Tyrolean family. J Mol Neurosci. 2009;39(3):346–53. PubMed PMID: 19757205.
189. Dai X, Gao Y, Xu Z, Cui X, Liu J, Li Y, et al. Identification of a novel genetic locus on chromosome 8p21.1-q11.23 for idiopathic basal ganglia calcification. Am J Med Genet B Neuropsychiatr Genet Off Publ Int Soc Psychiatr Genet. 2010;153B(7):1305–10. PubMed PMID: 20552677.
190. Wang C, Li Y, Shi L, Ren J, Patti M, Wang T, et al. Mutations in SLC20A2 link familial idiopathic basal ganglia calcification with phosphate homeostasis. Nat Genet. 2012;44(3): 254–6. PubMed PMID: 22327515.
191. Nicolas G, Pottier C, Maltete D, Coutant S, Rovelet-Lecrux A, Legallic S, et al. Mutation of the PDGFRB gene as a cause of idiopathic basal ganglia calcification. Neurology. 2013;80(2):181–7. PubMed PMID: 23255827.
192. Keller A, Westenberger A, Sobrido MJ, Garcia-Murias M, Domingo A, Sears RL, et al. Mutations in the gene encoding PDGF-B cause brain calcifications in humans and mice. Nat Genet. 2013;45(9):1077–82. PubMed PMID: 23913003.
193. Nicolas G, Pottier C, Charbonnier C, Guyant-Marechal L, Le Ber I, Pariente J, et al. Phenotypic spectrum of probable and genetically-confirmed idiopathic basal ganglia calcification. Brain. 2013;136(Pt 11):3395–407. PubMed PMID: 24065723.
194. Yamada M, Tanaka M, Takagi M, Kobayashi S, Taguchi Y, Takashima S, et al. Evaluation of SLC20A2 mutations that cause idiopathic basal ganglia calcification in Japan. Neurology. 2014;82(8):705–12. PubMed PMID: 24463626.
195. Zhu M, Zhu X, Wan H, Hong D. Familial IBGC caused by SLC20A2 mutation presenting as paroxysmal kinesigenic dyskinesia. Parkinsonism Relat Disord. 2014;20(3):353–4. PubMed PMID: 24411498.
196. Manyam BV. What is and what is not 'Fahr's disease'. Parkinsonism Relat Disord. 2005;11(2):73–80. PubMed PMID: 15734663.
197. Lemos RR, Ferreira JB, Keasey MP, Oliveira JR. An update on primary familial brain calcification. Int Rev Neurobiol. 2013;110:349–71. PubMed PMID: 24209445.
198. Yamada M, Asano T, Okamoto K, Hayashi Y, Kanematsu M, Hoshi H, et al. High frequency of calcification in basal ganglia on brain computed tomography images in Japanese older adults. Geriatr Gerontol Int. 2013;13(3):706–10. PubMed PMID: 23279700.
199. Nicolas G, Richard AC, Pottier C, Verny C, Durif F, Roze E, et al. Overall mutational spectrum of SLC20A2, PDGFB and PDGFRB in idiopathic basal ganglia calcification. Neurogenetics. 2014;15(3):215–6. PubMed PMID: 24770784.
200. Forstl H, Krumm B, Eden S, Kohlmeyer K. Neurological disorders in 166 patients with basal ganglia calcification: a statistical evaluation. J Neurol. 1992;239(1):36–8. PubMed PMID: 1541967.
201. Li X, Yang HY, Giachelli CM. Role of the sodium-dependent phosphate cotransporter, Pit-1, in vascular smooth muscle cell calcification. Circ Res. 2006;98(7):905–12. PubMed PMID: 16527991.

202. Mahy N, Prats A, Riveros A, Andres N, Bernal F. Basal ganglia calcification induced by excitotoxicity: an experimental model characterised by electron microscopy and X-ray microanalysis. Acta Neuropathol. 1999;98(3):217–25. PubMed PMID: 10483777.
203. Ramonet D, Pugliese M, Rodriguez MJ, de Yebra L, Andrade C, Adroer R, et al. Calcium precipitation in acute and chronic brain diseases. J Physiol Paris. 2002;96(3–4):307–12. PubMed PMID: 12445910.
204. Bottger P, Pedersen L. Mapping of the minimal inorganic phosphate transporting unit of human PiT2 suggests a structure universal to PiT-related proteins from all kingdoms of life. BMC Biochem. 2011;12:21. PubMed PMID: 21586110. Pubmed Central PMCID: 3126765.
205. Villa-Bellosta R, Ravera S, Sorribas V, Stange G, Levi M, Murer H, et al. The Na+–Pi cotransporter PiT-2 (SLC20A2) is expressed in the apical membrane of rat renal proximal tubules and regulated by dietary Pi. Am J Physiol Renal Physiol. 2009;296(4):F691–9. PubMed PMID: 19073637. Pubmed Central PMCID: 2670642.
206. Villa-Bellosta R, Sorribas V. Compensatory regulation of the sodium/phosphate cotransporters NaPi-IIc (SCL34A3) and Pit-2 (SLC20A2) during Pi deprivation and acidosis. Pflugers Arch. 2010;459(3):499–508. PubMed PMID: 19841935.
207. Uckert W, Willimsky G, Pedersen FS, Blankenstein T, Pedersen L. RNA levels of human retrovirus receptors Pit1 and Pit2 do not correlate with infectibility by three retroviral vector pseudotypes. Hum Gene Ther. 1998;9(17):2619–27. PubMed PMID: 9853528.
208. Hsu SC, Sears RL, Lemos RR, Quintans B, Huang A, Spiteri E, et al. Mutations in SLC20A2 are a major cause of familial idiopathic basal ganglia calcification. Neurogenetics. 2013;14(1):11–22. PubMed PMID: 23334463. Pubmed Central PMCID: 4023541.
209. Zhang Y, Guo X, Wu A. Association between a novel mutation in SLC20A2 and familial idiopathic basal ganglia calcification. PLoS One. 2013;8(2):e57060. PubMed PMID: 23437308. Pubmed Central PMCID: 3577762.
210. Beck L, Leroy C, Beck-Cormier S, Forand A, Salaun C, Paris N, et al. The phosphate transporter PiT1 (Slc20a1) revealed as a new essential gene for mouse liver development. PLoS One. 2010;5(2):e9148. PubMed PMID: 20161774. Pubmed Central PMCID: 2818845.
211. Liu L, Sanchez-Bonilla M, Crouthamel M, Giachelli C, Keel S. Mice lacking the sodium-dependent phosphate import protein, PiT1 (SLC20A1), have a severe defect in terminal erythroid differentiation and early B cell development. Exp Hematol. 2013;41(5):432–43.e7. PubMed PMID: 23376999. Pubmed Central PMCID: 3948150. Epub 2013/02/05. eng.
212. Heldin CH, Ostman A, Ronnstrand L. Signal transduction via platelet-derived growth factor receptors. Biochim Biophys Acta. 1998;1378(1):F79–113. PubMed PMID: 9739761. Epub 1998/09/18. eng.
213. Hutchins JB, Jefferson VE. Developmental distribution of platelet-derived growth factor in the mouse central nervous system. Brain Res Dev Brain Res. 1992;67(2):121–35. PubMed PMID: 1324805. Epub 1992/06/19. eng.
214. Soriano P. Abnormal kidney development and hematological disorders in PDGF beta-receptor mutant mice. Genes Dev. 1994;8(16):1888–96. PubMed PMID: 7958864. Epub 1994/08/15. eng.
215. Sanchez-Contreras M, Baker MC, Finch NA, Nicholson A, Wojtas A, Wszolek ZK, et al. Genetic screening and functional characterization of PDGFRB mutations associated with basal ganglia calcification of unknown etiology. Hum Mutat. 2014;35(8):964–71. PubMed PMID: 24796542. Pubmed Central PMCID: 4107018.
216. Tallquist MD, French WJ, Soriano P. Additive effects of PDGF receptor beta signaling pathways in vascular smooth muscle cell development. PLoS Biol. 2003;1(2):E52. PubMed PMID: 14624252. Pubmed Central PMCID: 261889. Epub 2003/11/19. eng.
217. Hellstrom M, Gerhardt H, Kalen M, Li X, Eriksson U, Wolburg H, et al. Lack of pericytes leads to endothelial hyperplasia and abnormal vascular morphogenesis. J Cell Biol. 2001;153(3):543–53. PubMed PMID: 11331305. Pubmed Central PMCID: 2190573. Epub 2001/05/02. eng.

218. Daneman R, Zhou L, Kebede AA, Barres BA. Pericytes are required for blood-brain barrier integrity during embryogenesis. Nature. 2010;468(7323):562–6. PubMed PMID: 20944625. Pubmed Central PMCID: 3241506. Epub 2010/10/15. eng.
219. Armulik A, Genove G, Mae M, Nisancioglu MH, Wallgard E, Niaudet C, et al. Pericytes regulate the blood-brain barrier. Nature. 2010;468(7323):557–61. PubMed PMID: 20944627. Epub 2010/10/15. eng.
220. Nicolas G, Jacquin A, Thauvin-Robinet C, Rovelet-Lecrux A, Rouaud O, Pottier C, et al. A de novo nonsense PDGFB mutation causing idiopathic basal ganglia calcification with laryngeal dystonia. Eur J Hum Genet. 2014;22(10):1236–8. PubMed PMID: 24518837.
221. Nicolas G, Rovelet-Lecrux A, Pottier C, Martinaud O, Wallon D, Vernier L, et al. PDGFB partial deletion: a new, rare mechanism causing brain calcification with leukoencephalopathy. J Mol Neurosci. 2014;53(2):171–5. PubMed PMID: 24604296.

Chapter 15
Genetics of Restless Legs Syndrome (RLS)

Eva C. Schulte and Juliane Winkelmann

Abstract Restless legs syndrome (RLS) is a complex genetic disease characterized by dysesthesias primarily affecting the lower limbs, which are precipitated by rest and classically occur at night. Movement of the affected extremity leads to prompt symptom relief. Genetically, RLS is a complex disorder with a heritability of up to 60 %. While linkage analyses were largely unsuccessful, genome-wide association studies (GWAS) have identified six genomic loci, to date, which harbor common genetic variants associated with an increased risk for RLS. At least one of these regions also harbors rare variants, which contribute to the genetic architecture of the disease. The first functional follow-up studies in the post-GWAS era have implicated expression alterations and forebrain development as well as dysfunctional iron metabolism as the possible downstream effects of the RLS-associated genetic alterations.

Keywords Restless legs syndrome • Genetics • Genes • Post-GWAS • GWAS • Functional follow-up

Introduction

Restless legs syndrome (RLS) is a frequent neurologic disorder characterized by (1) dysesthesias affecting the legs, (2) triggered by periods of rest or inactivity, (3) relieved by movement, and (4) occurring mostly during the evening and at night.

E.C. Schulte, MD, PhD
Neurologische Klinik und Poliklinik, Klinikum rechts der Isar, Technische Universität München, Munich 81675, Germany

Neurologische Klinik und Poliklinik, Institut für Humangenetik, Helmholtz Zentrum München, Munich 81675, Germany

J. Winkelmann, MD (✉)
Neurologische Klinik und Poliklinik, Klinikum rechts der Isar, Technische Universität München, Munich 81675, Germany

Institute of Neurogenomics, Helmholtz Zentrum München, Munich, Germany

Munich Cluster for Systems Neurology (SyNergy), Munich, Germany
e-mail: winkelmann@lrz.tu-muenchen.de

S.A. Schneider, J.M.T. Brás (eds.), *Movement Disorder Genetics*,
DOI 10.1007/978-3-319-17223-1_15

These four characteristics represent the four essential criteria of the current diagnostic criteria set forth by the International RLS Study Group (IRLSSG) [1]. Supportive criteria such as (1) a positive treatment response to dopaminergic drugs, (2) the presence of periodic limb movements (PLMs), and (3) a positive family history further lend credibility to a diagnosis. Lastly, associated features such as (1) a progressive and fluctuating natural clinical course of disease, (2) subjective sleep disturbances, or (3) an unremarkable neurologic examination in primary forms of the disease complete the current diagnostic criteria [1]. Consequences of leg discomfort and restlessness are severe disturbances in sleep architecture and quality, depression, anxiety, and possibly also increased cardiovascular risk [2, 3]. Diagnosis is made solely based on the medical history reported by the patient as currently no specific diagnostic tools such as biomarkers are available. Severe presentations of RLS can include other body regions (such as the arms [4], the stomach [5], or the bladder) and painful or cramp-like sensations [6, 7].

Age- and sex-dependent prevalences between 5.4 and 14.2 % in adult populations of European descent render RLS one of the most common neurologic disorders overall [8–11]. In populations of Asian, Indian, and African descent, prevalences are lower ranging from around 0.5 % in people in Singapore [12] and 1.1–5 % in Japan [13, 14] to 3.2 % in Turkey [15]. However, a female preponderance (female-to-male ratio approx. 1.4:1.0 [16]) is found in most populations examined so far. The cause for this overrepresentation of females in the RLS patient population is unclear to date. The fact that brother-brother pairs have a higher RLS correlation than brother-sister or sister-sister pairs [17] argues that nongenetic factors could be responsible for the increased prevalence of RLS among women.

Although the pathophysiologic factors underlying disease development are just starting to be uncovered, it is well established that sensory and motor symptoms can be alleviated by dopaminergic (levodopa and dopamine agonists), opioidergic, and—sometimes—antiepileptic drugs (e.g., pregabalin [18], gabapentin [19] and gabapentin enacarbil [20]). Additionally, it has been shown that some individuals with RLS benefit from oral [21] and intravenous [22] iron substitution. At present, the mechanism of action of any of these treatments with regard to RLS has yet to be established.

RLS as a Genetic Disorder

The beginning of RLS genetics dates back to 1923 when German neurologist Hermann Oppenheim first described RLS as a "hereditary disorder" in his *Textbook of Nerve Disorders* [23]. Swedish neurologist, Karl Ekbom, who in 1945 rendered the first "modern" description and coined the name of "restless legs syndrome," also noted a familial aggregation [24]. He estimated "one-third" of all RLS cases to be hereditary and described families with an apparent autosomal-dominant pattern of inheritance [24]. Subsequently, the late 1970s and 1980s gave rise to the first systematic evaluations of single families with RLS [25–29].

In order to better understand the different roles genetic factors can play in RLS, it is important to recognize that RLS can be a primary disorder or secondary to a number of other medical conditions such as iron deficiency, pregnancy, and renal failure. When compared to its prevalence in the general population, RLS has also been reported to occur more frequently in a number of different conditions ranging from neurologic diseases such as amyotrophic lateral sclerosis [30], Parkinson's disease [31], and multiple sclerosis [32] to rheumatoid arthritis [33], as well as celiac [34–36] and Crohn's disease [37]. If the underlying condition can be treated, RLS symptoms also improve.

Primary RLS, on the other hand, can be subdivided further into familial and idiopathic forms. A positive family history as defined by at least one affected first-degree relative is reported by 40–90 % of patients [38–41]. To date, apart from the age of onset, there is no way to differentiate these two forms based solely on clinical features [39, 41]. In 232 individuals with idiopathic or primary RLS, however, individuals with a positive family history had a younger age of onset (35.5 vs. 47.2 years, $p < 0.05$) [41]. Complex segregation analysis in 238 patients and 537 first-degree relatives revealed two distinct groups of individuals with familial RLS—those with an age of onset below the age of 30 in whom a single major gene acting in an autosomal-dominant fashion with an additional multifactorial component served as the best model and those with an age of onset above the age of 30 in whom no major gene seemed to contribute to disease development [42]. A second study utilizing complex segregation analysis to model the RLS trait in 590 individuals belonging to 77 pedigrees also saw a single-locus autosomal-dominant model with sex as a covariate and an allele frequency of 0.077 and complete penetrance as the best fit only when considering RLS as a dichotomous trait. When age of onset was considered, the single-major-gene model was rejected [43].

Next to an assessment of family histories, twin studies can be used to further investigate the heritable component of a disease and to evaluate the contribution of genotype and environment interactions to a phenotype. The larger the difference in concordance rates between monozygotic (MZ) and dizygotic (DZ) twins, the larger the genetic contribution to a given trait. With regard to RLS, only three twin studies have been published. The first one investigated 12 MZ twin pairs of whom 10 (83 %) were concordant for RLS [44]. For one, this study is hampered by the small size and the fact that only monozygotic twins were included. Secondly, recruitment bias could be an issue as the twins were recruited through a newsletter advertisement calling specifically for twins with RLS instead of a general twin registry as in the second study. Here, the presence of RLS symptoms was assessed by self-administered questionnaire in 933 female MZ and 1,004 all-female DZ twin pairs from the St Thomas' UK Adult Twin Registry. As expected, concordance rates were higher for MZ (61 %) than DZ (45 %) twins, and heritability for RLS was estimated to be 54 %. A collection of additive genetic effects combined with unique environmental influence proved to be the best approximation in multifactorial liability threshold modeling [45]. In the Canadian Restless Legs Syndrome Twin Study, when examined by self-administered questionnaire or telephone interview, of 140 MZ twin pairs, 11 pairs were concordant and 19 pairs were discordant for

RLS. Among 132 DZ twin pairs, only two were concordant, but 22 were discordant for RLS, yielding concordance rates of 53.7 and 15.4 % respectively. Interestingly, these authors also found a high correlation of age of onset ($r=0.915$, $p=0.001$) and severity scores ($r=0.764$, $p=0.01$) among the twin pairs, supporting a role of genetic factors as important determinants. Here, heritability was estimated to be 69.4 % [46].

Taken together the twin studies lend further support to the perception of RLS as a highly heritable disease. At the same time, concordance rates among MZ twins fell short of 100 % arguing for the existence of epigenetic or environmental factors.

Genetic factors play a role in bringing about RLS in all of these cases—though likely to a very different extent. Classically, RLS has been considered to be a complex genetic disorder. In symptomatic or secondary RLS, this may simply mean that individuals who develop RLS due to an underlying condition possess genetic variants conferring increase susceptibility to RLS but without an additional insult such as another predisposing medical condition; these individuals would never develop symptoms of RLS. On the other end of the spectrum, in familial RLS, mono- or oligogenic forms may exist in which, in the most extreme scenario, only one genetic alteration would be sufficient to cause disease. Complex segregation analysis demonstrated that in individuals with an age of onset younger than 30 years, one major genetic factor inherited in an autosomal-dominant fashion likely produces the RLS phenotype [42]. However, it is unclear whether this means that there is a single genetic variant in a single gene, different variants in a single gene, or different variants in different genes in the affected individuals. Further, as discussed below in more details, variable expressivity even within a single family, incomplete penetrance, the existence of phenocopies, and genetic heterogeneity further characterize the genetics of RLS.

Family Studies of RLS

The large heritability estimates and the occurrence of large pedigrees with RLS prompted the first systematic family studies in the 1980s [27, 28, 40, 47]. Here, it was noted that in most pedigrees, the recurring pattern of transmission seemed to be autosomal dominant [27, 28]. This observation was later substantiated by the systematic evaluation of the pattern of inheritance in 300 individuals with RLS [41]. Under the assumption of a single causative gene playing a role in familial RLS, linkage analyses were used to identify genomic regions shared by affected individuals from a family.

To date, a total of seven such genomic loci have been identified (Table 15.1). In all but one, a model of autosomal-dominant inheritance with reduced penetrance yielded the highest LOD scores [6, 17, 53–58]. For RLS-1, however, the first RLS linkage locus identified in a French-Canadian family on chromosome 12q12–21, an autosomal-recessive model with a high allele frequency of 0.25, resulting in a pseudodominant mode of inheritance, represented the best fit [55, 59].

Table 15.1 Linkage regions in RLS

Chr	Region (hg19)	Peak marker	Size (Mb)	Max LOD	Model	Replication status	Reference
12q12–21	94176800-104264737	*D12S1044*	10.09	3.59	Auto rec	+	[47]
		94176800			Pseudodominant		
14q13–21	34459194-47133518	*D14S288*	12.68	3.23	Auto dom	+	[7]
		43171519	(1.3)				
9p24–22	516800-19680020	*D9S286*	19.18	3.9	Auto dom	+	[17]
		8043378	(16.60)	3.22	Model-free		
9p21	22340644-ca. 3225000	*D9S147E*	9.9	3.6	Auto dom	–	[48]
		31044744					
2q33	197566845-208825061	*D2S325*	11.26	5.5	Auto dom	(+)	[49]
		207978881	(0.045)		Reduced pen (0.7)		
20p13	82754-5315186	*D20S849*	5.2	3.86	Auto dom	(+)	[50]
		5142034	(4.5)		Reduced pen (0.7)		
16p12	22758479-23312075	Several	1.18	3.5	Auto dom	(+)	[51]
					Reduced pen (0.8)		
19p13	0-2518075	*D19S878*	2.5	3.59	Auto dom	–	[52]
		2310697					

For the size of the linkage region, first the originally reported size is given and, secondly, if pertinent, the best current approximation after additional fine-mapping and replication studies + replicated with significant LOD score, (+) replicated with LOD score suggestive of linkage, – not replicated

Next to the seven linkage regions that were found to have genome-wide significant LOD scores above the conventional threshold of 3.3, a total of 21 linkage regions on 14 chromosomes have also been reported with LOD scores ranging between 1.00 and 2.61 [6, 17, 49, 54–56]. For a more in-depth discussion of the RLS linkage loci, please cf. [60].

Despite this plethora of evidence supporting the existence of single genetic variants of strong effect that play a role in familial RLS, it is also important to realize that most of these loci where only found in single or—in the best case—a few families leaving many more families where the underlying genetic factors remain obscure.

The recurrent finding in the family studies was that of genetic heterogeneity and complexity in RLS. Interestingly, a large German RLS family in whom linkage analysis argued for the existence of two independent linkage loci on chromosomes 4 and 17 also exists, possibly reflecting an oligogenic mode of inheritance in this family (Winkelmann J et al., unpublished observation). Also, replication of the above loci has proven very difficult [49–52, 57, 59, 61], and the maximum LOD scores found fall short of the maximum attainable scores projected by the pedigree structure. Overall, linkage studies in RLS have failed to the extent that no underlying genetic factor could be identified for any of the above loci, even when the most up-to-date technologies such as targeted next-generation sequencing were employed to resolve the regions [62, 63].

Candidate Gene Association Studies

Over the past two decades, several candidate gene studies have been performed in RLS. Because dopaminergic drugs are one of the mainstays of treatment, an involvement of dopaminergic pathways in the pathophysiology of RLS has long been projected. Accordingly, in one of the first association studies in RLS, SNPs in eight genes playing a role in dopaminergic neurotransmission were examined for possible association with the RLS phenotype in 92 cases and 182 controls. However, no association of any of the tested genetic variants with the RLS phenotype was observed [48]. Next to the dopaminergic system, the iron metabolism has long been implicated in RLS. However, no SNP located within any of 111 iron-related genes ± 4 Mb showed a replicable association with the RLS phenotype in three case/control samples totaling to 2,425 cases and 3,285 general population controls [64]. In summary, candidate association studies—in parallel to the linkage analyses—have been unsuccessful in identifying genetic factors involved in RLS.

Genome-Wide Association Studies

To date, three genome-wide association studies (GWAS) have been performed for RLS and one for RLS and periodic limb movements in sleep (PLMS) (Tables 15.2 and 15.3). The PLMS GWAS was carried out under the deCODE Genetics umbrella and included 306 cases with RLS and PLMS and 15,664 controls from Iceland in

Table 15.2 Study characteristics of GWAS performed for RLS

Genome-wide sample (cases/controls)	Origin	SNP array	Replication sample(s) (cases/controls)	Origin	Lead SNPs	Candidate gene	Replication status	Reference
306/15,633	Iceland	Human Hap300 and Hap300-duo+	123/1,233	Iceland	rs3923809	*BTBD9*	+	[65]
		Bead, Illumina	188/662	USA				
401/1,644	Germany	500 K, Affymetrix	903/891	Germany	rs2300478	*MEIS1*	+	[66]
			255/287	Canada	rs9296249	*BTBD9*	+	
					rs1026732	*MAP2K5/SKOR1*	+	
628/1,644	Germany	500 K, Affymetrix (n=401+1,644)	1,271/1,901	Germany	rs4626664	*PTPRD*	+	[67]
		Genome-wide human SNP 5.0	279/368	Czech Republic	rs1975197	*PTPRD*	+	
		Array, Affymetrix (n=227)	285/842	Canada				
954/1,814	Germany and Austria	Genome-wide human SNP 5.0	1,236/1,471	Germany and Austria	rs2300478	*MEIS1*	+	[68]
		Array, Affymetrix (cases)	1,104/1,065	Germany and Austria	rs9357271	*BTBD9*	+	
		Genome-wide human SNP 6.0	351/597	Czech Republic	rs1975197	*PTPRD*	+	
		Array, Affymetrix (controls)	141/360	Finland	rs12593813	*MAP2K5/SKOR1*	+	
			182/768	France	rs6747972	Intergenic	–	
			285/285	Canada	rs3104767	*TOX3/BC034767*	–	
			556/1,208	USA				

For a more detailed description of results, also see Table 15.3
+ statistically significant in independent population, – not (yet) replicated

Table 15.3 RLS GWAS loci [68]

Locus	Chr	LD block (Mb)	Lead SNP	Risk allele	Risk allele freq (cases/controls)	P_{joint}	Odds ratio (95 % CI)
MEIS1	2	66.57–66.64	rs2300478	G	0.35/0.24	3.40×10^{-49}	1.68 (1.57–1.81)
MAP2K5/SKOR1	15	65.25–65.94	rs12593813	G	0.75/0.68	1.37×10^{-22}	1.41 (1.32–1.52)
BTBD9	6	37.82–38.79	rs9357271	T	0.82/0.76	7.75×10^{-22}	1.47 (1.35–1.47)
TOX3/BC034767	16	51.07–51.21	rs3104767	G	0.65/0.58	9.40×10^{-19}	1.35 (1.27–1.43)
Intergenic	2	67.88–68.00	rs6747972	A	0.47/0.44	9.03×10^{-11}	1.23 (1.16–1.31)
PTPRD	9	8.80–8.88	rs1975197	A	0.19/0.16	3.49×10^{-10}	1.29 (1.19–1.40)

the genome-wide phase. An intronic variant in *BTBD9* within a linkage disequilibrium (LD) block on chromosome 6p21.2 showed genome-wide significant association ($p_{nominal} = 2 \times 10^{-9}$, OR = 1.8) and was replicated in a second Icelandic and a US-American sample (combined sample (617 cases/17,528 controls): $p_{nominal} = 3 \times 10^{-14}$, OR = 1.7). Moreover, the major allele of the lead SNP (rs3923809) was also associated with an increase in PLMS of approximately 3/h as well as a 13 % decrease in serum iron per allele when tested in 965 individuals [69].

Simultaneously, the first RLS GWAS, which included 401 German cases and 1,644 general population controls in the genome-wide phase as well as 903 German cases and 891 controls and 255 Canadian cases and 287 controls in the replication samples, also showed association to the same SNP and the same 115 kb LD block on chromosome 6p containing intron 5 of *BTBD9*. However, on chromosome 2p, an association signal located within a 32 kb LD block containing intron 8 and exon 9 of *MEIS1* was more strongly associated with the RLS phenotype in all individuals included in the genome-wide phase as well as the combined sample (rs2300478, $p_{nominal} = 3.41 \times 10^{-28}$, OR = 1.74). Fine-mapping and haplotype analysis in the German replication sample revealed a haplotype associated with RLS with an increased OR of up to 2.75 (95 % CI: 2.23–3.41) ($p_{nominal} = 5.87 \times 10^{-20}$, frequency in cases 0.231 vs. 0.102 in controls). A third association signal of genome-wide significance was located within a 48 kb locus on chromosome 15q spanning the 3′ end of *MAP2K5* as well as *SKOR1* (formerly called *LBXCOR1*) (combined $p_{nominal} = 6.09 \times 10^{-17}$) [70].

A GWAS-based analysis of the RLS-3 locus encompassing 31 Mb on chromosome 9p23–24 in 628 cases and 1,644 general population controls revealed two independent ($r^2 = 0$) SNPs within two independent LD blocks in intron 8 (rs4626664) and intron 10 (rs1975197) of the 5′ untranslated region (UTR) of *PTPRD* which were replicated in a sample of 1,835 cases and 3,111 controls from Germany, the Czech Republic, and Canada. When combined with the genome-wide discovery sample, both SNPs surpassed thresholds for genome-wide significance (rs4626664: $p_{nominal} = 5.91 \times 10^{-10}$, OR = 1.44; rs1975197: $p_{nominal} = 5.81 \times 10^{-9}$, OR = 1.31). No variants in any of the 35 coding and 10 noncoding exons of *PTPRD* could be identified in nine affected individuals from an RLS-3-linked family, and the common variants in *PTPRD* only explain a minor portion of the original RLS-3 linkage signal [71].

An increased sample size of 922 cases and 1,526 controls in the genome-wide phase and a multinational replication sample of 3,935 cases and 5,754 controls of European descent revealed two new loci of genome-wide significance: an intergenic region on chromosome 2p14 approximately 1.3 Mb downstream of *MEIS1* (rs6747972, $p_{nominal} = 9.03 \times 10^{-11}$, OR = 1.23) as well as a locus on chromosome 16q12.1 encompassing an LD block of 140 kb containing both the 5′-end of *TOX3* and the noncoding RNA *BC034767* (rs3104767, $p_{nominal} = 9.4 \times 10^{-19}$, OR = 1.35) [72].

While the two most recent loci still await replication in independent studies, the first four loci have been replicated in independent case/control samples [65–67]. In individuals with secondary RLS due to end-stage renal insufficiency, the lead SNPs in *BTBD9* were also associated with increased susceptibility to RLS in a combined German/Greek sample of 341 dialysis patients with RLS and 836 without RLS, while *MEIS1* lead SNPs showed significant association only in the German sample [68]. A single association study in a non-European population corroborated the link between the intronic variants in *BTBD9* (rs3923809 and rs9296249) and RLS in the Korean population [73]. To date, no GWAS in non-European populations or considering specific endophenotypes have been performed for RLS.

Single SNPs at the RLS-associated loci identified by the above studies bear effect sizes between 1.22 and 1.77 and risk allele frequencies between 0.19 and 0.82 (Table 15.3) [72]. Although the conferred risk is large when compared to common variants associated with other complex traits, when taken together, the most significant SNPs at these loci only explain about 6.8 % of the heritability of RLS [72]. Arguing for—most likely—both the existence of additional independent RLS-related variants within these loci as well as a number of additional loci. It is also important to realize that the lead SNPs may not be identical to the causal genetic variants at these loci, which makes functional follow-up studies indispensible in order to utilize genetic variants to inform the pathophysiology of RLS.

Following Up on GWAS

The link between the most likely candidate genes at the associated GWAS loci and RLS is not readily apparent. Functionally, most of the candidate genes highlighted by the GWAS are not well characterized. Transcriptional regulation especially in developmental processes in the nervous system seems to be the largest common denominator.

MEIS1

The transcription factor *MEIS1* belongs to the family of highly conserved TALE homeobox genes and interacts with PBX and HOX proteins to increase the affinity and specificity of HOX proteins [74] as well as *CREB1* [75] in DNA binding. In *Xenopus laevis*, *meis1* is known to be involved in neural crest development [76]. Murine Meis1 is essential for proximo-distal limb patterning [77] and plays a role in the Hox transcriptional regulatory network that specifies spinal motor neuron pool identity and connectivity [78]. In the CNS of the adult mouse, it is known to be expressed in cerebellar granule cells, the forebrain, and the substantia nigra. While *MEIS1* was initially identified in the context of acute myeloid leukemia [79, 80], in recent years, a role in murine heart development has also been recognized [81], and SNPs in intron 8 (but in weak LD with the known RLS SNPs) play a role in determining atrioventricular conduction velocity as reflected by the length of the PR interval of the electrocardiogram in both Europeans and African-Americans [82, 83]. *Meis1−/−* mice develop ocular and vascular defects, fail to produce megakaryocytes, and display extensive hemorrhaging. They also die by embryonic day 14.5 [84]. *Meis1−/+* mice, however, survive into adulthood and exhibit hyperactivity reminiscent of the human RLS phenotype [85].

A second independent association signal is located in an intergenic region approximately 1.3 Mb downstream of *MEIS1* and potentially possesses long-range regulatory function with *MEIS1* and *ETAA1* as potential target genes [72].

Several rare non-synonymous variants in *MEIS1* have been identified in RLS patients. However, coding variants in *MEIS1* are very rare in general (13 out of approximately 4,250 individuals with a non-synonymous variant in the NHLBI-ESP exomes [86]), possibly owing to the fact that *MEIS1* represents one of the most highly conserved genes in the human genome, and, therefore, remain ambiguous with regard to possible causality of the RLS phenotype [87–90]. On the whole, however, non-synonymous variants with MAF <0.1 % were found significantly more frequently in individuals with RLS compared to the general population [90]. Functional annotation using an in vivo complementation assay in zebra fish further revealed that variants harboring a loss of *MEIS1* function were significantly enriched in individuals with RLS [90]. The same study also identified a low-frequency variant in the 3′ untranslated region (UTR) of *MEIS1* (rs11693221; $MAF_{cases} = 13.55$ % vs. $MAF_{controls} = 3.58$ %; $p = 1.27 \times 10^{-89}$, OR=4.42) associated with RLS [90]. Yet, at present, it cannot be determined whether this or any other variant tagged by rs11693221 represents the causal factor underlying this association signal. What does become clear, though, is the fact that, at the *MEIS1* locus, an allelic series of genetic variants of different frequencies and different effect sizes contributes to the genetic framework of RLS.

Since the publication of the first GWAS, which identified common variants in *MEIS1* as susceptibility factors for RLS, three studies have been reported which examine the functional differences brought about by the RLS-associated intronic variants. In the first, a significant decrease in *MEIS1* mRNA and protein expression was found in lymphoblastoid cell lines and brain tissue (pons and thalamus) from homozygous carriers of the risk haplotype when compared to homozygous carriers of the non-risk haplotype [89]. In a second study, knockdown of the *MEIS1* orthologue *unc-62* by RNA interference in *Caenorhabditis elegans* was related to increased ferritin expression and an extended life span. In thalamus but not in pons samples of RLS patients homozygous for the *MEIS1* risk haplotype ($n = 9$), ferritin light and heavy chains as well as divalent metal transporter 1 (*DMT1*) mRNA and protein expression were significantly increased when compared to RLS patients carrying the protective haplotype ($n = 7$). Several other key players in the iron metabolism such as transferrin, the transferrin receptors 1 and 2, aconitase 1, iron-responsive element binding protein 2, ceruloplasmin, hepcidin, and ferroportin were unchanged [91]. The authors argue that these data are in support of a disruption of physiological iron transport into the brain and—in conjunction with the also observed decrease of MEIS1 expression in in vitro cell models of iron deprivation—provide a functional link between the RLS gene *MEIS1* and the iron metabolism, which is believed to play a role in RLS pathogenesis [91]. In the third study, it was shown that the risk allele of the best-associated SNP (rs12469063) in *MEIS1* from the GWAS reduces enhancer activity in the *Meis1* expression domain of the ganglionic eminences, which constitute the primordial basal ganglia, in mouse embryos at E12.5 [85]. In vitro studies suggest that CREB1 binds more strongly to this enhancer when the risk allele is present [85].

MAP2K5/SKOR1

Another locus encompasses both mitogen-activated protein kinase *MAP2K5* and transcriptional corepressor, *SKOR1*. MAPK pathways are highly conserved among different species and are activated in response to signals that mediate the transduction of extracellular signals to the cytoplasmic nuclear effectors [92]. More specifically, MAP2K5 phosphorylates and activates ERK5 in response to oxidative stress, hyperosmolarity, and growth factors. It is expressed in the heart and skeletal muscle and critical in muscle cell differentiation [92]. Interestingly, the MAP2K5/ERK5 pathway has also been implicated in neuroprotection of dopaminergic neurons [93]. Not much is known about the physiologic function of SKOR1. It acts as a transcriptional corepressor of homeobox gene *LBX1*, which has been recognized as a factor in the development of pain and touch relay via sensory pathways in the dorsal horn of the spinal cord [94]. The genomic locus comprising *MAP2K5* and SKOR1 was shown to harbor nine blood-based *cis*-eSNPs, that is, common variants that are located within ± 500 kb of the lead SNP, which alter blood-based gene expression [95]. None of these affected the expression of SKOR1, and only two affected the expression of MAP2K5, while seven altered expression of *CALML4*, thus highlighting the possibility that other genes in the vicinity of the current candidate genes at a given locus could also play a role in RLS pathophysiology [95].

BTBD9

BTBD9 belongs to the group of BTB (POZ) domain-containing proteins, which are involved in formation of the limbs and cell fate determination in the developing *Drosophila melanogaster* [96, 97]. Moreover, BTB (POZ) domain proteins are recognized in transcription repression, cytoskeleton regulation, tetramerization and gating of ion channels, and ubiquitin-dependent protein degradation [97]. *Btbd9* is widely expressed in the mouse with CNS expression in the thalamus, hypothalamus, cortex, cerebellum, hippocampus, caudate, and subthalamic nuclei in addition to pan-spinal expression [98].

The functional knockout of *Drosophila BTBD9* homologue *dBTBD9/CG1826* in two excision lines termed "wanderlust (wlst) 1 and 2" carrying large deletions in the *dBTBD9* locus was associated with changes of sleep architecture. Nighttime sleep in *dBTBD9*^{wlst1}&^{2} flies was fragmented with decreased length alongside increased number of sleep bouts. Also, the amount of wake time after sleep onset was increased in the mutant flies. The same sleep phenotype was observed when *dBTBD9* was knocked down by RNAi in a large subset of all dopaminergic neurons and could be rescued by treating the flies with dopamine D2 receptor agonist pramipexole. *dBTBD9*^{wlst1}&^{2} flies were also hyperlocomotive when enclosed within a restricted space with an increase in the time spent moving with fewer pauses. Further, a 50 % reduction in brain dopamine levels was found in *dBTBD9*^{wlst1}&^{2} flies arguing for a mechanistic link between dBTBD9 and dopaminergic neurotransmitter pathways [99].

Recently, the first murine knockout of Btbd9 was reported [100]. When analyzed for RLS-specific phenotypes, *Btbd9*$^{-/-}$ mice showed motor restlessness with respect to voluntary and total activity and changes in sleep architecture with increased awake time and arousals from sleep alongside a decrease in slow-wave sleep as well as increased serum iron levels and increased levels of the serotonin metabolite 5-HIAA in the striatum when compared to wild-type mice. Levels of iron and neurotransmitters dopamine and serotonin as well as a number of their metabolites in the striatum were unchanged [101]. Both *Btbd9*$^{-/-}$ and *Btbd9*$^{+/-}$ mice also had a decreased response time to thermal sensory stimuli possibly limited to the rest phase [101]. This is interesting in light of the fact that in humans with RLS thermal hypoesthesia has been reported to differentiate secondary RLS with small-fiber neuropathy from primary RLS [102]. Btbd9$^{-/-}$ mice also showed significant impairment in presynaptic activity as well as enhanced long-term potentiation and cued and contextual fear memory [100]. In an inbred strain of mice, *Btbd9* gene expression has also been correlated with midbrain iron concentrations [103], and *Btbd9* was hypothesized to play a role in iron homeostasis [104]. Taken together, the loss of BTBD9 homologue function in both fruit flies and mice recapitulates several aspects of the human RLS phenotype, especially with regard to sleep architecture. These novel animal models will certainly be important in further elucidating the GWAS-based findings in RLS.

TOX3

TOX3 is a member of the high-mobility box group family of non-histone chromatin proteins and interacts with CREB and CBP in mediating calcium-dependent transcription in neurons [105]. It is highly expressed in the human frontal and occipital cortex, the cerebellum, and the retina [106] as well as the salivary glands and the trachea [72] and is known to harbor forebrain-specific enhancers [107]. An intronic SNP in the same region of *TOX3* in low LD with the lead RLS SNP ($r^2 \sim 0.1$) also represents a susceptibility factor for breast cancer [108]. Within the same LD block, *BC034767* is a projected noncoding RNA expressed in the testes [72]; beyond this no additional characteristics are known. Both genes await investigation with regard to RLS.

PTPRD

Protein tyrosine phosphatase receptor type delta, *PTPRD*, harbored another association signal identified in the GWAS [71, 72]. Interestingly, the lead SNPs are located in the 5′ UTR within LD blocks overlapping the previously identified RLS-3 linkage region although it only explains a small part of the linkage signal. No rare coding variants which segregate with the RLS phenotype could be identified in a total of 24 probands from families linking to the RLS-3 locus [71, 109]. Two low-frequency variants in *PTPRD* (c.551–4 C>G and p.Pro278Pro (c.834 T>G)) were nominally associated with the RLS phenotype in a large case/control sample consisting of 3,262 cases and 2,944 general population controls but did not withstand correction for multiple testing. Yet, a Taiwanese study of 993 individuals with end-stage renal disease also found an association between an intronic variant in *PTPRD* (rs4626664) and RLS ($p_{corrected}=0.03$; OR = 1.52) [110].

Notably, the lead SNPs are found in an isoform of *PTPRD* that is expressed predominantly in developing and adult brain tissues [111, 112]. *Ptprd* knockout mice show defects in axonal guidance and motorneuron patterning during embryonic development [113]. Within the surge of GWAS, SNPs in *PTPRD* have also been recognized as susceptibility factors for plasma homocysteine levels [114], type II diabetes in specific populations [115, 116], and coronary artery disease [117], which could potentially be interesting in the context of an increased risk for cardiovascular diseases in individuals with RLS found in a number of studies [118].

Structural alterations and genomic instability in *PTPRD* have also been implicated in the pathophysiology of neuroblastomas [119, 120] and attention-deficit hyperactivity disorder [121]. Despite the fact that a role in neuronal development and function has been recognized, the direct link between genetic variants found in *PTPRD* and RLS remains to be established.

Moreover, although these genes represent the most likely candidates at the given loci, one can also not exclude that other genetic variants in high LD with the lead SNPs play a role or that the SNPs hold long-range regulatory function on other genes. Accordingly, ongoing efforts to functionally link the identified genes to the RLS phenotype will be important to better inform the nature of the observed associations.

Future Directions in RLS Genetics

Both family and association studies have implicated candidate genomic regions and candidate genes in RLS. However, no single genetic variant has to date been shown to be sufficient to induce the development of the RLS phenotype. Identification of a truly causal variant would be very beneficial in that it would greatly facilitate pathophysiologic studies and would provide an entry point into the establishment of specific animal models of RLS. Yet, one of the most common findings in the majority of studies throughout the past two decades has been that of genetic heterogeneity. In the most extreme case, this could mean that there are no "causal" alleles for RLS and that the RLS phenotype is always the result of several genetic factors acting in concert although the large pedigrees at first glance might suggest otherwise. In the context of linkage analyses, genetic heterogeneity is reflected by the fact that overall only very few RLS families actually link to the described loci and a number of families exist in whom no significant linkage signal could be identified even though family structure was suited to do so or in whom more than one linkage signal was present [Winkelmann J et al., unpublished]. With respect to genome-wide association studies, genetic heterogeneity is exemplified by the fact that the currently identified association signals only account for approximately 6.8 % of the projected heritability although they confer relatively large risk increases [72]. Increasing GWAS sample sizes will likely uncover more and more of the currently missing heritability. Yet, it is highly unlikely that GWAS, the way we understand them today, will be able to identify the remainder of genetic factors contributing to the RLS phenotype.

RLS is a genetically complex disease, and this complexity is probably not only marked by locus heterogeneity but also by the range of different variants likely to be involved. These might include variants present at a range of different frequencies in the population—common, rare, and everything in between. They will also include different types of variants such as coding and noncoding variants along with structural variation of stronger or weaker effect on the phenotype either acting together to cause the phenotype in an oligo- or polygenic way or as genetic modifiers. Here, it is interesting to note that RLS genetics research has yet to see the first successful application of next-generation sequencing technologies to, for example, better examine the role of rare or noncoding genetic variants or to resolve the linkage regions that have been described.

It seems, moreover, possible that additional layers of biology such as epigenetic phenomena could play a role in RLS. Investigations into the transcriptomics, methylomics, proteomics, and metabolomics of RLS could not only begin to answer these questions but could also make a valuable contribution to the search for biomarkers for application in diagnostics and therapy. In this context, the definition and assessment of endophenotypes in RLS (i.e., individuals with high vs. low ferritin levels or response to certain drugs such as pregabalin) could prove valuable.

References

1. Allen RP, Picchietti D, Hening WA, Trenkwalder C, Walters AS, Montplaisi J, et al. Restless legs syndrome: diagnostic criteria, special considerations, and epidemiology. A report from the restless legs syndrome diagnosis and epidemiology workshop at the National Institutes of Health. Sleep Med. 2003;4:101–19.
2. Winkelman JW, Shahar E, Sharief I, Gottlieb DJ. Association of restless legs syndrome and cardiovascular disease in the Sleep Heart Health Study. Neurology. 2008;70:35–42.
3. Winkelmann J, Prager M, Lieb R, Pfister H, Spiegel B, Wittchen HU, et al. "Anxietas tibiarum". Depression and anxiety disorders in patients with restless legs syndrome. J Neurol. 2005;252:67–71.
4. Michaud M, Chabli A, Lavigne G, Montplaisir J. Arm restlessness in patients with restless legs syndrome. Mov Disord. 2000;15:289–93.
5. Perez-Diaz H, Iranzo A, Rye DB, Santamaria J. Restless abdomen: a phenotypic variant of restless legs syndrome. Neurology. 2011;77:1283–6.
6. Bonati MT, Ferini-Strambi L, Aridon P, Oldani A, Zucconi M, Casari G. Autosomal dominant restless legs syndrome maps on chromosome 14q. Brain. 2003;126:1485–92.
7. Hornyak M, Sohr M, Busse M, Study G. Evaluation of painful sensory symptoms in restless legs syndrome: experience from two clinical trials. Sleep Med. 2011;12:186–9.

8. Allen RP, Walters AS, Montplaisir J, Hening W, Myers A, Bell TJ, et al. Restless legs syndrome prevalence and impact: REST general population study. Arch Intern Med. 2005;165:1286–92.
9. Berger K, Luedemann J, Trenkwalder C, John U, Kessler C. Sex and the risk of restless legs syndrome in the general population. Arch Intern Med. 2004;164:196–202.
10. Bjorvatn B, Leissner L, Ulfberg J, Gyring J, Karlsborg M, Regeur L, et al. Prevalence, severity and risk factors of restless legs syndrome in the general adult population in two Scandinavian countries. Sleep Med. 2005;6:307–12.
11. Hogl B, Kiechl S, Willeit J, Saletu M, Frauscher B, Seppi K, et al. Restless legs syndrome: a community-based study of prevalence, severity, and risk factors. Neurology. 2005;64:1920–4.
12. Tan EK. Restless legs syndrome and Parkinson's disease: is there an etiologic link? J Neurol. 2006;253 Suppl 7:VII33–7.
13. Kageyama T, Kabuto M, Nitta H, Kurokawa Y, Taira K, Suzuki S, et al. Prevalence of use of medically prescribed hypnotics among adult Japanese women in urban residential areas. Psychiatry Clin Neurosci. 1998;52:69–74.
14. Mizuno S, Miyaoka T, Inagaki T, Horiguchi J. Prevalence of restless legs syndrome in non-institutionalized Japanese elderly. Psychiatry Clin Neurosci. 2005;59:461–5.
15. Sevim S, Dogu O, Camdeviren H, Bugdayci R, Sasmaz T, Kaleagasi H, et al. Unexpectedly low prevalence and unusual characteristics of RLS in Mersin, Turkey. Neurology. 2003;61:1562–9.
16. Lazzarini A, Walters AS, Hickey K, Coccagna G, Lugaresi E, Ehrenberg BL, et al. Studies of penetrance and anticipation in five autosomal-dominant restless legs syndrome pedigrees. Mov Disord. 1999;14:111–6.
17. Chen S, Ondo WG, Rao S, Li L, Chen Q, Wang Q. Genomewide linkage scan identifies a novel susceptibility locus for restless legs syndrome on chromosome 9p. Am J Hum Genet. 2004;74:876–85.
18. Garcia-Borreguero D, Larrosa O, Williams AM, Albares J, Pascual M, Palacios JC, et al. Treatment of restless legs syndrome with pregabalin: a double-blind, placebo-controlled study. Neurology. 2010;74:1897–904.
19. Garcia-Borreguero D, Larrosa O, de la Llave Y, Verger K, Masramon X, Hernandez G. Treatment of restless legs syndrome with gabapentin: a double-blind, cross-over study. Neurology. 2002;59:1573–9.
20. Kushida CA, Becker PM, Ellenbogen AL, Canafax DM, Barrett RW, Group XPS. Randomized, double-blind, placebo-controlled study of XP13512/GSK1838262 in patients with RLS. Neurology. 2009;72:439–46.
21. Wang J, O'Reilly B, Venkataraman R, Mysliwiec V, Mysliwiec A. Efficacy of oral iron in patients with restless legs syndrome and a low-normal ferritin: a randomized, double-blind, placebo-controlled study. Sleep Med. 2009;10:973–5.
22. Allen RP, Adler CH, Du W, Butcher A, Bregman DB, Earley CJ. Clinical efficacy and safety of IV ferric carboxymaltose (FCM) treatment of RLS: a multi-centred, placebo-controlled preliminary clinical trial. Sleep Med. 2011;12:906–13.
23. Oppenheim H. Lehrbuch der Nervenkrankheiten. Berlin: S. Karger; 1923.
24. Ekbom KA. Restless legs. Acta Med Scand. 1945;158:1–123.
25. Boghen D, Peyronnard JM. Myoclonus in familial restless legs syndrome. Arch Neurol. 1976;33:368–70.
26. Montagna P, Coccagna G, Cirignotta F. Familial restless legs syndrome: long-term follow-up. In: Guilleminault C, Lugaresi E, editors. Sleep/wake disorders: natural history, epidemiology, and long-term evolution. New York: Raven; 1983. p. 231–5.
27. Trenkwalder C, Seidel VC, Gasser T, Oertel WH. Clinical symptoms and possible anticipation in a large kindred of familial restless legs syndrome. Mov Disord. 1996;11:389–94.
28. Walters AS, Picchietti D, Hening W, Lazzarini A. Variable expressivity in familial restless legs syndrome. Arch Neurol. 1990;47:1219–20.
29. Walters A, Hening W, Cote L, Fahn S. Dominantly inherited restless legs with myoclonus and periodic movements of sleep: a syndrome related to endogenous opiates? Adv Neurol. 1986;43:309–19.

30. Lo Coco D, Piccoli F, La Bella V. Restless legs syndrome in patients with amyotrophic lateral sclerosis. Mov Disord. 2010;25:2658–61.
31. Ondo WG, Vuong KD, Jankovic J. Exploring the relationship between Parkinson disease and restless legs syndrome. Arch Neurol. 2002;59:421–4.
32. Schurks M, Bussfeld P. Multiple sclerosis and restless legs syndrome: a systematic review and meta-analysis. Eur J Neurol. 2013;20:605–15.
33. Hening WA, Caivano CK. Restless legs syndrome: a common disorder in patients with rheumatologic conditions. Semin Arthritis Rheum. 2008;38:55–62.
34. Manchanda S, Davies CR, Picchietti D. Celiac disease as a possible cause for low serum ferritin in patients with restless legs syndrome. Sleep Med. 2009;10:763–5.
35. Moccia M, Pellecchia MT, Erro R, Zingone F, Marelli S, Barone DG, et al. Restless legs syndrome is a common feature of adult celiac disease. Mov Disord. 2010;25:877–81.
36. Weinstock LB, Walters AS, Mullin GE, Duntley SP. Celiac disease is associated with restless legs syndrome. Dig Dis Sci. 2010;55:1667–73.
37. Weinstock LB, Bosworth BP, Scherl EJ, Li E, Iroku U, Munsell MA, et al. Crohn's disease is associated with restless legs syndrome. Inflamm Bowel Dis. 2010;16:275–9.
38. Bassetti CL, Mauerhofer D, Gugger M, Mathis J, Hess CW. Restless legs syndrome: a clinical study of 55 patients. Eur Neurol. 2001;45:67–74.
39. Montplaisir J, Boucher S, Poirier G, Lavigne G, Lapierre O, Lesperance P. Clinical, polysomnographic, and genetic characteristics of restless legs syndrome: a study of 133 patients diagnosed with new standard criteria. Mov Disord. 1997;12:61–5.
40. Walters AS, Hickey K, Maltzman J, Verrico T, Joseph D, Hening W, et al. A questionnaire study of 138 patients with restless legs syndrome: the 'Night-Walkers' survey. Neurology. 1996;46:92–5.
41. Winkelmann J, Wetter TC, Collado-Seidel V, Gasser T, Dichgans M, Yassouridis A, et al. Clinical characteristics and frequency of the hereditary restless legs syndrome in a population of 300 patients. Sleep. 2000;23:597–602.
42. Winkelmann J, Muller-Myhsok B, Wittchen HU, Hock B, Prager M, Pfister H, et al. Complex segregation analysis of restless legs syndrome provides evidence for an autosomal dominant mode of inheritance in early age at onset families. Ann Neurol. 2002;52:297–302.
43. Mathias RA, Hening W, Washburn M, Allen RP, Lesage S, Wilson AF, et al. Segregation analysis of restless legs syndrome: possible evidence for a major gene in a family study using blinded diagnoses. Hum Hered. 2006;62:157–64.
44. Ondo WG, Vuong KD, Wang Q. Restless legs syndrome in monozygotic twins: clinical correlates. Neurology. 2000;55:1404–6.
45. Desai AV, Cherkas LF, Spector TD, Williams AJ. Genetic influences in self-reported symptoms of obstructive sleep apnoea and restless legs: a twin study. Twin Res. 2004;7:589–95.
46. Xiong L, Jang K, Montplaisir J, Levchenko A, Thibodeau P, Gaspar C, et al. Canadian restless legs syndrome twin study. Neurology. 2007;68:1631–3.
47. Walters AS, Wagner ML, Hening WA, Grasing K, Mills R, Chokroverty S, et al. Successful treatment of the idiopathic restless legs syndrome in a randomized double-blind trial of oxycodone versus placebo. Sleep. 1993;16:327–32.
48. Desautels A, Turecki G, Montplaisir J, Ftouhi-Paquin N, Michaud M, Chouinard VA, et al. Dopaminergic neurotransmission and restless legs syndrome: a genetic association analysis. Neurology. 2001;57:1304–6.
49. Kemlink D, Polo O, Montagna P, Provini F, Stiasny-Kolster K, Oertel W, et al. Family-based association study of the restless legs syndrome loci 2 and 3 in a European population. Mov Disord. 2007;22:207–12.
50. Kock N, Culjkovic B, Maniak S, Schilling K, Muller B, Zuhlke C, et al. Mode of inheritance and susceptibility locus for restless legs syndrome, on chromosome 12q. Am J Hum Genet. 2002;71:205–8. author reply 208.
51. Liebetanz KM, Winkelmann J, Trenkwalder C, Putz B, Dichgans M, Gasser T, et al. RLS3: fine-mapping of an autosomal dominant locus in a family with intrafamilial heterogeneity. Neurology. 2006;67:320–1.

52. Winkelmann J, Lichtner P, Putz B, Trenkwalder C, Hauk S, Meitinger T, et al. Evidence for further genetic locus heterogeneity and confirmation of RLS-1 in restless legs syndrome. Mov Disord. 2006;21:28–33.
53. Levchenko A, Provost S, Montplaisir JY, Xiong L, St-Onge J, Thibodeau P, et al. A novel autosomal dominant restless legs syndrome locus maps to chromosome 20p13. Neurology. 2006;67:900–1.
54. Levchenko A, Montplaisir JY, Asselin G, Provost S, Girard SL, Xiong L, et al. Autosomal-dominant locus for Restless Legs Syndrome in French-Canadians on chromosome 16p12.1. Mov Disord. 2009;24:40–50.
55. Desautels A, Turecki G, Montplaisir J, Sequeira A, Verner A, Rouleau GA. Identification of a major susceptibility locus for restless legs syndrome on chromosome 12q. Am J Hum Genet. 2001;69:1266–70.
56. Pichler I, Marroni F, Volpato CB, Gusella JF, Klein C, Casari G, et al. Linkage analysis identifies a novel locus for restless legs syndrome on chromosome 2q in a South Tyrolean population isolate. Am J Hum Genet. 2006;79:716–23.
57. Lohmann-Hedrich K, Neumann A, Kleensang A, Lohnau T, Muhle H, Djarmati A, et al. Evidence for linkage of restless legs syndrome to chromosome 9p: are there two distinct loci? Neurology. 2008;70:686–94.
58. Skehan EB, Abdulrahim MM, Parfrey NA, Hand CK. A novel locus for restless legs syndrome maps to chromosome 19p in an Irish pedigree. Neurogenetics. 2012;13:125–32.
59. Desautels A, Turecki G, Montplaisir J, Xiong L, Walters AS, Ehrenberg BL, et al. Restless legs syndrome: confirmation of linkage to chromosome 12q, genetic heterogeneity, and evidence of complexity. Arch Neurol. 2005;62:591–6.
60. Schulte EC, Winkelmann J. Family and genome-wide association studies of restless legs syndrome. In: Shaw P, Thorpy M, Tafti M, editors. Genetics of sleep and sleep disorders. Cambridge: Cambridge University Press; 2013.
61. Levchenko A, Montplaisir JY, Dube MP, Riviere JB, St-Onge J, Turecki G, et al. The 14q restless legs syndrome locus in the French Canadian population. Ann Neurol. 2004;55:887–91.
62. Pichler I, Schwienbacher C, Zanon A, Fuchsberger C, Serafin A, Facheris MF, et al. Fine-mapping of restless legs locus 4 (RLS4) identifies a haplotype over the SPATS2L and KCTD18 genes. J Mol Neurosci. 2013;49:600–5.
63. Weissbach A, Siegesmund K, Bruggemann N, Schmidt A, Kasten M, Pichler I, et al. Exome sequencing in a family with restless legs syndrome. Mov Disord. 2012;27:1686–9.
64. Oexle K, Schormair B, Ried JS, Czamara D, Heim K, Frauscher B, et al. Dilution of candidates: the case of iron-related genes in restless legs syndrome. Eur J Hum Genet. 2013;21:410–4.
65. Kemlink D, Polo O, Frauscher B, Gschliesser V, Hogl B, Poewe W, et al. Replication of restless legs syndrome loci in three European populations. J Med Genet. 2009;46:315–8.
66. Vilarino-Guell C, Farrer MJ, Lin SC. A genetic risk factor for periodic limb movements in sleep. N Engl J Med. 2008;358:425–7.
67. Yang Q, Li L, Chen Q, Foldvary-Schaefer N, Ondo WG, Wang QK. Association studies of variants in MEIS1, BTBD9, and MAP2K5/SKOR1 with restless legs syndrome in a US population. Sleep Med. 2011;12:800–4.
68. Schormair B, Plag J, Kaffe M, Gross N, Czamara D, Samtleben W, et al. MEIS1 and BTBD9: genetic association with restless leg syndrome in end stage renal disease. J Med Genet. 2011;48:462–6.
69. Stefansson H, Rye DB, Hicks A, Petursson H, Ingason A, Thorgeirsson TE, et al. A genetic risk factor for periodic limb movements in sleep. N Engl J Med. 2007;357:639–47.
70. Winkelmann J, Schormair B, Lichtner P, Ripke S, Xiong L, Jalilzadeh S, et al. Genome-wide association study of restless legs syndrome identifies common variants in three genomic regions. Nat Genet. 2007;39:1000–6.
71. Schormair B, Kemlink D, Roeske D, Eckstein G, Xiong L, Lichtner P, et al. PTPRD (protein tyrosine phosphatase receptor type delta) is associated with restless legs syndrome. Nat Genet. 2008;40:946–8.

72. Winkelmann J, Czamara D, Schormair B, Knauf F, Schulte EC, Trenkwalder C, et al. Genome-wide association study identifies novel restless legs syndrome susceptibility loci on 2p14 and 16q12.1. PLoS Genet. 2011;7:e1002171.
73. Kim MK, Cho YW, Shin WC, Cho JW, Shon YM, Kim JH, et al. Association of restless legs syndrome variants in Korean patients with restless legs syndrome. Sleep. 2013;36:1787–91.
74. Azcoitia V, Aracil M, Martinez AC, Torres M. The homeodomain protein Meis1 is essential for definitive hematopoiesis and vascular patterning in the mouse embryo. Dev Biol. 2005;280:307–20.
75. Wang Z, Iwasaki M, Ficara F, Lin C, Matheny C, Wong SH, et al. GSK-3 promotes conditional association of CREB and its coactivators with MEIS1 to facilitate HOX-mediated transcription and oncogenesis. Cancer Cell. 2010;17:597–608.
76. Maeda R, Mood K, Jones TL, Aruga J, Buchberg AM, Daar IO. Xmeis1, a protooncogene involved in specifying neural crest cell fate in Xenopus embryos. Oncogene. 2001;20:1329–42.
77. Mercader N, Leonardo E, Azpiazu N, Serrano A, Morata G, Martinez C, et al. Conserved regulation of proximodistal limb axis development by Meis1/Hth. Nature. 1999;402:425–9.
78. Dasen JS, Tice BC, Brenner-Morton S, Jessell TM. A Hox regulatory network establishes motor neuron pool identity and target-muscle connectivity. Cell. 2005;123:477–91.
79. Moskow JJ, Bullrich F, Huebner K, Daar IO, Buchberg AM. Meis1, a PBX1-related homeobox gene involved in myeloid leukemia in BXH-2 mice. Mol Cell Biol. 1995;15:5434–43.
80. Nakamura T, Largaespada DA, Shaughnessy Jr JD, Jenkins NA, Copeland NG. Cooperative activation of Hoxa and Pbx1-related genes in murine myeloid leukaemias. Nat Genet. 1996;12:149–53.
81. Stankunas K, Shang C, Twu KY, Kao SC, Jenkins NA, Copeland NG, et al. Pbx/Meis deficiencies demonstrate multigenetic origins of congenital heart disease. Circ Res. 2008;103:702–9.
82. Pfeufer A, van Noord C, Marciante KD, Arking DE, Larson MG, Smith AV, et al. Genome-wide association study of PR interval. Nat Genet. 2010;42:153–9.
83. Smith JG, Magnani JW, Palmer C, Meng YA, Soliman EZ, Musani SK, et al. Genome-wide association studies of the PR interval in African Americans. PLoS Genet. 2011;7:e1001304.
84. Hisa T, Spence SE, Rachel RA, Fujita M, Nakamura T, Ward JM, et al. Hematopoietic, angiogenic and eye defects in Meis1 mutant animals. EMBO J. 2004;23:450–9.
85. Spieler D, Kaffe M, Knauf F, Bessa J, Tena JJ, Giesert F, et al. Restless legs syndrome-associated intronic common variant in Meis1 alters enhancer function in the developing telencephalon. Genome Res. 2014;24:592–603.
86. N. G. E. S. P. (ESP). Exome variant server. 2012. Available: http://evs.gs.washington.edu/EVS/.
87. Schulte EC, Knauf F, Kemlink D, Schormair B, Lichtner P, Gieger C, et al. Variant screening of the coding regions of MEIS1 in patients with restless legs syndrome. Neurology. 2011;76:1106–8.
88. Vilarino-Guell C, Chai H, Keeling BH, Young JE, Rajput A, Lynch T, et al. MEIS1 p.R272H in familial restless legs syndrome. Neurology. 2009;73:243–5.
89. Xiong L, Catoire H, Dion P, Gaspar C, Lafreniere RG, Girard SL, et al. MEIS1 intronic risk haplotype associated with restless legs syndrome affects its mRNA and protein expression levels. Hum Mol Genet. 2009;18:1065–74.
90. Schulte EC, Kousi M, Tan PL, Tilch E, Knauf F, Lichtner P, et al. Targeted resequencing and systematic in vivo functional testing identifies rare variants in MEIS1 as significant contributors to restless legs syndrome. Am J Hum Genet. 2014;95:85–95.
91. Catoire H, Dion PA, Xiong L, Amari M, Gaudet R, Girard SL, et al. Restless legs syndrome-associated MEIS1 risk variant influences iron homeostasis. Ann Neurol. 2011;70:170–5.
92. Dinev D, Jordan BW, Neufeld B, Lee JD, Lindemann D, Rapp UR, et al. Extracellular signal regulated kinase 5 (ERK5) is required for the differentiation of muscle cells. EMBO Rep. 2001;2:829–34.
93. Cavanaugh JE, Jaumotte JD, Lakoski JM, Zigmond MJ. Neuroprotective role of ERK1/2 and ERK5 in a dopaminergic cell line under basal conditions and in response to oxidative stress. J Neurosci Res. 2006;84:1367–75.

94. Gross MK, Dottori M, Goulding M. Lbx1 specifies somatosensory association interneurons in the dorsal spinal cord. Neuron. 2002;34:535–49.
95. Schulte EC, Schramm K, Schurmann C, Lichtner P, Herder C, Roden M, et al. Blood cis-eQTL analysis fails to identify novel association signals among Sub-threshold candidates from genome-wide association studies in restless legs syndrome. PLoS One. 2014;9:e98092.
96. Godt D, Couderc JL, Cramton SE, Laski FA. Pattern formation in the limbs of Drosophila: bric a brac is expressed in both a gradient and a wave-like pattern and is required for specification and proper segmentation of the tarsus. Development. 1993;119:799–812.
97. Stogios PJ, Downs GS, Jauhal JJ, Nandra SK, Prive GG. Sequence and structural analysis of BTB domain proteins. Genome Biol. 2005;6:R82.
98. Lein ES, Hawrylycz MJ, Ao N, Ayres M, Bensinger A, Bernard A, et al. Genome-wide atlas of gene expression in the adult mouse brain. Nature. 2007;445:168–76.
99. Freeman A, Pranski E, Miller RD, Radmard S, Bernhard D, Jinnah HA, et al. Sleep fragmentation and motor restlessness in a drosophila model of restless legs syndrome. Curr Biol. 2012;22:1142–8.
100. DeAndrade MP, Zhang L, Doroodchi A, Yokoi F, Cheetham CC, Chen HX, et al. Enhanced hippocampal long-term potentiation and fear memory in Btbd9 mutant mice. PLoS One. 2012;7:e35518.
101. DeAndrade MP, Johnson Jr RL, Unger EL, Zhang L, van Groen T, Gamble KL, et al. Motor restlessness, sleep disturbances, thermal sensory alterations and elevated serum iron levels in Btbd9 mutant mice. Hum Mol Genet. 2012;21:3984–92.
102. Bachmann CG, Rolke R, Scheidt U, Stadelmann C, Sommer M, Pavlakovic G, et al. Thermal hypoaesthesia differentiates secondary restless legs syndrome associated with small fibre neuropathy from primary restless legs syndrome. Brain. 2010;133:762–70.
103. Jellen LC, Beard JL, Jones BC. Systems genetics analysis of iron regulation in the brain. Biochimie. 2009;91:1255–9.
104. Jones LC, Earley CJ, Allen RP, Jones BC. Of mice and men, periodic limb movements and iron: how the human genome informs the mouse genome. Genes Brain Behav. 2008;7:513–4.
105. Yuan SH, Qiu Z, Ghosh A. TOX3 regulates calcium-dependent transcription in neurons. Proc Natl Acad Sci U S A. 2009;106:2909–14.
106. Dittmer S, Kovacs Z, Yuan SH, Siszler G, Kogl M, Summer H, et al. TOX3 is a neuronal survival factor that induces transcription depending on the presence of CITED1 or phosphorylated CREB in the transcriptionally active complex. J Cell Sci. 2011;124:252–60.
107. Nord AS, Blow MJ, Attanasio C, Akiyama JA, Holt A, Hosseini R, et al. Rapid and pervasive changes in genome-wide enhancer usage during mammalian development. Cell. 2013;155:1521–31.
108. Easton DF, Pooley KA, Dunning AM, Pharoah PD, Thompson D, Ballinger DG, et al. Genome-wide association study identifies novel breast cancer susceptibility loci. Nature. 2007;447:1087–93.
109. Yang Q, Li L, Yang R, Shen GQ, Chen Q, Foldvary-Schaefer N, et al. Family-based and population-based association studies validate PTPRD as a risk factor for restless legs syndrome. Mov Disord. 2011;26:516–9.
110. Lin CH, Chen ML, Wu VC, Li WY, Sy HN, Wu SL, et al. Association of candidate genetic variants with restless legs syndrome in end stage renal disease: a multicenter case-control study in Taiwan. Eur J Neurol. 2014;21:492–8.
111. Pulido R, Krueger NX, Serra-Pages C, Saito H, Streuli M. Molecular characterization of the human transmembrane protein-tyrosine phosphatase delta. Evidence for tissue-specific expression of alternative human transmembrane protein-tyrosine phosphatase delta isoforms. J Biol Chem. 1995;270:6722–8.
112. Sato M, Takahashi K, Nagayama K, Arai Y, Ito N, Okada M, et al. Identification of chromosome arm 9p as the most frequent target of homozygous deletions in lung cancer. Genes Chromosomes Cancer. 2005;44:405–14.
113. Uetani N, Chagnon MJ, Kennedy TE, Iwakura Y, Tremblay ML. Mammalian motoneuron axon targeting requires receptor protein tyrosine phosphatases sigma and delta. J Neurosci. 2006;26:5872–80.

114. Malarstig A, Buil A, Souto JC, Clarke R, Blanco-Vaca F, Fontcuberta J, et al. Identification of ZNF366 and PTPRD as novel determinants of plasma homocysteine in a family-based genome-wide association study. Blood. 2009;114:1417–22.
115. Below JE, Gamazon ER, Morrison JV, Konkashbaev A, Pluzhnikov A, McKeigue PM, et al. Genome-wide association and meta-analysis in populations from Starr County, Texas, and Mexico City identify type 2 diabetes susceptibility loci and enrichment for expression quantitative trait loci in top signals. Diabetologia. 2011;54:2047–55.
116. Tsai FJ, Yang CF, Chen CC, Chuang LM, Lu CH, Chang CT, et al. A genome-wide association study identifies susceptibility variants for type 2 diabetes in Han Chinese. PLoS Genet. 2010;6:e1000847.
117. Saade S, Cazier JB, Ghassibe-Sabbagh M, Youhanna S, Badro DA, Kamatani Y, et al. Large scale association analysis identifies three susceptibility loci for coronary artery disease. PLoS One. 2011;6:e29427.
118. Walters AS, Rye DB. Review of the relationship of restless legs syndrome and periodic limb movements in sleep to hypertension, heart disease, and stroke. Sleep. 2009;32:589–97.
119. Molenaar JJ, Koster J, Zwijnenburg DA, van Sluis P, Valentijn LJ, van der Ploeg I, et al. Sequencing of neuroblastoma identifies chromothripsis and defects in neuritogenesis genes. Nature. 2012;483:589–93.
120. Stallings RL, Nair P, Maris JM, Catchpoole D, McDermott M, O'Meara A, et al. High-resolution analysis of chromosomal breakpoints and genomic instability identifies PTPRD as a candidate tumor suppressor gene in neuroblastoma. Cancer Res. 2006;66:3673–80.
121. Elia J, Gai X, Xie HM, Perin JC, Geiger E, Glessner JT, et al. Rare structural variants found in attention-deficit hyperactivity disorder are preferentially associated with neurodevelopmental genes. Mol Psychiatry. 2010;15:637–46.

Chapter 16
Genetics of Hereditary Spastic Paraplegias (HSP)

Rebecca Schüle and Ludger Schöls

Abstract Hereditary spastic paraplegias (HSP) are a group of degenerative disorders of the spinal cord that lead to a progressive spastic gait disturbance marked by lower limb spasticity and weakness. Genetically, HSPs are among the most heterogeneous Mendelian diseases and can be inherited following autosomal dominant, autosomal recessive, and X-chromosomal modes of inheritance. More than 80 genes and gene loci have been identified so far and require next-generation sequencing approaches for comprehensive genetic testing. In this chapter we discuss clinical aspects of HSP including differential diagnostics, typical presentation of common HSPs, limitations of genotype-phenotype correlation, and overlap with genetic disorders that cause progressive spasticity but are not categorized as HSP-like spastic ataxias, slow variants of amyotrophic lateral sclerosis, spastic variants of peripheral neuropathies, and adult-onset variants of leukodystrophies. In consideration of the complexity of this field, we propose an algorithm for a time- and cost-efficient strategy for genetic diagnostics in HSP.

Keywords Hereditary spastic paraplegia (HSP) • Spastic paraplegia gene (SPG) • Axonopathy • Upper motor neuron disease • Motor neuron degeneration

Clinical Characteristics of Hereditary Spastic Paraplegias

Hereditary spastic paraplegia (HSP) comprises a group of degenerative disorders of the spinal cord characterized by spastic gait, lower limb spasticity and weakness as clinical hallmarks. Frequently, additional signs of corticospinal tract dysfunction are

R. Schüle, MD (✉)
Department of Neurodegenerative Disease – Movement Disorder Genomics, University of Tübingen Center for Neurology, Tübingen 72076, Germany
e-mail: rebecca.schuele-freyer@uni-tuebingen.de

L. Schöls, MD (✉)
Department of Neurology and Hertie Institute for Clinical Brain Research, University of Tübingen, Tübingen 72076, Germany
e-mail: ludger.schoels@uni-tuebingen.de

S.A. Schneider, J.M.T. Brás (eds.), *Movement Disorder Genetics*,
DOI 10.1007/978-3-319-17223-1_16

present including increased muscle stretch reflexes, Babinski sign (extensor plantar response), and clonus. As a rule lower limbs are more severely and often earlier affected than the upper limbs, but electrophysiologically affection of the upper limbs can be demonstrated in about 1/3 of HSP patients [1]. HSP commonly also affects other long fiber tracts of the spinal cord like the dorsal columns and central tracts controlling bladder function, resulting in a decrease of the vibration sense and urge incontinence or bladder voiding. This complex of symptoms characterizes "pure" HSP [2]. In contrast, in "complicated" forms of HSP, additional parts of the nervous system are involved including the cerebrum, cerebellum, extrapyramidal circuits, peripheral nerves, and cranial nerves. This leads to "complicating" signs and symptoms like mental retardation, dementia, psychosis, epilepsy, ataxia, dysarthria, dysphagia, dystonia, parkinsonism, tremor, optic atrophy, retinopathy, hearing loss, sensory deficits (extending vibration sense), muscle wasting, and loss of reflexes. Rarely, non-neurological systems are affected, leading to cataract, diabetes mellitus, skin abnormalities, or gastroesophageal reflux as further complicating symptoms.

Due to its neurodegenerative nature, HSP is a slowly progressive disorder. Age of onset varies largely from congenital forms starting at birth to onset in the 7th or even 8th decade. Some genotypes typically go along with onset in the first decade, but age of onset can vary substantially even within genotypes. This is best documented for the most common genotype, SPG4, where onset may vary from the 1st year of life to the 8th decade even within one family carrying the same mutation. Similarly, progression of the disease is highly variable and may prevent walking from early childhood in the most severe cases. On the other hand, walking ability may be well-preserved for 50 years and more into the disease in other cases of HSP. Factors determining this high variability in age of onset and progression are only marginally understood as outlined in more detail in the genotype-phenotype paragraph below.

Prevalence estimates of HSP typically range between 4 and 10 per 100,000 [3, 4] but most likely underestimate the true prevalence due to misdiagnoses as the disease entity is not well known and the diagnosis of HSP can be proven only by genetic tools developed only recently.

Pre-genetic Diagnostic Workup

The core symptoms of HSP, spastic gait and spastic paraparesis, are unspecific features that may result from many different etiologies. Especially in the absence of a positive family history, HSP therefore remains a diagnosis of exclusion. Differential diagnosis of HSP thus requires a careful workup to exclude structural, inflammatory, metabolic, or other hereditary causes. MRI imaging of the brain and spinal cord is needed to exclude bilateral structural brain lesions (e.g., butterfly glioma) as well as spinal cord compression due to cervical or thoracic disk herniation, tumor, hemorrhage, or abscess. Additionally, malformations like meningomyelocele and tethered cord syndrome need to be excluded. Furthermore vascular disorders like spinal arteriovenous malformation should be considered. Metabolic disorders causing spasticity of the lower limbs include vitamin B12 and vitamin E deficiency and

Table 16.1 Differential workup of HSP

Diagnostic test	Differential diagnosis
Cranial MRI	Bilateral structural lesions
	Leukodystrophies
	Arnold-Chiari malformation
MRI of the spinal cord	Myelon compression due to cervical myelopathy and tumor
	Hemorrhage and abscess
	Arteriovenous malformation
	Myelomeningocele
	Tethered cord
	Syringomyelia
Blood tests	Vitamin B12 deficiency
	Very long-chain fatty acids (adrenomyeloneuropathy)
	Lysosomal enzymes incl. galactosylceramidase (Krabbe disease)
	TPHA (neurosyphilis)
	HTLV1 (tropical spastic paraparesis)
	HIV (AIDS)
Cerebrospinal fluid	Myelitis (cell count, oligoclonal bands)
Neurophysiology	
Motor evoked potentials	Amyotrophic lateral sclerosis
Nerve conduction studies	Primary lateral sclerosis
Electromyography	Spastic variants of Charcot-Marie-Tooth disease (HMSN type V)
Levodopa test	Dopamine-responsive dystonia (DRD)

copper deficiency as well as lysosomal storage disorders. Some of the latter may even manifest late in adulthood and can present with rather unremarkable brain MRIs like adrenomyeloneuropathy or Krabbe disease [5]. Inflammatory disorders resembling HSP include multiple sclerosis as well as (para)infectious myelitis (*Treponema pallidum*, HIV, HTLV1/2). Additionally, a number of other hereditary neurodegenerative diseases can present with HSP-like phenotypes, including some forms of hereditary ataxias, Charcot-Marie-Tooth disease (CMT), amyotrophic lateral sclerosis (ALS), and dopamine-responsive dystonia (DRD). We will devote a later paragraph of this chapter to these hereditary HSP mimics.

A suggestion for the differential workup of HSP is given in Table 16.1.

Genetic Subtypes of HSP

Hereditary Spastic Paraplegia Genes (SPG 1–72)

HSPs are among the most heterogeneous Mendelian diseases and can be inherited following autosomal-dominant, autosomal-recessive, and X-chromosomal modes of inheritance. Additionally almost half of all cases are apparently sporadic, and it is currently unknown whether these forms are also monogenetic in origin or whether they have more complex disease etiologies.

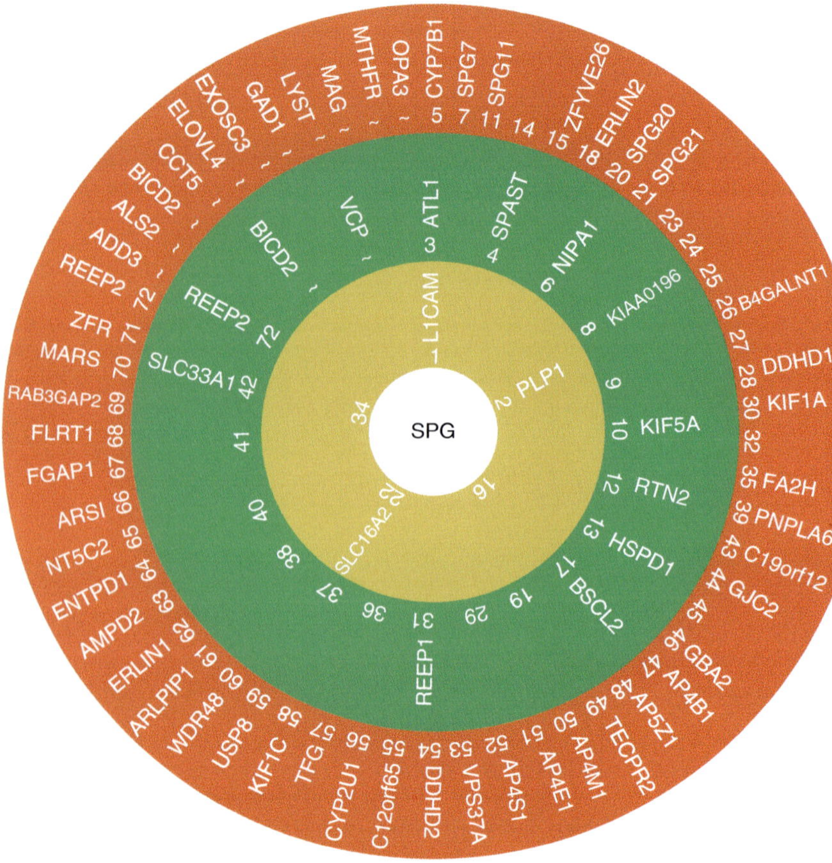
SPG
1 L1CAM
2 PLP1
16
22 SLC16A2
34
3 ATL1
4 SPAST
6 NIPA1
8 KIAA0196
9
10 KIF5A
12 RTN2
13 HSPD1
17 BSCL2
19
29
31 REEP1
36
37
38
40
41
42 SLC33A1
72 REEP2
~ BICD2
~ VCP
5 CYP7B1
7 SPG7
11 SPG11
14
15 ZFYVE26
18 ERLIN2
20 SPG20
21 SPG21
23
24
25
26 B4GALNT1
27
28 DDHD1
30 KIF1A
32
35 FA2H
39 PNPLA6
43 C19orf12
44 GJC2
45
46 GBA2
47 AP4B1
48 AP5Z1
49 TECPR2
50 AP4M1
51 AP4E1
52 AP4S1
53 VPS37A
54 DDHD2
55 C12orf65
56 CYP2U1
57 TFG
58 KIF1C
59 USP8
60 WDR48
61 ARLPIP1
62 ERLIN1
63 AMPD2
64 ENTPD1
65 NT5C2
66 ARSI
67 FGAP1
68 FLRT1
69 RAB3GAP2
70 MARS
71 ZFR
72 REEP2
~ ADD3
~ ALS2
~ BICD2
~ CCT5
~ ELOVL4
~ EXOSC3
~ GAD1
~ LYST
~ MAG
~ MTHFR
~ OPA3

Fig. 16.1 HSP genes

Currently there are at least 83 HSP loci and 68 HSP genes known, about three quarters of which have been identified within the past 5 years (Fig. 16.1) [6]. HSP loci are termed SPG 1–72 (SPG = spastic paraplegia gene) according to the HUGO gene nomenclature committee; however, not all HSP genes have received an SPG number.

Autosomal-Dominant HSP

About 40 % of HSP cases report an autosomal-dominant family history with affected family members in at least two generations. Mutations in any of the known 13 autosomal-dominant HSP genes explain about 70 % of dominant cases (Table 16.2).

SPG4, caused by mutations in the *SPAST* gene, accounts for roughly 50 % of autosomal-dominant HSP families and is by far the most common subtype of

Table 16.2 Autosomal-dominant HSP genes and phenotypes

				Phenotype				
Locus	Gene	Frequency	Mutation types	Age of onset	Typical presentation	Rare manifestations	MRI	Reference
SPG3	*ATL1*	6 % AD HSP Up to 39 % with onset in childhood	Missense, truncating Some cases with incomplete penetrance. Some de novo mutations	Childhood (rare: up to 5th decade)	Pure, slow progression	Distal amyotrophy (Silver syndrome), optic atrophy	Normal	[7, 8]
SPG4	*SPAST*	40–50 % AD HSP	Missense, truncating, splice site, indels, (multi)-exonic deletion or duplication Disease modifiers: c.334G>A and c.1157A>G. Some cases with incomplete penetrance	1st–8th decade. Intrafamilial variability can be considerable	Pure	Dementia, cerebellar ataxia, hand tremor, neuropathy, seizures	Most cases: normal cranial MRI Mild cerebellar and spinal cord atrophy, white matter lesions or thinning of corpus callosum may occur	[9, 10]
SPG6	*NIPA1*	< 1 % HSP	Missense	1st–4th decade	Pure	Epilepsy, neuropathy	Normal	[11]
SPG8	*KIAA0196*	Up to 4 % AD HSP	Missense	2nd–6th decade	Pure, frequent progression to wheelchair dependence	Distal amyotrophy	Brain normal, atrophy of the thoracic spinal cord	[12]
SPG10	*KIF5A*	3 % of AD HSP	Missense in kinesin motor domain	1st–6th decade	HSP with (subclinical) neuropathy	Cognitive impairment, parkinsonism, Silver syndrome, deafness, retinitis pigmentosa	Normal	[13, 14]

(continued)

Table 16.2 (continued)

				Phenotype				
Locus	Gene	Frequency	Mutation types	Age of onset	Typical presentation	Rare manifestations	MRI	Reference
SPG12	*RTN2*	Rare	Missense, truncating, gene deletion	1st–4th decade	Pure		Brain normal, atrophy of the spinal cord	[15]
SPG13	*HSPD1*	Rare	Missense	2nd–7th decade	Pure	Allelic disease: AR: hypomyelinating leukodystrophy		[16]
SPG17	*BSCL2*	Rare, about 30 families published	2 missense mutations in exon 3	2nd decade (range: 1st–7th decade), incomplete penetrance	Pure HSP or Silver syndrome (HSP with amyotrophy of intrinsic hand muscles)	Allelic diseases AD: Charcot-Marie-Tooth disease type 2, distal hereditary motor neuropathy (dHMN) type V AR: Berardinelli-Seip congenital lipodystrophy type 2	Brain normal, atrophy of the spinal cord	[17]
SPG31	*REEP1*	3 % HSP 8 % pure HSP 7 % AD HSP negative for SPG4	Missense, truncating, splice site, indels, 3'-UTR, (multi)-exonic duplication	1st–8th decade	Pure	Neuropathy, Silver syndrome, cerebellar ataxia, tremor, dementia	Normal	

(SPG33)	*ZFYVE27*	1 family	Missense, but allele frequency of G191V > 1‰ in controls	50	Pure			[18]
SPG42	*SLC33A1*	1 family	Missense. Incomplete penetrance	1st–5th decade	Pure	Muscle wasting in lower limbs	Normal	[19]
SPG72	*REEP2*	2 families	AD + AR inheritance! Missense, splice site	Childhood	Pure			[20]

HSP. SPG4 is characterized by a variable age at onset ranging from early childhood to the 8th decade even within families sharing the same mutation, with a mean age at onset of just over 30 years of age. The majority of SPG4 cases have pure HSP with rather frequent neurogenic bladder disturbance (~70 %) and affection of the dorsal columns (~50 %). Motor evoked potentials are often normal even when there is clinically definite involvement of the corticospinal tracts [1]. Some cases with complicated SPG4 have been reported that feature cognitive deficits, upper limb involvement, thin corpus callosum, or other complicating signs and symptoms. Mutation types in SPG4 included missense, nonsense and splice site mutations, small insertions and deletions, and large genomic deletions. It is important to note that the latter mutations, which account for about one fifth of SPG4 cases, cannot usually be detected by Sanger sequencing. State-of-the-art diagnostic testing in SPG4 therefore needs to include a method to screen for macro-deletions like multiplex ligation-dependent probe amplification (MLPA) [9].

SPG3 typically presents as childhood-onset (<10 years) pure HSP with very slow progression and may be equally common as SPG4 in this age group. However cases with an onset as late as the 5th decade have been reported [21]. In adult-onset cases, SPG3 contributes less than 10 %. The phenotypic spectrum of SPG3 is broad and also involves very severe childhood-onset cases with pseudobulbar palsy, severe tetraparesis, motor axonal neuropathy and variably cognitive impairment, TCC, or optic atrophy. Furthermore ATL1 mutation also causes hereditary sensory neuropathy I (HSN1D), a severe mutilating sensory axonal neuropathy. Missense mutations in ATL1 are the predominant mutation type in both SPG3 and HSN1D.

SPG10 (KIF5A) and *SPG31* (REEP1) both contribute about 5–10 % to SPG4-negative autosomal-dominant HSPs. With a broad age-at-onset spectrum reaching from childhood to late adulthood, they can both manifest as pure or variably complicated HSP. In SPG10, amyotrophy and cognitive deficits are the most frequent complicating features, and most patients with complicated SPG10 feature an axonal sensorimotor peripheral neuropathy. Additionally parkinsonism, deafness, and retinitis pigmentosa have been described in single cases. SPG31 can present with a Silver syndrome-like phenotype with severe hand muscle atrophy and axonal peripheral neuropathy; occurrence of both pure and complicated phenotypes within the same family has been reported.

Autosomal-Recessive HSP

With at least 52 known genes, autosomal-recessive HSP are extremely genetically heterogeneous, and most recessive HSP genes explain less than 1 % of cases (Table 16.3). Among the autosomal-recessive HSP subtypes that can present as pure HSP, SPG5 and SPG7 are the most common although both forms can also be complicated by additional symptoms.

SPG5 accounts for about 16 % of pure autosomal-recessive HSPs [22]. SPG5 mutation carriers develop the first symptoms in early adolescence (range early

Table 16.3 Autosomal-recessive HSP genes and phenotypes

Locus	Gene	Frequency	Mutation types	Phenotype				Reference
				Age of onset	Typical presentation	Rare manifestations	MRI	
SPG5	*CYP7B1*	16 % pure AR HSP ~3 % S HSP	Missense, truncating	Childhood–adulthood	Pure or complicated (afferent ataxia, optic atrophy)	Behavioral abnormalities	Normal or white matter changes and cerebellar vermian atrophy	[22, 23]
SPG7	*SPG7*	1.5–7 % S/AR HSP	Missense, truncating	Adulthood	Pure or complicated (cerebellar ataxia, optic atrophy)	Upper limb involvement, supranuclear gaze palsy, cognitive deficits	Normal or cerebellar atrophy	[24]
SPG11	*SPG11*	~20 % AR HSP	Truncating	Adolescence	Complicated (cognitive deficits, dysarthria, amyotrophy, axonal sensorimotor neuropathy)	Cerebellar ataxia, parkinsonism, ALS-like phenotype	TCC, white matter changes, cortical atrophy	[25]
SPG15	*ZFYVE25*	<3 % AR HSP	Truncating	Adolescence	Complicated (cognitive deficits, dysarthria, amyotrophy, axonal sensorimotor neuropathy; Kjellin syndrome (pigmentary maculopathy)	Parkinsonism, Kjellin syndrome (pigmentary maculopathy)	TCC, white matter changes, cortical atrophy	[26]
SPG18	*ERLIN2*	Rare	Truncating	Childhood	Complicated (severe cognitive impairment, dysarthria, contractures)		Normal	[27]
SPG20	*SPG20*	Frequent in Old Order Amish population	Truncating	Infancy/childhood	Troyer syndrome: complicated (mild cognitive impairment, dysarthria, distal amyotrophy, short stature)		White matter changes	[28]

(continued)

Table 16.3 (continued)

Locus	Gene	Frequency	Mutation types	Phenotype: Age of onset	Phenotype: Typical presentation	Phenotype: Rare manifestations	Phenotype: MRI	Reference
SPG21	*SPG21*	Frequent in Old Order Amish population	Missense, truncating	Adolescence/ adulthood	Mast syndrome: complicated (severe cognitive impairment, psychosis, dysarthria, cerebellar dysfunction)		Thin corpus callosum, cortical and cerebellar atrophy, white matter changes	[29]
SPG26	*B4GALNT1*	Rare	Truncating >> missense	Childhood/ adolescence	Complicated (cognitive deficits, cerebellar ataxia, dysarthria, peripheral neuropathy) Early disease onset, mental retardation, slow progression with additional variability like ataxia, peripheral neuropathy, and extrapyramidal features	Psychosis, autism, cataract, amyotrophy	Cortical atrophy, white matter changes	[30]
SPG28	*DDHD1*	Rare	Truncating	Adolescence	Pure	Cerebellar signs, axonal neuropathy	Normal	[31]
SPG30	*KIF1A*	Rare	Missense	Adolescence/ young adulthood	Complicated (peripheral neuropathy, mild cerebellar ataxia) Allelic disorders: HSAN (caused by truncating mutations)		Cerebellar atrophy	[32]
SPG35/ FAHN	*FA2H*	1–2 % AR/S HSP	Missense, truncating	Childhood–adulthood	Complicated (cognitive impairment, optic atrophy, ophthalmoplegia, dysarthria, cerebellar ataxia, seizures, dystonia) Allelic disorders: NBIA, leukodystrophy		Iron deposition in the globus pallidus, TCC, white matter changes, cerebral and cerebellar atrophy	[33]

SPG39	*PNPLA6*	Rare	Missense > truncating	Childhood/ adolescence	Complicated (cerebellar ataxia, motor neuropathy) Allelic disorders: Gordon-Holmes syndrome, Boucher-Neuhäuser syndrome		Cerebellar atrophy	[34]
SPG43/ MPAN	*C19orf12*	Rare	Missense, in-frame deletions	Childhood	Complicated (optic atrophy, psychiatric symptoms, extrapyramidal involvement (dystonia, parkinsonism, peripheral neuropathy)	ALS-like phenotype	Iron deposition in the globus pallidus and substantia nigra	[35]
SPG44	*GJC2*	Rare	Missense	Adulthood	Complicated (dysarthria, cerebellar ataxia, mild cognitive impairment) Allelic disorders: Pelizaeus-Merzbacher-like disease	Hearing loss, seizures	Hypomyelination	[36]
SPG46	*GBA2*	Rare	Truncating > missense	Adolescence/ adulthood	Complicated (cerebellar ataxia, cognitive deficits, cataract, axonal neuropathy)	Hearing loss, testicular hypotrophy, dystonia, external ophthalmoparesis	TCC, cerebral and cerebellar atrophy, hummingbird sign (midbrain atrophy)	[37, 38]
SPG47	*AP4B1*	Rare	Truncating	Infancy	Complicated (severe cognitive deficits, epilepsy, neonatal hypotonia, microcephaly, short stature		TCC, white matter changes	[39, 40]
SPG48	*AP5Z1*	Rare	Truncating	Infancy to adulthood	Pure or complicated (cognitive deficits)		Normal or TCC, white matter changes	[41]

(continued)

Table 16.3 (continued)

Locus	Gene	Frequency	Mutation types	Phenotype				Reference
				Age of onset	Typical presentation	Rare manifestations	MRI	
SPG49	*TECPR2*	Rare	Truncating	Infancy	Complicated (severe cognitive deficits, seizures, dysarthria, spastic tetraparesis, gastroesophageal reflux, short stature, dysmorphic features		TCC, cerebellar vermian atrophy, cortical atrophy	[42]
SPG50	*AP4M1*	Rare	Truncating	Infancy	Complicated (severe cognitive deficits, neonatal hypotonia, microcephaly, short stature)		White matter changes, cerebellar atrophy	[39]
SPG51	*AP4E1*	Rare	Truncating		Complicated (severe cognitive deficits, epilepsy, neonatal hypotonia, microcephaly, short stature)		White matter changes, cerebellar atrophy	[39, 43]
SPG52	*AP4S1*	Rare	Truncating	Infancy	Complicated (severe cognitive deficits, neonatal hypotonia, microcephaly, short stature)		Unknown	[39]
SPG53	*VPS37A*	Rare	Missense	Infancy	Complicated (cognitive deficits, spastic tetraparesis, kyphosis)	Hearing impairment	Normal	[44]
SPG54	*DDHD2*	Rare	Truncating >> missense	Childhood	Complicated (cognitive deficits, dysarthria, dysphagia, short stature)	Optic atrophy, saccadic eye pursuit, facial dysmorphism	TCC, white matter changes	[45, 46]
SPG55	*C12orf65*	Rare	Truncating	Childhood	Complicated (optic atrophy, peripheral neuropathy)		Normal	[47–49]

SPG56	*CYP2U1*	Rare	Missense, truncating	Infancy to childhood	Pure or complicated (cognitive deficits, dystonia, axonal neuropathy)		Normal or TCC and white matter changes, globus pallidus hypointensities	[31]
SPG57	*TFG*	1 family	Missense	Infancy	Complicated (optic atrophy, neuropathy)		Normal	[50]
SPG58	*KIF1C*	Rare	Missense, truncating	Infancy to adulthood	Complicated (cerebellar ataxia, extrapyramidal involvement (dystonia, chorea), demyelinating peripheral neuropathy)	Mild cognitive deficits, hypodontia, deafness Mild dominant phenotype!	White matter changes, cerebral and vermian cerebellar atrophy	[6, 51]
SPG59	*USP8*	1 family	Missense	Infancy	Pure	Nystagmus, mild cognitive deficits	Normal	[6]
SPG60	*WDR48*	1 family	In-frame deletion	Infancy	Complicated (mild cognitive deficits, nystagmus, peripheral neuropathy)		Normal	[6]
SPG61	*ARL6IP1*	1 family	Truncating	Infancy	Complicated (mutilating acropathy, sensorimotor neuropathy)		Normal	[6]
SPG62	*ERLIN1*	Rare	Missense, truncating	Childhood	Pure	Amyotrophy, mild cognitive deficits	Normal	[6]
SPG63	*AMPD2*	1 family	Truncating	Infancy	Pure	Short stature, amyotrophy	TCC, white matter changes	[6]

(continued)

Table 16.3 (continued)

Locus	Gene	Frequency	Mutation types	Phenotype: Age of onset	Phenotype: Typical presentation	Phenotype: Rare manifestations	Phenotype: MRI	Reference
SPG64	*ENTPD1*	Rare	Missense, truncating	Infancy	Complicated (cognitive deficits)	Behavioral abnormalities, cataracts	White matter changes	[6]
SPG65	*NT5C2*	Rare	Truncating	Infancy	Complicated (mild cognitive deficits)	Optic atrophy, amyotrophy, short stature	TCC +/– mild white matter changes	[6]
SPG66	*ARSI*	1 family	Truncating	Infancy	Complicated (mild cognitive deficits, severe sensorimotor peripheral neuropathy)		TCC, cerebellar hypoplasia, colpocephaly	[6]
SPG67	*PGAP1*	1 family	Truncating	Infancy	Complicated (cognitive deficits, amyotrophy)		TCC, hypoplasia of cerebellar vermis, hypomyelination	[6]
SPG68	*FLRT1*	1 family	Stop loss	infancy	Complicated (nystagmus, optic atrophy, peripheral neuropathy)		Normal	[6]
SPG69	*RAB3GAP2*	1 family	Truncating	Infancy	Complicated (dysarthria, deafness, congenital cataract)		Normal	[6]
SPG70	*MARS*	1 family	Missense	Infancy	Complicated (cognitive deficits, amyotrophy)	Cerebellar signs, nephrotic syndrome	n.a.	[6]
SPG71	*ZFR*	1 family	Missense	Infancy	Pure	–	TCC	[6]

n.a. not available; rare, frequency <1 %, *MPAN* mitochondrial membrane-associated neurodegeneration childhood–4th decade). SPG5 is characterized by frequent and rather severe dorsal column affection with loss of vibration and joint position sense in the lower limbs and gait ataxia. Evoked potentials with prolonged latencies or absent cortical potentials indicate widespread but often subclinical central involvement; the peripheral nervous system as a rule is not involved in SPG5. MRIs can be normal or show pancerebellar atrophy and white matter changes especially at later disease stages. SPG5 is caused by loss-of-function mutation in the 7α-hydroxylase gene *CYP7B1*, implicating cholesterol metabolism in the pathogenesis of HSP.

SPG7 can present as either pure or complicated adult-onset (mean ~30 years) HSP with mostly slow progression. Complicated cases commonly present with cerebellar ataxia, cerebellar atrophy, or both. Additional complicating features include optic atrophy, at least subclinically present in the majority of cases [52] and axonal peripheral neuropathy. Mitochondrial phenotypes with external ophthalmoplegia, dysphagia, and proximal myopathy in addition to spastic paraplegia or spastic ataxia have also been repeatedly reported, and indeed clonal expansion of mitochondrial DNA mutations was identified in these cases [53] [54].

SPG11 and SPG15 present with a rather characteristic phenotype and are clinically indistinguishable from each other. Core features that are present in the majority of patients with SPG11 and SPG15 comprise lower-limb-predominant spastic tetraparesis with pseudobulbar dysarthria, severe Silver syndrome-like hand muscle atrophy, moderate cognitive impairment and thin corpus callosum (TCC), white matter changes, and cortical atrophy on MRI [55, 56]. Additionally, extrapyramidal motor involvement (parkinsonism, dystonia), cerebellar ataxia, and sensorimotor peripheral neuropathy have been described among other more rare manifestations. SPG11 mutations that cause typical complicated HSP have also been found to cause a juvenile-onset form of autosomal-recessive ALS [57].

Although numerous recessive HSP genes can cause an SPG11-like phenotype or at least components of the phenotypic spectrum (e.g., SPG21, SPG35, SPG46, SPG48, SPG54, and many others), SPG11 is by far the most common gene in this constellation and explains about two thirds of recessive patients with spastic paraplegia accompanied by cognitive deficits and TCC. SPG15 is considerably rarer and accounts for about 3 % of cases with this phenotype.

The mutation mechanism in SPG11 and SPG15 is loss of function. Accordingly, all mutations in these two genes that have been linked to HSP or ALS are truncating changes including nonsense mutations, splice mutations, and small insertions or deletions. Due to the large size of both genes, missense mutations are a rather frequent incidental finding, but pathogenicity of those has not been established so far.

X-Linked HSP

Only three X-chromosomal HSP genes have been described so far: *L1CAM*, *PLP1*, and *SLC16A2*. They all cause complicated forms of HSP, the phenotypic details of which are listed in Table 16.4. Some PLP1 mutations, especially when leading to

Table 16.4 X-chromosomal HSP genes and phenotypes

Locus	Gene/ protein	Frequency	Mutation types	Phenotype				Reference
				Age of onset	Typical presentation	Rare manifestations	MRI	
SPG1	L1CAM	Unknown. Predictive value of adducted thumbs: 50 %	Missense, nonsense, splice site, indels, (multi)-exonic deletion or duplication	Infancy	Phenotypic spectrum: SPG1, spastic paraplegia with moderate cognitive impairment MASA[a] CRASH[b] HSAS[c]	Association with Hirschsprung's disease	Variable Normal Hydrocephalus Corpus callosum dysplasia Cerebellar hypoplasia Bilateral absence of the pyramids	[58]
SPG2	PLP1	Unknown	Majority: duplication, deletion of whole gene or exons ~30 %: missense, nonsense, splice site, indels	Childhood (up to 4th decade)	Phenotypic spectrum: SPG2, uncomplicated spastic paraplegia Pelizaeus-Merzbacher disease (PMD): nystagmus, initial hypotonia, spastic quadriparesis, ataxia, cognitive impairment	Dystonia, athetosis, neuropathy Female carriers may manifest mild to moderate signs	Variable Normal (SPG2) Diffuse T2-hyperintense leukoencephalopathy (PMD) +/– thin corpus callosum	[59]

SPG22	SLC16A2	Unknown, > 100 families reported	Missense, nonsense, frameshift, (multi)- exonic deletions	Infancy	Allan-Herndon-Dudley syndrome: severe mental retardation, dysarthric or absent speech, central hypotonia with poor head control, spastic quadriplegia Increased serum triiodothyronine (T3), low thyroxine (T4)	Ataxia, dystonic and athetoid movements	Hypomyelination improving with age	[60, 61]

[a]*MASA* mental retardation, adducted thumbs, shuffling gait, and aphasia
[b]*CRASH* syndrome: corpus callosum hypoplasia, retardation, adducted thumbs, spastic paraplegia, and hydrocephalus
[c]*HSAS* hydrocephalus with stenosis of the aqueduct of Sylvius

the absence of the protein or affecting certain *PLP1*-specific domains, lead to less severe or even pure phenotypes. Women carrying *PLP1* mutations are rather commonly affected with a mild carrier phenotype.

Apparently Sporadic HSP

Data on the genetic background of apparently sporadic cases of hereditary spastic paraplegia is extremely sparse. We know from systematic screenings of the SPG4 and SPG7 genes and from our own experience with large HSP patient cohorts (GeNeMove cohort) that at least a subset of apparently sporadic cases is caused by mutations in autosomal or X-chromosomal HSP genes. SPG4 has been found in 6–12 % of sporadic HSP cases [62, 63]; de novo mutations as well as reduced penetrance explain the lack of positive family history in some of these cases. Mutations in SPG7 occur in about 4–7 % of sporadic HSPs, [64]. In 31 sporadic adult-onset upper motor neuron disease cases, a single REEP1 variant was identified [65]. For the other HSP genes, systematic studies in sporadic cohorts are lacking. In our own cohort (GeNeMove cohort, 228 sporadic HSP cases), SPG5 and SPG11 each contribute about 3 %, and about 75 % of cases remain genetically unsolved. Increasing availability of high-throughput screening methods like whole-exome sequencing and panel testing will hopefully clarify the contribution of Mendelian inheritance patterns to sporadic HSP within the next few years.

Overlapping Phenotypes

Hereditary Ataxias with Spasticity

Spastic ataxias are an increasingly recognized group of hereditary disorders, which combine core features of both groups, hereditary spastic paraplegias and hereditary ataxias. Some of them like SPG7 have been classified as spastic paraplegias and consequently received a SPG number, whereas others were primarily regarded as ataxic disorders. The most prevalent ataxia subtypes that can go along with prominent spasticity are Friedreich's ataxia (FRDA), autosomal-recessive ataxia of Charlevoix-Saguenay (ARSACS), and spinocerebellar ataxias type 1, type 3, and type 7 (SCA1, SCA3, SCA7) (Table 16.5) (also see Chaps. 11 and 12). FRDA is the most common autosomal-recessive ataxia in the Western world. Typically, FRDA presents with afferent ataxia due to degeneration of the dorsal root ganglia. Dorsal root ganglia degeneration also results in loss of stretch reflexes in most patients and suppresses spasticity despite severe degeneration of the corticospinal tract in almost all patients. However, some patients, especially adult-onset cases, have increased reflexes and prominent spasticity [66].

Table 16.5 Overlapping genes and phenotypes

Locus	Gene/ protein	Mode of inheritance	Age of onset	Phenotype	MRI features
Hereditary ataxias					
SCA1[a]	ATXN1	AD	30–40 years (range: 1st–8th decade)	Cerebellar ataxia +/– spasticity	Cerebellar and pontine atrophy
SCA3[a]	ATXN3	AD	30–40 years (range: 1st–8th decade)	Cerebellar ataxia +/– spasticity +/– neuropathy +/– dystonia +/– parkinsonism	Cerebellar and pontine atrophy
SCA7[a]	ATXN7	AD	30–40 years (range: 1st–8th decade)	Cerebellar ataxia, macular degeneration, spasticity	Cerebellar and pontine atrophy
ARSACS[b]	SACS	AR	1–20 years	Spastic ataxia, neuropathy	Cerebellar atrophy. Hypointense stripes in the central pons
Friedreich ataxia	FXN	AR	~ Puberty (range 3–70 years)	Afferent ataxia, sensory neuropathy, corticospinal tract degeneration +/– diabetes +/– ardiomyopathy	Spinal cord atrophy
Hereditary neuropathies/Charcot-Marie-Tooth disease with spasticity					
CMT2A	MFN2	AD, (AR)	Childhood–adulthood	Axonal neuropathy, optic atrophy, pyramidal signs	Normal
HSAN2B	FAM134B	AR	Childhood–adulthood	Axonal neuropathy with mutilating acropathy	Normal
CMTX1	GJB1	XR	Infancy/childhood	Axonal-demyelinating neuropathy, rarely CNS involvement, hearing loss	Normal
Slowly progressive amyotrophic lateral sclerosis (ALS)					
IAHSP	ALS2	AR	Infancy/childhood	Ascending spastic tetraparesis, pseudobulbar palsy	Normal or cortical atrophy
ALS12	OPTN	AR/AD	4th–6th decade	Slowly progressive ALS	Normal

(continued)

Table 16.5 (continued)

Locus	Gene/ protein	Mode of inheritance	Age of onset	Phenotype	MRI features
VCP	VCP	AD	6th decade	Complicated HSP (Paget's disease of the bone) Allelic disease: frontotemporal dementia, inclusion body myopathy and Paget's disease of the bone (IBMPFD), ALS with or without frontotemporal dementia	Normal
Adult-onset leukodystrophies					
Krabbe disease	GALC	AR	Up to 7th decade	Spasticity > neuropathy (demyelinating) >> ataxia, dysarthria	Mild white matter hyperintensities of the corticospinal tract that may extend to optic radiation and posterior parts of the corpus callosum
X-linked adrenoleukodystrophy/ adrenomyeloneuropathy	ABCD1	X-linked	Up to 7th decade (especially in female carriers)	Spasticity > ataxia, bladder disturbance, neuropathy. Adrenal dysfunction in males. Cognitive impairment restricted to cerebral form	Normal. Mild cerebellar atrophy may occur. White matter lesions indicate conversion into cerebral form
Alexander disease	GFAP	AD	Up to 8th decade	Bulbar dysfunction (dysarthria, dysphagia), spasticity, cerebellar ataxia, palatal myoclonus	Atrophy and T2-hyperintensities of the medulla oblongata. Spinal cord atrophy
Dopa-responsive dystonias					
AD DRD	GCH1	AD	Usually childhood, rarely adulthood	Focal or generalized dystonia, parkinsonism, diurnal fluctuation, L-dopa responsive	Normal

AR DRD	TH	AR	1st decade	1. Progressive hypokinetic rigid syndrome, generalized dystonia, good response to L-dopa	Normal
				2. Complex encephalopathy, autonomic disturbances, limited response to L-dopa, hyperphenylalaninemia	
AR DRD	*SPR*	AR	1st decade	Dystonia, cognitive deficits, seizures, variably oculomotor apraxia, chorea, and other movement disorders	Normal

[a]*SCA1* spinocerebellar ataxia type 1
[b]*ARSACS* autosomal-recessive spastic ataxia type Charlevoix-Saguenay

ARSACS is not restricted to the Quebec region where it has been described originally but is a rather common type of recessive ataxia worldwide. ARSACS shows a rather characteristic combination of spasticity, cerebellar ataxia, peripheral neuropathy, and streaky T2 hypodensities of the central pons on MRI [67].

SCA1, SCA3, and SCA7 are autosomal dominantly inherited ataxias caused by CAG trinucleotide repeat expansions in coding regions of the respective genes. Clinical features accompanying ataxia are variable including slowing of saccadic eye movements, spasticity and peripheral neuropathy, and in the case of SCA7 characteristic retinal degeneration. Typical findings on MRI include cerebellar and pontine atrophy [68].

Hereditary Neuropathies/Charcot-Marie-Tooth Disease with Spasticity

When a lower limb pyramidal syndrome occurs in combination with peripheral nerve involvement, it can be clinically impossible to draw a clear line between complicated HSP and Charcot-Marie-Tooth disease (CMT), and this diagnostic line might even be crossed within a family. There are a number of HSPs that are known to sometimes cause CMT-like phenotypes, including SPG17 (*BSCL2*), *BICD2-related* HSP, SPG3, complicated forms of SPG10 and SPG31, SPG39, and others. On the flip side, there are some forms of CMT that are frequently associated with spasticity and therefore need to be considered in the differential diagnosis of HSP. Mutations in the outer mitochondrial membrane GTPase *MFN2* are the most common cause of axonal CMT (~20 %) and are frequently accompanied by optic atrophy, vocal cord paralysis, and pyramidal features. *CCT5* mutations cause sensory neuropathy with spastic paraplegia and a childhood-onset autosomal-recessive disorder with severe mutilating acropathy; *FAM134B* mutations can be associated with a similar phenotype. X-linked CMT1X, caused by mutations in *GJB1*, typically presents with sensorimotor peripheral neuropathy, cerebellar ataxia, and spastic paraparesis or tetraparesis. Rarely, pyramidal features can be associated with dominant mutations in *DYNC1H1* and *NEFL*.

Slowly Progressive Amyotrophic Lateral Sclerosis (ALS)

Amyotrophic lateral sclerosis (ALS) and HSPs naturally share a great deal of clinical overlap, and it is especially the slowly progressive, upper motor neuron (UMN)-predominant forms of ALS that can present clinically with an HSP-like phenotype. Just as there are some genetic subtypes of HSP that can mimic ALS, i.e., some forms of SPG3, Silver syndrome in SPG17, or SPG11, there are several ALS genes particularly commonly associated with a slowly progressive HSP-like phenotype. Homozygous and compound heterozygous mutations in the alsin-2 gene *ALS2* lead to a childhood-onset motoneuron disease that commonly commences in the lower limbs and later develops into spastic tetraparesis with pseudobulbar palsy. Autosomal-dominant *OPTN* mutations can also lead to a slowly progressive UMN-predominant syndrome. Mutations in the *VCP* gene, primarily known to cause frontotemporal dementia, inclusion body myopathy, and Paget's disease of the bone (IBMPFD), have now been described to cause ALS as well as HSP phenotypes inherited in an autosomal-dominant manner (see also Chap. 17).

Leukodystrophies

Further phenocopies of HSP are leukodystrophies like Krabbe disease, metachromatic leukodystrophy (MLD), vanishing white matter disease, Alexander disease, cerebrotendinous xanthomatosis, hereditary diffuse leukoencephalopathy with axonal spheroids (HDLS), adult polyglucosan body disease, and the adrenomyeloneuropathy (AMN) variant of X-linked adrenoleukodystrophy (X-ALD) [69]. With adult onset especially AMN, Krabbe disease and Alexander disease present with prominent spasticity (Table 16.5) [5]. Most female carriers of X-ALD/AMN mutations develop signs and symptoms of myelopathy and/or peripheral neuropathy between 40 and 60 years of age [70]. Although most of them show some abnormality in very long-chain acid metabolism, the only reliable diagnostic tool in females with suspected AMN is genetic testing of the *ABCD1* gene. Krabbe disease may manifest as late as the 7th decade and then typically presents as "pure HSP" with discrete white matter alterations on MRI [5, 71]. Alexander disease is caused by heterozygous mutations in the *GFAP gene*, but despite autosomal-dominant inheritance, family history is often negative due to frequent occurrence of de novo mutations. Alexander disease should especially be considered when spasticity is accompanied by ataxia and palatal myoclonus as well as pontomedullary signal alterations on T2-weighted images on MRI [72].

Dopa-Responsive Dystonias

Dopamine-responsive dystonia (DRD), first described in 1976 by Segawa and therefore commonly termed Segawa's disease, comprises a group of childhood-onset progressive movement disorders with typical diurnal fluctuation of dystonia worsening in the evening and an often dramatic and sustained response to treatment with L-dopa. They are caused by disturbances in dopamine synthesis. In autosomal-dominant DRD, the GTP cytohydrolase I gene *GCH1* is mutated, leading to a lack of the tyrosine hydroxylase cofactor tetrahydrobiopterin. Tetrahydrobiopterin synthesis is also affected by mutations in the sepiapterin reductase gene *SPR*, leading to an autosomal-recessive form of DRD. Mutations in the tyrosine hydroxylase gene itself (*TH*) also cause autosomal-recessive DRD. It has been demonstrated repeatedly that misdiagnosis of children with dopamine-responsive dystonia as hereditary spastic paraplegia is not uncommon, a fact that is all the more noteworthy considering the available treatment option of DRD with dopamine. We therefore recommend considering an experimental treatment course with L-dopa in every case of childhood-onset genetically unsolved suspected HSP. (DRD is also discussed in Chap. 7.)

Genotype-Phenotype Correlation and Phenotypic Variability

The past decade has witnessed numerous attempts to define clear genotype-phenotype correlations in HSP. With each gene that has been discovered, we have tried to describe the associated phenotype in detail and delineate what sets this particular HSP apart from the other forms of HSP. What we have learned however is that HSP does not play by our rules. There may be phenotypic clusters for some genotypes, and we have tried to describe them in the preceding paragraphs. SPG4 has a pure phenotype, SPG3 starts early, SPG7 is a late-onset spastic ataxia with slow progression, and the presence of TCC and cognitive impairment calls for SPG11 testing. But exceptions are common, and predicting the genotype in an individual patient is therefore often of limited success. This has important implications for diagnostic testing as we will detail in the following paragraph. And it also poses a huge challenge – and a unique opportunity – for genetic research to improve our understanding of the factors that modify severity and phenotypic spectrum of HSPs. One of the few examples identified so far is the intragenic polymorphisms S44L and P45Q in the *SPAST* gene (SPG4) that lead to alterations in spastin phosphorylation and result in a more severe phenotype if inherited with a classical *SPG4* mutation *in trans* [73].

Diagnostic Algorithm

The sheer number of HSP genes and the lack of specificity of genotype-phenotype correlations impede traditional gene-by-gene diagnostic testing strategies in HSP. Modern genetic techniques allow parallel sequencing of many genes or even the whole exome or genome as time- and cost-effective alternatives to conventional Sanger sequencing and are of particular usefulness in diagnostic testing of highly heterogeneous diseases like HSPs.

We propose a stepwise diagnostic algorithm for HSP that takes into account specific phenotypes, mode of inheritance, and frequency of genotypes as well as specific types of mutations like genomic deletions (Fig. 16.2). Initially, alternative etiologies of spasticity need to be carefully excluded for all patients as they may allow for causative therapies. In the second step, the following four

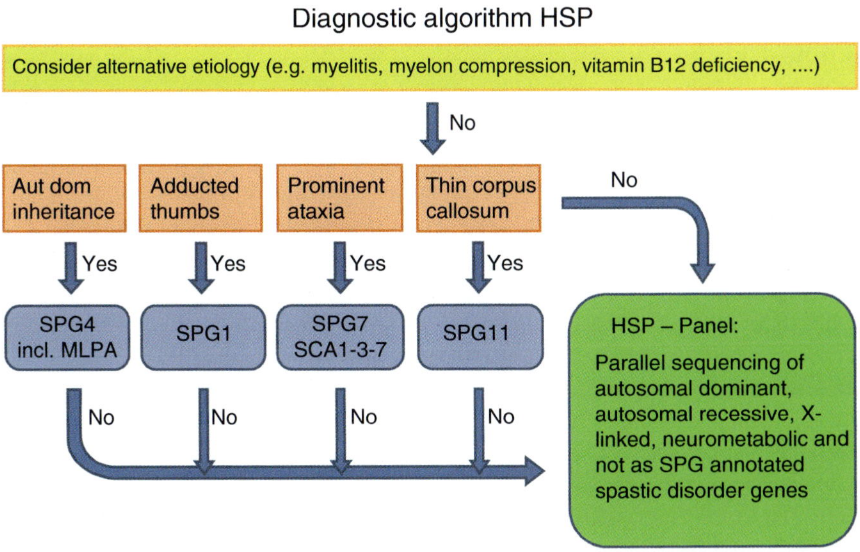

Fig. 16.2 HSP algorithm for genetic diagnostics

constellations should be considered: (1) If the family history is autosomal dominant, analysis of SPG4 should be initiated including MLPA as first-line diagnostic test. This will provide a definitive diagnosis in 50 % of families. (2) If spastic paraplegia is accompanied by cerebellar ataxia and family history is compatible with autosomal-recessive inheritance, SPG7 is the most frequent diagnosis. Additionally, the autosomal-dominant SCA1, SCA3, and SCA7 should be excluded. Testing for repeat expansion in these genes is comparatively fast and low-priced, and these mutation types would be missed using most next-generation sequencing techniques. (3) In patients with a thin corpus callosum on MRI, mutations in SPG11 are the most likely cause [25], and specific testing should be initiated. Finally (4), adducted thumbs are a rather specific phenotypic marker of SGP1.

In all other cases and if the abovementioned tests yielded negative results, we recommend next-generation sequencing-based screening of all remaining HSP genes, either by targeted HSP panel or by clinical grade whole-exome sequencing. As all but the SPG4 gene contribute to less than 10 % to the total of HSP cases and the majority of HSP genes account for less than 1 %, this approach is cost-effective considering the highly competitive cost of both methods in the range of conventional diagnostic testing of two to three HSP genes.

At our center we have successfully implemented this proposed strategy and use an HSP panel for broad screening of HSP genes. In our experience this strategy leads to a definite genetic diagnosis in about 70 % of dominant and almost half of autosomal-recessive cases. Novel HSP genes and/or mutations in noncoding areas of HSP genes as well as copy-number variations likely explain this diagnostic gap.

High-Throughput Genetic Testing: Targeted Panel Versus Whole-Exome Sequencing

Disease-specific panels on the one hand and whole-exome sequencing on the other hand differ in the way sample DNA is amplified prior to next-generation sequencing. For the HSP panel, sequences of HSP genes and further spasticity-related genes are specifically enriched using custom-designed enrichment protocols. This allows for analysis of >95 % of the targeted sequence with >20fold coverage, which is commonly considered sufficient for diagnostic testing. The "gaps" with lower than desired coverage can then be closed by conventional sequencing. Technical costs for an HSP panel are currently about one third of the cost for whole-exome sequencing, but prices increase substantially for diagnostic application if missing sequences have to be completed and suspicious variants are confirmed by Sanger sequencing.

In research-grade whole-exome sequencing, typically coverage of the exome of about 50- to 100fold is aimed at. Although this may seem high, coverage is not uniform across the exome with the currently available capture kits, and only about 80 % of the exome are covered above 20fold. Clinical-grade whole-exome sequencing therefore targets higher mean coverage at the expense of higher per-sample costs. Whole-exome sequencing is however far more flexible than disease panels as data can be reanalyzed at any time. Considering that about one third of dominant and more than half of recessive HSPs are currently not explained by mutations in known genes and that the last year alone has seen the discovery of >20 new HSP genes, this flexibility has decisive advantages in terms of the cost-effectiveness and may be even the longer-term diagnostic yield.

Both approaches are currently limited in their applicability to detect copy-number variations. Although this is technically possible for both methods, standardization is difficult, and the sensitivity is currently below that of established methods like MLPA or high-resolution array CGH.

We currently apply HSP panel testing for diagnostic purposes as we value the high diagnostic dependability of this technique for known HSP genes. For research applications we use whole-exome and/or genome sequencing as the higher flexibility in data analysis outweighs the technical limitations in regard to coverage uniformity.

Technical advances and a shift to whole genome sequencing with its naturally more uniform coverage and higher reliability in detecting copy-number variations may overcome many of these current limitations. The major challenge for all of these techniques however remains the interpretation of the huge number of variants with unknown significance detected by parallel sequencing of many genes. To ameliorate this problem, huge databases are required which provide large numbers of exome or genome sequences from different ethnical populations as well as most complete lists of (1) clearly disease-related mutations and (2) suspect variants with the respective phenotypes.

References

1. Karle KN, Schule R, Klebe S, Otto S, Frischholz C, Liepelt-Scarfone I, et al. Electrophysiological characterisation of motor and sensory tracts in patients with hereditary spastic paraplegia (HSP). Orphanet J Rare Dis. 2013;8:158. PubMed Pubmed Central PMCID: 3852552.
2. Harding AE. Classification of the hereditary ataxias and paraplegias. Lancet. 1983;1(8334):1151–5. PubMed Epub 1983/05/21. eng.
3. Schule R, Schols L. Genetics of hereditary spastic paraplegias. Semin Neurol. 2011;31(5):484–93. PubMed Epub 2012/01/24. eng.
4. Erichsen AK, Koht J, Stray-Pedersen A, Abdelnoor M, Tallaksen CM. Prevalence of hereditary ataxia and spastic paraplegia in southeast Norway: a population-based study. Brain. 2009;132(Pt 6):1577–88. PubMed PMID: 19339254.
5. Muller Vom Hagen J, Karle KN, Schule R, Krageloh-Mann I, Schols L. Leukodystrophies underlying cryptic spastic paraparesis: frequency and phenotype in 76 patients. Eur J Neurol. 2014;21(7):983–8. PubMed PMID: 24698313.
6. Novarino G, Fenstermaker AG, Zaki MS, Hofree M, Silhavy JL, Heiberg AD, et al. Exome sequencing links corticospinal motor neuron disease to common neurodegenerative disorders. Science. 2014;343(6170):506–11.
7. Durr A, Camuzat A, Colin E, Tallaksen C, Hannequin D, Coutinho P, et al. Atlastin1 mutations are frequent in young-onset autosomal dominant spastic paraplegia. Arch Neurol. 2004;61(12):1867–72.
8. Hedera P. Spastic paraplegia 3A. In: Pagon RA, Adam MP, Ardinger HH, Wallace SE, Amemiya A, Bean LJH, et al., editors. GeneReviews® [Internet]. Seattle (WA): University of Washington, Seattle; 1993–2015.
9. Beetz C, Nygren AO, Schickel J, Auer-Grumbach M, Burk K, Heide G, et al. High frequency of partial SPAST deletions in autosomal dominant hereditary spastic paraplegia. Neurology. 2006;67(11):1926–30. PubMed Epub 2006/10/13. eng.
10. Durr A, Tallaksen C, Depienne C. Spastic paraplegia 4. In: Pagon RA, Adam MP, Ardinger HH, Bird TD, Dolan CR, Fong CT, et al., editors. GeneReviews® [Internet]. Seattle (WA): University of Washington, Seattle; 1993–2015.
11. Svenstrup K, Moller RS, Christensen J, Budtz-Jorgensen E, Gilling M, Nielsen JE. NIPA1 mutation in complex hereditary spastic paraplegia with epilepsy. Eur J Neurol. 2011;18(9):1197–9.
12. Valdmanis PN, Meijer IA, Rouleau GA. Spastic paraplegia 8. In: Pagon RA, Adam MP, Ardinger HH, Bird TD, Dolan CR, Fong CT, et al., editors. GeneReviews® [Internet]. Seattle (WA): University of Washington, Seattle; 1993–2015.
13. Schule R, Kremer BP, Kassubek J, Auer-Grumbach M, Kostic V, Klopstock T, et al. SPG10 is a rare cause of spastic paraplegia in European families. J Neurol Neurosurg Psychiatry. 2008;79(5):584–7.
14. Goizet C, Boukhris A, Mundwiller E, Tallaksen C, Forlani S, Toutain A, et al. Complicated forms of autosomal dominant hereditary spastic paraplegia are frequent in SPG10. Hum Mutat. 2009;30(2):E376–85.
15. Montenegro G, Rebelo AP, Connell J, Allison R, Babalini C, D'Aloia M, et al. Mutations in the ER-shaping protein reticulon 2 cause the axon-degenerative disorder hereditary spastic paraplegia type 12. J Clin Invest. 2012;122(2):538–44.
16. Hansen JJ, Durr A, Cournu-Rebeix I, Georgopoulos C, Ang D, Nielsen MN, et al. Hereditary spastic paraplegia SPG13 is associated with a mutation in the gene encoding the mitochondrial chaperonin Hsp60. Am J Hum Genet. 2002;70(5):1328–32.
17. Ito D. BSCL2-related neurologic disorders/seipinopathy. In: Pagon RA, Adam MP, Ardinger HH, Bird TD, Dolan CR, Fong CT, et al., editors. GeneReviews® [Internet]. Seattle (WA): University of Washington, Seattle; 1993–2015.
18. Martignoni M, Riano E, Rugarli EI. The role of ZFYVE27/protrudin in hereditary spastic paraplegia. Am J Hum Genet. 2008;83(1):127–8; author reply 8–30.

19. Lin P, Li J, Liu Q, Mao F, Li J, Qiu R, et al. A missense mutation in SLC33A1, which encodes the acetyl-CoA transporter, causes autosomal-dominant spastic paraplegia (SPG42). Am J Hum Genet. 2008;83(6):752–9.
20. Esteves T, Durr A, Mundwiller E, Loureiro JL, Boutry M, Gonzalez MA, et al. Loss of association of REEP2 with membranes leads to hereditary spastic paraplegia. Am J Hum Genet. 2014;94(2):268–77.
21. Namekawa M, Ribai P, Nelson I, Forlani S, Fellmann F, Goizet C, et al. SPG3A is the most frequent cause of hereditary spastic paraplegia with onset before age 10 years. Neurology. 2006;66(1):112–4. PubMed Epub 2006/01/13. eng.
22. Tsaousidou MK, Ouahchi K, Warner TT, Yang Y, Simpson MA, Laing NG, et al. Sequence alterations within CYP7B1 implicate defective cholesterol homeostasis in motor-neuron degeneration. Am J Hum Genet. 2008;82(2):510–5. PubMed Pubmed Central PMCID: 2426914.
23. Schule R, Brandt E, Karle KN, Tsaousidou M, Klebe S, Klimpe S, et al. Analysis of CYP7B1 in non-consanguineous cases of hereditary spastic paraplegia. Neurogenetics. 2009;10(2):97–104.
24. Casari G, De Fusco M, Ciarmatori S, Zeviani M, Mora M, Fernandez P, et al. Spastic paraplegia and OXPHOS impairment caused by mutations in paraplegin, a nuclear-encoded mitochondrial metalloprotease. Cell. 1998;93(6):973–83.
25. Stevanin G, Santorelli FM, Azzedine H, Coutinho P, Chomilier J, Denora PS, et al. Mutations in SPG11, encoding spatacsin, are a major cause of spastic paraplegia with thin corpus callosum. Nat Genet. 2007;39(3):366–72. PubMed Epub 2007/02/27. eng.
26. Hanein S, Martin E, Boukhris A, Byrne P, Goizet C, Hamri A, et al. Identification of the SPG15 gene, encoding spastizin, as a frequent cause of complicated autosomal-recessive spastic paraplegia, including Kjellin syndrome. Am J Hum Genet. 2008;82(4):992–1002.
27. Alazami AM, Adly N, Al Dhalaan H, Alkuraya FS. A nullimorphic ERLIN2 mutation defines a complicated hereditary spastic paraplegia locus (SPG18). Neurogenetics. 2011;12:333–6.
28. Patel H, Cross H, Proukakis C, Hershberger R, Bork P, Ciccarelli FD, et al. SPG20 is mutated in Troyer syndrome, an hereditary spastic paraplegia. Nat Genet. 2002;31(4):347–8.
29. Simpson MA, Cross H, Proukakis C, Pryde A, Hershberger R, Chatonnet A, et al. Maspardin is mutated in mast syndrome, a complicated form of hereditary spastic paraplegia associated with dementia. Am J Hum Genet. 2003;73(5):1147–56.
30. Boukhris A, Schule R, Loureiro JL, Lourenco CM, Mundwiller E, Gonzalez MA, et al. Alteration of ganglioside biosynthesis responsible for complex hereditary spastic paraplegia. Am J Hum Genet. 2013;93(1):118–23.
31. Tesson C, Nawara M, Salih MA, Rossignol R, Zaki MS, Al Balwi M, et al. Alteration of Fatty-Acid-metabolizing enzymes affects mitochondrial form and function in hereditary spastic paraplegia. Am J Hum Genet. 2012;91(6):1051–64.
32. Klebe S, Azzedine H, Durr A, Bastien P, Bouslam N, Elleuch N, et al. Autosomal recessive spastic paraplegia (SPG30) with mild ataxia and sensory neuropathy maps to chromosome 2q37.3. Brain. 2006;129(Pt 6):1456–62.
33. Dick KJ, Eckhardt M, Paisan-Ruiz C, Alshehhi AA, Proukakis C, Sibtain NA, et al. Mutation of FA2H underlies a complicated form of hereditary spastic paraplegia (SPG35). Hum Mutat. 2010;31(4):E1251–60.
34. Synofzik M, Gonzalez MA, Lourenco CM, Coutelier M, Haack TB, Rebelo A, et al. PNPLA6 mutations cause Boucher-Neuhauser and Gordon Holmes syndromes as part of a broad neurodegenerative spectrum. Brain. 2014;137(Pt 1):69–77.
35. Landoure G, Zhu PP, Lourenco CM, Johnson JO, Toro C, Bricceno KV, et al. Hereditary spastic paraplegia type 43 (SPG43) is caused by mutation in C19orf12. Hum Mutat. 2013;34(10):1357–60.
36. Orthmann-Murphy JL, Salsano E, Abrams CK, Bizzi A, Uziel G, Freidin MM, et al. Hereditary spastic paraplegia is a novel phenotype for GJA12/GJC2 mutations. Brain. 2009;132(Pt 2):426–38.

37. Hammer MB, Eleuch-Fayache G, Schottlaender LV, Nehdi H, Gibbs JR, Arepalli SK, et al. Mutations in GBA2 cause autosomal-recessive cerebellar ataxia with spasticity. Am J Hum Genet. 2013;92:245–51.
38. Martin E, Schule R, Smets K, Rastetter A, Boukhris A, Loureiro JL, et al. Loss of function of glucocerebrosidase GBA2 is responsible for motor neuron defects in hereditary spastic paraplegia. Am J Hum Genet. 2013;92(2):238–44.
39. Abou Jamra R, Philippe O, Raas-Rothschild A, Eck SH, Graf E, Buchert R, et al. Adaptor protein complex 4 deficiency causes severe autosomal-recessive intellectual disability, progressive spastic paraplegia, shy character, and short stature. Am J Hum Genet. 2011;88(6):788–95.
40. Bauer P, Leshinsky-Silver E, Blumkin L, Schlipf N, Schroder C, Schicks J, et al. Mutation in the AP4B1 gene cause hereditary spastic paraplegia type 47 (SPG47). Neurogenetics. 2012;13(1):73–6.
41. Slabicki M, Theis M, Krastev DB, Samsonov S, Mundwiller E, Junqueira M, et al. A genome-scale DNA repair RNAi screen identifies SPG48 as a novel gene associated with hereditary spastic paraplegia. PLoS Biol. 2010;8(6):e1000408.
42. Oz-Levi D, Ben-Zeev B, Ruzzo EK, Hitomi Y, Gelman A, Pelak K, et al. Mutation in TECPR2 Reveals a Role for Autophagy in Hereditary Spastic Paraparesis. Am J Hum Genet. 2012;91(6):1065–72.
43. Moreno-De-Luca A, Helmers SL, Mao H, Burns TG, Melton AM, Schmidt KR, et al. Adaptor protein complex-4 (AP-4) deficiency causes a novel autosomal recessive cerebral palsy syndrome with microcephaly and intellectual disability. J Med Genet. 2011;48(2):141–4.
44. Zivony-Elboum Y, Westbroek W, Kfir N, Savitzki D, Shoval Y, Bloom A, et al. A founder mutation in Vps37A causes autosomal recessive complex hereditary spastic paraparesis. J Med Genet. 2012;49(7):462–72.
45. Schuurs-Hoeijmakers JH, Geraghty MT, Kamsteeg EJ, Ben-Salem S, de Bot ST, Nijhof B, et al. Mutations in DDHD2, Encoding an Intracellular Phospholipase A(1), Cause a Recessive Form of Complex Hereditary Spastic Paraplegia. Am J Hum Genet. 2012;91:1073–81.
46. Gonzalez M, Nampoothiri S, Kornblum C, Oteyza AC, Walter J, Konidari I, et al. Mutations in phospholipase DDHD2 cause autosomal recessive hereditary spastic paraplegia (SPG54). Eur J Hum Genet. 2013;21(11):1214–8.
47. Shimazaki H, Takiyama Y, Ishiura H, Sakai C, Matsushima Y, Hatakeyama H, et al. A homozygous mutation of C12orf65 causes spastic paraplegia with optic atrophy and neuropathy (SPG55). J Med Genet. 2012;49(12):777–84.
48. Spiegel R, Mandel H, Saada A, Lerer I, Burger A, Shaag A, et al. Delineation of C12orf65-related phenotypes: a genotype-phenotype relationship. Eur J Hum Genet. 2014;22(8):1019–25.
49. Tucci A, Liu YT, Preza E, Pitceathly RD, Chalasani A, Plagnol V, et al. Novel C12orf65 mutations in patients with axonal neuropathy and optic atrophy. J Neurol Neurosurg Psychiatry. 2014;85(5):486–92.
50. Beetz C, Johnson A, Schuh AL, Thakur S, Varga RE, Fothergill T, et al. Inhibition of TFG function causes hereditary axon degeneration by impairing endoplasmic reticulum structure. Proc Natl Acad Sci U S A. 2013;110(13):5091–6.
51. Caballero Oteyza A, Battaloglu E, Ocek L, Lindig T, Reichbauer J, Rebelo AP, et al. Motor protein mutations cause a new form of hereditary spastic paraplegia. Neurology. 2014;82:2007–16.
52. Klebe S, Depienne C, Gerber S, Challe G, Anheim M, Charles P, et al. Spastic paraplegia gene 7 in patients with spasticity and/or optic neuropathy. Brain. 2012;135(Pt 10):2980–93. PubMed Pubmed Central PMCID: 3470714. Epub 2012/10/16. eng.
53. Pfeffer G, Gorman GS, Griffin H, Kurzawa-Akanbi M, Blakely EL, Wilson I, et al. Mutations in the SPG7 gene cause chronic progressive external ophthalmoplegia through disordered mitochondrial DNA maintenance. Brain. 2014;137(Pt 5):1323–36. PubMed Pubmed Central PMCID: 3999722.
54. Wedding IM, Koht J, Tran GT, Misceo D, Selmer KK, Holmgren A, et al. Spastic paraplegia type 7 is associated with multiple mitochondrial DNA deletions. PLoS One. 2014;9(1):e86340. PubMed Pubmed Central PMCID: 3899233.

55. Stevanin G, Azzedine H, Denora P, Boukhris A, Tazir M, Lossos A, et al. Mutations in SPG11 are frequent in autosomal recessive spastic paraplegia with thin corpus callosum, cognitive decline and lower motor neuron degeneration. Brain. 2008;131(Pt 3):772–84. PubMed Epub 2007/12/15. eng.
56. Hehr U, Bauer P, Winner B, Schule R, Olmez A, Koehler W, et al. Long-term course and mutational spectrum of spatacsin-linked spastic paraplegia. Ann Neurol. 2007;62(6):656–65. PubMed Epub 2007/12/11. eng.
57. Daoud H, Zhou S, Noreau A, Sabbagh M, Belzil V, Dionne-Laporte A, et al. Exome sequencing reveals SPG11 mutations causing juvenile ALS. Neurobiol Aging. 2012;33(4):839.e5–9. PubMed Epub 2011/12/14. Eng.
58. Schrander-Stumpel C, Vos YJ. L1 syndrome. In: Pagon RA, Adam MP, Ardinger HH, Bird TD, Dolan CR, Fong CT, et al., editors. GeneReviews® [Internet]. Seattle (WA): University of Washington, Seattle; 1993–2015.
59. Hobson GM, Kamholz J. PLP1-related disorders. In: Pagon RA, Adam MP, Ardinger HH, Bird TD, Dolan CR, Fong CT, et al., editors. GeneReviews® [Internet]. Seattle (WA): University of Washington, Seattle; 1993–2015.
60. Dumitrescu AM, Liao XH, Best TB, Brockmann K, Refetoff S. A novel syndrome combining thyroid and neurological abnormalities is associated with mutations in a monocarboxylate transporter gene. Am J Hum Genet. 2004;74(1):168–75.
61. Dumitrescu AM, Fu J, Dempsey MA, Refetoff S. MCT8-specific thyroid hormone cell-membrane transporter deficiency. In: Pagon RA, Adam MP, Ardinger HH, Bird TD, Dolan CR, Fong CT, et al., editors. GeneReviews® [Internet]. Seattle (WA): University of Washington, Seattle; 1993–2015.
62. Depienne C, Tallaksen C, Lephay JY, Bricka B, Poea-Guyon S, Fontaine B, et al. Spastin mutations are frequent in sporadic spastic paraparesis and their spectrum is different from that observed in familial cases. J Med Genet. 2006;43(3):259–65. PubMed Pubmed Central PMCID: 2563242. Epub 2005/08/02. eng.
63. Brugman F, Veldink JH, Franssen H, de Visser M, de Jong JM, Faber CG, et al. Differentiation of hereditary spastic paraparesis from primary lateral sclerosis in sporadic adult-onset upper motor neuron syndromes. Arch Neurol. 2009;66(4):509–14. PubMed Epub 2009/04/15. eng.
64. Brugman F, Scheffer H, Wokke JH, Nillesen WM, de Visser M, Aronica E, et al. Paraplegin mutations in sporadic adult-onset upper motor neuron syndromes. Neurology. 2008;71(19):1500–5. PubMed Epub 2008/09/19. eng.
65. de Bot ST, Veldink JH, Vermeer S, Mensenkamp AR, Brugman F, Scheffer H, et al. ATL1 and REEP1 mutations in hereditary and sporadic upper motor neuron syndromes. J Neurol. 2012;260:869–75. PubMed Epub 2012/10/31. Eng.
66. Bhidayasiri R, Perlman SL, Pulst SM, Geschwind DH. Late-onset Friedreich ataxia: phenotypic analysis, magnetic resonance imaging findings, and review of the literature. Arch Neurol. 2005;62(12):1865–9. PubMed PMID: 16344344.
67. Synofzik M, Soehn AS, Gburek-Augustat J, Schicks J, Karle KN, Schule R, et al. Autosomal recessive spastic ataxia of Charlevoix Saguenay (ARSACS): expanding the genetic, clinical and imaging spectrum. Orphanet J Rare Dis. 2013;8:41. PubMed Pubmed Central PMCID: 3610264. Epub 2013/03/19. eng.
68. Schols L, Bauer P, Schmidt T, Schulte T, Riess O. Autosomal dominant cerebellar ataxias: clinical features, genetics, and pathogenesis. Lancet Neurol. 2004;3(5):291–304. PubMed PMID: 15099544.
69. Ahmed RM, Murphy E, Davagnanam I, Parton M, Schott JM, Mummery CJ, et al. A practical approach to diagnosing adult onset leukodystrophies. J Neurol Neurosurg Psychiatry. 2014;85(7):770–81. PubMed PMID: 24357685.
70. Engelen M, Barbier M, Dijkstra IM, Schur R, de Bie RM, Verhamme C, et al. X-linked adrenoleukodystrophy in women: a cross-sectional cohort study. Brain. 2014;137(Pt 3):693–706. PubMed PMID: 24480483.

71. Debs R, Froissart R, Aubourg P, Papeix C, Douillard C, Degos B, et al. Krabbe disease in adults: phenotypic and genotypic update from a series of 11 cases and a review. J Inherit Metab Dis. 2013;36(5):859–68. PubMed PMID: 23197103.
72. Pareyson D, Fancellu R, Mariotti C, Romano S, Salmaggi A, Carella F, et al. Adult-onset alexander disease: a series of eleven unrelated cases with review of the literature. Brain. 2008;131(Pt 9):2321–31. PubMed PMID: 18684770.
73. Svenson IK, Kloos MT, Gaskell PC, Nance MA, Garbern JY, Hisanaga S, et al. Intragenic modifiers of hereditary spastic paraplegia due to spastin gene mutations. Neurogenetics. 2004;5(3):157–64. PubMed PMID: 15248095.
74. Kumar KR, Blair NF, Vandebona H, Liang C, Ng K, Sharpe DM, et al. Targeted next generation sequencing in SPAST-negative hereditary spastic paraplegia. J Neurol. 2013;260(10):2516–22. PubMed PMID: 23812641.

Chapter 17
Genetics of ALS

Russell Lewis McLaughlin, Kevin Patrick Kenna, and Orla Hardiman

Abstract Amyotrophic lateral sclerosis (ALS) is genetically heterogeneous, with extensive phenotypic diversity and overlap with related clinical phenotypes. Although many genes have been identified that are mutated in ALS with many more implicated in the disease, the genetic cause for a large proportion of ALS risk remains to be discovered. The underlying biological mechanisms that converge on ALS are only partially understood but it is likely that aberrant RNA processing and protein homeostasis play central roles. Future research into the undiscovered genetic contribution to ALS will shed further light on these pathogenic mechanisms, as well as providing a complete catalog of the causes of the disease, which will, hopefully, contribute towards the development of a cure for this devastating condition.

Keywords Amyotrophic lateral sclerosis (ALS) • Neurodegenerative disease • Sporadic amyotrophic lateral sclerosis (sALS) • Familial ALS (fALS) • Linkage mapping • SOD1 mutations • Optineurin (OPTN) • Ubiquilin 2 (UBQLN2) • Chromosome 9 open reading frame 72 (C9orf72) • Genome-wide association study (GWAS) • Autosomal dominant inheritance

Amyotrophic lateral sclerosis (ALS) is a neurodegenerative disease characterized by progressive loss of upper and lower motor neurons. The lifetime risk for developing ALS is approximately 1 in 400 [1–3] in populations of European extraction; yet, owing to its short duration (affected individuals usually die within 3–5 years of symptom onset), the prevalence of the disease is relatively low (around 4–6 per

R.L. McLaughlin, BSc, HDip, PhD (✉)
Population Genetics Laboratory, Smurfit Institute of Genetics, Trinity College Dublin, College Green, Dublin 2, Ireland
e-mail: mclaugr@tcd.ie

K.P. Kenna, BSc, PhD
Ocular Genetics Unit, Smurfit Institute of Genetics, Trinity College Dublin, College Green, Dublin 2, Ireland

O. Hardiman, BSc, MD
Academic Unit of Neurology, Trinity College Dublin, Trinity Biomedical Sciences Institute, Dublin 2, Ireland

S.A. Schneider, J.M.T. Brás (eds.), *Movement Disorder Genetics*,
DOI 10.1007/978-3-319-17223-1_17

100,000 person-years) [4]. The disease is heterogeneous in nature, with variability in age at onset (typically 40–70 years), site of onset (first symptoms in muscles innervated by spinal or bulbar motor neurons), presence of extra-motor involvement (cognitive and behavioral changes), and disease duration. There is currently no cure for ALS; the only treatment is riluzole, which can prolong survival by a few months.

Up to 50 % of people with ALS have evidence of cognitive or behavioral impairment, and approximately 15 % of cases fulfill the criteria for frontotemporal dementia (FTD) [5]. The pathological hallmark of ALS is ubiquitinated inclusions in the cytoplasm of motor neurons, a major component of which is the protein TAR DNA-binding protein 43 (TDP-43) [6]. Similar TDP-43-positive inclusions are observed in some forms of FTD, indicating that ALS and FTD exist on a spectrum of disease. Initial symptoms for ALS vary, but typically begin in one anatomical region, initially spreading to adjacent regions in a manner that is believed to be reflected by focal spread of pathology from distinct neuroanatomical regions along anatomical pathways to neighboring cells [7].

In 5–15 % of cases, a family history of ALS is evident (familial ALS or fALS) [8, 9]; the remainder of cases are considered to be sporadic (sporadic ALS or sALS). However, even without a family history of ALS, sALS kindreds often exhibit aggregation of neurological and neuropsychiatric phenotypes, indicating that genetic risk factors with potentially pleiotropic effects may play a role in pathogenesis in these cases [9]. Furthermore, estimates of heritability – the proportion of phenotypic variance attributable to genetic variation – are high (twin-based heritability estimates are 38–78 %), evidencing a clear role for inherited risk factors in otherwise unexplained cases of sALS [10]. For this reason, the distinction between fALS and at least some cases of sALS is considered by some to be artificial, in that inherited risk factors cause the disease even in sporadic cases. Moreover, misclassification of some cases of sALS can occur as a consequence of insufficient pedigree size for ascertainment of multiple affected members, early death from other causes, misclassification of disease in preceding generations, or incomplete penetrance of disease-causing mutations. It has been shown that pedigree size and reduced penetrance have a substantial effect on the rate of observed familiality in a disease with heritable cause [11]. Genetic risk factors are therefore an active area of research in both familial and apparently sporadic forms of ALS.

Because ALS is most likely to be a spectrum rather than a single disease entity, it is unlikely that there is a single unifying pathogenic mechanism, and for this reason the discovery of the underlying genetic risk factors is a challenge. A large number of genes have been studied in ALS; Fig. 17.1 shows the genomic location of every gene that has received sufficient attention to warrant inclusion in the ALS online genetics database (ALSoD), an online repository of genetic research in ALS [12]. Several of these genes are also mutated in FTD, providing evidence of genetic overlap that supports the clinical and pathological overlap between the two diseases (Fig. 17.2). For many of the genes in Fig. 17.1, evidence for a true role in ALS varies and many of the genetic variants that have been described as potential causes of ALS are actually present in unaffected individuals at too high a frequency to be considered pathogenic [15]. Discretion is therefore important in the interpretation of the extant literature on ALS genetics, as many more genes have been implicated

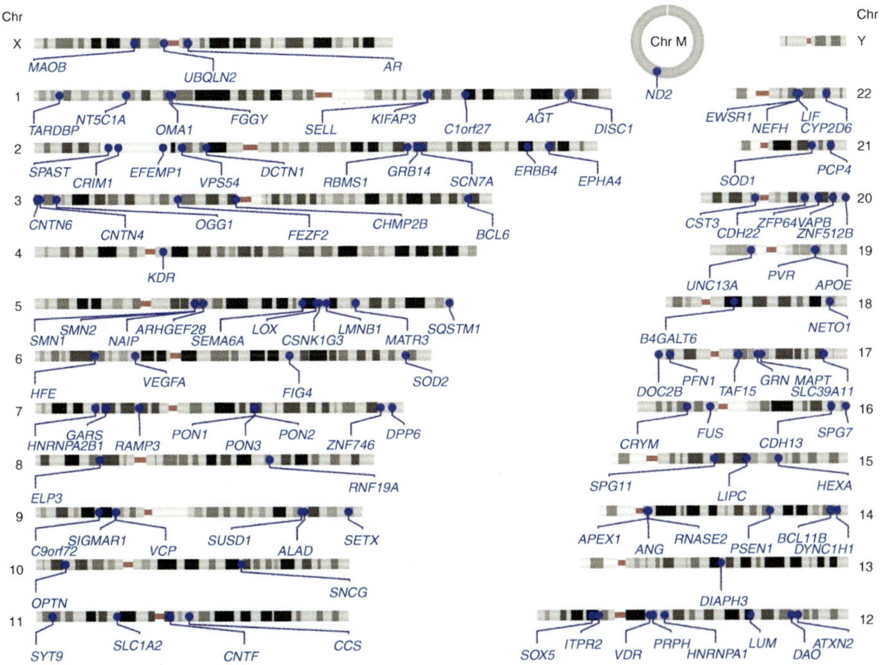

Fig. 17.1 Genomic locations of genes that have been studied in the biology of ALS. A complete account of every mutation that has been studied in the biology of ALS, regardless of quality of evidence for pathogenicity, is provided in the ALS online genetics database (ALSoD) [12]. Note that the mitochondrial genome (Chr M) is not drawn to scale with the remainder of the genome

than are likely to be causative of ALS (and currently known). Table 17.1 describes 18 genes in which mutations have shown evidence of Mendelian inheritance, segregating with affected members of ALS pedigrees, therefore being considered bona fide ALS genes, although of these only a small number cause what would be considered "typical ALS."

Inherited Risk Factors

Before large-scale population-based methods were a feasible approach for the discovery of ALS genes, the use of fALS kindreds in linkage mapping was the principal method of choice. In 1993, the first ALS-causing mutations were discovered in *SOD1* (encoding superoxide dismutase 1) [32]. This was a major breakthrough as it permitted the generation of the first credible transgenic rodent model of ALS, the *SOD1* G93A mouse, which in turn has driven most of the research concerning the translational biology of ALS over the past 15 years. However, more recent research has suggested that that the pathology of *SOD1* related ALS differs from the majority of sporadic disease, as the pathology of mutant *SOD1* is not associated with deposition of TDP-43, a hallmark of classical ALS and most forms of

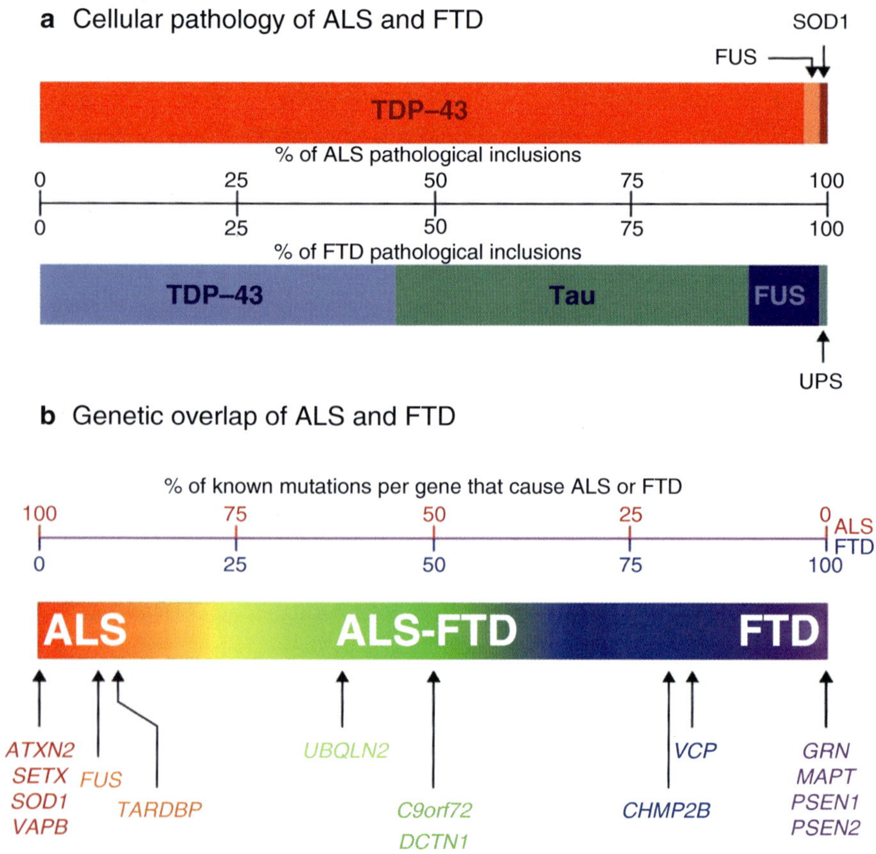

Fig. 17.2 Cytopathological and genetic overlap between ALS and FTD (Adapted from Ling et al. [13] including data from the ALS online genetics database [12] and the Alzheimer Disease and Frontotemporal Dementia Mutation Database [14]). (**a**) The proportion of ALS and FTD cases whose cellular pathology is driven by inclusions positive for major ALS and FTD proteins is shown. A large proportion of ALS and FTD cases overlap in terms of cellular pathology, with TDP-43-positive and FUS-positive inclusions observed in both. (**b**) The percentage of the known mutations in an array of ALS and FTD genes that cause the two diseases (note that this does not denote the proportion of disease *cases* caused by particular mutations) is shown. Proportions are based on approximations from the ALS and FTD mutation databases and expert opinion derived from the extant literature [13]

FTD. Moreover, the epidemiology of *SOD1* mutations varies across populations; while rare in Irish [37] and Dutch [38] populations, *SOD1* mutations account for up to 23 % of familial ALS in the United States [39] and 18 % in Italy [40]. Since the initial discovery that *SOD1* mutations cause ALS, 177 mutations in the gene have been associated with ALS etiology, with both autosomal dominant and autosomal recessive transmission. However, the evidence for pathogenicity varies for these mutations and some may represent incidental findings of benign polymorphisms [41]. Characteristic phenotypes have been described in association with

Table 17.1 Genes associated with familial ALS

Gene	Year	Mutations	Model	Gene function	Phenotype	Refs.
ALS2	2001	27	AR	Guanine exchange factor	jALS, jPLS, iHSP	[16, 17]
ANG	2004	29	AD	Ribonuclease	ALS, PD	[18]
C9orf72	2011	1	AD	Guanine exchange factor	ALS, ALS-FTD, PD	[19, 20]
DAO	2010	2	AD	Oxidation of D-amino acids	ALS, SCA2	[21]
DCTN1	2003	6	AD	Microtubule transport	DHMN-7B, PS, ALS, ALS-FTD	[22]
ERBB4	2013	2	AD	Receptor tyrosine kinase	ALS	[23]
FUS	2009	77	AD, AR	RNA-binding protein	ALS, ALS-FTD, jALS, ETM4	[24, 25]
HNRNPA1	2013	1	AD	Heterogeneous nuclear ribonucleoprotein	ALS, MSP	[26]
MATR3	2014	4	AD	RNA-binding protein	ALS, MPD2, MSP	[27]
OPTN	2010	37	AD, AR	TNFα signaling regulator	ALS, GLC1E	[28]
PFN1	2012	4	AD	Actin-binding protein	ALS	[29]
SETX	2004	8	AD	DNA/RNA helicase	jALS, AOA2	[30]
SIGMAR1	2011	1	AR	Transmembrane receptor	jALS	[31]
SOD1	1993	177	AD, AR	Superoxide dismutase	ALS	[32]
TARDBP	2008	50	AD	DNA/RNA-binding protein	ALS, ALS-FTD	[33]
UBQLN2	2011	6	XD	Ubiquitin signaling	ALS, ALS-FTD	[34]
VAPB	2004	2	AD	Membrane protein	ALS, SMA	[35]
VCP	2010	7	AD	ATP-binding protein	ALS, IBMPFD	[36]

Mutation counts are based on those reported in the ALS Online Genetics Database
AD autosomal dominant, *AOA2* ataxia with oculomotor apraxia type 2, *AR* autosomal recessive, *DHMN-7B* distal hereditary motor neuropathy type 7b, *ETM4* essential tremor type 4, *GLC1E* glaucoma type 1e, *IBMPFD* inclusion body myopathy with Paget's disease and FTD, *iHSP* infantile hereditary spastic paraplegia, *jALS* juvenile ALS, *jPLS* juvenile primary lateral sclerosis, *MPD2* distal myopathy 2, *MSP* multisystem proteinopathy, *PD* Parkinson's disease, *PS* Perry syndrome, *SCA2* spinocerebellar ataxia type 2, *SMA* spinal muscular atrophy, *XD* X-linked dominant

some mutations of undoubted pathogenicity. For example, while homozygous carriers of the D90A mutation [42] and H46R carriers [43] exhibit a very long disease course (in excess of 10 years from symptom onset), A4V carriers typically die within a year of symptom onset [39].

For almost a decade, *SOD1* remained the only gene in which mutations were known to cause ALS. In 2001, advances in linkage mapping and candidate gene resequencing led to the discovery of five new genes in quick succession: *ALS2* (encoding alsin) [16, 17], *DCTN1* (dynactin subunit 1) [22], *ANG* (angiogenin) [18], *SETX* (senataxin) [30], and *VAPB* (vesicle-associated membrane-associated protein B) [35]. However, with the possible exception of *ANG*, none of these genes was associated with typical ALS, and both *ANG* and *DCTN1* are considered by many to be susceptibility genes rather than single genes of major effect. Moreover, the population frequency of putative pathogenic variants for all five genes is less than 1 % of all fALS. Likewise, *DAO* (D-amino acid oxidase) [21] and *SIGMAR1* (sigma non-opioid intracellular receptor 1) [31], discovered later in 2010 and 2011, have received little attention since their initial publication as mutations in these genes are likely to represent a very small proportion of all ALS.

Two major discoveries, one in 2008 (*TARDBP*, encoding TAR DNA-binding protein 43 or TDP-43) [33] and the second in 2009 (*FUS*, encoding fused in sarcoma) [24, 25], represented a major advance in the genetics of ALS. Jointly, these discoveries opened major new approaches to understanding the neurobiology of ALS, as both are genes that are involved in RNA trafficking and processing [44]. The discovery of mutations in *TARDBP* was of particular importance, given that cytoplasmic accumulation of its protein product, TDP-43, had been shown 2 years earlier to be the major pathological hallmark of ALS and FTD [6]. With the exception of Sardinia [45], however, mutations in this gene are a relatively rare cause of ALS, indicating that the physiological signature of ubiquitinated TDP-43-positive inclusions is generally a consequence of a convergent pathological mechanism as opposed to direct perturbation of TDP-43 function through *TARDBP* mutation.

The following year, *OPTN* (optineurin) was discovered as a cause of an autosomal recessive form of ALS in Japanese families through a combination of homozygosity mapping and candidate gene resequencing [28]. Like many ALS genes, *OPTN* is pleiotropic: mutations also cause primary open-angle glaucoma, and the locus has been implicated in the etiology of Paget's disease of the bone [46]. A similar pleiotropic phenotype is observed for *VCP* (vasolin-containing protein; Table 17.1), another gene discovered in 2010, and *SQSTM1*, a gene that has been implicated in ALS but currently without supporting evidence of familial segregation. Taken together, these findings indicate a clinical overlap between some forms of Paget's disease and ALS [47]. *OPTN* mutations have been shown not to be a common cause of ALS in European populations [37, 48], further underscoring the population specificity and ethnic differentiation of the frequencies of ALS-causing mutations.

In 2011, *UBQLN2* (ubiquilin 2) mutations were discovered in X-linked dominant ALS [34]. In these cases, transmission cannot be male to male because males, who carry one X and one Y sex chromosome, necessarily inherit their X chromosome from the mother (females carry two copies of the X chromosome and no Y chromosome). *UBQLN2* mutations in ALS are rare [49, 50], but the potential importance of the ubiquitin signaling pathway in motor neuron degeneration highlights the central role that the gene may come to play in our understanding of the pathogenic mechanisms underlying ALS.

The discovery of an ALS-causing mutation in *C9orf72* (chromosome 9 open reading frame 72) in 2011 represented a major milestone in ALS genetics research [19, 20]. Its location on chromosome 9p21 had been known to be an important ALS locus for several years following evidence from familial linkage [51] and genome-wide association studies [52–54]. Extensive sequencing by many groups failed to identify credible pathogenic variants within the locus until a combination of elegant work using segregation analysis coupled with extensive next-generation sequencing of the region eventually led to the discovery of a hexanucleotide repeat expansion in the 1st intron or promoter region (depending on transcript variant) of the gene. Typically, an unaffected individual would carry three repeats of the hexanucleotide sequence GGGGCC, but in the cases of repeat expansion carriers, an excess of 30 repeats appears to be sufficient to cause ALS, with most mutation-carrier patients harboring hundreds or thousands of repeats. The mutation appears to have derived from a single European founder [55], and allelic heterogeneity in terms of the length of the repeat expansion indicates inherent instability of the sequence.

With an unstable expanded repeat sequence, there can be a propensity for the size of the repeat expansion to increase in subsequent generations. This is a principle known as anticipation, and there is some evidence to suggest that this may be the case in *C9orf72*-mediated ALS, with consecutive generations exhibiting younger age of onset [56]. However, inherent difficulties in accurately measuring the length of the repeat expansion, coupled with somatic mosaicism of the repeat expansion length (rendering convenient tissues like blood inappropriate for accurate genetic testing), complicate a straightforward interpretation of this finding. It has also been suggested that variation in the length of the repeat expansion may confer the clinical variation observed within repeat expansion carriers, as the mutation is also observed in FTD, Alzheimer's disease, Parkinson's disease, and Lewy body dementia [57]. A much broader ALS-FTD phenotype has also been associated with the repeat expansion in *C9orf72*, comprising a range of neuropsychiatric conditions including psychosis, bipolar affective disorder, and obsessive-compulsive disorder [9, 58, 59].

Since the discovery of the *C9orf72* repeat expansion as a major cause of ALS, a substantial body of work has been generated, describing the clinical characteristics of mutation carriers, its population genetics, and its likely role in the cellular pathology of ALS. The *C9orf72* repeat expansion currently represents the most common known cause of ALS in populations of European extraction, explaining up to 40 % of fALS and 7 % of sALS, depending on the population studied [60]. Conversely, the variant is rare in populations of non-European extraction. In European populations, the observation that a fALS gene is present in a high percentage of apparently sporadic ALS reinforces the indefinite nature of the distinction between the two forms of the disease. *C9orf72* repeat expansions are also present in up to 25 % of familial FTD of European extraction [60], providing the strongest genetic basis to date for the clinical overlap between the two diseases. This is further reinforced by a significantly higher extent of comorbid FTD in ALS patients with the repeat expansion than in patients without it [61].

More recently implicated genes in fALS etiology include *PFN1* (profilin 1) [29], *ERBB4* (v-erb-a erythroblastic leukemia viral oncogene homolog 4) [23], *HNRNPA1* (heterogeneous nuclear ribonucleoprotein A1) [26], and *MATR3* (matrin 3) [27]. Owing to their recent discovery as fALS genes, it remains to be determined exactly how important each of these genes is in its pathophysiology. *PFN1* mutations have been shown to be a rare cause of ALS [62] but the discovery of ALS mutations in this gene may be an important event in our understanding of the biology of ALS as it implicates disruption of the cytoskeleton as a novel disease mechanism. The same is true for *ERBB4* mutations, which implicate the neuregulin pathway. *HNRNPA1* mutations are observed in multisystem proteinopathy, providing further evidence of overlap between ALS and other clinical syndromes. A similar pleiotropic phenotype is observed in carriers of mutations in *VCP* and *MATR3* [27], which is also a TDP-43 interactor and an RNA- and DNA-binding protein, so an understanding of the role of this gene in ALS biology is likely to shed further light on convergent underlying disease mechanisms.

Non-inherited Risk Factors

ALS may not be an entirely genetic disease, and some level of environmental contribution, or gene × environment interaction, may play a role. Non-inherited risk can also derive from genetic factors. For most of the genes listed in Table 17.1, affected individuals inherit the ALS-causing mutations from their parents. However, mutations can also arise spontaneously (termed de novo mutations) and would therefore not be observed in the non-germ cells of parents of affected individuals. The parents would also not be expected to manifest the disease. Examples of de novo mutations have been observed in *SOD1* [63] and *FUS* [64, 65], with the latter often exhibiting an aggressive, early-onset, and short disease course [66]. A de novo *FUS* mutation has even been observed in a case of apparently familial ALS [67], highlighting the potential for the coincidence of two independent causes of ALS in the same fALS pedigree.

A systematic search for undiscovered de novo mutations was published in 2013, using exome sequencing (high-throughput sequencing of the entire protein-coding portion of the genome) in ALS trios [68]. In this study, the unaffected parents of ALS patients were sequenced along with the patients themselves with the assumption that, in these cases, a de novo mutation is the cause of ALS in the affected offspring. In any given parent-offspring trio (affected or unaffected by ALS), the expected number of de novo mutations in the exome of the offspring is roughly 1 [69], and directly implicating these rare events in ALS is accordingly challenging. Nevertheless, the authors used functional evidence to indicate a role for de novo mutations in *SS18L1* (synovial sarcoma translocation gene on chromosome 18-like 1; also known as *CREST*) in ALS etiology, as well as forwarding suggestive evidence for a number of other de novo mutations.

Although the twin-based heritability of ALS is high (38–78 %) [10], heritability estimates describing the proportion of phenotypic variance of ALS attributable to common genetic variation are lower (two independent studies estimate this to be

11.0–12.7 % [70] and 17.1–24.9 % [71]). Therefore, although a large component of ALS risk is heritable, much of this heritability is unlikely to be due to common genetic variation. This suggests that the portion of ALS risk accounted for by undiscovered genetic risk factors may be explained, in part, by de novo mutations. Many of the undiscovered heritable risk factors are, however, likely to be due to rare mutations which are not well captured by common genetic variation. The discovery of the undetermined causes of ALS is therefore the focus of intensive research in the international research community.

Other Genes and Missing Heritability

Even without evidence of segregation of mutations within a pedigree, a gene can still be associated with disease. If the risk allele of a mutation (or a nearby benign polymorphism) is present at much higher frequency in a population-based cohort of sALS patients than a corresponding cohort of unaffected individuals or if there is functional evidence to support the role of a mutation in the pathological mechanisms underlying ALS, then the gene is considered to be involved in its etiology. Usually, these mutations would be associated with ALS in sporadic cohorts and they can be discovered through a variety of methodologies. Table 17.2 details some of the major genes to be associated with sALS by these methods.

One gene of particular importance in Table 17.2 is *SQSTM1* [96, 97], which encodes the protein p62, a major component of pathological protein aggregates in ALS. Although evidence of segregation has not yet been observed in pedigrees, the finding that mutations in *SQSTM1* account for around 1 % of ALS cases provides, like *TARDBP* and TDP-43, data relating causative genetic lesions to underlying protein pathology. Another important gene is *ATXN2* (ataxin 2). In this gene, a polyglutamine repeat expansion in exon 1 causes spinocerebellar ataxia (SCA), but intermediate-length repeat expansions (27–33 repeats) are associated with ALS [72]. *ATXN2* repeat expansions of this length are, however, present in the general population at a frequency of around 2.4 %, implying that this mutation exerts its effect with incomplete penetrance. 5.5 % of ALS patients harbor repeat expansions of intermediate length, indicating that this allele size range increases disease risk around 2.3-fold [72].

Taken together, Tables 17.1 and 17.2 present a large list of genes implicated in ALS, which may lead to the conclusion that the underlying genetic etiology of the condition is well understood. However, with the exception of *C9orf72*, and depending on population, each gene detailed in Tables 17.1 and 17.2 contributes very little to the overall percentage of cases of ALS. For example, in Ireland, only around 10 % of cases of ALS (sALS and fALS combined) can be explained by established genetic mutations in ALS-associated genes [37]. However, heritability estimates indicate that genetic risk factors play a role in a significant proportion of the unexplained cases – an observation termed *missing heritability*. One method that has dominated the search for the missing heritability of ALS (and a huge number of other diseases) in recent years is the genome-wide association study (GWAS).

Table 17.2 Genes associated with sporadic ALS

Gene	Year	Method	Details	Refs.
ATXN2	2010	CG association testing	Intermediate CAG repeat expansions associated with ALS risk; longer expansions cause SCA	[72]
CABIN1	2013	GWAS	Association with disease susceptibility in single-marker analyses	[73]
CAMK1G	2013	GWAS	Association with disease susceptibility in single-marker analyses	[73]
CHMP2B	2006	CG resequencing	Rare heterozygous mutations identified among ALS patients	[74, 75]
CRMP4	2013	CG resequencing	Rare missense mutation higher frequency in ALS than controls; specific to France	[76]
DPP6	2008	GWAS	Association with disease susceptibility in single-marker and CNV analyses	[77–79]
ELP3	2009	GWAS	Association with disease susceptibility in single-marker analyses. Supportive evidence from a *Drosophila* mutagenesis screen	[80]
FIG4	2009	CG resequencing	Rare heterozygous mutations identified among ALS patients	[81]
FGGY	2007	GWAS	Association with disease susceptibility in single-marker analyses	[82]
ITPR2	2007	GWAS	Association with disease susceptibility in single-marker analyses	[83]
KIFAP3	2009	GWAS	Association with patient survival in single-marker analyses	[84]
MAPT	2001	CG association testing	Association with susceptibility to the Guam ALS-PDC	[85]
NIPA1	2010	GWAS/CG resequencing	Association between disease susceptibility and deletions/polyalanine repeat expansions	[77, 86]
NEFH	1999	CG resequencing	Supported by additional reports of mutation carriers among ALS cases	[87]
PARK7	2005	CG resequencing	Homozygous mutation carriers identified among patients with ALS-PDC	[88]
PON1-3	2006	CG association testing	Associations with disease risk but original studies did not account for multiple testing	[89–93]
SPG4	2005	CG resequencing	Heterozygous mutation identified among an individual with atypical ALS	[94]
SPG11	2010	CG resequencing	Mutations observed in homozygous configuration among patients with autosomal recessive juvenile ALS	[95]
SUSD2	2013	GWAS	Association with disease susceptibility in single-marker analyses	[73]
SQSTM1	2011	CG resequencing	Excess in the frequency of rare variants among cases. Supported by additional reports of mutation carriers among ALS cases	[96, 97]
TAF15	2011	CG resequencing	Mutations observed among fALS cases	[98]
UNC13A	2009	GWAS	Associations with disease risk and patient survival	[52]

ALS-PDC ALS-parkinsonism-dementia complex, *CG* candidate gene, *CNV* copy number variant, *GWAS* genome-wide association study, *SCA* spinocerebellar ataxia

A GWAS involves the simultaneous genotyping of hundreds of thousands of genetic markers (usually single nucleotide polymorphisms or SNPs) in a large cohort of individuals exhibiting a particular trait (for example, ALS), and, if it is a case-control study, a large cohort of control individuals not displaying the trait. The genetic markers act as proxies for nearby genetic variation (for example, disease-causing mutations) by virtue of the fact that the genome is inherited as a block-like mosaic of the haplotypes observed in an individual's parents, and neighboring alleles are usually inherited together (they are *linked*). Neighboring alleles are linked because genetic recombination only occurs periodically on a chromosome, so two positions that are physically close on a chromosome are less likely to be separated by recombination than distant positions. Therefore, if an allele of a particular genetic marker is observed significantly more frequently in, for example, ALS cases, than in controls, the genetic locus surrounding the marker is implicated in the disease.

Because a GWAS conducts many hundreds of thousands of independent statistical tests, the experiment must have an extremely low level for alpha – the size of the p-value required for a result to be considered statistically significant – in order that truly significant results stand out from those that simply represent chance variation instead of systematic case-control effects. Because of this, unless effect sizes are large, the cohort sample sizes required to attain such extreme p-values number into the thousands. The extreme stringency required for alpha is often referred to as the *multiple testing problem* and it represented a major issue the early efforts of GWAS in ALS [78, 82, 83], whose sample sizes were too low to detect significant case-control associations. These studies did, however, indicate the extent of the expected heterogeneity within the undiscovered genetic causes of ALS, and the problem of small cohort sizes would come to be addressed later by much larger GWAS that were made possible through international collaboration [52, 54, 70, 99]. However, these larger studies have, to date, still only identified a small handful of significantly, and replicably, associated loci. Nevertheless, they proved invaluable in the identification of *C9orf72* as a major risk locus [52–54], and ongoing efforts are likely to continue to contribute to our understanding of the etiology of ALS.

Apart from the *C9orf72* locus, other notable loci implicated in ALS by GWAS include chromosomes 19p13.3 (representing *UNC13A* as a risk locus and as a modifier of disease duration) [52], 1p34.1 [99], 17q11.2 [70], 1q32.2 (*CAMK1G*), and 22q11.23 (*CABIN1* and *SUSD2*). The latter three loci were recently implicated in a GWAS of Han Chinese ALS patients [73] and had not previously been implicated in studies involving patients of European descent, indicating the utility of extending GWAS to worldwide ethnic groups. Although many of the loci implicated by GWAS represent excellent candidate genes for ALS etiology with strong supporting evidence, determining the causative genetic lesion in each case has not been trivial and is the focus of ongoing research.

A potential confounder in the search for novel genetic loci involved in ALS is the population differentiation observed in the frequency of ALS-causing mutations. If an undiscovered locus contributes differently to disease risk in different populations, this can mask the size of the observed effect if case and control cohorts are imbalanced in terms of their representation from each population (termed *population stratification*). Although large-scale international GWAS usually carefully control for this possibility, parallel studies involving single populations can serve to detect population-specific risk loci, particularly when a founder effect may play a major role. Furthermore, there is evidence that genetic admixture protects against ALS, with lower mortality rates observed in populations of mixed ancestry, indicating that undiscovered causes of ALS may act through recessive or oligogenic mechanisms [100]. The oligogenic basis for ALS has been supported by the observation of co-inheritance of mutations in more than one ALS gene in some ALS patients [101], providing a possible explanation for much of the missing heritability and incomplete penetrance observed in ALS. However, formally searching for the co-inheritance of novel risk loci by methods such as GWAS is extremely difficult, due to the number of combinations of potential loci to test (known as the *curse of dimensionality*). This can be ameliorated by reducing the number of loci tested using prior knowledge; to this end, an understanding of the underlying biological mechanisms contributing to ALS pathophysiology is extremely useful.

Biological Mechanisms

Although the biological mechanisms underpinning ALS etiology are still incompletely understood, functional and structural similarities in ALS genes and proteins and their converging biological pathways point to a range of common mechanisms that may explain the unifying pathological processes and represent targets for therapeutic intervention. In general, the fact that Mendelian ALS typically exhibits autosomal dominant inheritance suggests that unless haploinsufficiency (loss of function in a single copy of a gene being enough to cause disease) is a feature of most fALS-related genes, the disease is not simply a matter of loss in normal gene functioning. It is also the case that the toxicity of most ALS mutations is an independent attribute of the mutation itself rather than a perturbation of the gene in which the variant occurs.

In vitro and in vivo models of various human ALS mutations suggest that toxicity is usually more likely to reflect gain of function than loss of function effects. For example, many ALS mutations of *SOD1* do not appear to influence the normal enzymatic activity of the encoded protein and knocking out the gene in mice does not recapitulate the ALS-like phenotypes observed with transgenic overexpression of certain human mutations [102]. *SOD1* mutations, which were initially suspected to exert their effects through loss of superoxide dismutase activity, act through a toxic gain of function [103]. Mutant SOD1 protein misfolds [104] and may propagate the misfolding of wild-type SOD1 [105]. Misfolded SOD1 protein aggregates in the cell and brings about a stress response called the unfolded protein response, stalling protein translation and ultimately leading to cell apoptosis and microglial activation [106, 107].

In general, ALS genes tend to be ubiquitously expressed and participate in a diverse array of biological processes. Many ALS genes have a role in RNA processing, suggesting that this may play a crucial part in the etiology of the disease. The structurally similar proteins FUS and TDP-43 (encoded by the ALS genes *FUS and TARDBP*) both share a function in pre-mRNA splicing, RNA transport, and RNA translation [106]. Aggregation of TDP-43 into cytoplasmic stress granules during cellular stress results in a simultaneous gain-of-function and loss-of-function effect that may have downstream effects on RNA processing, leading to cell vulnerability. The gain-of-function aggregation in the cytoplasm results in a depletion of nuclear TDP-43 (the loss-of-function effect), resulting in aberrant processing of its many thousands of RNA targets [108], potentially leading to perturbed cellular processes and cell death. However, exactly why this results in such cell-specific pathology is still uncertain [109].

Proteins encoded by many ALS-associated genes, including *TARDBP*, *SOD1*, *FUS*, *OPTN*, and *UBQLN2*, often localize to ubiquitinated neuronal inclusions within mutation carriers [110]. This could be an indication that toxicity is simply the result of generic gains in protein aggregation propensity. Conversely, protein aggregation may not represent a primary disease process but instead simply a non-pathogenic feature of ALS pathobiology. There is some indication that dysregulated protein homeostasis is a convergent feature of ALS, as ubiquilin 2 (*UBQLN2*), p62 (*SQSTM1*), optineurin (*OPTN*), and vasolin-containing protein 1 (*VCP*) are all involved in proteostasis [109]. The presence of ubiquilin 2 pathology, even in individuals not harboring *UBQLN2* mutations, supports the potential role of the protein degradation pathway as a convergent pathological mechanism [34]. Again, how this leads to cell-specific degeneration, however, is unclear [109].

Impaired axonal maintenance may play a role in the etiology of ALS and this is reflected in some of the mutations observed in fALS. Vesicle-associated membrane-associated protein B (*VAPB*) interacts with EPHA4 protein to mediate cytoskeletal arrangements crucial to axonal integrity, and mutations in profilin-1 (*PFN1*) inhibit axonal outgrowth, potentially exacerbating denervation of muscles [106]. Such a mechanism is biologically plausible given that the primary disease process in ALS is the loss of innervation at the neuromuscular junction through retraction of the axon and failure of compensatory axonal reinnervation [106].

The *C9orf72* repeat expansion represents the most common ALS mutation identified to date, but despite extensive screening, no other mutations disrupting *C9orf72* function have been shown to contribute to ALS etiology. The exact pathological mechanism by which the *C9orf72* repeat expansion elicits disease is not fully understood, but three major possible mechanisms play a role. The first is haploinsufficiency, whereby loss of transcription of the mutated copy of the gene results in lower expression and subsequent pathogenic loss of function. This is supported by a 50 % reduction in *C9orf72* mRNA levels when one copy of the gene contains the expanded allele [19] and functional evidence suggesting that knockdown of the C9orf72 protein invokes an ALS-like phenotype in zebra fish [111]. The second mechanism is generation of toxic repetitive mRNA sequences during transcription [112] resulting in sequestration of mRNA-binding proteins reminiscent of the loss-of-function mechanisms described earlier for TDP-43-mediated toxicity. Finally, secondary structures formed by the GC-rich repeat expansion result in translation of repetitive protein sequences independent of any AUG start codon, by a process known as repeat-associated RNA-encoded non-ATG translation (RAN translation). In this case, all three reading frames of the repeat expansion are translated, resulting in the pathological accumulation of poly-GA, poly-GP, and poly-GR aggregates, as well as, possibly, some poly-PR and poly-PA from *C9orf72* antisense transcripts [113, 114]. It is possible that these pathological inclusions play a role in disrupted protein homeostasis or protein-mediated cytotoxicity.

Despite extensive study, the pathobiological mechanisms leading to selective motor neuron death in ALS are not completely understood. However, it is probable that the majority of mutations act through some kind of toxic gain-of-function process, resulting in RNA toxicity, aberrant RNA metabolism, protein aggregation, aberrant proteostasis, impaired axonal maintenance, or a combination of some or all of these. However, some loss-of-function effects are observed, for example, in recessively inherited *ALS2*-mediated disease. Taken together it should therefore perhaps be anticipated that a complete understanding of ALS pathogenesis will involve a diverse array of mechanisms, that loss and gain of function effects will be relevant, but that gain of function effects may prove the most important. On the question of the existence of final common disease pathways, it remains too early to do more than speculate, but the genotype-phenotype correlations observed with certain ALS gene mutations argue that some heterogeneity should be expected and that a set of convergent pathways is more likely than one single unifying mechanism.

Towards a Complete Understanding and Better Treatment

Extensive genetic heterogeneity, pleiotropy, variable penetrance, variable pedigree size, late age of onset, and rarity of mutations all conspire to confound the straightforward discovery of ALS risk loci and the interpretation of their biological significance. Nevertheless, modern advances in technology and analytical methodologies, coupled with an understanding that progress is best made through large-scale international collaboration, enable large-scale studies such as genome-wide association studies and next-generation sequencing projects, which are likely to continue to shed light on the genetic causes of ALS. In particular, exome and genome sequencing of affected members of ALS pedigrees have yielded a number of novel ALS genes recently, and application of these methodologies to further pedigrees and population-based cohorts will help to define the missing heritability of ALS.

Currently, established ALS genes can explain up to two-thirds of fALS cases and 11 % of sALS cases [47] (these estimates vary depending on population). In-depth understanding of the underlying genetic causes of ALS provides insight into the biological mechanisms underlying its etiology, and a better understanding will inevitably assist towards finding the convergent pathogenic mechanisms. This will aid the development of novel therapeutic strategies and biomarkers for improved and earlier intervention and better outlook for patients.

However, given its heterogeneous nature and its multiple genetic causes, there is a growing opinion that ALS should be viewed as a clinicopathological syndrome, rather than a single disease, with multiple upstream pathological causes converging on a related set of clinical disease features [109]. With this in mind, patient categorization based on genetics and tailored therapies may improve the outcome of pharmacological intervention, as patients belonging to distinct etiological subgroups may respond only to specific therapeutic strategies. This principle is already in effect in a cohort of *SOD1*-positive ALS patients, in which antisense oligonucleotide therapies are being tested as a potential therapeutic intervention [115].

In order for such strategies to become commonplace, routine genetic testing of ALS patients is required. Genetic testing is not, however, universally practiced as part of the clinical management of ALS patients, and opinions differ on which genes should be included in the test panel constituting a standard ALS screen and whether testing should be restricted just to fALS patients or offered to all patients and their relatives [116]. Furthermore, the complexities involved in measuring the size of the expanded allele in the pathogenic *C9orf72* repeat expansion often render the results of tests for this particular variant of ALS inconsistent between laboratories [117]. The variable penetrance of risk alleles such as the *ATXN2* repeat expansion adds complexity in the interpretation of genetic testing and counseling for ALS [118], an issue further complicated by the uncertain nature of the pathogenicity of many ALS-associated alleles [15]. It has therefore been suggested that all of these issues are taken into account in the decision to offer genetic testing to a patient and that the complexities and uncertainties are clearly discussed with patients and their relatives [116].

In conclusion, ALS is genetically heterogeneous, with extensive phenotypic diversity and overlap with related clinical phenotypes. Although many genes have been identified that are mutated in ALS with many more implicated in the disease, the genetic cause for a large proportion of ALS risk remains to be discovered. The underlying biological mechanisms that converge on ALS are only partially understood but it is likely that aberrant RNA processing and protein homeostasis play central roles. Future research into the undiscovered genetic contribution to ALS will shed further light on these pathogenic mechanisms, as well as providing a complete catalog of the causes of the disease, which will, hopefully, contribute towards the development of a cure for this devastating condition.

References

1. Chiò A, Mora G, Calvo A, Mazzini L, Bottacchi E, Mutani R, PARALS. Epidemiology of ALS in Italy: a 10-year prospective population-based study. Neurology. 2009;72(8):725–31.
2. Alonso A, Logroscino G, Jick SS, Hernán MA. Incidence and lifetime risk of motor neuron disease in the United Kingdom: a population-based study. Eur J Neurol. 2009;16(6):745–51.
3. Johnston CA, Stanton BR, Turner MR, Gray R, Blunt AH, Butt D, Ampong MA, Shaw CE, Leigh PN, Al-Chalabi A. Amyotrophic lateral sclerosis in an urban setting: a population based study of inner city London. J Neurol. 2006;253(12):1642–3.

4. Traynor BJ, Codd MB, Corr B, Forde C, Frost E, Hardiman O. Incidence and prevalence of ALS in Ireland, 1995–1997: a population-based study. Neurology. 1999;52(3):504–9.
5. Elamin M, Bede P, Byrne S, Jordan N, Gallagher L, Wynne B, O'Brien C, Phukan J, Lynch C, Pender N, Hardiman O. Cognitive changes predict functional decline in ALS: a population-based longitudinal study. Neurology. 2013;80(17):1590–7.
6. Neumann M, Sampathu DM, Kwong LK, Truax AC, Micsenyi MC, Chou TT, Bruce J, Schuck T, Grossman M, Clark CM, McCluskey LF, Miller BL, Masliah E, Mackenzie IR, Feldman H, Feiden W, Kretzschmar HA, Trojanowski JQ, Lee VM. Ubiquitinated TDP-43 in frontotemporal lobar degeneration and amyotrophic lateral sclerosis. Science. 2006;314(5796):130–3.
7. Kanouchi T, Ohkubo T, Yokota T. Can regional spreading of amyotrophic lateral sclerosis motor symptoms be explained by prion-like propagation? J Neurol Neurosurg Psychiatry. 2012;83(7):739–45.
8. Byrne S, Walsh C, Lynch C, Bede P, Elamin M, Kenna K, McLaughlin R, Hardiman O. Rate of familial amyotrophic lateral sclerosis: a systematic review and meta-analysis. J Neurol Neurosurg Psychiatry. 2011;82(6):623–7.
9. Byrne S, Heverin M, Elamin M, Bede P, Lynch C, Kenna K, MacLaughlin R, Walsh C, Al Chalabi A, Hardiman O. Aggregation of neurologic and neuropsychiatric disease in amyotrophic lateral sclerosis kindreds: a population-based case–control cohort study of familial and sporadic amyotrophic lateral sclerosis. Ann Neurol. 2013;74(5):699–708.
10. Al-Chalabi A, Fang F, Hanby MF, Leigh PN, Shaw CE, Ye W, Rijsdijk F. An estimate of amyotrophic lateral sclerosis heritability using twin data. J Neurol Neurosurg Psychiatry. 2010;81:1324–6.
11. Al-Chalabi A, Lewis CM. Modelling the effects of penetrance and family size on rates of sporadic and familial disease. Hum Herid. 2011;71(4):281–8.
12. Abel O, Powell JF, Andersen PM, Al-Chalabi A. ALSoD: a user-friendly online bioinformatics tool for amyotrophic lateral sclerosis genetics. Hum Mutat. 2012;33(9):1345–51.
13. Ling SC, Polymenidou M, Cleveland DW. Converging mechanisms in ALS and FTD: disrupted RNA and protein homeostasis. Neuron. 2013;79(3):416–38.
14. Cruts M, Theuns J, Van Broeckhoven C. Locus-specific mutation databases for neurodegenerative brain diseases. Hum Mutat. 2012;33(9):1340–4.
15. Kenna KP, McLaughlin RL, Hardiman O, Bradley DG. Using reference databases of genetic variation to evaluate the potential pathogenicity of candidate disease variants. Hum Mutat. 2013;34(6):836–41.
16. Hadano S, Hand CK, Osuga H, Yanagisawa Y, Otomo A, Devon RS, Miyamoto N, Showguchi-Miyata J, Okada Y, Singaraja R, Figlewicz DA, Kwiatkowski T, Hosler BA, Sagie T, Skaug J, Nasir J, Brown Jr RH, Scherer SW, Rouleau GA, Hayden MR, Ikeda JE. A gene encoding a putative GTPase regulator is mutated in familial amyotrophic lateral sclerosis 2. Nat Genet. 2001;29(2):166–73.
17. Yang Y, Hentati A, Deng HX, Dabbagh O, Sasaki T, Hirano M, Hung WY, Ouahchi K, Yan J, Azim AC, Cole N, Gascon G, Yagmour A, Ben-Hamida M, Pericak-Vance M, Hentati F, Siddique T. The gene encoding alsin, a protein with three guanine nucleotide exchange factor domains, is mutated in a form of recessive amyotrophic lateral sclerosis. Nat Genet. 2001;29(2):160–5.
18. Greenway MJ, Andersen PM, Russ C, Ennis S, Cashman S, Donaghy C, Patterson V, Swingler R, Kieran D, Prehn J, Morrison KE, Green A, Acharya KR, Brown Jr RH, Hardiman O. ANG mutations segregate with familial and 'sporadic' amyotrophic lateral sclerosis. Nat Genet. 2006;38(4):411–3.
19. DeJesus-Hernandez M, Mackenzie IR, Boeve BF, Boxer AL, Baker M, Rutherford NJ, Nicholson AM, Finch NA, Flynn H, Adamson J, Kouri N, Wojtas A, Sengdy P, Hsiung GY, Karydas A, Seeley WW, Josephs KA, Coppola G, Geschwind DH, Wszolek ZK, Feldman H, Knopman DS, Petersen RC, Miller BL, Dickson DW, Boylan KB, Graff-Radford NR, Rademakers R. Expanded GGGGCC hexanucleotide repeat in noncoding region of C9ORF72 causes chromosome 9p-linked FTD and ALS. Neuron. 2011;72(2):245–56.

20. Renton AE, Majounie E, Waite A, Simón-Sánchez J, Rollinson S, Gibbs JR, Schymick JC, Laaksovirta H, van Swieten JC, Myllykangas L, Kalimo H, Paetau A, Abramzon Y, Remes AM, Kaganovich A, Scholz SW, Duckworth J, Ding J, Harmer DW, Hernandez DG, Johnson JO, Mok K, Ryten M, Trabzuni D, Guerreiro RJ, Orrell RW, Neal J, Murray A, Pearson J, Jansen IE, Sondervan D, Seelaar H, Blake D, Young K, Halliwell N, Callister JB, Toulson G, Richardson A, Gerhard A, Snowden J, Mann D, Neary D, Nalls MA, Peuralinna T, Jansson L, Isoviita VM, Kaivorinne AL, Hölttä-Vuori M, Ikonen E, Sulkava R, Benatar M, Wuu J, Chiò A, Restagno G, Borghero G, Sabatelli M, ITALSGEN Consortium, Heckerman D, Rogaeva E, Zinman L, Rothstein JD, Sendtner M, Drepper C, Eichler EE, Alkan C, Abdullaev Z, Pack SD, Dutra A, Pak E, Hardy J, Singleton A, Williams NM, Heutink P, Pickering-Brown S, Morris HR, Tienari PJ, Traynor BJ. A hexanucleotide repeat expansion in C9ORF72 is the cause of chromosome 9p21-linked ALS-FTD. Neuron. 2011;72(2):257–68.
21. Mitchell J, Paul P, Chen HJ, Morris A, Payling M, Falchi M, Habgood J, Panoutsou S, Winkler S, Tisato V, Hajitou A, Smith B, Vance C, Shaw C, Mazarakis ND, de Belleroche J. Familial amyotrophic lateral sclerosis is associated with a mutation in D-amino acid oxidase. Proc Natl Acad Sci U S A. 2010;107(16):7556–61.
22. Puls I, Jonnakuty C, LaMonte BH, Holzbaur EL, Tokito M, Mann E, Floeter MK, Bidus K, Drayna D, Oh SJ, Brown Jr RH, Ludlow CL, Fischbeck KH. Mutant dynactin in motor neuron disease. Nat Genet. 2003;33(4):455–6.
23. Takahashi Y, Fukuda Y, Yoshimura J, Toyoda A, Kurppa K, Moritoyo H, Belzil VV, Dion PA, Higasa K, Doi K, Ishiura H, Mitsui J, Date H, Ahsan B, Matsukawa T, Ichikawa Y, Moritoyo T, Ikoma M, Hashimoto T, Kimura F, Murayama S, Onodera O, Nishizawa M, Yoshida M, Atsuta N, Sobue G, Fifita JA, JaCALS, Williams KL, Blair IP, Nicholson GA, Gonzalez-Perez P, Brown Jr RH, Nomoto M, Elenius K, Rouleau GA, Fujiyama A, Morishita S, Goto J, Tsuji S. ERBB4 mutations that disrupt the neuregulin-ErbB4 pathway cause amyotrophic lateral sclerosis type 19. Am J Hum Genet. 2013;97(5):900–5.
24. Kwiatkowski Jr TJ, Bosco DA, Leclerc AL, Tamrazian E, Vanderburg CR, Russ C, Davis A, Gilchrist J, Kasarskis EJ, Munsat T, Valdmanis P, Rouleau GA, Hosler BA, Cortelli P, de Jong PJ, Yoshinaga Y, Haines JL, Pericak-Vance MA, Yan J, Ticozzi N, Siddique T, McKenna-Yasek D, Sapp PC, Horvitz HR, Landers JE, Brown Jr RH. Mutations in the FUS/TLS gene on chromosome 16 cause familial amyotrophic lateral sclerosis. Science. 2009;323(5918): 1205–8.
25. Vance C, Rogelj B, Hortobágyi T, De Vos KJ, Nishimura AL, Sreedharan J, Hu X, Smith B, Ruddy D, Wright P, Ganesalingam J, Williams KL, Tripathi V, Al-Saraj S, Al-Chalabi A, Leigh PN, Blair IP, Nicholson G, de Belleroche J, Gallo JM, Miller CC, Shaw CE. Mutations in FUS, an RNA processing protein, cause familial amyotrophic lateral sclerosis type 6. Science. 2009;323(5918):1208–11.
26. Kim HJ, Kim NC, Wang YD, Scarborough EA, Moore J, Diaz Z, MacLea KS, Freibaum B, Li S, Molliex A, Kanagaraj AP, Carter R, Boylan KB, Wojtas AM, Rademakers R, Pinkus JL, Greenberg SA, Trojanowski JQ, Traynor BJ, Smith BN, Topp S, Gkazi AS, Miller J, Shaw CE, Kottlors M, Kirschner J, Pestronk A, Li YR, Ford AF, Gitler AD, Benatar M, King OD, Kimonis VE, Ross ED, Weihl CC, Shorter J, Taylor JP. Mutations in prion-like domains in hnRNPA2B1 and hnRNPA1 cause multisystem proteinopathy and ALS. Nature. 2013; 495(7442):467–73.
27. Johnson JO, Pioro EP, Boehringer A, Chia R, Feit H, Renton AE, Pliner HA, Abramzon Y, Marangi G, Winborn BJ, Gibbs JR, Nalls MA, Morgan S, Shoai M, Hardy J, Pittman A, Orrell RW, Malaspina A, Sidle KC, Fratta P, Harms MB, Baloh RH, Pestronk A, Weihl CC, Rogaeva E, Zinman L, Drory VE, Borghero G, Mora G, Calvo A, Rothstein JD, ITALSGEN Consortium, Drepper C, Sendtner M, Singleton AB, Taylor JP, Cookson MR, Restagno G, Sabatelli M, Bowser R, Chiò A, Traynor BJ. Mutations in the Matrin 3 gene cause familial amyotrophic lateral sclerosis. Nat Neurosci. 2014;17(5):664–6.
28. Maruyama H, Morino H, Ito H, Izumi Y, Kato H, Watanabe Y, Kinoshita Y, Kamada M, Nodera H, Suzuki H, Komure O, Matsuura S, Kobatake K, Morimoto N, Abe K, Suzuki N, Aoki M, Kawata A, Hirai T, Kato T, Ogasawara K, Hirano A, Takumi T, Kusaka H,

Hagiwara K, Kaji R, Kawakami H. Mutations of optineurin in amyotrophic lateral sclerosis. Nature. 2010;465(7295):223–6.

29. Wu CH, Fallini C, Ticozzi N, Keagle PJ, Sapp PC, Piotrowska K, Lowe P, Koppers M, McKenna-Yasek D, Baron DM, Kost JE, Gonzalez-Perez P, Fox AD, Adams J, Taroni F, Tiloca C, Leclerc AL, Chafe SC, Mangroo D, Moore MJ, Zitzewitz JA, Xu ZS, van den Berg LH, Glass JD, Siciliano G, Cirulli ET, Goldstein DB, Salachas F, Meininger V, Rossoll W, Ratti A, Gellera C, Bosco DA, Bassell GJ, Silani V, Drory VE, Brown Jr RH, Landers JE. Mutations in the profilin 1 gene cause familial amyotrophic lateral sclerosis. Nature. 2012;488(7412):499–503.
30. Chen YZ, Bennett CL, Huynh HM, Blair IP, Puls I, Irobi J, Dierick I, Abel A, Kennerson ML, Rabin BA, Nicholson GA, Auer-Grumbach M, Wagner K, De Jonghe P, Griffin JW, Fischbeck KH, Timmerman V, Cornblath DR, Chance PF. DNA/RNA helicase gene mutations in a form of juvenile amyotrophic lateral sclerosis (ALS4). Am J Hum Genet. 2004;74(6):1128–35.
31. Al-Saif A, Al-Mohanna F, Bohlega S. A mutation in sigma-1 receptor causes juvenile amyotrophic lateral sclerosis. Ann Neurol. 2011;70(6):913–9.
32. Rosen DR, Siddique T, Patterson D, Figlewicz DA, Sapp P, Hentati A, Donaldson D, Goto J, O'Regan JP, Deng H, Rahmani Z, Krizus A, McKenna-Yasek D, Cayabyab A, Gaston SM, Berger R, Tanzi RE, Halperin JJ, Herzfeldt B, Van den Bergh R, Hung W, Bird T, Deng G, Mulder DW, Smyth C, Laing NG, Soriano E, Pericak–Vance MA, Haines J, Rouleau GA, Gusella JS, Horvitz HR, Brown Jr RH. Mutations in Cu/Zn superoxide dismutase gene are associated with familial amyotrophic lateral sclerosis. Nature. 1993;362(6415):59–62.
33. Sreedharan J, Blair IP, Tripathi VB, Hu X, Vance C, Rogelj B, Ackerley S, Durnall JC, Williams KL, Buratti E, Baralle F, de Belleroche J, Mitchell JD, Leigh PN, Al-Chalabi A, Miller CC, Nicholson G, Shaw CE. TDP-43 mutations in familial and sporadic amyotrophic lateral sclerosis. Science. 2008;319(5870):1668–72.
34. Deng HX, Chen W, Hong ST, Boycott KM, Gorrie GH, Siddique N, Yang Y, Fecto F, Shi Y, Zhai H, Jiang H, Hirano M, Rampersaud E, Jansen GH, Donkervoort S, Bigio EH, Brooks BR, Ajroud K, Sufit RL, Haines JL, Mugnaini E, Pericak-Vance MA, Siddique T. Mutations in UBQLN2 cause dominant X-linked juvenile and adult-onset ALS and ALS/dementia. Nature. 2011;47(7363):211–5.
35. Nishimura AL, Mitne-Neto M, Silva HC, Richieri-Costa A, Middleton S, Cascio D, Kok F, Oliveira JR, Gillingwater T, Webb J, Skehel P, Zatz M. A mutation in the vesicle-trafficking protein VAPB causes late-onset spinal muscular atrophy and amyotrophic lateral sclerosis. Am J Hum Genet. 2004;75(5):822–31.
36. Johnson JO, Mandrioli J, Benatar M, Abramzon Y, Van Deerlin VM, Trojanowski JQ, Gibbs JR, Brunetti M, Gronka S, Wuu J, Ding J, McCluskey L, Martinez-Lage M, Falcone D, Hernandez DG, Arepalli S, Chong S, Schymick JC, Rothstein J, Landi F, Wang YD, Calvo A, Mora G, Sabatelli M, Monsurrò MR, Battistini S, Salvi F, Spataro R, Sola P, Borghero G, ITALSGEN Consortium, Galassi G, Scholz SW, Taylor JP, Restagno G, Chiò A, Traynor BJ. Exome sequencing reveals VCP mutations as a cause of familial ALS. Neuron. 2010;68(5):857–64.
37. Kenna KP, McLaughlin RL, Byrne S, Elamin M, Heverin M, Kenny EM, Cormican P, Morris DW, Donaghy CG, Bradley DG, Hardiman O. Delineating the genetic heterogeneity of ALS using targeted high-throughput sequencing. J Med Genet. 2013;50(11):776–83.
38. van Es MA, Dahlberg C, Birve A, Veldink JH, van den Berg LH, Andersen PM. Large-scale SOD1 mutation screening provides evidence for genetic heterogeneity in amyotrophic lateral sclerosis. J Neurol Neurosurg Psychiatry. 2010;81(5):562–6.
39. Cudkowicz ME, McKenna-Yasek D, Sapp PE, Chin W, Geller B, Hayden DL, Schoenfeld DA, Hosler BA, Horvitz HR, Brown RH. Epidemiology of mutations in superoxide dismutase in amyotrophic lateral sclerosis. Ann Neurol. 1997;41(2):210–21.
40. Chiò A, Traynor BJ, Lombardo F, Fimognari M, Calvo A, Ghiglione P, Mutani R, Restagno G. Prevalence of SOD1 mutations in the Italian ALS population. Neurology. 2008;70(7):533–7.
41. Andersen PM. Amyotrophic lateral sclerosis associated with mutations in the CuZn superoxide dismutase gene. Curr Neurol Neurosci Rep. 2006;6(1):37–46.

42. Andersen PM, Forsgren L, Binzer M, Nilsson P, Ala-Hurula V, Keränen ML, Bergmark L, Saarinen A, Haltia T, Tarvainen I, Kinnunen E, Udd B, Marklund SL. Autosomal recessive adult-onset amyotrophic lateral sclerosis associated with homozygosity for Asp90Ala CuZn-superoxide dismutase mutation. A clinical and genealogical study of 36 patients. Brain. 1996;119(4):1153–72.
43. Muller FL, Liu Y, Jernigan A, Borchelt D, Richardson A, Van Remmen H. MnSOD deficiency has a differential effect on disease progression in two different ALS mutant mouse models. Muscle Nerve. 2008;38(3):1173–83.
44. Lagier-Tourenne C, Cleveland DW. Rethinking ALS: the FUS about TDP-43. Cell. 2009;136(6):1001–4.
45. Chiò A, Borghero G, Pugliatti M, Ticca A, Calvo A, Moglia C, Mutani R, Brunetti M, Ossola I, Marrosu MG, Murru MR, Floris G, Cannas A, Parish LD, Cossu P, Abramzon Y, Johnson JO, Nalls MA, Arepalli S, Chong S, Hernandez DG, Traynor BJ, Restagno G, Italian Amyotrophic Lateral Sclerosis Genetic (ITALSGEN) Consortium. Large proportion of amyotrophic lateral sclerosis cases in Sardinia due to a single founder mutation of the TARDBP gene. Arch Neurol. 2011;68(5):594–8.
46. Albagha OM, Visconti MR, Alonso N, Langston AL, Cundy T, Dargie R, Dunlop MG, Fraser WD, Hooper MJ, Isaia G, Nicholson GC, del Pino Montes J, Gonzalez-Sarmiento R, di Stefano M, Tenesa A, Walsh JP, Ralston SH. Genome-wide association study identifies variants at CSF1, OPTN and TNFRSF11A as genetic risk factors for Paget's disease of bone. Nat Genet. 2010;42(6):520–4.
47. Renton AE, Chiò A, Traynor BJ. State of play in amyotrophic lateral sclerosis genetics. Nat Neurosci. 2014;17(1):17–23.
48. Chiò A, Calvo A, Mazzini L, Cantello R, Mora G, Moglia C, Corrado L, D'Alfonso S, Majounie E, Renton A, Pisano F, Ossola I, Brunetti M, Traynor BJ, Restagno G, PARALS. Extensive genetics of ALS: a population-based study in Italy. Neurology. 2012;79(19):1983–9.
49. Millecamps S, Corcia P, Cazeneuve C, Boillée S, Seilhean D, Danel-Brunaud V, Vandenberghe N, Pradat PF, Le Forestier N, Lacomblez L, Bruneteau G, Camu W, Brice A, Meininger V, LeGuern E, Salachas F. Mutations in UBQLN2 are rare in French amyotrophic lateral sclerosis. Neurobiol Aging. 2012;33(4):839.e1–3.
50. McLaughlin RL, Kenna KP, Vajda A, Byrne S, Bradley DG, Hardiman O. UBQLN2 mutations are not a frequent cause of amyotrophic lateral sclerosis in Ireland. Neurobiol Aging. 2014;35(1):267.e9–11.
51. Morita M, Al-Chalabi A, Andersen PM, Hosler B, Sapp P, Englund E, Mitchell JE, Habgood JJ, de Belleroche J, Xi J, Jongjaroenprasert W, Horvitz HR, Gunnarsson LG, Brown Jr RH. A locus on chromosome 9p confers susceptibility to ALS and frontotemporal dementia. Neurology. 2006;66(6):839–44.
52. van Es MA, Veldink JH, Saris CG, Blauw HM, van Vught PW, Birve A, Lemmens R, Schelhaas HJ, Groen EJ, Huisman MH, van der Kooi AJ, de Visser M, Dahlberg C, Estrada K, Rivadeneira F, Hofman A, Zwarts MJ, van Doormaal PT, Rujescu D, Strengman E, Giegling I, Muglia P, Tomik B, Slowik A, Uitterlinden AG, Hendrich C, Waibel S, Meyer T, Ludolph AC, Glass JD, Purcell S, Cichon S, Nöthen MM, Wichmann HE, Schreiber S, Vermeulen SH, Kiemeney LA, Wokke JH, Cronin S, McLaughlin RL, Hardiman O, Fumoto K, Pasterkamp RJ, Meininger V, Melki J, Leigh PN, Shaw CE, Landers JE, Al-Chalabi A, Brown Jr RH, Robberecht W, Andersen PM, Ophoff RA, van den Berg LH. Genome-wide association study identifies 19p13.3 (UNC13A) and 9p21.2 as susceptibility loci for sporadic amyotrophic lateral sclerosis. Nat Genet. 2009;41(10):1083–7.
53. Laaksovirta H, Peuralinna T, Schymick JC, Scholz SW, Lai SL, Myllykangas L, Sulkava R, Jansson L, Hernandez DG, Gibbs JR, Nalls MA, Heckerman D, Tienari PJ, Traynor BJ. Chromosome 9p21 in amyotrophic lateral sclerosis in Finland: a genome-wide association study. Lancet Neurol. 2010;9(10):978–85.
54. Shatunov A, Mok K, Newhouse S, Weale ME, Smith B, Vance C, Johnson L, Veldink JH, van Es MA, van den Berg LH, Robberecht W, Van Damme P, Hardiman O, Farmer AE, Lewis

CM, Butler AW, Abel O, Andersen PM, Fogh I, Silani V, Chiò A, Traynor BJ, Melki J, Meininger V, Landers JE, McGuffin P, Glass JD, Pall H, Leigh PN, Hardy J, Brown Jr RH, Powell JF, Orrell RW, Morrison KE, Shaw PJ, Shaw CE, Al-Chalabi A. Chromosome 9p21 in sporadic amyotrophic lateral sclerosis in the UK and seven other countries: a genome-wide association study. Lancet Neurol. 2010;9(10):986–94.

55. Mok K, Traynor BJ, Schymick J, Tienari PJ, Laaksovirta H, Peuralinna T, Myllykangas L, Chiò A, Shatunov A, Boeve BF, Boxer AL, DeJesus-Hernandez M, Mackenzie IR, Waite A, Williams N, Morris HR, Simón-Sánchez J, van Swieten JC, Heutink P, Restagno G, Mora G, Morrison KE, Shaw PJ, Rollinson PS, Al-Chalabi A, Rademakers R, Pickering-Brown S, Orrell RW, Nalls MA, Hardy J. Chromosome 9 ALS and FTD locus is probably derived from a single founder. Neurobiol Aging. 2012;33(1):209.e3–8.
56. Boeve BF, Boylan KB, Graff-Radford NR, DeJesus-Hernandez M, Knopman DS, Pedraza O, Vemuri P, Jones D, Lowe V, Murray ME, Dickson DW, Josephs KA, Rush BK, Machulda MM, Fields JA, Ferman TJ, Baker M, Rutherford NJ, Adamson J, Wszolek ZK, Adeli A, Savica R, Boot B, Kuntz KM, Gavrilova R, Reeves A, Whitwell J, Kantarci K, Jack Jr CR, Parisi JE, Lucas JA, Petersen RC, Rademakers R. Characterization of frontotemporal dementia and/or amyotrophic lateral sclerosis associated with the GGGGCC repeat expansion in C9ORF72. Brain. 2012;135(3):765–83.
57. Cooper-Knock J, Shaw PJ, Kirby J. The widening spectrum of C9ORF72-related disease; genotype/phenotype correlations and potential modifiers of clinical phenotype. Acta Neuropathol. 2014;127(3):333–45.
58. Meisler MH, Grant AE, Jones JM, Lenk GM, He F, Todd PK, Kamali M, Albin RL, Lieberman AP, Langenecker SA, McInnis MG. C9ORF72 expansion in a family with bipolar disorder. Bipolar Disord. 2013;15(3):326–32.
59. Calvo A, Moglia C, Canosa A, Cistaro A, Valentini C, Carrara G, Soldano E, Ilardi A, Bersano E, Bertuzzo D, Brunetti M, Ossola I, Restagno G, Chiò A. Amyotrophic lateral sclerosis/frontotemporal dementia with predominant manifestations of obsessive-compulsive disorder associated to GGGGCC expansion of the c9orf72 gene. J Neurol. 2012;259(12): 2723–5.
60. Majounie E, Renton AE, Mok K, Dopper EG, Waite A, Rollinson S, Chiò A, Restagno G, Nicolaou N, Simon-Sanchez J, van Swieten JC, Abramzon Y, Johnson JO, Sendtner M, Pamphlett R, Orrell RW, Mead S, Sidle KC, Houlden H, Rohrer JD, Morrison KE, Pall H, Talbot K, Ansorge O, Chromosome 9-ALS/FTD Consortium, French research network on FTLD/FTLD/ALS, ITALSGEN Consortium, Hernandez DG, Arepalli S, Sabatelli M, Mora G, Corbo M, Giannini F, Calvo A, Englund E, Borghero G, Floris GL, Remes AM, Laaksovirta H, McCluskey L, Trojanowski JQ, Van Deerlin VM, Schellenberg GD, Nalls MA, Drory VE, Lu CS, Yeh TH, Ishiura H, Takahashi Y, Tsuji S, Le Ber I, Brice A, Drepper C, Williams N, Kirby J, Shaw P, Hardy J, Tienari PJ, Heutink P, Morris HR, Pickering-Brown S, Traynor BJ. Frequency of the C9orf72 hexanucleotide repeat expansion in patients with amyotrophic lateral sclerosis and frontotemporal dementia: a cross-sectional study. Lancet Neurol. 2012;11(4):323–40.
61. Byrne S, Elamin M, Bede P, Shatunov A, Walsh C, Corr B, Heverin M, Jordan N, Kenna K, Lynch C, McLaughlin RL, Iyer PM, O'Brien C, Phukan J, Wynne B, Bokde AL, Bradley DG, Pender N, Al-Chalabi A, Hardiman O. Cognitive and clinical characteristics of patients with amyotrophic lateral sclerosis carrying a C9orf72 repeat expansion: a population-based cohort study. Lancet Neurol. 2012;11(3):232–40.
62. Lattante S, Le Ber I, Camuzat A, Brice A, Kabashi E. Mutations in the PFN1 gene are not a common cause in patients with amyotrophic lateral sclerosis and frontotemporal lobar degeneration in France. Neurobiol Aging. 2013;34(6):1709.e1–2.
63. Alexander MD, Traynor BJ, Miller N, Corr B, Frost E, McQuaid S, Brett FM, Green A, Hardiman O. "True" sporadic ALS associated with a novel SOD-1 mutation. Ann Neurol. 2002;52(5):680–3.
64. DeJesus-Hernandez M, Kocerha J, Finch N, Crook R, Baker M, Desaro P, Johnston A, Rutherford N, Wojtas A, Kennelly K, Wszolek ZK, Graff-Radford N, Boylan K, Rademakers

R. De novo truncating FUS gene mutation as a cause of sporadic amyotrophic lateral sclerosis. Hum Mutat. 2010;31(5):E1377–89.
65. Chiò A, Calvo A, Moglia C, Ossola I, Brunetti M, Sbaiz L, Lai SL, Abramzon Y, Traynor BJ, Restagno G. A de novo missense mutation of the FUS gene in a "true" sporadic ALS case. Neurobiol Aging. 2011;32(3):553.e23–26.
66. Conte A, Lattante S, Zollino M, Marangi G, Luigetti M, Del Grande A, Servidei S, Trombetta F, Sabatelli M. P525L FUS mutation is consistently associated with a severe form of juvenile amyotrophic lateral sclerosis. Neuromuscular Disord. 2012;22(1):73–5.
67. Calvo A, Moglia C, Canosa A, Brunetti M, Barberis M, Traynor BJ, Carrara G, Valentini C, Restagno G, Chiò A. A de novo nonsense mutation of the FUS gene in an apparently familial amyotrophic lateral sclerosis case. Neurobiol Aging. 2014;35(6):1513.e7–11.
68. Chesi A, Staahl BT, Jovičić A, Couthouis J, Fasolino M, Raphael AR, Yamazaki T, Elias L, Polak M, Kelly C, Williams KL, Fifita JA, Maragakis NJ, Nicholson GA, King OD, Reed R, Crabtree GR, Blair IP, Glass JD, Gitler AD. Exome sequencing to identify de novo mutations in sporadic ALS trios. Nat Neurosci. 2013;16(7):581–855.
69. Neale BM, Kou Y, Liu L, Ma'ayan A, Samocha KE, Sabo A, Lin CF, Stevens C, Wang LS, Makarov V, Polak P, Yoon S, Maguire J, Crawford EL, Campbell NG, Geller ET, Valladares O, Schafer C, Liu H, Zhao T, Cai G, Lihm J, Dannenfelser R, Jabado O, Peralta Z, Nagaswamy U, Muzny D, Reid JG, Newsham I, Wu Y, Lewis L, Han Y, Voight BF, Lim E, Rossin E, Kirby A, Flannick J, Fromer M, Shakir K, Fennell T, Garimella K, Banks E, Poplin R, Gabriel S, DePristo M, Wimbish JR, Boone BE, Levy SE, Betancur C, Sunyaev S, Boerwinkle E, Buxbaum JD, Cook Jr EH, Devlin B, Gibbs RA, Roeder K, Schellenberg GD, Sutcliffe JS, Daly MJ. Patterns and rates of exonic de novo mutations in autism spectrum disorders. Nature. 2012;485(7397):242–5.
70. Fogh I, Ratti A, Gellera C, Lin K, Tiloca C, Moskvina V, Corrado L, Sorarù G, Cereda C, Corti S, Gentilini D, Calini D, Castellotti B, Mazzini L, Querin G, Gagliardi S, Del Bo R, Conforti FL, Siciliano G, Inghilleri M, Saccà F, Bongioanni P, Penco S, Corbo M, Sorbi S, Filosto M, Ferlini A, Di Blasio AM, Signorini S, Shatunov A, Jones A, Shaw PJ, Morrison KE, Farmer AE, Van Damme P, Robberecht W, Chiò A, Traynor BJ, Sendtner M, Melki J, Meininger V, Hardiman O, Andersen PM, Leigh NP, Glass JD, Overste D, Diekstra FP, Veldink JH, van Es MA, Shaw CE, Weale ME, Lewis CM, Williams J, Brown RH, Landers JE, Ticozzi N, Ceroni M, Pegoraro E, Comi GP, D'Alfonso S, van den Berg LH, Taroni F, Al-Chalabi A, Powell J, Silani V, SLAGEN Consortium Collaborators. A genome-wide association meta-analysis identifies a novel locus at 17q11.2 associated with sporadic amyotrophic lateral sclerosis. Hum Mol Genet. 2014;23(8):2220–31.
71. Keller MF, Ferrucci L, Singleton AB, Tienari PJ, Laaksovirta H, Restagno G, Chiò A, Traynor BJ, Nalls MA. Genome-wide analysis of the heritability of amyotrophic lateral sclerosis. JAMA Neurol. 2014;71(9):1123–34. doi:10.1001/jamaneurol.2014.1184.
72. Elden AC, Kim HJ, Hart MP, Chen-Plotkin AS, Johnson BS, Fang X, Armakola M, Geser F, Greene R, Lu MM, Padmanabhan A, Clay-Falcone D, McCluskey L, Elman L, Juhr D, Gruber PJ, Rüb U, Auburger G, Trojanowski JQ, Lee VM, Van Deerlin VM, Bonini NM, Gitler AD. Ataxin-2 intermediate-length polyglutamine expansions are associated with increased risk for ALS. Nature. 2010;466(7310):1069–75.
73. Deng M, Wei L, Zuo X, Tian Y, Xie F, Hu P, Zhu C, Yu F, Meng Y, Wang H, Zhang F, Ma H, Ye R, Cheng H, Du J, Dong W, Zhou S, Wang C, Wang Y, Wang J, Chen X, Sun Z, Zhou N, Jiang Y, Liu X, Li X, Zhang N, Liu N, Guan Y, Han Y, Han Y, Lv X, Fu Y, Yu H, Xi C, Xie D, Zhao Q, Xie P, Wang X, Zhang Z, Shen L, Cui Y, Yin X, Cheng H, Liang B, Zheng X, Lee TM, Chen G, Zhou F, Veldink JH, Robberecht W, Landers JE, Andersen PM, Al-Chalabi A, Shaw C, Liu C, Tang B, Xiao S, Robertson J, Zhang F, van den Berg LH, Sun L, Liu J, Yang S, Ju X, Wang K, Zhang X. Genome-wide association analyses in Han Chinese identify two new susceptibility loci for amyotrophic lateral sclerosis. Nat Genet. 2013;45(6):697–700.
74. Cox LE, Ferraiuolo L, Goodall EF, Heath PR, Higginbottom A, Mortiboys H, Hollinger HC, Hartley JA, Brockington A, Burness CE, Morrison KE, Wharton SB, Grierson AJ, Ince PG,

Kirby J, Shaw PJ. Mutations in CHMP2B in lower motor neuron predominant amyotrophic lateral sclerosis (ALS). PLoS One. 2010;5(3):e9872.

75. Parkinson N, Ince PG, Smith MO, Highley R, Skibinski G, Andersen PM, Morrison KE, Pall HS, Hardiman O, Collinge J, Shaw PJ, Fisher EM, MRC Proteomics in ALS Study, FReJA Consortium. ALS phenotypes with mutations in CHMP2B (charged multivesicular body protein 2B). Neurology. 2006;67(6):1074–7.
76. Blasco H, Bernard-Marissal N, Vourc'h P, Guettard YO, Sunyach C, Augereau O, Khederchah J, Mouzat K, Antar C, Gordon PH, Veyrat-Durebex C, Besson G, Andersen PM, Salachas F, Meininger V, Camu W, Pettmann B, Andres CR, Corcia P, French ALS Study Group. A rare motor neuron deleterious missense mutation in the DPYSL3 (CRMP4) gene is associated with ALS. Hum Mutat. 2013;34(7):953–60.
77. Blauw HM, Al-Chalabi A, Andersen PM, van Vught PW, Diekstra FP, van Es MA, Saris CG, Groen EJ, van Rheenen W, Koppers M, Van't Slot R, Strengman E, Estrada K, Rivadeneira F, Hofman A, Uitterlinden AG, Kiemeney LA, Vermeulen SH, Birve A, Waibel S, Meyer T, Cronin S, McLaughlin RL, Hardiman O, Sapp PC, Tobin MD, Wain LV, Tomik B, Slowik A, Lemmens R, Rujescu D, Schulte C, Gasser T, Brown Jr RH, Landers JE, Robberecht W, Ludolph AC, Ophoff RA, Veldink JH, van den Berg LH. A large genome scan for rare CNVs in amyotrophic lateral sclerosis. Hum Mol Genet. 2010;19(20):4091–9.
78. Cronin S, Berger S, Ding J, Schymick JC, Washecka N, Hernandez DG, Greenway MJ, Bradley DG, Traynor BJ, Hardiman O. A genome-wide association study of sporadic ALS in a homogenous Irish population. Hum Mol Genet. 2008;17(5):768–74.
79. van Es MA, van Vught PW, Blauw HM, Franke L, Saris CG, Van den Bosch L, de Jong SW, de Jong V, Baas F, van't Slot R, Lemmens R, Schelhaas HJ, Birve A, Sleegers K, Van Broeckhoven C, Schymick JC, Traynor BJ, Wokke JH, Wijmenga C, Robberecht W, Andersen PM, Veldink JH, Ophoff RA, van den Berg LH. Genetic variation in DPP6 is associated with susceptibility to amyotrophic lateral sclerosis. Nat Genet. 2008;40(1):29–31.
80. Simpson CL, Lemmens R, Miskiewicz K, Broom WJ, Hansen VK, van Vught PW, Landers JE, Sapp P, Van Den Bosch L, Knight J, Neale BM, Turner MR, Veldink JH, Ophoff RA, Tripathi VB, Beleza A, Shah MN, Proitsi P, Van Hoecke A, Carmeliet P, Horvitz HR, Leigh PN, Shaw CE, van den Berg LH, Sham PC, Powell JF, Verstreken P, Brown Jr RH, Robberecht W, Al-Chalabi A. Variants of the elongator protein 3 (ELP3) gene are associated with motor neuron degeneration. Hum Mol Genet. 2009;18(3):472–81.
81. Chow CY, Landers JE, Bergren SK, Sapp PC, Grant AE, Jones JM, Everett L, Lenk GM, McKenna-Yasek DM, Weisman LS, Figlewicz D, Brown RH, Meisler MH. Deleterious variants of FIG4, a phosphoinositide phosphatase, in patients with ALS. Am J Hum Genet. 2009;84(1):85–8.
82. Dunckley T, Huentelman MJ, Craig DW, Pearson JV, Szelinger S, Joshipura K, Halperin RF, Stamper C, Jensen KR, Letizia D, Hesterlee SE, Pestronk A, Levine T, Bertorini T, Graves MC, Mozaffar T, Jackson CE, Bosch P, McVey A, Dick A, Barohn R, Lomen-Hoerth C, Rosenfeld J, O'connor DT, Zhang K, Crook R, Ryberg H, Hutton M, Katz J, Simpson EP, Mitsumoto H, Bowser R, Miller RG, Appel SH, Stephan DA. Whole-genome analysis of sporadic amyotrophic lateral sclerosis. N Engl J Med. 2007;357(8):775–88.
83. van Es MA, Van Vught PW, Blauw HM, Franke L, Saris CG, Andersen PM, Van Den Bosch L, de Jong SW, van't Slot R, Birve A, Lemmens R, de Jong V, Baas F, Schelhaas HJ, Sleegers K, Van Broeckhoven C, Wokke JH, Wijmenga C, Robberecht W, Veldink JH, Ophoff RA, van den Berg LH. ITPR2 as a susceptibility gene in sporadic amyotrophic lateral sclerosis: a genome-wide association study. Lancet Neurol. 2007;6(10):869–77.
84. Landers JE, Melki J, Meininger V, Glass JD, van den Berg LH, van Es MA, Sapp PC, van Vught PW, McKenna-Yasek DM, Blauw HM, Cho TJ, Polak M, Shi L, Wills AM, Broom WJ, Ticozzi N, Silani V, Ozoguz A, Rodriguez-Leyva I, Veldink JH, Ivinson AJ, Saris CG, Hosler BA, Barnes-Nessa A, Couture N, Wokke JH, Kwiatkowski Jr TJ, Ophoff RA, Cronin S, Hardiman O, Diekstra FP, Leigh PN, Shaw CE, Simpson CL, Hansen VK, Powell JF, Corcia P, Salachas F, Heath S, Galan P, Georges F, Horvitz HR, Lathrop M, Purcell S, Al-Chalabi A, Brown Jr RH. Reduced expression of the Kinesin-Associated Protein 3

(KIFAP3) gene increases survival in sporadic amyotrophic lateral sclerosis. Proc Natl Acad Sci U S A. 2009;106(22):9004–9.

85. Poorkaj P, Tsuang D, Wijsman E, Steinbart E, Garruto RM, Craig UK, Chapman NH, Anderson L, Bird TD, Plato CC, Perl DP, Weiderholt W, Galasko D, Schellenberg GD. TAU as a susceptibility gene for amyotropic lateral sclerosis-parkinsonism dementia complex of Guam. Arch Neurol. 2001;58(11):1871–8.
86. Blauw HM, van Rheenen W, Koppers M, Van Damme P, Waibel S, Lemmens R, van Vught PW, Meyer T, Schulte C, Gasser T, Cuppen E, Pasterkamp RJ, Robberecht W, Ludolph AC, Veldink JH, van den Berg LH. NIPA1 polyalanine repeat expansions are associated with amyotrophic lateral sclerosis. Hum Mol Genet. 2012;21(11):2497–502.
87. Al-Chalabi A, Andersen PM, Nilsson P, Chioza B, Andersson JL, Russ C, Shaw CE, Powell JF, Leigh PN. Deletions of the heavy neurofilament subunit tail in amyotrophic lateral sclerosis. Hum Mol Genet. 1999;8(2):157–64.
88. Annesi G, Savettieri G, Pugliese P, D'Amelio M, Tarantino P, Ragonese P, La Bella V, Piccoli T, Civitelli D, Annesi F, Fierro B, Piccoli F, Arabia G, Caracciolo M, Cirò Candiano IC, Quattrone A. DJ-1 mutations and parkinsonism-dementia-amyotrophic lateral sclerosis complex. Ann Neurol. 2005;58(5):803–7.
89. Cronin S, Greenway MJ, Prehn JH, Hardiman O. Paraoxonase promoter and intronic variants modify risk of sporadic amyotrophic lateral sclerosis. J Neurol Neurosurg Psychiatry. 2007;78(9):984–6.
90. Saeed M, Siddique N, Hung WY, Usacheva E, Liu E, Sufit RL, Heller SL, Haines JL, Pericak-Vance M, Siddique T. Paraoxonase cluster polymorphisms are associated with sporadic ALS. Neurology. 2006;67(5):771–6.
91. Slowik A, Tomik B, Wolkow PP, Partyka D, Turaj W, Malecki MT, Pera J, Dziedzic T, Szczudlik A, Figlewicz DA. Paraoxonase gene polymorphisms and sporadic ALS. Neurology. 2006;67(5):766–70.
92. van Blitterswijk M, Blokhuis A, van Es MA, van Vught PW, Rowicka PA, Schelhaas HJ, van der Kooi AJ, de Visser M, Veldink JH, van den Berg LH. Rare and common paraoxonase gene variants in amyotrophic lateral sclerosis patients. Neurobiol Aging. 2012;33(8):1845.e1–3.
93. Wills AM, Cronin S, Slowik A, Kasperaviciute D, Van Es MA, Morahan JM, Valdmanis PN, Meininger V, Melki J, Shaw CE, Rouleau GA, Fisher EM, Shaw PJ, Morrison KE, Pamphlett R, Van den Berg LH, Figlewicz DA, Andersen PM, Al-Chalabi A, Hardiman O, Purcell S, Landers JE, Brown Jr RH. A large-scale international meta-analysis of paraoxonase gene polymorphisms in sporadic ALS. Neurology. 2009;73(1):16–24.
94. Meyer T, Schwan A, Dullinger JS, Brocke J, Hoffmann KT, Nolte CH, Hopt A, Kopp U, Andersen P, Epplen JT, Linke P. Early-onset ALS with long-term survival associated with spastin gene mutation. Neurology. 2005;65(1):141–3.
95. Orlacchio A, Babalini C, Borreca A, Patrono C, Massa R, Basaran S, Munhoz RP, Rogaeva EA, St George-Hyslop PH, Bernardi G, Kawarai T. SPATACSIN mutations cause autosomal recessive juvenile amyotrophic lateral sclerosis. Brain. 2010;133(2):591–8.
96. Fecto F, Yan J, Vemula SP, Liu E, Yang Y, Chen W, Zheng JG, Shi Y, Siddique N, Arrat H, Donkervoort S, Ajroud-Driss S, Sufit RL, Heller SL, Deng HX, Siddique T. SQSTM1 mutations in familial and sporadic amyotrophic lateral sclerosis. Arch Neurol. 2011;68(11):1440–6.
97. Rubino E, Rainero I, Chiò A, Rogaeva E, Galimberti D, Fenoglio P, Grinberg Y, Isaia G, Calvo A, Gentile S, Bruni AC, St George-Hyslop PH, Scarpini E, Gallone S, Pinessi L, TODEM Study Group. SQSTM1 mutations in frontotemporal lobar degeneration and amyotrophic lateral sclerosis. Neurology. 2012;79(15):1556–62.
98. Ticozzi N, Vance C, Leclerc AL, Keagle P, Glass JD, McKenna-Yasek D, Sapp PC, Silani V, Bosco DA, Shaw CE, Brown Jr RH, Landers JE. Mutational analysis reveals the FUS homolog TAF15 as a candidate gene for familial amyotrophic lateral sclerosis. Am J Med Genet B Neuropsychiatr Genet. 2011;156B(3):285–90.
99. ALSGEN Consortium, Ahmeti KB, Ajroud-Driss S, Al-Chalabi A, Andersen PM, Armstrong J, Birve A, Blauw HM, Brown RH, Bruijn L, Chen W, Chio A, Comeau MC, Cronin S, Diekstra FP, Soraya Gkazi A, Glass JD, Grab JD, Groen EJ, Haines JL, Hardiman O, Heller

S, Huang J, Hung WY, ITALSGEN Consortium, Jaworski JM, Jones A, Khan H, Landers JE, Langefeld CD, Leigh PN, Marion MC, McLaughlin RL, Meininger V, Melki J, Miller JW, Mora G, Pericak-Vance MA, Rampersaud E, Robberecht W, Russell LP, Salachas F, Saris CG, Shatunov A, Shaw CE, Siddique N, Siddique T, Smith BN, Sufit R, Topp S, Traynor BJ, Vance C, van Damme P, van den Berg LH, van Es MA, van Vught PW, Veldink JH, Yang Y, Zheng JG. Age of onset of amyotrophic lateral sclerosis is modulated by a locus on 1p34.1. Neurobiol Aging. 2013;34(1):357.e7–19.
100. Zaldivar T, Gutierrez J, Lara G, Carbonara M, Logroscino G, Hardiman O. Reduced frequency of ALS in an ethnically mixed population: a population-based mortality study. Neurology. 2009;72(19):1640–5.
101. van Blitterswijk M, van Es MA, Hennekam EA, Dooijes D, van Rheenen W, Medic J, Bourque PR, Schelhaas HJ, van der Kooi AJ, de Visser M, de Bakker PI, Veldink JH, van den Berg LH. Evidence for an oligogenic basis of amyotrophic lateral sclerosis. Hum Mol Genet. 2012;21(17):3776–84.
102. Shibata N. Transgenic mouse model for familial amyotrophic lateral sclerosis with superoxide dismutase-1 mutation. Neuropathology. 2001;21(1):82–92.
103. Bruijn LI, Houseweart MK, Kato S, Anderson KL, Anderson SD, Ohama E, Reaume AG, Scott RW, Cleveland DW. Aggregation and motor neuron toxicity of an ALS-linked SOD1 mutant independent from wild-type SOD1. Science. 1998;281(5384):1851–4.
104. Hart PJ. Pathogenic superoxide dismutase structure, folding, aggregation and turnover. Curr Opin Chem Biol. 2006;10(2):131–8.
105. Grad LI, Guest WC, Yanai A, Pokrishevsky E, O'Neill MA, Gibbs E, Semenchenko V, Yousefi M, Wishart DS, Plotkin SS, Cashman NR. Intermolecular transmission of superoxide dismutase 1 misfolding in living cells. Proc Natl Acad Sci U S A. 2011;108(39):16398–403.
106. Robberecht W, Philips T. The changing scene of amyotrophic lateral sclerosis. Nat Rev Neurosci. 2013;14(4):248–64.
107. Saxena S, Cabuy E, Caroni P. A role for motoneuron subtype-selective ER stress in disease manifestations of FALS mice. Nat Neurosci. 2009;12(5):627–36.
108. Lagier-Tourenne C, Polymenidou M, Hutt KR, Vu AQ, Baughn M, Huelga SC, Clutario KM, Ling SC, Liang TY, Mazur C, Wancewicz E, Kim AS, Watt A, Freier S, Hicks GG, Donohue JP, Shiue L, Bennett CF, Ravits J, Cleveland DW, Yeo GW. Divergent roles of ALS-linked proteins FUS/TLS and TDP-43 intersect in processing long pre-mRNAs. Nat Neurosci. 2012;15(11):1488–97.
109. Talbot K. Amyotrophic lateral sclerosis: cell vulnerability or system vulnerability? J Anat. 2014;224(1):45–51.
110. Al-Chalabi A, Jones A, Troakes C, King A, Al-Sarraj S, van den Berg LH. The genetics and neuropathology of amyotrophic lateral sclerosis. Acta Neuropathol. 2012;124(3):339–52.
111. Ciura S, Lattante S, Le Ber I, Latouche M, Tostivint H, Brice A, Kabashi E. Loss of function of C9orf72 causes motor deficits in a zebrafish model of amyotrophic lateral sclerosis. Ann Neurol. 2013;74(2):180–7.
112. Donnelly CJ, Zhang PW, Pham JT, Haeusler AR, Mistry NA, Vidensky S, Daley EL, Poth EM, Hoover B, Fines DM, Maragakis N, Tienari PJ, Petrucelli L, Traynor BJ, Wang J, Rigo F, Bennett CF, Blackshaw S, Sattler R, Rothstein JD. RNA toxicity from the ALS/FTD C9ORF72 expansion is mitigated by antisense intervention. Neuron. 2013;80(2):415–28.
113. Ash PE, Bieniek KF, Gendron TF, Caulfield T, Lin WL, Dejesus-Hernandez M, van Blitterswijk MM, Jansen-West K, Paul 3rd JW, Rademakers R, Boylan KB, Dickson DW, Petrucelli L. Unconventional translation of C9ORF72 GGGGCC expansion generates insoluble polypeptides specific to c9FTD/ALS. Neuron. 2013;77(4):639–46.
114. Mori K, Weng SM, Arzberger T, May S, Rentzsch K, Kremmer E, Schmid B, Kretzschmar HA, Cruts M, Van Broeckhoven C, Haass C, Edbauer D. The C9orf72 GGGGCC repeat is translated into aggregating dipeptide-repeat proteins in FTLD/ALS. Science. 2013;339(6125):1335–8.
115. Miller TM, Pestronk A, David W, Rothstein J, Simpson E, Appel SH, Andres PL, Mahoney K, Allred P, Alexander K, Ostrow LW, Schoenfeld D, Macklin EA, Norris DA, Manousakis G, Crisp M, Smith R, Bennett CF, Bishop KM, Cudkowicz ME. An antisense oligonucleotide

against SOD1 delivered intrathecally for patients with SOD1 familial amyotrophic lateral sclerosis: a phase 1, randomised, first-in-man study. Lancet Neurol. 2013;12(5):435–42.
116. Chiò A, Battistini S, Calvo A, Caponnetto C, Conforti FL, Corbo M, Giannini F, Mandrioli J, Mora G, Sabatelli M, ITALSGEN Consortium, Ajmone C, Mastro E, Pain D, Mandich P, Penco S, Restagno G, Zollino M, Surbone A. Genetic counselling in ALS: facts, uncertainties and clinical suggestions. J Neurol Neurosurg Psychiatry. 2014;85(5):478–85.
117. Akimoto C, Volk AE, van Blitterswijk M, Van den Broeck M, Leblond CS, Lumbroso S, Camu W, Neitzel B, Onodera O, van Rheenen W, Pinto S, Weber M, Smith B, Proven M, Talbot K, Keagle P, Chesi A, Ratti A, van der Zee J, Alstermark H, Birve A, Calini D, Nordin A, Tradowsky DC, Just W, Daoud H, Angerbauer S, DeJesus-Hernandez M, Konno T, Lloyd-Jani A, de Carvalho M, Mouzat K, Landers JE, Veldink JH, Silani V, Gitler AD, Shaw CE, Rouleau GA, van den Berg LH, Van Broeckhoven C, Rademakers R, Andersen PM, Kubisch C. A blinded international study on the reliability of genetic testing for GGGGCC-repeat expansions in C9orf72 reveals marked differences in results among 14 laboratories. J Med Genet. 2014;51(6):419–24.
118. Gellera C, Ticozzi N, Pensato V, Nanetti L, Castucci A, Castellotti B, Lauria G, Taroni F, Silani V, Mariotti C. ATAXIN2 CAG-repeat length in Italian patients with amyotrophic lateral sclerosis: risk factor or variant phenotype? Implication for genetic testing and counseling. Neurobiol Aging. 2012;33(8):1847.e15–21.

Chapter 18
Genetics of Mitochondrial Disease with Focus on Movement Disorders

Josef Finsterer and Salma Majid Wakil

Abstract There is increasing awareness that mitochondrial disorders with involvement of the central nervous system may also manifest with movement disorders. Movement disorders most frequently manifesting in mitochondrial disorders are ataxia, parkinsonism, dystonia, choreoathetosis, cerebral palsy, and non-Parkinson's tremor. More rarely, myoclonus, restless leg syndrome, tic disorders, or stereotypy disorders were described in mitochondrial disorders. Syndromic as well as nonsyndromic mitochondrial disorders may present with movement disorders. Frequently, the movement disorder is not the only clinical manifestation but one among others. It may be the dominant phenotypic feature or an ancillary manifestation. Clinical manifestations other than movement disorders may result from additional affection of the central nervous system, the eyes, the ears, the endocrine organs, the heart, the guts, the kidneys, the skin, or the bone marrow. Genes most frequently mutated in mitochondrial movement disorders are POLG1, twinkle, tRNAs, and respiratory chain complex I subunit genes. Treatment of movement disorders in mitochondrial disorders is not at variance from treatment of movement disorders in other patients, but therapy may be less beneficial than in non-mitochondrial patients.

Keywords Mitochondrial disorder • Central nervous system • Movement disorders • Parkinson • Ataxia • Athetosis • Chorea • Dystonia • Tremor • Cerebral palsy

Abbreviations

ACO2	Aconitase-2 gene
ADCK3	AarF domain containing kinase-3
ANT1	ADP/ATP translokase-1

J. Finsterer, MD, PhD (✉)
Krankenanstalt Rudolfstiftung (KAR), Vienna 1180, Austria
e-mail: fifigs1@yahoo.de

S.M. Wakil, PhD
Department of Genetics, King Faisal Specialist Hospital and Research Center, Riyadh 11211, Saudi Arabia

S.A. Schneider, J.M.T. Brás (eds.), *Movement Disorder Genetics*,
DOI 10.1007/978-3-319-17223-1_18

ARSAL	Autosomal recessive spastic ataxia with leukoencephalopathy
CABC1	Chaperone activity of bc1 complex gene (synonymous with ADCK3)
CNS	Central nervous system
CoQ	Coenzyme Q
COX	Cytochrome c oxidase
CPEO	Chronic progressive external ophthalmoplegia
CSF	Cerebrospinal fluid
DDS	Deafness diabetes syndrome
DNA	Desoxynucleic acid
DYTCA	Dystonia cerebellar ataxia syndrome
HSD10	Hydroxysteroid dehydrogenase 10
IMMP2L	Inner mitochondrial membrane peptidase-2-like
IOSCA	Infantile-onset spinocerebellar ataxia
LHON	Leber's hereditary optic neuropathy
MELAS	Mitochondrial encephalomyopathy, lactic acidosis, and stroke-like episodes
MERRF	Myoclonic epilepsy with ragged-red fibers syndrome
MHBD	2-Methyl-3-hydroxybutyryl-CoA dehydrogenase
MID	Mitochondrial disorder
MILS	Maternally inherited Leigh syndrome
MPV17	Mitochondrial inner membrane protein
MR1	Myofibrillogenesis regulator 1 gene
MRI	Magnetic resonance imaging
mtDNA	Mitochondrial DNA
MTS	Mitochondria-targeted sequence
NARP	Neuropathy, ataxia, retinitis pigmentosa syndrome
nDNA	Nuclear DNA
PCH	Pontocerebellar hypoplasia
POLG1	Polymerase gamma-1
RARS2	Mitochondrial arginyl-transfer RNA synthetase gene
RCC	Respiratory chain complex
SANDO	Sensory ataxia neuropathy dysarthria and ophthalmoplegia
TACO1	Translational activator of cytochrome-c-oxidase gene
tRNA	Transfer ribonucleic acid
UPDRS	Unified Parkinson's Disease Rating Scale

Introduction

Mitochondrial disorders (MIDs) are usually multisystem disorders either already at onset of the clinical manifestations or sooner or later during the disease course [1]. One of the organs frequently affected in MIDs is the central nervous system (CNS) [2].

Among the various CNS manifestations, movement disorders are the ones less well appreciated. This chapter wants to highlight the genetic background of those MIDs which go along with clinical manifestations of a movement disorder and, if reported, the management of these patients.

Methods

Data for this chapter were collected by searches of MEDLINE, Current Contents, and PubMed and of references from relevant articles using the search terms "mitochondrial DNA," "nuclear DNA," "deletion," "multiple deletions," "POLG1," and "twinkle" in combination with "mitochondrial disorder," "respiratory chain," "mitochondrial cytopathy," "MELAS," "MERRF," "CPEO," "NARP," "MILS," "LHON," "IOSCA," "SANDO," and "Leigh syndrome." Considered were articles about humans, animals, and cell cultures published in English between 1966 and 2014 and investigated in randomized (blinded or open label) clinical trials, longitudinal studies, case series, or case reports. All age groups and both sexes were included. Excluded were abstracts or reports about meetings. Papers matching these criteria were studied and discussed for their suitability to be included in this chapter.

Definition of Movement Disorders

Movement disorders comprise a huge spectrum of diseases, which go along with abnormal movements [3]. Movement disorders include akathisia (inability to sit still), akinesia (lack of movement), associated movements (mirror movements or homolateral synkinesias), athetosis (contorted torsion or twisting), ataxia (lack of coordination of movements), ballism (violent involuntary rapid and irregular movements), bradykinesia (slow movement), cerebral palsy (static encephalopathy), chorea (rapid involuntary movement), dyskinesia (abnormal, involuntary movement), dystonia (sustained torsion), blepharospasm, writer's cramps, spasmodic torticollis (twisting of head and neck), dopamine-responsive dystonia (hereditary progressive dystonia with diurnal fluctuation or Segawa's disease), essential tremor, geniospasm (episodic involuntary up and down movements of the chin or lower lips), myoclonus (brief, involuntary twitching of a muscle or a group of muscles), mirror movements (involuntary movements on one side of the body mirroring voluntary movements of the other side), Parkinson's disease, paroxysmal kinesigenic dyskinesia, restless leg syndrome, spasms, stereotypic movement disorder, stereotype (repetition), Tic disorders (involuntary, compulsive repetitive, stereotyped movements), and tremor (oscillations) [3].

Parkinson's Syndrome (Parkinsonism)

POLG1 Mutations

Since recent years, it is well established that polymerase γ-1 (POLG1) mutations are occasionally associated with levodopa-responsive parkinsonism [4]. Even polymorphisms within the POLG1 gene seem to predispose for Parkinson's syndrome, at least in the Chinese population [4]. The fact that POLG1 mutations are more frequently associated with parkinsonism than mutations in other MID causing genes was confirmed by a number of cases with parkinsonism carrying a POLG1 mutation [5].

In a 48-year-old female carrying a POLG1 mutation manifesting as multisystem MID, parkinsonism was a dominant phenotypic feature [6]. In a Brazilian family carrying a POLG1 mutation, three family members were clinically affected. One patient presented with chronic progressive external ophthalmoplegia (CPEO), polyneuropathy, cardiomyopathy, and parkinsonism with onset at the age of 20 [7]. The oldest brother of the index case had a similar phenotype. An older sister presented with CPEO and depression [7]. Parkinsonism in the index patient improved under pramipexole 3 mg/day [7]. In a compound heterozygote for a POLG1 mutation, orthostatic tremor evolved into levodopa-responsive parkinsonism [8]. In addition to parkinsonism, the patient presented with autosomal recessive CPEO [8]. In a 71-year-old male with CPEO, ptosis, hypoacusis, dysarthria, dysphagia, polyneuropathy, migraine, myopathy, cardiomyopathy, symmetric rigidity, and tremor, manifestations of parkinsonism were assessed as 26 on the Unified Parkinson's Disease Rating Scale (UPDRS) part III [9]. Carbidopa/levodopa in a dosage of 75/300 mg/day reduced the UPDRS score to 14 [9]. Since the patient did not tolerate this medication over a longer period, it was switched to clonazepam with success [9]. A male patient with CPEO developed bradykinesia, rigidity, and camptocormia in the third decade [10]. Parkinsonism in this patient was only partially responsive to dopaminergic replacement [10]. His father and brother presented with a similar phenotype, which was attributed to a POLG1 mutation in all of them [10]. Mutations in the POLG1 gene, which manifest as Alpers syndrome in children, may cause parkinsonism in addition to ataxia, CPEO, polyneuropathy, and hypoacusis in elderly patients (see also section "Ataxia") [11]. In a large family with parkinsonism and CPEO, multiple mitochondrial DNA (mtDNA) deletions due to a POLG1 mutation were found to be causative [12]. A patient carrying an ADP/ATP translocase 1 (ANT1) and POLG1 mutation presented with parkinsonism in addition to CPEO, sensory and cerebellar ataxia, polyneuropathy, and depression (see also section "Ataxia") [13]. The mutations were associated with multiple mtDNA deletions [13]. Parkinsonism due to POLG1 mutations may not only occur together with CPEO [9] but also with other movement disorders. Early-onset parkinsonism and polyneuropathy may be another phenotypic expression of a POLG1 mutation [14]. Parkinsonism due to POLG1 mutations may be additionally associated with premature ovarian failure [15].

Occasionally, POLG1 mutations may cause only marked nigrostriatal degeneration without overt clinical parkinsonism [16]. In these patients, structural abnormalities may be found in the thalamus and the cerebellum [16]. On the cellular level, dopaminergic nigral neurons of patients with POLG1 encephalopathy show increased mtDNA depletion compared to patients with idiopathic Parkinson's disease [16]. There are some indications that a CAG-repeat number of 6–9 or 12–14 predisposes for the development of Parkinson's disease at least in some populations [17, 18]. The normal poly-Q tract in exon 2 of the POLG1 gene has 10–11 CAG repeats. POLG1 mutation-related parkinsonism may be differentiated from idiopathic Parkinson's disease by means of the neuromelatonin MRI [5].

Other Genes

Not only POLG1 mutations may go along with parkinsonism but also mutations in other genes encoding mitochondrial proteins, tRNAs, or rRNAs, such as C10orf2 (twinkle, encodes for the twinkle helicase, a functional partner of the polymerase γ [19]), MPV17, MT-TI (tRNA(Ile)), 12S-rRNA, MT-TL (tRNA(Leu)), and tRNA(Ile). In an Italian family carrying a twinkle gene mutation, the index patient developed parkinsonism at the age of 82 in addition to ptosis, ophthalmoplegia, and hypoacusis since childhood [20]. Parkinsonism responded only moderately to levodopa. The 79-year-old sister of the index patient had developed resting and postural tremor and rigor (plastic hypertonia) since the age of 76 [20]. In a 74-year-old male with ptosis, CPEO, progressive left-sided weakness, mild proximal myopathy, exercise intolerance, predominantly left-sided parkinsonism with hypomimia, mild resting tremor, and moderate bradykinesia were found [9]. He scored 10 on the UPDRS part III [9]. The phenotype was attributed to a mutation in the twinkle gene [9]. In a 65-year-old male with polyneuropathy, ptosis, CPEO, diabetes, exercise intolerance, steatohepatopathy, depression, and gastrointestinal dysmotility, parkinsonism was a further phenotypic feature of the underlying mutation in the MPV17 gene [21]. The MPV17 mutation caused multiple mtDNA deletions without indication for mtDNA depletion [21]. In a single Italian family carrying a mutation in the mitochondrial 12S-rRNA gene, the phenotype was characterized by deafness, polyneuropathy, and parkinsonism [22]. The mutation resulted in depletion of mitochondrial glutathione and combined respiratory chain complex (RCC) II/III deficiency [22]. Administration of gentamicin dramatically increased the number of apoptotic cells in this family [22]. In a 55-year-old Japanese female with dementia, tetraspasticity, CPEO, myopathy, deafness, and diabetes, carrying an MT-TL (tRNA(Leu)) mutation, parkinsonism was diagnosed at the age of 55 [23]. Her 48-year-old brother had similar manifestations of the mutation, but instead of parkinsonism, he presented with ataxia (see also section "Ataxia") [23]. Cerebral MRI showed supra- and infratentorial atrophy and periventricular hyperintensities [23]. Pyruvate and lactate were elevated in the serum. Parkinsonism may also occur in patients carrying MT-TI (tRNA(Ile)) gene mutations [24]. Parkinsonism in these patients may go along with developmental retardation and hypogonadism [24]. In a neonate with episodes of truncal hypertonia and apnea progressing to a hypokinetic-rigid syndrome characterized by hypokinesia, tremor, head lag, absent suck and gag reflexes, hyperreflexia, ankle and jaw clonus, and autonomic dysfunction, mtDNA depletion was detected in the muscle homogenate [25]. Respiratory chain enzymology demonstrated decreased RCCIV activity [25]. Treatment with pyridoxal phosphate, tetrahydrobiopterin, and levodopa was ineffective [25]. The underlying genetic defect could not be detected. In a study of 32 patients with idiopathic Parkinson's disease, the mtDNA deletion mt.4977del was found in 15 patients and thus much more frequent than in the control group [26].

Ataxia

Cerebellar or sensory ataxia is a frequent phenotypic manifestation of MIDs with cerebral or peripheral nerve involvement [27, 28]. Ataxia may develop in syndromic as well as nonsyndromic MIDs. Among the syndromic MIDs, ataxia is a dominant phenotypic feature in infantile-onset spinocerebellar ataxia (IOSCA), pontocerebellar hypoplasia (PCH), Alpers syndrome, sensory ataxia neuropathy dysarthria and ophthalmoplegia (SANDO), autosomal recessive spastic ataxia with leukoencephalopathy (ARSAL) syndrome, dystonia and cerebellar ataxia (DYTCA) syndrome, Ekbom syndrome, and Leigh syndrome.

Syndromic MIDs

In two Korean patients with IOSCA due to a compound heterozygote mutation in the twinkle gene, the phenotype additionally included polyneuropathy and myopathy [29]. The nDNA mutation secondarily caused multiple mtDNA deletions [29]. Since the age of 15 months, the two children additionally developed athetosis, hypoacusis, and intellectual decline (see also section "Athetosis") [29]. In another family, two members presented with IOSCA due to another twinkle mutation [30]. In addition to ataxia, the two patients developed polyneuropathy, athetosis, seizures, hypoacusis, and ophthalmoplegia (see also section "Athetosis") [30]. Twinkle mutations may not only cause IOSCA but also Alpers syndrome. In two infants with early-onset encephalopathy, muscle hypotonia, athetosis, sensory neuropathy, ataxia, hypoacusis, CPEO, intractable epilepsy, and hepatopathy, reminiscent to Alpers syndrome, the phenotype was caused by mutations in the twinkle gene (see also section "Athetosis") [19]. The mutations secondarily caused mtDNA depletion in the liver [19]. In Alpers syndrome due to POLG1 mutations, ataxia may be found in addition to parkinsonism, CPEO, polyneuropathy, and hypoacusis (see also section "Parkinson's syndrome (parkinsonism)") [11]. In a female child carrying a MT-TK (tRNA(Lys)) mutation, the phenotype was classified as Leigh syndrome with progressive ataxia, myoclonus, seizures, and cognitive decline (see also section "Myoclonus") [31].

Cerebral MRI showed T2 hyperintensities in the putamen and the posterior medulla. Cerebrospinal fluid (CSF) lactate was elevated and muscle biopsy showed COX-negative fibers [31]. Ataxia and polyneuropathy were the dominant phenotypic features in another patient with Leigh syndrome due to a mutation in the mitochondrial ATP6 gene [32]. Adult-onset ataxia, polyneuropathy, and pyramidal dysfunction were the clinical manifestations in two families carrying other ATP6 mutations [33]. Mutations in the ATP6 gene were responsible for Leigh syndrome, initially manifesting with ataxia and dysarthria [34]. In Leigh syndrome due to a ND6 mutation, the patient presented with dystonia, ataxia, optic atrophy, and epilepsy (see also section "Dystonia") [35]. Sensory ataxia is a typical feature of the clinical presentation in SANDO syndrome due to twinkle mutations [36]. However, SANDO with sensory neuropathy, dysarthria, and CPEO may be also due to POLG1 mutations [37]. In a patient with SANDO, manifesting as polyneuropathy with sensory ataxia, gait disturbance with falls, blurred vision, CPEO, tremor, and dementia, the causative mutation was located in the POLG1 gene (see also section "Non-Parkinson's tremor") [38]. In two siblings with DYTCA syndrome and neuropathy, the phenotype could be attributed to a homozygous missense mutation in exon2 of the COX20 gene (see also section "Dystonia") [39]. Ataxia is also a dominant clinical feature of PCH. In a patient with PCH type 6, the phenotype included cerebellar and cerebral atrophy, microcephaly, epilepsy, dystonia, optic atrophy, thinning of the corpus callosum, and lactic acidosis (see also section "Dystonia") [40]. The phenotype was attributed to a mutation in the RARS2 gene, which encodes the mitochondrial arginyl-tRNA synthetase, a protein essential for translation of mitochondrially synthesized proteins [40]. Mutations in the mitochondrial methionyl-tRNA synthetase 2 (MARS2) gene have been recently shown to cause autosomal recessive spastic ataxia with leukoencephalopathy (ARSAL) in humans [41]. Affected patients not only presented with reduced MARS2 activity but also reduced RCCI activity [41]. Cerebellar ataxia is a key feature of Ekbom syndrome additionally manifesting with photomyoclonus, skeletal deformities and lipoma (see also section "Restless leg syndrome") [42]. Ekbom syndrome is due to mutations in the mitochondrial tRNA(Lys) gene [42].

Nonsyndromic MIDs

Cerebellar or sensory ataxia is not only a typical feature of the clinical presentation in syndromic but also in nonsyndromic MIDs. Nonsyndromic MIDs with ataxia may be due to mtDNA mutations or nDNA mutations.

mtDNA Mutations

In a family in which two members were affected by a nonsyndromic, multisystem MID, a 48-year-old male presented with dementia, quadruspasticity, CPEO, myopathy, deafness, diabetes, and additionally ataxia [23]. The MID was due to a mutation in the mitochondrial MT-TL (tRNA(Leu)) gene [23]. In an adult male carrying an MT-TE (tRNA(Glu)) mutation, the phenotype was characterized by early-onset cataract, progressive paraparesis, and ataxia [43]. Muscle biopsy showed COX-deficient fibers, and biochemical investigations revealed a RCCI defect [43]. Rarely, ataxia may be found in patients carrying the MERRF mutation m.8344A > G [44]. The dominant feature of the phenotype, however, may be CNS demyelination and demyelinating polyneuropathy, associated with palpitations, tinnitus, bilateral 6th nerve palsy, and flaccid quadruparesis [44]. Ataxia has been also reported in a patient carrying a mutation in the tRNA(Pro) gene [45]. He additionally presented with retinitis pigmentosa, dysarthria, hypoacusis, and leukoencephalopathy [45]. In two patients carrying a tRNA(Ser) mutation, cerebellar ataxia was part of the phenotype in addition to myoclonus, epilepsy, and progressive hypoacusis (see also section "Myoclonus") [46]. Cerebellar ataxia, in addition to hypogonadism, and chorioretinal dystrophy were the dominant clinical manifestations of a mtDNA deletion resulting in deficiency of RCCI [47]. In patients with cerebellar ataxia due to mtDNA mutations, the cell density was decreased in the cerebellum, suggesting that the olivary-cerebellum is particularly vulnerable to mtDNA mutations [27].

nDNA Mutations

Sensory and cerebellar ataxia was part of the multisystem phenotype in a patient with parkinsonism, CPEO, polyneuropathy, and depression (see also section "Parkinson's syndrome (parkinsonism)") [13]. The phenotype was due to mutations in the ANT1 and POLG1 genes [13]. Ataxia in nonsyndromic, multisystem MIDs may be also caused by mutations in the OPA1 gene [48]. Additionally, these patients present with color vision deficit, muscle hypotonia, gastrointestinal dysmotility, dysphagia, and severe, early-onset optic atrophy [48]. Ataxia together with late-onset, progressive optic atrophy and myopathy may be the clinical manifestations of mutations in the gene encoding the flavoprotein subunit of RCCII [49]. Ataxia was part of the phenotype in six patients carrying mutations in the CABC1/ADCK3 gene [50]. In addition to ataxia, all patients presented with cerebellar ataxia, epilepsy, and myopathy and some of them with dystonia, spasticity, tremor, migraine, and cognitive impairment (see also section "Dystonia") [50]. Ataxia was one among several other features in a consanguineous Israeli Bedouin family carrying a mutation in the UQCRQ gene (see also section "Dystonia") [51]. Furthermore, ataxia can be a phenotypic feature in primary coenzyme-Q deficiency [52]. In a study of 4 patients carrying mutations in the ADCK3/CABC1 gene, the phenotype was characterized by progressive cerebellar ataxia and epilepsy [52]. In two siblings from a consanguineous Pakistani family, cerebellar ataxia and severe myoclonus could be attributed to a mutation in the ADCK3/CABC1 gene, encoding a mitochondrial protein involved in the CoQ metabolism (see also section "Myoclonus") [53]. The mutation resulted in primary coenzyme-Q deficiency, and supplementation of CoQ was followed by marked clinical improvement [53]. Ataxia was also the dominant manifestation in a patient with CPEO who carried a twinkle mutation [36]. Even polymorphisms in one of the RCCI genes may be associated spinocerebellar ataxia [54].

Dystonia

Dystonia is characterized by sustained muscle contractions causing twisting or repetitive movements or abnormal postures [3]. It may manifest focally, segmentally, regionally, or in a generalized distribution. Focal dystonia includes blepharospasm, oromandibular dystonia, hemifacial spasm, cervical dystonia, spasmodic dysphonia, writer's cramps, or pelvic floor dystonia. Dystonia as a manifestation of MID has been described in syndromic and nonsyndromic MIDs.

Syndromic MIDs

Among the syndromic MIDs, dystonia may be particularly found in Leber's hereditary optic neuropathy (LHON) for which the acronym LDYT has been coined [55]. LDYT may be due to mutations in the ND3, ND4, or ND6 genes, respectively [55]. In a large Dutch family with LHON, the phenotype additionally included spastic dystonia [56]. Causative mutations were found in the mitochondrial ND4 and ND6 genes, respectively [56]. In a five-generation Belgian family with 12 affected subjects, a mutation in the ND6 gene manifested with a broad phenotypic heterogeneity, ranging from progressive myoclonic epilepsy, dystonia, and hypokinetic-rigid syndrome to migraine, LHON, optic atrophy, hypoacusis, and diabetes [57]. Activity of RCCI was mildly reduced on muscle biopsy [57]. In a 17-year-old female, LHON was accompanied by spasticity, dystonia, and dysarthria [58]. Biochemical investigations revealed an RCCI defect [58]. Rarely, dystonia may be part of the phenotype in Leigh syndrome caused by a mutation in the ND6 gene [35]. The patient additionally presented with ataxia, optic atrophy, and epilepsy (see also section "Ataxia") [35]. In a patient with Leigh syndrome due to a mutation in the ND3 gene, dystonia was an additional phenotypic characteristic [59]. Dystonia in addition to slowly progressive cognitive decline and visual impairment was also the clinical manifestation of a homozygous mutation in the TACO1 gene in five individuals from a consanguineous family [60]. The disorder was classified as Leigh syndrome after cerebral MRI had shown bilaterally symmetric lesions of the basal ganglia [60]. Dystonia is also a typical phenotypic feature of deafness-dystonia syndrome (DDS), also known as Mohr-Tranebjaerg syndrome [61]. DDS is characterized by early-onset deafness, dystonia, cortical blindness, spasticity, and dementia [62]. DDS is due to mutations in the TIMM8a gene on chromosome X, which encodes a protein responsible for the transport and sorting of proteins to the inner mitochondrial membrane [61]. In a Turkish family with DYTCA syndrome, two affected siblings additionally presented with sensory neuropathy (see also section "Ataxia") [39]. Dystonia manifested as torticollis in the affected female and regional leg dystonia in the affected male [39]. Biochemical investigations revealed a RCCIV defect and CoQ deficiency [39]. The phenotype was due to a homozygous missense mutation in exon 2 of the COX20 gene [39]. A mutation in the COX20 gene was also the cause of ataxia and muscle hypotonia in another patient with a RCCIV defect [63]. In a patient with progressive cerebellar and cerebral atrophy, microcephaly, and epilepsy, PCH type 6 was diagnosed [40]. Additional manifestations usually described in types 2 and 4, such as dystonia, optic atrophy, thinning of the corpus callosum, and lactic acidosis, were also present [40]. The phenotype was attributed to a mutation in the RARS2 gene, which encodes the mitochondrial arginyl-tRNA synthetase, a protein essential for translation of mitochondrially synthesized proteins [40]. Dystonia is a typical phenotypic manifestation of paroxysmal non-kinesigenic dyskinesia (PNKD), which is due to mutations in the myofibrillogenesis regulator 1 (MR1) gene (see also sections "Athetosis" and "Chorea") [64].

Nonsyndromic MIDs

Slowly progressive dystonia with cognitive impairment and striatal lesions may be the dominant clinical feature in patients carrying mutations in the ND6 gene [65]. Muscle biopsy in these patients may show deficiency of RCCI [65]. Progressive generalized dystonia was the main clinical presentation of a patient carrying a mutation in the ND6 gene [66]. He also showed bilateral striatal necrosis on MRI [66]. Dystonia was part of the phenotype also in four patients and two of their siblings carrying mutations in the CABC1/ADCK3 gene [50]. In addition to dystonia all patients presented with cerebellar ataxia, epilepsy, and myopathy and some of them with spasticity, tremor, migraine, and cognitive impairment (see also section "Ataxia") [50]. Muscle biopsy showed lipid accumulation, mitochondrial proliferation, and COX-negative fibers. RCC activities and CoQ were decreased [50]. In a consanguineous Israeli Bedouin family a mutation in the UQCRQ gene, encoding the ubiquinol-c-reductase complex III subunit 7, caused a nonlethal phenotype characterized by severe psychomotor retardation, dystonia, athetosis, ataxia, muscle hypotonia, and dementia (see also sections "Ataxia" and "Athetosis") [51]. There was mild lactic acidosis, hyperintense putamen and hypointense caudate and lentiform nuclei on MRI and RCCIII deficiency on muscle biopsy in affected individuals [51]. In three Korean children, a mutation in the ND3 gene manifested with childhood-onset, progressive generalized dystonia and in one of them with stroke-like episodes [67]. In a single patient, a mutation in the NDUFV1 gene manifested clinically with CPEO, cerebellar ataxia, spasticity, and dystonia [68]. Muscle biopsy revealed a RCCI defect. Ketogenic diet had a beneficial effect on CPEO but not on the other manifestations [68]. In a patient with adult-onset dystonia, spasticity, and myopathy, a heteroplasmic missense mutation in the ND1 gene was causative [69]. Dystonia due to fumarase deficiency was part of the phenotype in two siblings of consanguineous parents [70]. They additionally presented with progressive encephalopathy, leukopenia, and neutropenia [70]. A causative missense mutation was found in the fumarase gene [70].

Athetosis

Athetosis is a clinical characteristic of MIDs with CNS involvement but less frequently appreciated than ataxia, parkinsonism, or dystonia. Usually, athetosis is associated with chorea. In a Korean family carrying a twinkle mutation, two family members (infants) manifested as infantile-onset spinocerebellar ataxia (IOSCA) (see also section "Ataxia") [29]. They developed normally until the age of 18 months and then developed athetosis, ataxia, hypoacusis, axonal polyneuropathy, and intellectual decline afterwards [29]. Muscle biopsy showed multiple mtDNA mutations [29]. In another family with IOSCA, two members presented with ataxia, polyneuropathy, athetosis, seizures, hypoacusis, and ophthalmoplegia (see also section "Ataxia") [30]. The phenotype was due to a novel twinkle mutation [30]. In a study of eight individuals from two unrelated families with a nonsyndromic, multisystem MID presenting with athetosis, truncal hypotonia, epilepsy, developmental delay, psychomotor retardation, optic and retinal atrophy, and visual loss, extensive diagnostic workup revealed progressive prominent cerebellar atrophy, thinning of the corpus callosum, cortical atrophy, and demyelination [71]. The cause of the abnormalities was a mutation in the ACO2 gene encoding the mitochondrial aconitase, a component of the Krebs cycle [71]. Paroxysmal non-kinesigenic dyskinesia (PNKD) is an autosomal dominant movement disorder characterized by attacks of dystonia, chorea, and athetosis (see also sections "Dystonia" and "Chorea"). The disorder is due to mutations in the MR1 gene [64]. Three isoforms of the gene product exist, MR1M, located on the Golgi apparatus, endoplasmatic reticulum, and plasma membrane, and MR1L and MR1S, both located in the mitochondrial matrix [64]. The two latter are imported via the N-terminal mitochondrial-targeting sequence (MTS) [64]. Athetosis was part of the phenotype also in two infants with early-onset encephalopathy, muscle hypotonia, sensory neuropathy, ataxia, hypoacusis, CPEO, intractable epilepsy, and hepatopathy (see also section "Ataxia") [19]. The phenotype was classified as Alpers syndrome due to mutations in the twinkle gene [19]. Dystonia was one among several other features in a consanguineous Israeli Bedouin family carrying a mutation in the UQCRQ gene resulting in RCCIII deficiency (see also section "Dystonia") [51].

Chorea

Chorea is a rather rare clinical manifestation of MIDs. Frequently, it is associated with athetosis. Patients with hydroxysteroid dehydrogenase 10 (HSD10) deficiency may manifest with X-linked, metabolic acidosis, mental retardation, refractory epilepsy, and choreoathetosis [72]. HSD10 is a mitochondrial multifunctional enzyme encoded by the HSD17B10 gene on chromosome X [72]. Mutations in this gene result in elevated levels of 2-methyl-3-hydroxybutyrate and tiglylglycine in the urine organic acid profile [72]. Choreoathetosis was also a phenotypic feature of 2-methyl-3-hydroxybutyryl-CoA dehydrogenase (MHBD) deficiency in an infant with moderately delayed psychomotor development during the first year of life and progressive deterioration of mental and motor skills since the age of 2 years [73]. The patient developed marked restlessness, absence of directed hand movements, and marked hypotonia [73]. Urinary investigations revealed marked elevation of 2-methyl-3-hydroxybutyrate and tiglylglycine [73]. Biochemical investigations showed a mitochondrial β-oxidation defect, which improved upon dietary isoleucine restriction [73]. Chorea is also a typical phenotypic manifestation of paroxysmal non-kinesigenic dyskinesia (PNKD), which is due to mutations in the MR1 gene (see also section "Athetosis") [64]. In a 30-month-old male, Leigh syndrome presented with failure to thrive, lethargy, hypotonia, choreoathetosis, lactic acidemia, and basal ganglia hypodensities on cerebral CT scan [74]. Activity of the PDH complex and RCCI was reduced to 25 and 13 %, respectively [74].

Cerebral Palsy

Cerebral palsy (static encephalopathy) is a permanent, nonprogressive movement disorder characterized by physical disability to carry out certain body movements; sensory disturbances, particularly depth perception; and communication disability [3]. In one third of the patients, cognitive decline and epilepsy are part of the phenotype [3]. Other subtypes present with quadruspasticity and some with poor coordination [3]. Cerebral palsy has been only rarely reported in patients with MID. In a study of 44 patients with lactic acidosis, one patient presented with cerebral palsy and mental retardation due to a mitochondrial tRNA mutation [75]. Cerebral palsy was part of the phenotype also in an infant with PCH [76]. The causative mutation could not be detected. In two children aged 10 and 13 years, nonsyndromic, multisystem MID was initially misdiagnosed as cerebral palsy [77]. The causative mutation has not been reported [77]. Cerebral palsy was additionally observed in two girls with PDH deficiency due to a mutation in the E1-alpha gene [78]. One of the girls additionally presented with quadriplegia, microcephaly, hypocalcemia, and seizures [78]. Cerebral palsy was additionally described in a family with Leigh syndrome due to a NARP mutation [79]. In another patient cerebral palsy was associated with a RCCI defect [80]. In 14 patients with basal ganglia calcification, a typical finding in CNS involvement in MIDs, some patients presented with cerebral palsy [81]. Repeatedly it has been described that cerebral palsy had been misdiagnosed in patients who actually suffered from a multisystem MID. In an infant with leukoencephalopathy and lactic acidosis, an MID due to COX deficiency was diagnosed, which initially was misdiagnosed as cerebral palsy [82].

Non-Parkinson's Tremor

Non-Parkinson's tremor is a rare phenotypic manifestation of MIDs. In a 70-year-old male with ptosis, CPEO and orthostatic tremor with a frequency of 17.5 Hz since the age of 40 years, the phenotype was caused by a novel twinkle mutation [83]. Nerve conduction studies and electromyography additionally revealed mild axonal neuropathy and myopathic features. Muscle biopsy confirmed the myopathic changes and revealed ragged-red fibers [83]. Resting tremor of the hands was one of the clinical manifestations in addition to polyneuropathy with sensory ataxia, gait disturbance with falls, blurred vision, CPEO, and dementia with deficits in registration and construction in a patient with SANDO due to a POLG1 mutation (see also section "Ataxia") [38]. POLG1 mutations may also manifest with palatal tremor and facial dyskinesia (see also section "Dyskinesia") [84]. Essential tremor is one of the most frequent movement disorders although there is little agreement concerning the pathogenetic background and diagnostic criteria [85]. In a study of patients with essential tremor, mtDNA deletions not affecting the D-loop or the COXI region were detected in some of these patients [85].

Myoclonus

Myoclonus is a typical phenotypic feature of syndromic or nonsyndromic MIDs with myoclonic epilepsy, such as patients with MERRF syndrome, but may also occur in MIDs without epilepsy [86]. Severe myoclonus was reported in two Pakistani siblings from consanguineous parents carrying a novel mutation in the ADCK3/CABC1 gene (see also section "Ataxia") [53]. The mutation resulted in primary coenzyme-Q deficiency and supplementation of CoQ was beneficial [53]. In a female child carrying a tRNA(Lys) mutation, the phenotype was classified as Leigh syndrome manifesting with progressive ataxia, myoclonus, seizures, and cognitive decline (see also section "Ataxia") [31]. Segmental myoclonus, which could be induced by chewing, was described in a patient with Leigh syndrome [87]. In two patients carrying a tRNA(Ser) mutation, myoclonus was part of the phenotype in addition to cerebellar ataxia, epilepsy, and progressive hypoacusis (see also section "Ataxia") [46]. One patient additionally developed myopathy with appropriate histological and biochemical abnormalities on muscle biopsy [46]. Myoclonus together with recurrent stroke-like episodes and seizures were the clinical manifestations of a ND5 mutation in a patient with MELAS/MERRF overlap syndrome [88].

Restless Leg Syndrome

Only few data are available about the prevalence of restless leg syndrome in MIDs. A recent study of patients with CPEO has shown that one third of these patients develops restless leg syndrome [89]. Restless leg syndrome together with blurred vision may be even the presenting manifestation of a MID [90]. Restless leg syndrome has been also found in patients with Ekbom syndrome characterized by cerebellar ataxia, photomyoclonus, skeletal deformities, and lipoma [42]. Ekbom syndrome is due to mutations in the mitochondrial tRNA(Lys) gene (see also section "Ataxia") [42].

Tic Disorders (Tic Phenotype)

Only few data are available about the prevalence of tic disorders in MIDs. Variations in the mitochondrial ribosomal protein L3 (MRPL3) gene have been shown to be associated with Tourette syndrome/chronic Tic phenotype [91]. Since disruption of the inner mitochondrial membrane peptidase 2-like (IMMP2L) gene by a chromosomal breakpoint has been recently described in a patient with Gilles de la Tourette syndrome, it cannot be excluded that mutations also in this gene cause tic phenotypes [92].

Stereotypic Movement Disorder

Only few data are available about the prevalence of stereotypic movement disorder in MIDs. In a male child carrying a tRNA(Lys) mutation, the phenotype was initially characterized by autism [31]. During his second year of life, he lost language skills and developed hyperactivity with toe-walking, abnormal reciprocal social interaction, restricted interests, self-injurious behavior, seizures, and stereotyped mannerisms [31]. Cerebral MRI and CSF lactate were normal. His sister presented with a Leigh-like phenotype but did not develop stereotypies so far (see also section "Ataxia"). Stereotypies in MIDs may be associated with mental retardation and may favorably respond to escitalopram [93].

Dyskinesia

Dyskinesia has been only rarely reported as a clinical manifestation of MID. POLG1 mutations may also manifest with palatal tremor and facial dyskinesia (see also section "Non-Parkinson's tremor") [84].

No reports have been published so far describing MIDs with clinical manifestations of akathisia, synkinesia, homolateral synkinesias, mirror movements, associated movements, geniospasm, paroxysmal kinesigenic dyskinesia, spasms, or ballism.

Discussion

This chapter shows that movement disorders in MIDs are more frequent than previously reported. Quite a number of cases, in which parkinsonism, ataxia, dystonia, athetosis, chorea, cerebral palsy, or tremor predominate, are in fact attributable to a MID. Frequently, not only a single movement disorder but several others may be simultaneously present in MIDs [29, 30]. In the majority of the cases, movement disorders represent not only the sole aspect of the phenotype. In addition to movement disorders, other CNS abnormalities may occur in MIDs with CNS involvement. Furthermore, other organs than the CNS are frequently affected in MIDs with movement disorders. Since there is a huge phenotypic heterogeneity within a family and between families, it is not unusual that the index patient is the only one with parkinsonism in a family with other members presenting with a completely different phenotype. Particularly MIDs, which manifest also with parkinsonism, often show extensive intra-familial phenotypic heterogeneity, such that an affected member may present with a movement disorder, whereas another does not present with a movement disorder at all, or that one family member has a single movement disorder, whereas other family members present with two or more. The movement disorder most frequently found in MIDs is ataxia, followed by parkinsonism and dystonia. MIDs with movement disorders are due to mutations in genes located in the mtDNA or the nDNA. These genes encode for proteins, tRNAs, or rRNAs involved in mitochondrial function, reproduction, and biogenesis. Genes most frequently mutated in MIDs with movement disorders are POLG1, twinkle, tRNAs, or RCCI-subunit genes. Parkinsonism in MIDs is most frequently due to a POLG1 mutation if associated with other neurological disease, in particular movement disorders. Treatment of movement disorders in MIDs is not at variance from treatment of movement disorders in non-MID patients. However, levodopa or dopamine-agonist therapy in MID-associated parkinsonism is often only marginally effective.

Conclusion

In patients with one or more movement disorders and other cerebral or non-cerebral abnormalities, MID should be suspected. Treatment of movement disorders in MIDs is not at variance from treatment of movement disorders in non-MID patients, but the therapeutic effect may be different in patients with MID and those without. Genes most frequently mutated in MIDs with movement disorders include POLG1, twinkle, tRNA, and RCCI-subunit genes. Despite increasing awareness about movement disorders as a manifestation of MIDs, knowledge about movement disorders in MIDs is still limited. Only case reports or family studies are available. This is why more information about movement disorders in MIDs is warranted.

References

1. Finsterer J. Inherited mitochondrial disorders. Adv Exp Med Biol. 2012;942:187–213.
2. Finsterer J. Central nervous system manifestations of mitochondrial disorders. Acta Neurol Scand. 2006;114:217–38.
3. Donaldson I, Marsden CD, Schneider S, Bhatia K. Marsden's book of movement disorders. Oxford: Oxford University Press; 2012. ISBN 978-0-19-261911-2.
4. Gui YX, Xu ZP, Lv W, Liu HM, Zhao JJ, Hu XY. Association of mitochondrial DNA polymerase γ gene POLG1 polymorphisms with parkinsonism in Chinese populations. PLoS One. 2012;7(12):e50086. doi:10.1371/journal.pone.0050086.

5. Mukai M, Sugaya K, Yabe I, Goto Y, Yokochi F, Miyamoto K, Cai H, Sasaki H, Matsubara S. Neuromelanin MRI in a family with mitochondrial parkinsonism harboring a Y955C mutation in POLG1. Parkinsonism Relat Disord. 2013;19:821–4.
6. BandettinidiPoggio M, Nesti C, Bruno C, Meschini MC, Schenone A, Santorelli FM. Dopamine-agonist responsive Parkinsonism in a patient with the SANDO syndrome caused by POLG mutation. BMC Med Genet. 2013;14:105.
7. Gurgel-Giannetti J, Camargos ST, Cardoso F, Hirano M, DiMauro S. POLG1 Arg953Cys mutation: expanded phenotype and recessive inheritance in a Brazilian family. Muscle Nerve. 2012;45:453–4.
8. Invernizzi F, Varanese S, Thomas A, Carrara F, Onofrj M, Zeviani M. Two novel POLG1 mutations in a patient with progressive external ophthalmoplegia, levodopa-responsive pseudo-orthostatic tremor and parkinsonism. Neuromuscul Disord. 2008;18:460–4.
9. Brandon BR, Diederich NJ, Soni M, Witte K, Weinhold M, Krause M, Jackson S. Autosomal dominant mutations in POLG and C10orf2: association with late onset chronic progressive external ophthalmoplegia and Parkinsonism in two patients. J Neurol. 2013;260:1931–3.
10. Dolhun R, Presant EM, Hedera P. Novel polymerase gamma (POLG1) gene mutation in the linker domain associated with parkinsonism. BMC Neurol. 2013;13:92. doi:10.1186/1471-2377-13-92.
11. Remes AM, Hinttala R, Kärppä M, Soini H, Takalo R, Uusimaa J, Majamaa K. Parkinsonism associated with the homozygous W748S mutation in the POLG1 gene. Parkinsonism Relat Disord. 2008;14:652–4.
12. Hudson G, Schaefer AM, Taylor RW, Tiangyou W, Gibson A, Venables G, Griffiths P, Burn DJ, Turnbull DM, Chinnery PF. Mutation of the linker region of the polymerase gamma-1 (POLG1) gene associated with progressive external ophthalmoplegia and Parkinsonism. Arch Neurol. 2007;64:553–7.
13. Galassi G, Lamantea E, Invernizzi F, Tavani F, Pisano I, Ferrero I, Palmieri L, Zeviani M. Additive effects of POLG1 and ANT1 mutations in a complex encephalomyopathy. Neuromuscul Disord. 2008;18:465–70.
14. Davidzon G, Greene P, Mancuso M, Klos KJ, Ahlskog JE, Hirano M, DiMauro S. Early-onset familial parkinsonism due to POLG mutations. Ann Neurol. 2006;59:859–62.
15. Pagnamenta AT, Taanman JW, Wilson CJ, Anderson NE, Marotta R, Duncan AJ, Bitner-Glindzicz M, Taylor RW, Laskowski A, Thorburn DR, Rahman S. Dominant inheritance of premature ovarian failure associated with mutant mitochondrial DNA polymerase gamma. Hum Reprod. 2006;21:2467–73.
16. Tzoulis C, Tran GT, Schwarzlmüller T, Specht K, Haugarvoll K, Balafkan N, Lilleng PK, Miletic H, Biermann M, Bindoff LA. Severe nigrostriatal degeneration without clinical parkinsonism in patients with polymerase gamma mutations. Brain. 2013;136:2393–404.
17. Balafkan N, Tzoulis C, Müller B, Haugarvoll K, Tysnes OB, Larsen JP, Bindoff LA. Number of CAG repeats in POLG1 and its association with Parkinson disease in the Norwegian population. Mitochondrion. 2012;12:640–3.
18. Anvret A, Westerlund M, Sydow O, Willows T, Lind C, Galter D, Belin AC. Variations of the CAG trinucleotide repeat in DNA polymerase γ (POLG1) is associated with Parkinson's disease in Sweden. Neurosci Lett. 2010;485:117–20.
19. Hakonen AH, Isohanni P, Paetau A, Herva R, Suomalainen A, Lönnqvist T. Recessive Twinkle mutations in early onset encephalopathy with mtDNA depletion. Brain. 2007;130:3032–40.
20. Kiferle L, Orsucci D, Mancuso M, Lo Gerfo A, Petrozzi L, Siciliano G, Ceravolo R, Bonuccelli U. Twinkle mutation in an Italian family with external progressive ophthalmoplegia and parkinsonism: a case report and an update on the state of art. Neurosci Lett. 2013;556:1–4.
21. Garone C, Rubio JC, Calvo SE, Naini A, Tanji K, Dimauro S, Mootha VK, Hirano M. MPV17 mutations causing adult-onset multisystemic disorder with multiple mitochondrial DNA deletions. Arch Neurol. 2012;69:1648–51.
22. Muyderman H, Sims NR, Tanaka M, Fuku N, Raghupathi R, Thyagarajan D. The mitochondrial T1095C mutation increases gentamicin-mediated apoptosis. Mitochondrion. 2012;12:465–71.

23. Hara K, Yamamoto M, Anegawa T, Sakuta R, Nakamura M. Mitochondrial encephalomyopathy associated with parkinsonism and a point mutation in the mitochondrial tRNA(Leu)(UUR)) gene. Rinsho Shinkeigaku. 1994;34:361–5.
24. Martikainen MH, Kytövuori L, Majamaa K. Juvenile parkinsonism, hypogonadism and Leigh-like MRI changes in a patient with m.4296G>A mutation in mitochondrial DNA. Mitochondrion. 2013;13:83–6.
25. Moran MM, Allen NM, Treacy EP, King MD. "Stiff neonate" with mitochondrial DNA depletion and secondary neurotransmitter defects. Pediatr Neurol. 2011;45:403–5.
26. Taravari A, Panov S, Petrov I, Petrova V, Medziti F, Haliti G. Delta deletion 4977 in mitochondrial DNA in patients with idiopathic Parkinson's disease. Bratisl Lek Listy. 2014;115:7–13.
27. Lax NZ, Hepplewhite PD, Reeve AK, Nesbitt V, McFarland R, Jaros E, Taylor RW, Turnbull DM. Cerebellar ataxia in patients with mitochondrial DNA disease: a molecular clinicopathological study. J Neuropathol Exp Neurol. 2012;71:148–61.
28. Zeviani M, Simonati A, Bindoff LA. Ataxia in mitochondrial disorders. Handb Clin Neurol. 2012;103:359–72.
29. Park MH, Woo HM, Hong YB, Park JH, Yoon BR, Park JM, Yoo JH, Koo H, Chae JH, Chung KW, Choi BO, Koo SK. Recessive C10orf2 mutations in a family with infantile-onset spinocerebellar ataxia, sensorimotor polyneuropathy, and myopathy. Neurogenetics. 2014;15:171–82.
30. Dündar H, Ozgül RK, Yalnızoğlu D, Erdem S, Oğuz KK, Tuncel D, Temuçin CM, Dursun A. Identification of a novel Twinkle mutation in a family with infantile onset spinocerebellar ataxia by whole exome sequencing. Pediatr Neurol. 2012;46:172–7.
31. Graf WD, Marin-Garcia J, Gao HG, Pizzo S, Naviaux RK, Markusic D, Barshop BA, Courchesne E, Haas RH. Autism associated with the mitochondrial DNA G8363A transfer RNA(Lys) mutation. J Child Neurol. 2000;15:357–61.
32. Castagna AE, Addis J, McInnes RR, Clarke JT, Ashby P, Blaser S, Robinson BH. Late onset Leigh syndrome and ataxia due to a T to C mutation at bp 9,185 of mitochondrial DNA. Am J Med Genet A. 2007;143A:808–16.
33. Pfeffer G, Blakely EL, Alston CL, Hassani A, Boggild M, Horvath R, Samuels DC, Taylor RW, Chinnery PF. Adult-onset spinocerebellar ataxia syndromes due to MTATP6 mutations. J Neurol Neurosurg Psychiatry. 2012;83:883–6.
34. Wilson CJ, Wood NW, Leonard JV, Surtees R, Rahman S. Mitochondrial DNA point mutation T9176C in Leigh syndrome. J Child Neurol. 2000;15:830–3.
35. Leshinsky-Silver E, Shuvalov R, Inbar S, Cohen S, Lev D, Lerman-Sagie T. Juvenile Leigh syndrome, optic atrophy, ataxia, dystonia, and epilepsy due to T14487C mutation in the mtDNA-ND6 gene: a mitochondrial syndrome presenting from birth to adolescence. J Child Neurol. 2011;26:476–81.
36. Hudson G, Deschauer M, Busse K, Zierz S, Chinnery PF. Sensory ataxic neuropathy due to a novel C10Orf2 mutation with probable germline mosaicism. Neurology. 2005;64:371–3.
37. Van Goethem G, Martin JJ, Dermaut B, Löfgren A, Wibail A, Ververken D, Tack P, Dehaene I, Van Zandijcke M, Moonen M, Ceuterick C, De Jonghe P, Van Broeckhoven C. Recessive POLG mutations presenting with sensory and ataxic neuropathy in compound heterozygote patients with progressive external ophthalmoplegia. Neuromuscul Disord. 2003;13:133–42.
38. Lovan A, Ihtsham ul Haq, Balakrishnan N. Diagnostic challenges in movement disorders: Sensory Ataxia Neuropathy Dysarthria and Ophthalmoplegia (SANDO) syndrome. BMJ Case Rep. 2013;2013. pii:bcr2013010343. doi:10.1136/bcr-2013-010343.
39. Doss S, Lohmann K, Seibler P, Arns B, Klopstock T, Zühlke C, Freimann K, Winkler S, Lohnau T, Drungowski M, Nürnberg P, Wiegers K, Lohmann E, Naz S, Kasten M, Bohner G, Ramirez A, Endres M, Klein C. Recessive dystonia-ataxia syndrome in a Turkish family caused by a COX20 (FAM36A) mutation. J Neurol. 2014;261:207–12.
40. Glamuzina E, Brown R, Hogarth K, Saunders D, Russell-Eggitt I, Pitt M, de Sousa C, Rahman S, Brown G, Grunewald S. Further delineation of pontocerebellar hypoplasia type 6 due to mutations in the gene encoding mitochondrial arginyl-tRNA synthetase, RARS2. J Inherit Metab Dis. 2012;35:459–67.

41. Bayat V, Thiffault I, Jaiswal M, Tétreault M, Donti T, Sasarman F, Bernard G, Demers-Lamarche J, Dicaire MJ, Mathieu J, Vanasse M, Bouchard JP, Rioux MF, Lourenco CM, Li Z, Haueter C, Shoubridge EA, Graham BH, Brais B, Bellen HJ. Mutations in the mitochondrial methionyl-tRNA synthetase cause a neurodegenerative phenotype in flies and a recessive ataxia (ARSAL) in humans. PLoS Biol. 2012;10(3):e1001288. doi:10.1371/journal.pbio.1001288.
42. Träff J, Holme E, Ekbom K, Nilsson BY. Ekbom's syndrome of photomyoclonus, cerebellar ataxia and cervical lipoma is associated with the tRNA(Lys) A8344G mutation in mitochondrial DNA. Acta Neurol Scand. 1995;92:394–7.
43. Lax NZ, Gnanapavan S, Dowson SJ, Alston CL, He L, Polvikoski TM, Jaros E, O'Donovan DG, Yarham JW, Turnbull DM, Dean AF, Taylor RW. Early-onset cataracts, spastic paraparesis, and ataxia caused by a novel mitochondrial tRNAGlu (MT-TE) gene mutation causing severe complex I deficiency: a clinical, molecular, and neuropathologic study. J Neuropathol Exp Neurol. 2013;72:164–75.
44. Erol I, Alehan F, Horvath R, Schneiderat P, Talim B. Demyelinating disease of central and peripheral nervous systems associated with a A8344G mutation in tRNALys. Neuromuscul Disord. 2009;19:275–8.
45. Da Pozzo P, Cardaioli E, Malfatti E, Gallus GN, Malandrini A, Gaudiano C, Berti G, Invernizzi F, Zeviani M, Federico A. A novel mutation in the mitochondrial tRNA(Pro) gene associated with late-onset ataxia, retinitis pigmentosa, deafness, leukoencephalopathy and complex I deficiency. Eur J Hum Genet. 2009;17:1092–6.
46. Pulkes T, Liolitsa D, Eunson LH, Rose M, Nelson IP, Rahman S, Poulton J, Marchington DR, Landon DN, Debono AG, Morgan-Hughes JA, Hanna MG. New phenotypic diversity associated with the mitochondrial tRNA(SerUCN) gene mutation. Neuromuscul Disord. 2005;15:364–71.
47. Barrientos A, Casademont J, Genís D, Cardellach F, Fernández-Real JM, Grau JM, Urbano-Márquez A, Estivill X, Nunes V. Sporadic heteroplasmic single 5.5 kb mitochondrial DNA deletion associated with cerebellar ataxia, hypogonadotropic hypogonadism, choroidal dystrophy, and mitochondrial respiratory chain complex I deficiency. Hum Mutat. 1997;10:212–6.
48. Schaaf CP, Blazo M, Lewis RA, Tonini RE, Takei H, Wang J, Wong LJ, Scaglia F. Early-onset severe neuromuscular phenotype associated with compound heterozygosity for OPA1 mutations. Mol Genet Metab. 2011;103:383–7.
49. Birch-Machin MA, Taylor RW, Cochran B, Ackrell BA, Turnbull DM. Late-onset optic atrophy, ataxia, and myopathy associated with a mutation of a complex II gene. Ann Neurol. 2000;48:330–5.
50. Horvath R, Czermin B, Gulati S, Demuth S, Houge G, Pyle A, Dineiger C, Blakely EL, Hassani A, Foley C, Brodhun M, Storm K, Kirschner J, Gorman GS, Lochmüller H, Holinski-Feder E, Taylor RW, Chinnery PF. Adult-onset cerebellar ataxia due to mutations in CABC1/ADCK3. J Neurol Neurosurg Psychiatry. 2012;83:174–8.
51. Barel O, Shorer Z, Flusser H, Ofir R, Narkis G, Finer G, Shalev H, Nasasra A, Saada A, Birk OS. Mitochondrial complex III deficiency associated with a homozygous mutation in UQCRQ. Am J Hum Genet. 2008;82:1211–6.
52. Mollet J, Delahodde A, Serre V, Chretien D, Schlemmer D, Lombes A, Boddaert N, Desguerre I, de Lonlay P, de Baulny HO, Munnich A, Rötig A. CABC1 gene mutations cause ubiquinone deficiency with cerebellar ataxia and seizures. Am J Hum Genet. 2008;82:623–30.
53. Liu YT, Hersheson J, Plagnol V, Fawcett K, Duberley KE, Preza E, Hargreaves IP, Chalasani A, Laurá M, Wood NW, Reilly MM, Houlden H. Autosomal-recessive cerebellar ataxia caused by a novel ADCK3 mutation that elongates the protein: clinical, genetic and biochemical characterisation. J Neurol Neurosurg Psychiatry. 2014;85:493–8.
54. Simon DK, Zheng K, Velázquez L, Santos N, Almaguer L, Figueroa KP, Pulst SM. Mitochondrial complex I gene variant associated with early age at onset in spinocerebellar ataxia type 2. Arch Neurol. 2007;64:1042–4.
55. Wang K, Takahashi Y, Gao ZL, Wang GX, Chen XW, Goto J, Lou JN, Tsuji S. Mitochondrial ND3 as the novel causative gene for Leber hereditary optic neuropathy and dystonia. Neurogenetics. 2009;10:337–45.

56. De Vries DD, Went LN, Bruyn GW, Scholte HR, Hofstra RM, Bolhuis PA, van Oost BA. Genetic and biochemical impairment of mitochondrial complex I activity in a family with Leber hereditary optic neuropathy and hereditary spastic dystonia. Am J Hum Genet. 1996;58:703–11.
57. Dermaut B, Seneca S, Dom L, Smets K, Ceulemans L, Smet J, De Paepe B, Tousseyn S, Weckhuysen S, Gewillig M, Pals P, Parizel P, De Bleecker JL, Boon P, De Meirleir L, De Jonghe P, Van Coster R, Van Paesschen W, Santens P. Progressive myoclonic epilepsy as an adult-onset manifestation of Leigh syndrome due to m.14487T>C. J Neurol Neurosurg Psychiatry. 2010;81:90–3.
58. Abu-Amero KK, Bosley TM, Bohlega S, McLean D. Complex I respiratory defect in LHON plus dystonia with no mitochondrial DNA mutation. Br J Ophthalmol. 2005;89:1380–1.
59. Sarzi E, Brown MD, Lebon S, Chretien D, Munnich A, Rotig A, Procaccio V. A novel recurrent mitochondrial DNA mutation in ND3 gene is associated with isolated complex I deficiency causing Leigh syndrome and dystonia. Am J Med Genet A. 2007;143:33–41.
60. Seeger J, Schrank B, Pyle A, Stucka R, Lörcher U, Müller-Ziermann S, Abicht A, Czermin B, Holinski-Feder E, Lochmüller H, Horvath R. Clinical and neuropathological findings in patients with TACO1 mutations. Neuromuscul Disord. 2010;20:720–4.
61. Blesa JR, Solano A, Briones P, Prieto-Ruiz JA, Hernández-Yago J, Coria F. Molecular genetics of a patient with Mohr-Tranebjaerg Syndrome due to a new mutation in the DDP1 gene. Neuromolecular Med. 2007;9:285–91.
62. Binder J, Hofmann S, Kreisel S, Wöhrle JC, Bäzner H, Krauss JK, Hennerici MG, Bauer MF. Clinical and molecular findings in a patient with a novel mutation in the deafness-dystonia peptide (DDP1) gene. Brain. 2003;126:1814–20.
63. Szklarczyk R, Wanschers BF, Nijtmans LG, Rodenburg RJ, Zschocke J, Dikow N, van den Brand MA, Hendriks-Franssen MG, Gilissen C, Veltman JA, Nooteboom M, Koopman WJ, Willems PH, Smeitink JA, Huynen MA, van den Heuvel LP. A mutation in the FAM36A gene, the human ortholog of COX20, impairs cytochrome c oxidase assembly and is associated with ataxia and muscle hypotonia. Hum Mol Genet. 2013;22:656–67.
64. Ghezzi D, Viscomi C, Ferlini A, Gualandi F, Mereghetti P, DeGrandis D, Zeviani M. Paroxysmal non-kinesigenic dyskinesia is caused by mutations of the MR-1 mitochondrial targeting sequence. Hum Mol Genet. 2009;18:1058–64.
65. Raspall-Chaure M, Solano A, Vázquez E, Macaya-Ruiz A, del Toro-Riera M, Cabezuelo-Briones A, Montoya J, Andreu A, Roig-Quilis M. A patient with bilateral lesion in the striatum and slowly progressive dystonia secondary to T14487C mutation in the ND6 gene of complex I of the mitochondrial respiratory chain. Rev Neurol. 2004;39:1129–32.
66. Solano A, Roig M, Vives-Bauza C, Hernandez-Peña J, Garcia-Arumi E, Playan A, Lopez-Perez MJ, Andreu AL, Montoya J. Bilateral striatal necrosis associated with a novel mutation in the mitochondrial ND6 gene. Ann Neurol. 2003;54:527–30.
67. Chae JH, Lee JS, Kim KJ, Hwang YS, Bonilla E, Tanji K, Hirano M. A novel ND3 mitochondrial DNA mutation in three Korean children with basal ganglia lesions and complex I deficiency. Pediatr Res. 2007;61:622–4.
68. Laugel V, This-Bernd V, Cormier-Daire V, Speeg-Schatz C, de Saint-Martin A, Fischbach M. Early-onset ophthalmoplegia in Leigh-like syndrome due to NDUFV1 mutations. Pediatr Neurol. 2007;36:54–7.
69. Simon DK, Friedman J, Breakefield XO, Jankovic J, Brin MF, Provias J, Bressman SB, Charness ME, Tarsy D, Johns DR, Tarnopolsky MA. A heteroplasmic mitochondrial complex I gene mutation in adult-onset dystonia. Neurogenetics. 2003;4:199–205.
70. Bourgeron T, Chretien D, Poggi-Bach J, Doonan S, Rabier D, Letouzé P, Munnich A, Rötig A, Landrieu P, Rustin P. Mutation of the fumarase gene in two siblings with progressive encephalopathy and fumarase deficiency. J Clin Invest. 1994;93:2514–8.
71. Spiegel R, Pines O, Ta-Shma A, Burak E, Shaag A, Halvardson J, Edvardson S, Mahajna M, Zenvirt S, Saada A, Shalev S, Feuk L, Elpeleg O. Infantile cerebellar-retinal degeneration associated with a mutation in mitochondrial aconitase, ACO2. Am J Hum Genet. 2012;90:518–23.
72. Seaver LH, He XY, Abe K, Cowan T, Enns GM, Sweetman L, Philipp M, Lee S, Malik M, Yang SY. A novel mutation in the HSD17B10 gene of a 10-year-old boy with refractory epilepsy, choreoathetosis and learning disability. PLoS One. 2011;6:e27348. doi:10.1371/journal.pone.0027348.

73. Zschocke J, Ruiter JP, Brand J, Lindner M, Hoffmann GF, Wanders RJ, Mayatepek E. Progressive infantile neurodegeneration caused by 2-methyl-3-hydroxybutyryl-CoA dehydrogenase deficiency: a novel inborn error of branched-chain fatty acid and isoleucine metabolism. Pediatr Res. 2000;48:852–5.
74. Shenkman Z, Krichevski I, Elpeleg ON, Joseph A, Kadari A. Anaesthetic management of a patient with Leigh's syndrome. Can J Anaesth. 1997;44:1091–5.
75. Ueki I, Koga Y, Povalko N, Akita Y, Nishioka J, Yatsuga S, Fukiyama R, Matsuishi T. Mitochondrial tRNA gene mutations in patients having mitochondrial disease with lactic acidosis. Mitochondrion. 2006;6:29–36.
76. Salman MS, Blaser S, Buncic JR, Westall CA, Héon E, Becker L. Pontocerebellar hypoplasia type 1: new leads for an earlier diagnosis. J Child Neurol. 2003;18:220–5.
77. Mordekar SR, Baxter PS. 'Cerebral palsy' due to mitochondrial cytopathy. J Paediatr Child Health. 2004;40:714–5.
78. Lissens W, Vreken P, Barth PG, Wijburg FA, Ruitenbeek W, Wanders RJ, Seneca S, Liebaers I, De Meirleir L. Cerebral palsy and pyruvate dehydrogenase deficiency: identification of two new mutations in the E1alpha gene. Eur J Pediatr. 1999;158:853–7.
79. Fryer A, Appleton R, Sweeney MG, Rosenbloom L, Harding AE. Mitochondrial DNA 8993 (NARP) mutation presenting with a heterogeneous phenotype including 'cerebral palsy'. Arch Dis Child. 1994;71:419–22.
80. Tsao CY, Wright FS, Boesel CP, Luquette M. Partial NADH dehydrogenase defect presenting as spastic cerebral palsy. Brain Dev. 1994;16:393–5.
81. Billard C, Dulac O, Bouloche J, Echenne B, Lebon P, Motte J, Robain O, Santini JJ. Encephalopathy with calcifications of the basal ganglia in children. A reappraisal of Fahr's syndrome with respect to 14 new cases. Neuropediatrics. 1989;20:12–9.
82. Willis TA, Davidson J, Gray RG, Poulton K, Ramani P, Whitehouse W. Cytochrome oxidase deficiency presenting as birth asphyxia. Dev Med Child Neurol. 2000;42:414–7.
83. Milone M, Klassen BT, Landsverk ML, Haas RH, Wong LJ. Orthostatic tremor, progressive external ophthalmoplegia, and Twinkle. JAMA Neurol. 2013;70:1429–31.
84. Johansen KK, Bindoff LA, Rydland J, Aasly JO. Palatal tremor and facial dyskinesia in a patient with POLG1 mutation. Mov Disord. 2008;23:1624–6.
85. Yoo YM, Lee CJ, Lee U, Kim YJ. Mitochondrial DNA in patients with essential tremor. Neurosci Lett. 2008;434:29–34.
86. Ramelli GP, Gallati S, Weis J, Krähenbühl S, Burgunder JM. Point mutation tRNA(Ser(UCN)) in a child with hearing loss and myoclonus epilepsy. J Child Neurol. 2006;21:253–5.
87. Navarro-Otano J, Valls-Solé J, Guaita M, Santamaria J, Cardellach F, Muñoz E. Chewing-induced segmental myoclonus in a patient with Leigh syndrome. Mov Disord. 2013;28:1756–7.
88. Naini AB, Lu J, Kaufmann P, Bernstein RA, Mancuso M, Bonilla E, Hirano M, DiMauro S. Novel mitochondrial DNA ND5 mutation in a patient with clinical features of MELAS and MERRF. Arch Neurol. 2005;62:473–6.
89. Smits BW, Westeneng HJ, van Hal MA, van Engelen BG, Overeem S. Sleep disturbances in chronic progressive external ophthalmoplegia. Eur J Neurol. 2012;19:176–8.
90. Aitken H, Gorman G, McFarland R, Roberts M, Taylor RW, Turnbull DM. Clinical reasoning: blurred vision and dancing feet: restless legs syndrome presenting in mitochondrial disease. Neurology. 2009;72:e86–90.
91. Guo Y, Deng X, Zhang J, Su L, Xu H, Luo Z, Deng H. Analysis of the MRPL3, DNAJC13 and OFCC1 variants in Chinese Han patients with TS-CTD. Neurosci Lett. 2012;517:18–20.
92. Petek E, Schwarzbraun T, Noor A, Patel M, Nakabayashi K, Choufani S, Windpassinger C, Stamenkovic M, Robertson MM, Aschauer HN, Gurling HM, Kroisel PM, Wagner K, Scherer SW, Vincent JB. Molecular and genomic studies of IMMP2L and mutation screening in autism and Tourette syndrome. Mol Genet Genomics. 2007;277:71–81.
93. Kalapatapu RK. Escitalopram treatment of stereotypic movement disorder in an adolescent with mitochondrial disorder and mental retardation. J Child Adolesc Psychopharmacol. 2009;19:313–6.

Part II
Technical and Scientific Aspects of Genetic Testing

Chapter 19
Genetic Testing, Interpretation of Genetic Test Reports and Genetic Counseling for Clinicians

Robin L. Bennett

Abstract Genetic testing for hereditary movement disorders is complex. This chapter reviews the major patterns of inheritance of inherited movement disorders, clues in a family history to suggest an inherited movement disorder, and the pedigree symbols used to record a family history. Some of the common genetic counseling issues facing individuals and their families with hereditary movement disorders are discussed. Pre- and post-test genetic counseling is important in the evaluation of the individual and family with a potential inherited movement disorder.

Keywords Genetic testing • Interpretation of genetic test reports • Counseling • Genetic counseling • Patterns of inheritance • Pedigree • Anticipation • Genetic heterogeneity • Expressivity

Introduction

Genetic testing is becoming more routine to diagnose a growing number of hereditary movement disorders. With this clinical application of testing, the spectrum of the symptoms (*phenotype*) that define hereditary movement disorders is expanding; individuals with less classic disease symptoms are now diagnosed, whereas in the past, such individuals would have eluded diagnosis. Genetic testing can help distinguish the more rare inherited causes of movement disorders from the common sporadic forms which may be difficult to distinguish from neurological features alone. A classic example is Parkinson's disease where there are several different genes following various patterns of inheritance and there may be little obvious difference in the clinical symptoms [10]. This is referred to as *genetic heterogeneity*; multiple genes give rise to similar phenotypes such as with hereditary ataxias and some of the hereditary Parkinson's diseases [10]. There can also be the problem of *phenocopy* for conditions which are common; thus in the case of Parkinson's disease, a

R.L. Bennett, MS, LGC, ScD Hon
Division of Medical Genetics, Department of Medicine, University of Washington Medical Center, Seattle, WA 98195, USA
e-mail: robinb@uw.edu

S.A. Schneider, J.M.T. Brás (eds.), *Movement Disorder Genetics*,
DOI 10.1007/978-3-319-17223-1_19

family with several relatives with a SNCA-associated (PARK1) mutation may have a relative who does not have the familial mutation but has a diagnosis of Parkinson's disease.

Genetic testing for hereditary movement disorders may be offered throughout the life span, from newborn screening to pediatric and adolescent evaluations to adult-onset disorders and preconception and pregnancy testing. Therefore, it is important for clinicians to have a general understanding of genetic principles, how to document family history, and to recognize the importance of genetic counseling in conjunction with genetic testing.

Family History: The First Genetic Test

Documenting a three-or-more-generation family history is a first step in recognizing a possible hereditary movement disorder. Clinical genetic tests do not replace the importance of a family history. In fact, genetic testing must be interpreted in the context of family history. For example, if a genetic test is inconclusive or a pathogenic variant is not identified, the family history can inform the interpretation.

Family history clues to an inherited movement disorder include

- Relatives in one generation, or over more than one generation, with a neurological condition (e.g., seizures, ataxia, dystonia, uncontrolled movements)
- Earlier than typical age of onset of symptoms (often before age 40), particularly if symptoms begin in childhood or adolescence
- Progression of neurological symptoms
- Cognitive decline (e.g., dementia, intellectual disability, personality change)
- Multiple significant medical problems (e.g., hearing loss, vision loss, muscle weakness, ataxia, dysarthria)
- No obvious environmental factors (e.g., alcohol abuse, medication side effect, lead or mercury toxicity)
- No obvious occupational exposure (e.g. painter, working around batteries, furniture finishing)
- Parents related as close relatives (such as first cousins), which may be a clue to an autosomal recessively inherited condition

Family history forms are helpful for obtaining family history, but a multigenerational pedigree is a quick, concise, and graphic way to document the health history of many relatives [1]. The collection and interpretation of a family health history is not only a diagnostic tool, but it can also serve as a way of establishing rapport with the patient, demonstrating variability of the disease within the family (e.g., relatives may have different manifestations of the disease or varying severity of symptoms). A pedigree can also serve as an educational tool to educate the patient about the hereditary movement disorder and as a visual reminder of who else is at risk for the condition in the family and who in turn might benefit from genetic counseling and testing. Families may have misconceptions of how the disorder is inherited in the family (e.g., only the oldest child is affected in a family, or every other child is affected); a pedigree can be used to help debunk family lore [1]. Standard pedigree nomenclature for documenting family history is shown in Fig. 19.1.

Key information to record on a pedigree includes [4]

- Age and/or year of birth
- Age and cause of death (year if known)

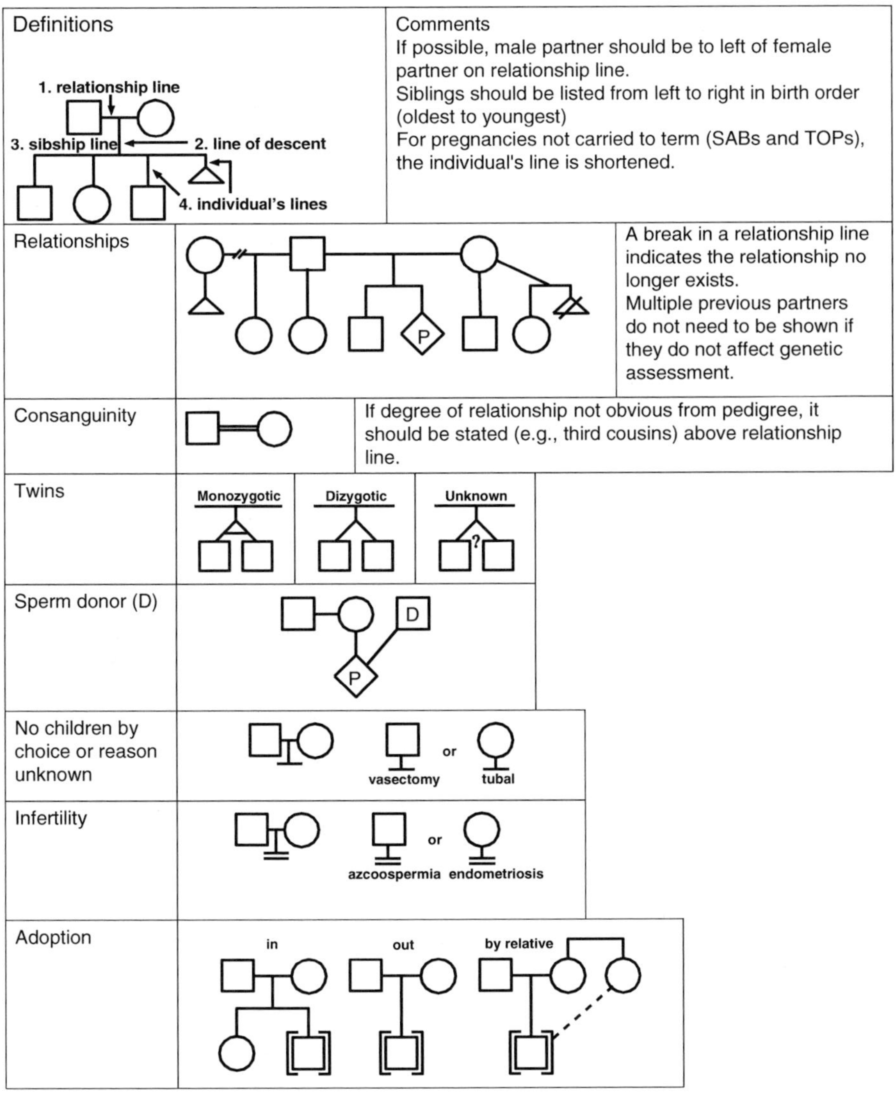

Fig. 19.1 Common pedigree symbols, definitions, and abbreviations (Adapted from Bennett et al. [4])

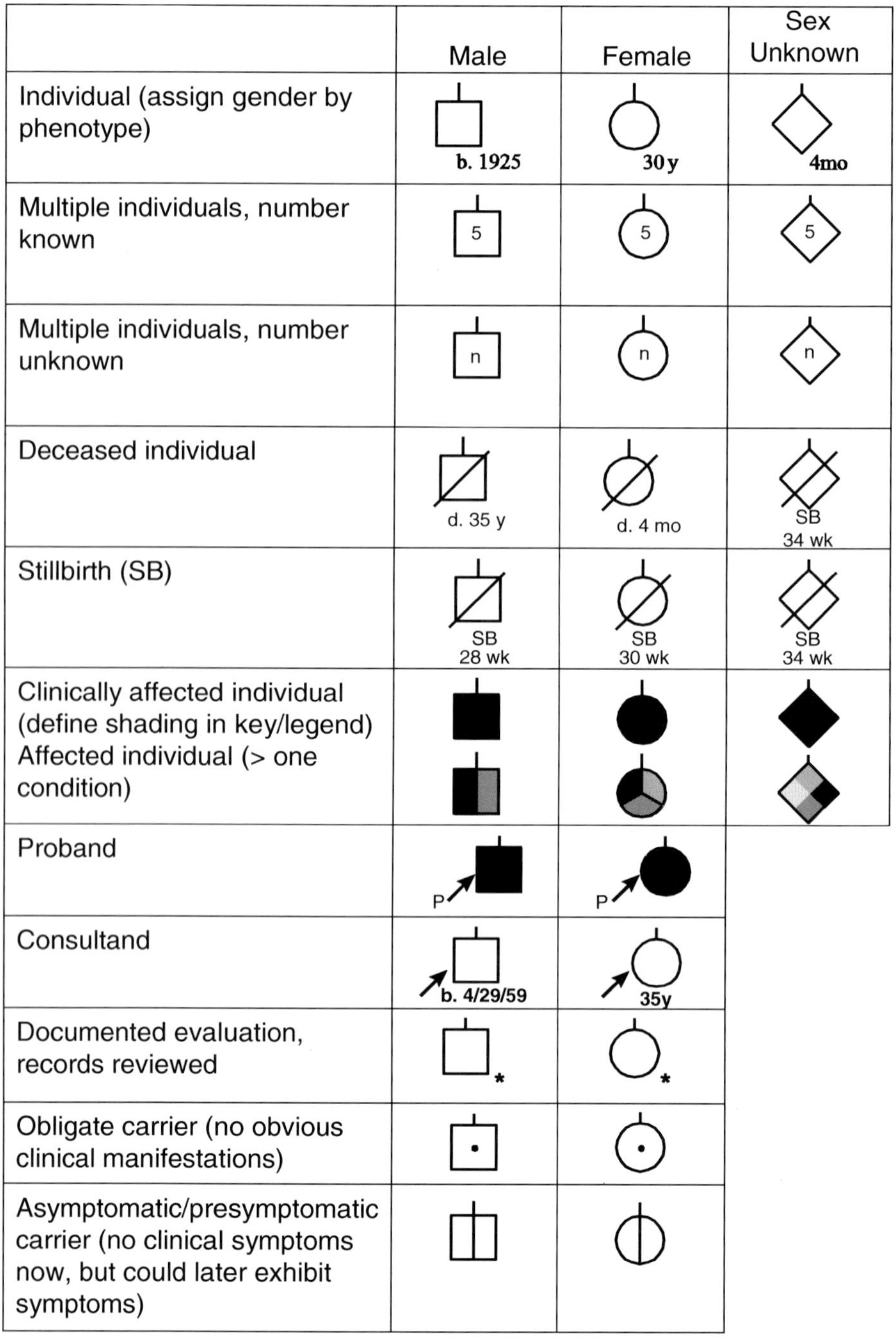

Fig. 19.1 (continued)

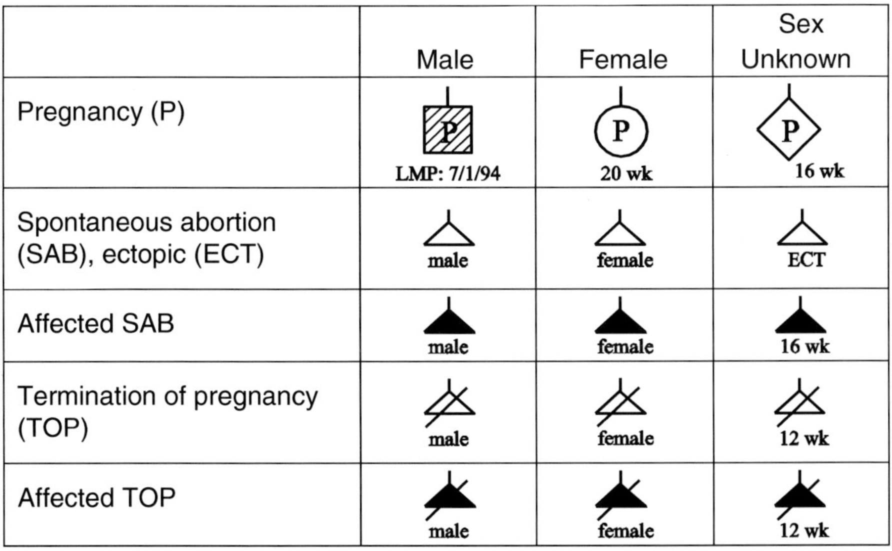

Fig. 19.1 (continued)

- Relevant health information and age of diagnosis (e.g., chorea, onset age 40 years)
- Ethnic background/country of origin for each grandparent
- Any consanguinity (with degree of relationship noted, such as first cousins)

Unless three generations of family history are recorded, it is difficult to observe patterns of inheritance; a good rule of thumb is two generations "up" (parents, grandparents, aunts and uncles) and two generations "down" (first cousins, children, and grandchildren). Distinguishing full siblings from half-siblings is also important. An arrow is used to point to the *proband* (the first affected person in the pedigree) or the *consultand* (the person who is seeking medical advice, who may be affected or not). Ancestry of the grandparents is noted because some genetic disorders are more common in certain populations (an example is Machado-Joseph/SCA3 in the Azores, DYT3 dystonia in Filipino or HDL2 in Black Africans) or there may be common *founder mutations* making certain pathogenic mutations more likely to be identified. For example, the autosomal dominant Parkinson *LLRK2* gene mutation G2019S is common in the Ashkenazi population and in North African Arabs, whereas the R1441G variant is more common in persons of Hispanic or Spanish descent [6, 11, 12]. The autosomal dominant *TOR1A* pathogenic mutation is associated with early-onset dystonia in the Ashkenazi population. If the parents of the person who is being evaluated for a movement disorder are closely related (such as first cousins), this can be a clue that an autosomal recessive movement disorder is in the differential diagnosis (see Table 19.1) [3, 8].

Family history is dynamic—children are born, relatives die, and relatives become affected with new diseases over time. It is important to update family history every few years. Noting who recorded the pedigree, the reason it was taken (e.g., family history of Huntington disease, family history of Parkinson's disease), and the date it was recorded is essential to note [4].

Patterns of Inheritance for Hereditary Movement Disorders

Movement disorders are inherited in many different patterns. Knowledge of these patterns can assist with differential diagnosis and of course be used for genetic counseling regarding chance of disease occurrence and recurrence. These basic inheritance patterns and examples of some of the hereditary movement disorders are summarized in Table 19.1.

Recognizing patterns of inheritance requires recognition of the *phenotype* (outward expression of the condition), which can be difficult for many reasons including *reduced penetrance* (not every person who has the pathogenic mutation(s) develops the condition) and *variable expressivity* (the relatives in the family may have very mild expression of the disease and therefore never be diagnosed with the hereditary movement disorders).

Autosomal Dominant

The majority of the currently recognized hereditary movement disorders follow this inheritance pattern. Autosomes refer to the 22 pairs of nonsex chromosomes, numbered from 1 to 22. With this pattern of vertical transmission, a person who has a disease-causing mutation has a 50:50 chance to pass the mutation to each son or daughter. Two major clues to autosomal dominant inheritance are recognition of the disease in more than one generation and male-to-male (i.e., father-to-son) transmission (mother-to-son transmission could be autosomal dominant or X linked). A person can have a new autosomal dominant deleterious mutation (the mutation occurred in the egg or sperm, and neither parent is affected) and thus be the first person with the disease in the family; their siblings would not be at risk for the disease, but he or she would have a 50 % chance to pass the mutation on to each son or daughter.

Gonadal mosaicism can occur with autosomal dominant conditions. This means that the mutation occurring in the testes or ovaries are mosaic for the pathogenic mutation and thus not all the progenitor cells have the mutation; the parent has no symptoms of the condition, but they are at risk to have children with the condition.

There are several autosomal dominant neurological disorders that show *anticipation*. This is where relatives with the disease have more severe manifestations and often earlier age at onset with each generation. A classic example of this is Huntington's disease. Anticipation in Huntington's disease is explained by instability in the CAG expansion which can expand over successive generations, and relatives with larger CAG repeats can have earlier onset of symptoms (Chap. 8). Other examples are HDL2 (Chap. 8) and some of the spinocerebellar ataxias (Chap. 11).

Table 19.1 Examples of inheritance patterns for several hereditary movement disorders, clues for recognizing patterns of inheritance, and variables that can mask recognition of these patterns

Inheritance pattern	Mode of transmission	Pedigree clues	Confounding factors	Disease examples
Autosomal dominant (AD)	50 % risk to each son/daughter (heterozygotes affected with disease)	Vertical transmission Male-male transmission Males/females affected (often with similar degree of clinical manifestations) Often variability in disease severity Homozygotes may be affected more severely than heterozygotes Homozygous state may be lethal	Reduced penetrance Can miss diagnosis in relatives if mild expression for disease New mutations may be mistaken for sporadic if small family size Gonadal mosaicism	Dopa-responsive dystonia DRPLA[a] Dystonia (early-onset primary dystonia) Huntington's disease Huntington's disease-like 2 Frontotemporal dementia with Parkinsonism-17 Neuroferritnopathy SOD-1 Related Amytrophic lateral sclerosis Spinocerebellar ataxias
Autosomal recessive (AR)	25 % risk to each son/daughter (homozygotes affected with disease) Parents "healthy" but mutation carriers (heterozygotes)	Usually one generation (horizontal transmission) Males/females affected Often seen in newborn, infancy, childhood Often inborn errors of metabolism May be more common in certain ethnic groups (e.g., Tay-Sachs disease and Ashkenazim) Sometimes parental consanguinity	May be mistaken as sporadic if small family size If carrier frequency high, can look like autosomal dominant	Ataxia-telangiectasia Ataxia with oculomotor apraxia Friedreich ataxia Hyperekplexia Lafora body disease Myoclonic epilepsy of Unverricht and Lundborg Neuroacanthocytosis Panthothenate kinase-associated neurodegeneration (PKAN) Parkin type of juvenile Parkinson's disease (Park2) Tyrosine hydroxylase-deficient DRD Wilson disease

(continued)

Table 19.1 (continued)

Inheritance pattern	Mode of transmission	Pedigree clues	Confounding factors	Disease examples
X-linked dominant (XLD)	Heterozygous women affected with 50:50 risk to have affected daughter/50:50 chance for affected male (though lethal)	No male-to-male transmission Often lethal in males so see paucity of males in pedigree May see multiple miscarriages (due to male fetal lethality) Females usually express condition but have milder symptoms than males	Small family size	Rett syndrome
X-linked (XL)	Women have 50 % chance for affected son/50 % chance for heterozygous daughter (usually unaffected)	No male-to-male transmission Males affected Females may be affected but often milder and/or with later onset than males	May be missed if paucity of females in female Lyonization	Adrenoleukodystrophy Fragile X syndrome Lesch-Nyan disease
Mitochondrial	0–100 %	No male transmission to offspring, only maternal transmission Highly variable clinical expression Often central nervous disorders Males and females affected, often in multiple generations	Generally considered rare	Mitochondrial encephalopathy with ragged-red fibers (MERRF) Mitochondrial encephalopathy, lactic acidosis, strokes (MELAS) Neuropathy with ataxia and retinitis pigmentosa (NARP)
Multifactorial	Based on empirical risk tables	Males and females affected No clear pattern Skips generations Few affected family members	May actually be single gene	Schizophrenia Bipolar disorder Epilepsy

[a]*DRPLA* Dentaorubral-pallidoluysian atrophy

Autosomal Recessive

To have an autosomal recessive condition, the individual would have two pathogenic mutations, one inherited from each parent. The couple who each carry a mutation have a 25 % chance with each pregnancy to have an affected son or daughter. The person with the condition will always pass one copy of the pathogenic mutation to each offspring, but he or she would only have an affected child if his or her partner carried a mutation in the same gene. Usually, the likelihood that the offspring of an affected parent will have a child affected with the same condition is less than 1 %. The unaffected sibling of a person with an autosomal recessive condition has a 2/3 chance to be a carrier, but to have an affected child, their partner must also carry a pathogenic mutation for the condition, thus the a priori chance to have an affected child is usually in the range of 1 %.

Although it is rare for the offspring or unaffected siblings of a person with an autosomal recessive condition to in turn have a child affected with the hereditary movement disorder, it is important that carrier testing be offered to their partner. Some populations have a high carrier frequency for certain autosomal recessive disorders. A clue to a possible recessive disorder in the family includes if the parents are close "blood relatives" (such as first cousins). This is referred to as *consanguinity*. People who are closely related are more likely to have the same genetic variants in common [3, 8].

There can be hundreds of pathogenic changes in a gene. If the person carries the same allele, then this is referred to as *homozygous*. If the person carries two different copies of the same gene, then this is *compound heterozygosity*. Usually, the disease severity is not affected by whether a person is homozygous or a compound heterozygote, but there are some diseases where certain mutations may be associated with variable disease severity.

X-linked

With this pattern, the pathogenic mutation occurs on the X chromosome. Women generally do not show symptoms because the gene on the other X chromosome functions normally. If she has a male offspring, there is a 50 % chance he will inherit the pathogenic mutation and thus be affected, and for a female offspring, there is 50 % chance that she has the pathogenic mutation, but she often has no symptoms or mild symptoms. Many X-linked conditions have a high rate of new mutation (if the males have limited reproductive fitness).

Mitochondrial Inheritance

Mitochondria have their own genome with a circular DNA molecule A single cell can have hundreds of mitochondria. With mitochondrial inheritance, women are affected and can pass the mutation to sons or daughters; but sons cannot pass the mitochondrial mutation to their children. Depending on the number of mitochondria that are randomly included in the cytoplasm during meiosis, it affects the offspring's mitochondrial DNA component. Thus, offspring of a woman with a mitochondrial disease can have marked variability in the disease expression, and the chance the offspring will be affected ranges from 0 to 100 %.

Mitochondrial diseases can be inherited from nuclear DNA (usually autosomal recessive disorders) or mitochondrial DNA. The understanding of this distinction is essential for genetic counseling regarding disease occurrence and recurrence risks.

Multifactorial and Polygenic Disorders

Multifactorial conditions have both environmental and genetic components. Multiple genes may play a role in the expression of the condition (polygenic inheritance). Many common neurological disorders have multiple genetic and environmental factors at the root of their expression. For these conditions, "chance has a memory," meaning the recurrence risk rises as the number of affected individuals within the family increases.

Genetic Counseling

The effects of a new diagnosis of an inherited movement disorder often ripple beyond the individual and extend to siblings, children, even grandchildren, the prior generation (parents, aunts, uncles), and distant cousins. Individuals with a new genetic diagnosis often have the similar emotional reactions at diagnosis as people with nongenetic disorders—grief, shock, denial, distress, depression, and anger. Reactions unique to a genetic diagnosis are parental guilt and survivor guilt (for relatives who test negative for the disorder). Alternatively, there are also many positive reactions to a confirmatory genetic diagnosis which can include relief at having a diagnosis (particularly if there has been a long diagnostic odyssey), increased appreciation of life, and empowerment (e.g., the ability to participate in research, enroll in disease-specific registries, or enroll in clinical trials, some of which specifically recruit gene mutation carriers) [2, 5, 7].

The permanent nature of genetic disease may bring a sense of fatalism or hopelessness accompanying the diagnosis or the results of genetic testing. Genetic disorders are chronic diseases—there may be a continual array of new health and physical challenges over a person's lifetime. The individual and the family may experience "chronic sorrow" for the healthy person who will never be. Results of genetic testing may alter the person's perception of health, self-concept, and self-esteem as well as their perceived genetic or social identity. A major difference in the diagnosis of an inherited movement disorder as compared to a nongenetic etiology is that the inherited disorder may alter reproductive options.

The diagnosis of a genetic condition may lead to alternation in reproductive plans for not just the initial person diagnosed with the condition but many other relatives. The religious and ethical belief systems of couples and their families may be challenged, particularly as couples wrestle with core values on how they regard life and health and their relationship to the couple's and their family's views on biological parenting. Often, the perceived parental role is threatened by finding out genetic carrier status. Couples at risk to have offspring with a neurogenetic disorder face difficult decisions about adoption, assisted reproductive technologies (including the use of donor egg or sperm including three-parent IVF which combines genes from three parents most recently approved of in England and preimplantation diagnosis), prenatal diagnosis and possible abortion of an affected fetus, or taking their spin at genetic roulette.

Genetic counselors are specifically trained to deal with the spectrum of scientific and psychosocial issues that are involved with genetic diagnosis and testing for individuals and their families as is evidenced by the definition of genetic counseling [13]:

Genetic counseling is the process of helping people understand and adapt to the medical, psychological, and family implications of genetic contributions to disease.

This process integrates

- Collection and interpretation of family and medical histories to assess the chance of disease occurrence or recurrence
- Education about inheritance, testing, management, prevention, resources, and research
- Counseling to promote informed choices and adaptation to the risk of the condition

Genetic counseling has a tradition of not directing patient decision-making (nondirective counseling), particularly with regard to reproductive choices and demonstrating respect for patient autonomy. The current approach to genetic counseling favors a psychosocial approach that emphasizes shared deliberation and decision-making between the counselor and the client. The process of genetic counseling can help people understand their options and make decisions that are appropriate in view of their perceptions of risk, religion, life beliefs, relationships, family beliefs, and life goals. This approach is designed to reduce the patient's anxiety, enhance the client's sense of control and mastery over life circumstances, increase his or her understanding of the genetic disorder and options for testing and disease management, and provide the client and family with the tools required to adjust to potential outcomes [2, 13].

The internet can help to locate a genetic counselor, e.g., www.nsgc.org for genetic counselors in the United States and www. cagc-accg.ca for genetic counselors in canada.

Approaches to Genetic Testing

It is always best to test the person in the family who is most severely affected (such as the youngest age at disease diagnosis or most severe symptoms). This is extremely important before testing unaffected at-risk relatives (presymptomatic testing; Table 19.2). If a disease-causing mutation is not identified in the affected person, there is no reason to test the unaffected relative because a definitive genetic

Table 19.2 Factors considered in selecting a genetic test

<table>
<tr><th>Test</th><th>Description</th><th>Example</th><th>Embryo or blastocyst (preimplantation genetic diagnosis)</th><th>Fetus (prenatal testing)</th><th>Child</th><th>Adult</th></tr>
<tr><td>Newborn screening</td><td>Targeted tests for recessive genetic disorders</td><td>Phenylketonuria, cystic fibrosis, sickle-cell anemia</td><td>Not applicable</td><td>Not applicable</td><td>Tests provided at birth vary by country and state or region</td><td>Not applicable</td></tr>
<tr><td rowspan="2">Diagnostic testing</td><td rowspan="2">Confirmatory test or differential diagnosis testing for a symptomatic individual</td><td rowspan="2">Ataxias dystonias</td><td colspan="2">Specimen type and limited available amount for sampling may restrict platform selection (e.g., WES or WGS versus SNP or STR typing)</td><td colspan="2" rowspan="2">Where treatment is desired, turnaround time may restrict platform selection</td></tr>
<tr><td colspan="2">Turnaround time necessary may restrict platform selection</td></tr>
<tr><td>Carrier testing</td><td>Targeted testing for asymptomatic individuals potentially carrying one or more recessive mutations</td><td>Cystic fibrosis, thalassaemias, Tay–Sachs disease</td><td colspan="2">Applied typically for rare diseases but applicable for other familial mutations</td><td>Carrier testing of minors is considered in the context of individual pediatric cases</td><td>According to standard of care</td></tr>
<tr><td>Predictive testing</td><td>Tests for variants causing or associated with diseases or disorders with a hereditary component, usually with adult-onset symptoms</td><td>Dementia, cardiovascular disease, diabetes</td><td colspan="3">Some have discouraged genetic testing of asymptomatic minors for adult-onset conditions</td><td>According to standard of care</td></tr>
</table>

Presymptomatic testing	Tests for variants causing or associated with diseases or disorders known to be inherited in the family, often with adult-onset symptoms	Huntington's disease, frontotemporal, dementia	Some have discouraged genetic testing of asymptomatic minors for adult-onset conditions			According to standard of care
			Interpretation of VUSs will depend on presenting phenotypes in the family			
Pharmacogenetics	Targeted tests for variants associated with pharmaceutical dosage choice or adverse reactions	DNA tests for abacavir, warfarin, carbamazepine	Application not currently conducted but theoretically feasible	Application not currently conducted but conceivably applicable for screening treatment approaches in utero	Pharmacogenetic testing is considered in context of individual pediatric cases	According to standard of care

Reprinted by permission from Macmillan Publishers Ltd: Katsanis and Katsanis [9], copyright 2013
SNP single-nucleotide polymorphism, *STR* short tandem repeat, *WES* whole-exome sequencing, *WGS* whole-genome sequencing, *VUS* variant of unknown significance

diagnosis has not been made. If an affected person is not available to test in the family, testing can be initiated on the patient who is unaffected; the problem is the interpretation of a normal test result; is this test normal because the person has not inherited a disease-causing mutation that is in the family, or is the person still at risk for the movement disorder because it is some other inherited movement disorder and thus the puzzle of the disease diagnosis has not been solved? Take the example of patient A, who is healthy but has a parent, aunt, and grandparent with ataxia. This pattern suggests that patient A is at 50 % risk for ataxia. If the affected parent is tested and diagnosed with SCA3, then accurate and reliable testing is available for patient A and patient A's siblings and extended family. If patient A is tested without testing an affected relative (perhaps testing for the common ataxias such as types 1, 2, 3, and 6); if patient A has CAG trinucleotide repeats in *ATXN3* within the normal range, it is still possible that patient A is at risk for one of the other inherited ataxias (of which there are many) (e.g., [14] reported a case describing this scenario).

Methods of genetic testing for inherited movement disorders is changing rapidly as are the number of diseases that can be tested for. If a patient had a negative genetic screen for movement disorders a few years ago, it is often reasonable to retest with new panels for inherited movement disorders. It is also important to update the family history with new information as this information may provide clues to new genetic tests that should be considered.

Types of Genetic Test and Interpreting Genetic Test Reports

There is no single type of genetic test that can be applied diagnostically to all hereditary movement disorders; but numerous methodologies for genetic testing are available (see Table 19.3). There are many different types of pathogenic mutations which can include single nucleotides, deletions, duplications, and trinucleotide repeat expansions. Different methodologies are needed to identify certain types of gene mutations, and different testing methodologies may be needed to identify mutations within the same gene. The descriptions of the various types of mutations are reviewed in detail in the disease-specific chapters. It is important to note that even whole genome and whole exome sequencing does not identify all types of mutations in all diseases. Patients often expect that genetic testing will always provide a definitive answer; informed consent before a patient is genetically tested is essential to assure that the patient has reasonable expectations about what questions genetic testing can address and what gaps still remain after testing.

Many labs provide genetic testing (and the internet can help to locate a lab which offers the gene-required test, e.g., www.geneclinics.org), and currently there is no standard report format required. Some simple but important genetic facts and terminology can be useful in interpreting these often lengthy and complex reports. First, the word *mutation* is not always used to refer to genetic variation that is "abnormal." Mutation implies a change in the gene. The mutation then may be described as

Table 19.3 Clinical genetic testing methodologies

Method	Common point mutations	Rare point mutations	Copy number variants	Uniparental disomy[a]	Balanced invertions translocationn	Repeat expansions	Analytical sensitivity[b,c]	Analytical specificity[b,d]	Turnaround time[b,e]	Cost[f]	Examples
Linkage analysis (commonly STRs)	X		X[g]				Low	Low	Low	Low	Historical familial mutation
FISH			X		X		Low	Low	Low	Low	Angelman's syndrome
Array CGH or virtual karyotyping			X	X			Average	Average	Average	Average	A new referral or challenging diagnostic case
Genome-wide SNP microarrays	X		X				Low	Low	Low	Low	Cardiovascular disease risk assessment
Target PCR	X	X[g]				X	High	High	Low	Low	Cystic fibrosis carrier testing
Sanger gene sequencing	X	X					High	High	Average–high	Average	Treacher Collins syndrome diagnosis
Southern blot or MLPA			X			X	High	High	High	Low	Fragile X syndrome
Panel or pathway sequencing	X	X					Average	Low	Average	Average	Long QT syndrome

(continued)

Table 19.3 (continued)

Method	Common point mutations	Rare point mutations	Copy number variants	Uniparental disomy[a]	Balanced invertions translocationn	Repeat expansions	Analytical sensitivity[b,c]	Analytical specificity[b,d]	Turnaround time[b,e]	Cost[f]	Examples
WES or WGS	X	X	X[h]				Low	Low	High	High	A new referral or challenging case to diagnose

Reprinted by permission from Macmillan Publishers Ltd: Katsanis and Katsanis [9], copyright 2013

CGH comparative genomic hybridization, *FISH* fluorescent *in situ* hybridization, *MLPA* multiplex ligation-dependent probe amplification, *SNP* single-nucleotide polymorphism, *STR* short tandem repeat, *WES* whole-exome sequencing, *WGS* whole-genome sequencing

[a]Familial mutations or genomic rearrangements can be assayed

[b]Categorical assignments in these columns are subjective and vary according to context of the tests being ordered and the laboratory conducting the tests. The 'low', 'average' and 'high' are presented to simplify and to compare platforms generally

[c]Low, <80 %; average, 80–98 %; high, >98 %

[d]Low, <80 %; average, 80–98 %; high, >98 %

[e]Low, <1 week; average, 1 week–1 month; high, >1 month

[f]Costs of the testing will widely vary from one laboratory to the next; however, these estimates are based on the charge of the test from a sampling of laboratories, not on the costs of consumables or the reimbursed amount. Low, less than US$400; average, $400–$2,000; high, >$2,000

[g]Uniparental disomy can be detected by any method if both parents are genotyped. However, only the indicated approaches will detect uniparental disomy in absence of the parental genetic samples

[h]Copy number variant detections are improving in next-generation sequencing applications but are more efficient in WGS than WES, although they are of limited reliability for clinical diagnostics

pathogenic, deleterious, disease causing, or abnormal. These categories can also be described with less certainty (such as possibly pathogenic, possibly deleterious, etc.). The gene variation may also be described as a variation of uncertain significance (VUS or VOUS). Finally, the normal variation may be described as wild type.

In providing genetic evaluation, it is always essential to obtain a copy of the actual genetic testing report. This cannot be emphasized enough.

Conclusion

Genetic testing provides powerful diagnostic tools for individuals with movement disorders. The tools of molecular genetics should be used in conjunction with documentation of family history and findings of physical examination. Pre- and post-test genetic counseling is important for individuals undergoing genetic testing. The goal of genetic counseling is to facilitate patient decision-making to promote informed choices and adaptation to the condition. The implications of a genetic test result reach beyond the first person tested in the family. Genetic counselors and other clinical genetic specialists are specifically trained to serve as a resource to health professionals and their patients with regard to genetic diagnosis and management and to provide psychological support for individuals and their families who face the many issues surrounding a diagnosis of a hereditary movement disorder.

References

1. Bennett RL. The practical guide to the genetic family history. Hoboken: Wiley-Blackwell; 2010.
2. Bennett RL. Genetic counseling. In: Runge MS, Patterson C, editors. Principles of molecular medicine. 2nd ed. Totowa: Humana Press; 2006. p. 46–52.
3. Bennett RL, Motulsky AG, Bittles AH, et al. Genetic counseling and screening of consanguineous couples and their offspring: recommendations of the National Society of Genetic Counselors. J Genet Couns. 2002;11(2):97–119.
4. Bennett RL, Steinhaus French KA, Resta RG, Doyle DL. Standardized human pedigree nomenclature: update and assessment of the recommendations of the National Society of Genetic Counselors. J Genet Couns. 2008;17(5):424–33.
5. Crozier S, Robertson N, Dale M. The psychological impact of predictive genetic testing for Huntington's disease: a systematic review of the literature. J Genet Couns. 2015;24:c29–39.
6. Goldwrum S, Di Fonzo A, Simons EJ, Rohe CF, Zini M, Canesi M, et al. The G6055A (G2019S) mutation in LRRK2 is frequent in both early and late onset Parkinson's disease and originates from a common ancestor. J Med Genet. 2005;42(11):e65.
7. Hagberg A, Winberg E, Bui TH. More appreciation of life or regretting the test? Experiences of living as a mutation carrier of Huntington's disease. J Genet Couns. 2011;20:10–79.
8. Hamamy H, Antonarakis SE, Cavallie-Sforza LL, Temtamy S, Romeo G, Kate LP, Bennett RL, Shaw A, et al. Consanguineous marriages, pearls and perils: Geneva International Consanguinity Workshop Report. Genet Med. 2011;13:841–7.
9. Katsanis SH, Katsanis N. Molecular genetic testing and the future of clinical genomics. Nat Rev Genet. 2013;14(6):415–26.

10. Klein C, Schlossmacher MG. The genetics of Parkinson disease: implications for neurological care. Nat Clin Pract Neurol. 2006;2(3):136–46.
11. Lesage S, Durr A, Tazir M, Lohmann E, Leutenneger AL, Janin S, et al. *LRRK2* G2019S as a cause of Parkinson's disease in Northern African Arabs. N Engl J Med. 2006;354:422–3.
12. Ozelius LJ, Senthil G, Saunders-Pullman R, Ohmann E, Deligtisch A, Tagliati M, et al. *LRRK2* G2019S as a cause of Parkinson's disease in Ashkenazi Jews. N Engl J Med. 2006;354: 424–5.
13. Resta RG, Biesecker BB, Bennett RL, et al. A new definition of genetic counseling: National Society of Genetic Counselor's Task Force report. J Genet Couns. 2006;15(2):77–83.
14. Schneider SA, van de Warrenburg BP, Hughes TD, Davis M, Sweeney M, Wood N, Quinn NP, Bhatia KP. Phenotypic homogeneity of the Huntington disease-like presentation in a SCA17 family. Neurology. 2006;67:1701–3.

Chapter 20
Genetic Testing: An Industrial Perspective

Dirk Hadaschik, Yasmin Singh, and Saskia Biskup

Abstract Modern genetic testing relies on a wide spectrum of cytogenetic and molecular genetic methods. The decision as to which method and application achieves the best diagnostic result is made by the medical expert based on a suspected diagnosis. Diverse processing steps have to be passed till a clinical diagnosis is finally secured, especially for genetically heterogeneous diseases like neuromuscular disorders. The accomplished diagnostic pipeline may be carried out by multiple processing units or in one centralized facility offering the whole sample workflow. The challenges for such diagnostic units are diverse. On one side, they have to generate and maintain a validated, standardized workflow meeting the highest quality requirements. Additionally, the ability to adjust to the changing field of genetic testing methods, to process urgent samples (e.g., from pregnant women), or to deal with uncommon sample material still has to be guaranteed. Here, we describe how methods for genetic testing are applied for diagnostics, the creation of a standardized sample workflow for next-generation sequencing (NGS)-based diagnostic gene panels, and how a high degree of automation and quality may be achieved while flexibility is retained.

Keywords Genetic testing • Sample workflow • Centralized unit • Automation • Next-generation sequencing • Diagnostic gene panels

Introduction

The elucidation of the human genome and the implementation of next-generation sequencing (NGS) have revolutionized the field of modern molecular diagnostic testing [1]. Since then, the applications for genetic testing are rapidly diversifying, and the resolution of the underlying molecular biology methods is constantly being refined.

D. Hadaschik, PhD
Tumor Diagnostics, CeGaT GmbH, Tuebingen 72076, Germany

Y. Singh, PhD
Project management, CeGaT GmbH, Tuebingen 72076, Germany

S. Biskup, MD, PhD (✉)
Executive board, CeGaT GmbH, Tuebingen 72076, Germany
e-mail: saskia.biskup@cegat.de

S.A. Schneider, J.M.T. Brás (eds.), *Movement Disorder Genetics*,
DOI 10.1007/978-3-319-17223-1_20

As a consequence, it is today possible to quickly and reliably detect virtually all genetic alterations in single genes, panels of genes, or even the whole genome. These developments do not only provide immense chances for the genetic testing market but also lead to major challenges. Genetic counselors, for example, experience a great rise in demand but also require expert and up-to-date knowledge about the advantages and limitations of the wide spectrum of modern genetic testing methods in order to find the best and most economic testing strategy. For diagnostic labs, a major challenge is to keep the pace implementing the constantly improving methods which inherently become more and more complex. Utilizing NGS, for example, does not only require expensive and complex apparatus like sequencers and liquid handling robots for sample and library preparation but also computational expertise to establish the required bioinformatics pipeline and server infrastructure for analyzing and storing the vast amount of sequencing data. Whole genome sequencing easily reveals hundreds of thousands to millions of genetic alterations in each newly analyzed case compared to the human reference genome. This enormous number complicates the identification of those variants which are responsible for the observed phenotype. For small labs, it is therefore extremely challenging to meet all these requirements to establish such genetic tests. Furthermore, before offering these to the public market, they need to be thoroughly and laboriously validated for sensitivity, specificity, precision, and reproducibility to obtain approval by the local authorities like the FDA or CAP-CLIA in the USA. Ordering tests from centralized units offering the complete workflow from sample preparation to NGS data analysis including the identification of potentially disease-causing variants and which operate in a highly regulated and controlled environment provides a cost-effective and reliable way to address these needs in the future and to ensure the necessary data quality. Here, we provide an overview over the genetic testing methods and their applications. We also further discuss which advantages centralized units may offer to health care providers and patients.

Genetic Testing Today

Altogether, for 2012, the size of the genetic testing market in the USA was estimated to be around US$6 billion [2], and this is predicted to rapidly increase to US$15–25 billion till the year 2021 [3]. In summary, this includes tests identifying carriers of recessive or dominant mutations, tests applied for newborn screening, invasive and noninvasive prenatal aneuploidy, and pharmacogenomic tests. Genetic tests commonly detect one or more types of genetic alterations in human DNA like single or multiple nucleotide variants (SNVs, MNVs), copy number variations (CNVs) like insertions and deletions (Indels), aneuploidies, chromosomal translocations, and gene fusions. If such genetic variants or mutated genes have been associated with the susceptibility, inheritance, development, or progression of genetic diseases, their identification may provide information for disease predisposition, prevention, monitoring, or potential treatment options. Genetic testing may also be useful to confirm or rule out a diagnosis or to identify asymptomatic carriers potentially harboring recessive mutations. In the hands of an experienced genetic counselor, such genetic information may also be the basis to evaluate the risk of a couple to pass on disease alleles to their offspring. Also, NGS-based noninvasive prenatal testing (NIPT) of fetal aneuploidies like trisomies of chromosomes 13, 18, or 21 is gaining more and more importance as such tests are more sensitive than other traditionally applied noninvasive tests based on ultrasound and confer less risk to the fetus than invasive tests like amniocentesis or choriocentesis [4]. In newborns, genetic tests have a long history for the detection of diseases like phenylketonuria. Finally, so-called pharmacogenetics will have a huge impact in the future by providing genetic information indicating whether certain drugs will be effective or ineffective for the treatment of diseases like cancer [5]. Increasing knowledge in this field will form the basis for the development of personalized therapies.

Genetic Testing Methods and Their Applications

The menu of cytogenetic and molecular genetic methods for the detection of genetic alterations is growing, and their resolution is constantly refined. This chapter aims to provide an overview over the most used methods and their applications with a special focus on NGS technology and its utilization for genetic testing. However, it is not intended to go into every technical detail. Which stepwise diagnostic strategy or single test is chosen by the medical practitioner or genetic counselor depends on how detailed the available patient information is, the family history, and the time requirements, which may be critical if the health complications prove to be substantial and acute. This requires good knowledge about what kind of information each test may provide and which limitations it possesses. In general, genetic tests can be divided into methods detecting mainly larger structural variants (>100 nts) and tests identifying SNVs, MNVs, and shorter CNVs.

Methods Detecting Large Structural Variants

Structural variants (SVs) are duplications, deletions, inversions, and translocations of chromosomal fragments larger than 100 nts [6]. The 1,000 genome project has shown that such germline SVs are responsible for a greater share of sequence differences between two individuals than SNPs [7] and that they may have substantial effects on gene expression [8].

Giemsa Banding

Metaphase chromosomes are incubated with Giemsa dye in order to stain AT-rich heterochromatic regions and less so GC-rich actively transcribed regions of the chromosome. The characteristic chromosomal banding is used to quickly and cost-effectively identify Indels (5–10 Mb) or genomic rearrangements like translocations, inversions, or reciprocal translocations [9, 10].

Fluorescent In Situ Hybridization (FISH)

Fluorescent in situ hybridization (FISH) utilizes fluorescently labeled DNA probes (>50 kb–2 Mb) to immunostain complementary chromosomal regions for microscopic detection [9]. This low-cost cytogenetic method is able to detect large Indels and translocations and can be multiplexed (multiprobe FISH). It is relatively labor intensive, provides only a low resolution image, and requires an a priori hypothesis of which chromosomal location may be affected in a clinical phenotype.

Comparative Genomic Hybridization (CGH)

Comparative genomic hybridization (CGH) has traditionally been used to identify CNVs with a resolution of 5–10 Mb. The patient DNA and a reference DNA are labeled with two different fluorescent dyes and are subsequently hybridized together to a spread of normal metaphase chromosomes. By fluorescent microscopy, chromosomal regions can be identified in the patient DNA which show lower or higher copy numbers than the reference.

Array Comparative Genomic Hybridization (aCGH)

Array comparative genomic hybridization (aCGH) is based on the CGH principle but provides a higher resolution. Again, a reference DNA and the patient DNA under investigation are labeled with two different fluorescent dyes and are subsequently competitively hybridized to numerous different probes immobilized on a microarray. By analyzing the ratio of the overlayed fluorescent signals, conclusions can be derived about which regions of the patient genome show gain or loss of DNA copies. The resolution of aCGH analysis depends on the size of the probes and the space between them on a chromosome. Probe size may vary greatly between 1 Mb–10 kb (BACs) to 45–85 nts on high-resolution CGH arrays [9, 11]. Besides the detection of submicroscopic medium- to large-size CNVs, this technology allows the identification of chromosomal rearrangements and uniparental disomy but not of balanced inversions and translocations which show no change in copy number [12].

Methods Detecting SNVs, MNVs, and Shorter CNVs

SNP Arrays

SNP arrays were originally developed to perform genome-wide linkage analysis in order to identify SNP markers which are associated with certain traits but which are not necessarily the cause of the phenotype. Such arrays may additionally be used to identify homozygous regions and loss of heterozygosity due to deletions or uniparental disomy and may in general confirm larger deletions and duplications [9].

So-called SNP-CGH arrays combine the ability to detect SNPs, CNVs, and unbalanced chromosomal translocations. Exome arrays detecting all reported SNPs within the coding regions of patients and normal individuals may be used for detection of variants that may be relevant for disease status [12].

Multiplex Ligation-Dependent Probe Amplification (MLPA)

For this molecular method, two oligonucleotides are designed in such a way that they anneal to adjacent genomic regions. Due to their close proximity, they can subsequently be ligated to each other. Both ligated oligonucleotides contain different artificial primer binding sites to which the forward and reverse primers anneal during the following PCR amplification. Multiplexing in one tube is possible if several ligation products of different sizes are ligated and amplified using the same PCR primer pair. As one primer is fluorescently labeled, the MLPA products can subsequently be resolved and quantified by capillary electrophoresis. By relating the MLPA results of a patient sample to those of a normal reference sample prepared in parallel, this technology allows the detection of SNVs, smaller-sized CNVs (e.g., deleted or duplicated exons), and aneuploidies. Balanced rearrangements like inversions or translocations are not identified by this method.

Polymerase Chain Reaction (PCR)

Polymerase chain reaction (PCR) is used to confirm the presence of SNVs or small CNVs. For this purpose, PCR primer design requires that at least one primer ends exactly at the mutated site. The unpaired last nucleotide at the 3′ end of the primer inhibits effectively the extension by the polymerase. Often, standards or a reference DNA known to be not mutated at the respective site are amplified in parallel to allow the calculation of the variant allele frequency. If the variant is heterozygous, the amount of completed amplicons is decreased to roughly 50 % of the reference. If the site of interest is duplicated, the relative amount of PCR product is roughly 200 %. The resulting PCR products can either be quantified by gel electrophoresis (limited cycle PCR) or more reliably by real-time PCR. PCR is relatively fast and cheap and can be easily performed on many samples in parallel. Furthermore, real-time PCR has a wide dynamic range, and its high sensitivity is ideal for variant detection. However, utilizing PCR often requires prior knowledge about the exact site of the variant. In that respect, it is used to screen for hot spots that are often mutated in a specific phenotype or to confirm known variants.

Sanger Sequencing

This method is a highly sensitive and specific diagnostic tool if the phenotype provides a clear indication for the analysis of a small single gene, e.g., to detect variants responsible for monogenic diseases. Another application may be the confirmation of mutations which have been previously detected by NGS or which are known to be present in close relatives [12]. After the gene or exon of interest has been amplified by PCR, the chain termination reaction is performed in the presence of an excess of normal unlabeled desoxynucleotides and fluorescently labeled didesoxynucleotides. The latter are blocked at the 3′ end, and their random incorporation into the nascent strand ensures the synthesis of DNA strands of different lengths which after denaturation can be electrophoretically separated by size in polymer-filled capillaries of Sanger sequencers. The four differently fluorescently labeled didesoxynucleotides at the end of each DNA molecule are detected when passing the end of the capillary. In the resulting electropherogram traces, SNVs with an allele frequency between 5 and 15 % may still be detected [13, 14], but NGS (see next section) is clearly superior in the detection of mosaicism. Sanger sequencing is also used to identify short Indels. However, this procedure is often insensitive with regard to structural variant detection [12].

Next-Generation Sequencing (NGS)

The recent improvements of NGS technologies from Illumina (Solexa), Life Technologies (IonTorrent), and Roche (454) led to a rapid decline in sequencing costs per base. These platforms are nowadays able to sequence from 100,000 to 2 billion DNA fragments in parallel and deliver relatively short sequences of 100–1,000 nts. In total, this leads to a sequencing output of 70 Mb–500 Gb per run, which may be doubled if paired-end sequencing is employed.

The short reads generated by NGS allow for the sensitive detection of SNVs, MNVs, and small-sized Indels. Though the latter is more difficult, great progress has been made developing better algorithms for short Indel calling [6]. As the amount of reads per sample can be individually scaled, NGS has an extremely high dynamic range. With increasing number of reads produced per sample, the amount of reads representing each nucleotide in the patient DNA (coverage) is rising, leading to a higher confidence and sensitivity of variant detection. This is extremely important for genetic analysis of tumor samples which are often very heterogeneous due to contamination with surrounding healthy tissue or because the tumor itself is subdivided into several subclones harboring differing mutations. By increasing the overall mean coverage to 1,000-fold, heterozygous variants may still be reliably detected in samples with as low as 20 % tumor content [15] and allele frequencies down to 2 % (personal communication). The high sensitivity of NGS also helps identify cases of mosaicism. However, larger structural variants (>100 nts) like chromosome translocations, inversions, and large Indels are intrinsically hard to detect with short NGS reads, and detection is nearly impossible adjacent to repeat regions which are often causal for chromosomal rearrangements [6]. Mate pair sequencing with short paired-end reads may be helpful to detect some structural variants within a range of 5–10 kb. Besides, third-generation sequencers allowing longer read lengths like those of Pacific Bioscience or nanopore-based single-molecule sequencers of Oxford Nanopores may prove to be more informative concerning identification of genomic structural variants or repetitive regions. Those may also provide haplotype information about variants in relatively close proximity on the same chromosome.

NGS Applications

By multiplexing several patient samples within one sequencing run, the sample throughput may be increased, and the costs per sample are lowered, which is desirable in a diagnostic setting. To further increase cost-efficiency, sequencing can be exclusively focused on a group of genes which are known to be involved in the development or progression of the observed disease or phenotype. For this purpose, the respective regions of the DNA are enriched by hybridization to oligonucleotide probes (which are either supplied in solution or immobilized onto microarrays) or by multiplex PCR prior to sequencing.

Whole Genome Sequencing

Whole genome sequencing provides the most complete picture of all variants present in the investigated genome. This is beneficial in case that only limited patient information is available for genetic diagnosis, for example, to identify the causes of rare or orphan diseases. Also, if other genetic tests fail to provide clues for the cause of a clinical phenotype, whole genome sequencing may help to elucidate the underlying mechanism. However, the many hundreds of thousands to millions of variants which are easily obtained using this approach are still hard to be interpreted. The pure sequencing costs are a few thousand Euros per genome; a genome suitable for diagnostic purposes costs Euros 4,000 upward. In addition to the sequencing costs, the analysis and medical interpretation of the data may cost another 4,000 or even 5,000 Euros. Taking also into account the expense and effort necessary to handle and store such large data sets makes exome sequencing often the more economical way to diagnose such patients.

Exome Sequencing

Exome sequencing focuses only on the protein coding regions accounting for approximately 1 % of the human genome. Compared to variants in noncoding regions, mutations in exons are often more revealing as effects on protein function or integrity are either known or may be predicted from the altered amino acid sequence and their functional consequences are often more obvious. The pure sequencing costs range from 500 to 3,500 Euros per exome; an exome suitable for diagnostic purposes costs Euro 1,500 upward. In addition to the sequencing costs, the analysis and medical interpretation of the data may cost another low four-digit

Euro amount. A full trio exome analysis, which includes examination of the index patient and both parents, can be conducted for approximately 6,000 Euros.

Diagnostic Panels

Diagnostic panels enable to sequence and analyze exclusively genes that are associated with a certain disease. This approach is particularly applied to genetically heterogeneous diseases. Compared to classical single-gene testing methods like Sanger sequencing, the probability of identifying the causative genetic variant is strongly enhanced. In comparison to whole genome or exome sequencing, the use of diagnostic gene panels allows increasing the coverage while reducing the overall amount of sequencing reads due to the smaller target region. This strongly enhances the diagnostic reliability of the results gained by panel sequencing. Therefore, exome analysis should only be conducted when no panel is available or for diseases with complex and diverse symptoms. Furthermore, the speed for sequencing and subsequent data analysis for variant detection is drastically faster for diagnostic panels resulting in an overall reduction in time. However, it is required that the list of candidate genes included in a diagnostic panel is updated on a regular basis according to the current literature. The costs for panel diagnostics are slightly below that of exome analyses.

Sample Workflow in Centralized Units (Panel Diagnostics for Neuromuscular Diseases at CeGaT)

The cause of neuromuscular diseases (NMDs) is most often genetic. Hundreds of disease-related genes harboring different types of mutations have been identified so far [16]. In order to deal with this great genetic complexity and to enhance the chances to detect the pathogenic mutation, a standardized sample workflow for panel diagnostics has been applied to patients with NMD. The developed NMD panel comprises in total 187 genes which are assigned to different subpanels depending on the clinical phenotype (such as spinal muscular atrophy, Charcot-Marie-Tooth and sensory neuropathies, myopathies, muscular dystrophies, myasthenic syndromes, and myotonias). In terms of a stepwise diagnostic procedure, the most common mutations are excluded by single gene testing prior to panel diagnostics. The conducted procedures include all steps from sample preparation to writing of the medical report (see Fig. 20.1).

In Step 1, received patient samples are being prepared for sequencing. Depending on the type of disease, this includes handling of different types of samples, usually blood but also fresh frozen tissue, formalin-fixed paraffin-embedded (FFPE) tissue, plasma, sputum, and others. After gDNA isolation and quality control, a shot-gun DNA library is prepared. For this purpose, gDNA is randomly sheared, and sequencing platform specific adapters are ligated to both ends of each DNA fragment. All DNA regions of interest are subsequently enriched after hybridization to a custom-made pool of

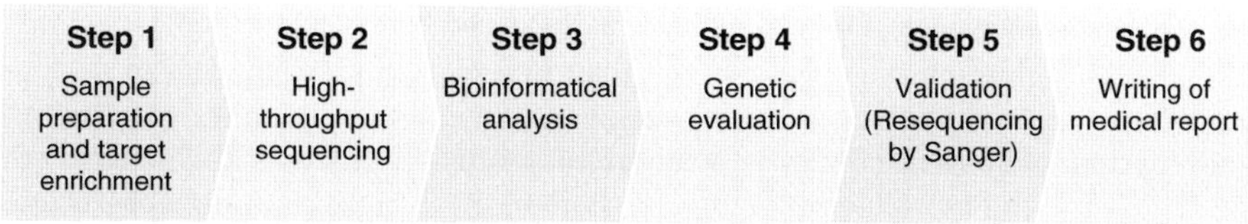

Fig. 20.1 Sample workflow for NGS-based diagnostic panels at CeGaT

probes ensuring that only disease-related genes are analyzed. For each library, individual barcodes are introduced into the adapters by PCR allowing to pool several samples from different patients in one NGS run (Step 2). The sequencing data are further processed using an established bioinformatics pipeline (Step 3). Here, the sequencing reads are assigned to the corresponding patient samples using their respective barcode (demultiplexing), adapters are clipped, reads are mapped to the reference genome, and variants are called and annotated. The detected genetic variants (SNVs, small Indels, and CNVs) are further evaluated by experts of the respective medical area (e.g., neuromuscular diseases) regarding their potential pathogenicity (Step 4). To validate the sequencing data, the identified potentially disease-causing variants are resequenced by Sanger (Step 5). The results are finally summarized in a medical report and directly sent to the clinician (Step 6).

Diagnostic results from 330 patients analyzed using the NMD panel were statistically evaluated. In 28 % of the cases, the genetic cause of the disease could be clearly identified by panel diagnostics, and in additional 20 % likely pathogenic variants were detected. Pathogenic mutations were found in 34 different genes, unclear variants in further 27 genes emphasizing the enormous genetic heterogeneity among NMD patients. Therefore, applying NGS-based diagnostic gene panels to NMD patients is strongly recommended. The same holds true for many other neurological diseases like ataxias, epilepsies, dementia, neurodegenerative diseases, movement disorders, neurometabolic diseases, and mitochondrial diseases as prominent examples.

Advantages of Centralized Units

Genetic testing comprises a multistep process that starts with a certain request and may end with a sequencing result or a clinical diagnosis. Providing all steps in one centralized facility is certainly both challenging and advantageous. In order to fulfill the high quality standards, each process has to be defined, validated, and regularly optimized. The possibility to perform all processing steps under one roof allows to thoroughly control each step and thereby to enhance the quality of the sample workflow. Thus, for example, exact barcoding of samples before sequencing ensures that sequencing results are assigned to the corresponding sample.

Modern molecular genetic testing methods like NGS require expensive and complex lab machines like robots and sequencers. Only if sufficient samples are available, these can be utilized to their full capacity, which is important for cost-efficient processing. Of note, using smaller-sized bench-top sequencers which allow to multiplex less samples per run than high-capacity sequencers leads to a large increase in sequencing costs per sample.

Preparing samples for NGS is a laborious multistep process. To increase the speed, quality, and reproducibility, it is recommended to highly automate the whole workflow on liquid handling robots. Besides, the implementation of a laboratory information management system (LIMS) recording all protocols used and their intermediate results is vital to track and quality control all samples while they pass through the different steps. A LIMS also allows to retrospectively identify deviations from the standard protocol if the final results are not satisfactory and thereby facilitates elimination of such mistakes.

Higher utilization of robots and high-capacity sequencers reduces the costs for offered services and subsequently leads to substantial cost savings for the health care providers, the health care system, and the patient. Furthermore, medical doctors and patients have a central access point for all upcoming questions regarding offered services, processing times, sending of samples, available methods, or interpretation of genetic results. The spatial proximity and the close teamwork of different departments also allow a high degree of flexibility to changing needs. This may include the demand for additional analysis, receiving of urgent patient samples, or adjustments of methods and equipment when required by technological progress. Those challenges might be harder to meet for small diagnostic labs.

A more time-efficient pipeline also delivers earlier diagnostic results for clinicians to secure or exclude a suspected diagnosis. Thereby, patients may benefit directly from earlier information about their disease, its prognosis, and the possibilities regarding targeted therapy. Many diseases are genetically and phenotypically heterogeneous and their diagnosis complex and difficult. These disorders are a challenge for small genetic laboratories. In order to secure a clinical diagnosis, a broad range of methods is required to be able to detect different types of mutations. For example, deletions and duplications in certain NMD-related genes are excluded prior to panel diagnostics. At the moment, the detection of CNVs by NGS is bioinformatically challenging, and therefore centralized units should offer additional methods for this purpose like MLPA or qPCR analysis while working at the same time on improved algorithms to detect CNVs from NGS data. The application of different approaches and the interpretation of the detected genetic variants also require qualified and experienced staff. On that account, the creation of an in-house database that collects information about detected variants and clinical phenotypes facilitates the genetic evaluation. It helps to discriminate between patient-specific variants and those with a high frequency in the normal population, which are most likely not causal for the investigated phenotype.

Conclusion

Small laboratories that offer genetic testing are faced with great challenges: on the one hand, they have to be able to offer a broad spectrum of methods, expensive equipment, and skilled staff not only for operating technical devices but also with knowledge and experience in bioinformatics analyses and interpretation of genetic data. On the other hand, flexibility is required for changing needs, e.g., to handle the continuous technical progress in this field and to deal with upcoming individual requests. At the same time, genetic testing also demands a high level of quality to ensure reliable diagnostic results. Standardized sample workflows enable fast and efficient processing, which is reflected in reduced costs for offered services. At the moment, whole genome sequencing is rather a research approach in diagnostics but a promising method in the future, and only centralized laboratories are able to sequence whole genomes for a reasonable amount of money. But the costs are still too high to use it in a routine diagnostic setting and the diagnostic reliability cannot be insured if the coverage per relevant base is not high enough. Ideally, there will be one single method to detect all types of relevant mutations within the human genome. NGS seems to be the obvious technology having the capacity to identify all types of genetic alterations in the near futute. As there is continuous progress in this field, it will ultimately replace currently available technologies including microarrays to detect copy number variations and other methods used for genetic testing (i.e., methods to detect repeats and epigenetic signatures). There will also be a need for the industry to adjust to this changing situation. Utilizing NGS for the analysis of diagnostic gene panels on the other hand provides for now a quick and cost-effective way to find the cause of genetically heterogeneous phenotypes like those found in neuromuscular diseases. As genetic counseling is at the beginning of each diagnostic procedure, it is the essential step to decide which diagnostic test is applied for the patient. In contrary to other countries, genetic counseling in Germany is not only mandatory prior to diagnostic testing but also has to be carried out by a clinician with further education in human genetics. This procedure is governed by the German Act of Gene Diagnostics or so-called Gendiagnostikgesetz. When considering that the genetic counselor is responsible for informing the patient about the applied diagnostic method, this is a reasonable settlement. Furthermore, the constant scientific development and the growing amount of generated data makes the proper interpretation of diagnostic reports more and more challenging. Yet, this issue has already been known before the application of genome-wide arrays and the introduction of NGS. Taken together, to ensure best possible patient care and to save costs for following diagnostics, counseling should be conducted in local medical practices by experienced and trained personnel, and the diagnostic genetic testing should then be passed to experienced centralized units.

Taken together, centralized facilities have the capacity to cope with all tasks that are necessary for high-quality genetic testing and thereby ensure the overall advantages for the health care system, clinicians, and patients.

References

1. Koboldt DC, Steinberg KM, Larson DE, Wilson RK, Mardis ER. The next-generation sequencing revolution and its impact on genomics. Cell. 2013;155:27–38.

2. Practice BTP. The Economic and Functional Impacts of Genetic and Genomic Clinical Laboratory Testing in the United States. 2012.
3. United Health, Center for Health Reform & Modernization. Personalized medicine: trends and prospects for the new science of genetic testing and molecular diagnostics; 2012. http://www.unitedhealthgroup.com/~/media/UHG/PDF/2012/UNH-Working-Paper-7.ashx
4. Norwitz ER, Levy B. Noninvasive prenatal testing: the future is now. Rev Obstet Gynecol. 2013;6(2):48–62.
5. Carr DF, Alfirevic A, Pirmohamed M. Pharmacogenomics: current state-of-the-art. Genes (Basel). 2014;5(2):430–43.
6. Raphael BJ. Chapter 6: structural variation and medical genomics. PLoS Comput Biol. 2012;8(12):e1002821.
7. Redon R, Ishikawa S, Fitch K, Feuk L, Perry G, et al. Global variation in copy number in the human genome. Nature. 2006;444:444–54.
8. Stranger BE, Forrest MS, Dunning M, Ingle CE, Beazley C, et al. Relative impact of nucleotide and copy number variation on gene expression phenotypes. Science. 2007;315:848–53.
9. Gijsbers AC, Ruivenkamp CA. Molecular karyotyping: from microscope to SNP arrays. Horm Res Paediatr. 2011;76(3):208–13.
10. Breman AM, Bi WM, Cheung SW. Prenatal diagnosis by array-based comparative genomic hybridization in the clinical laboratory setting. Beijing Da Xue Xue Bao. 2009;41(4):500–4.
11. Pearson PL. Historical development of analysing large-scale changes in the human genome. Cytogenet Genome Res. 2006;115(3–4):198–204.
12. Katsanis SH, Katsanis N. Molecular genetic testing and the future of clinical genomics. Nat Rev Genet. 2013;14:415–26.
13. Davidson CJ, Zeringer E, Champion KJ, Gauthier MP, Wang F, Boonyaratanakornkit J, Jones JR, Schreiber E. Improving the limit of detection for Sanger sequencing: a comparison of methodologies for KRAS variant detection. Biotechniques. 2012;53(3):182–8.
14. Tsiatis AC, Norris-Kirby A, Rich RG, Hafez MJ, Gocke CD, Eshleman JR, Murphy KM. Comparison of Sanger sequencing, pyrosequencing, and melting curve analysis for the detection of KRAS mutations: diagnostic and clinical implications. J Mol Diagn. 2010;12(4):425–32.
15. Gerstung M, Papaemmanuil E, Campbell PJ. Subclonal variant calling with multiple samples and prior knowledge. Bioinformatics. 2014;30(9):1198–204.
16. Laing NG. Genetics of neuromuscular disorders. Crit Rev Clin Lab Sci. 2012;49:33–48.

Chapter 21
Direct-to-Consumer DNA Genetic and Genomic Testing

Ronald J. Trent

Abstract Direct-to-consumer (DTC) DNA genetic and genomic testing refers to the provision of DNA testing services by a laboratory directly to the public. The DTC industry emerged in the early 2000s and offered a range of DNA testing options for medical and other applications. The DTC approach is possible because DNA can be transported by mail, and the expanding role of the Internet in everyday life allows products to be advertised widely. The media and some in the scientific community helped the industry by highlighting new discoveries in genetic knowledge which were research-in-progress although packaged as having immediate benefits to health and well-being. The DTC industry has undergone a number of changes and is at a defining moment as regulators and the courts are asking questions about the product for sale. The model of care exemplified by the DTC approach is attractive and likely to grow although the role of a medical practitioner in DTC DNA testing remains uncertain.

Keywords Direct-to-consumer • Genetics • Genomics • DNA test • Information • Ethical, legal and social implications • ELSI

Abbreviations

DTC	Direct-to-consumer
ELSI	Ethical legal social issues
HD	Huntington's disease
FDA	Food and Drug Administration
T2D	Type 2 diabetes
VUS	Variant of unknown significance
WGS	Whole genome sequencing

R.J. Trent, PhD, MBBS, DPhil, FRACP, FRCPA
Department of Medical Genomics and Sydney Medical School, University of Sydney, Royal Prince Alfred Hospital B65L6, Camperdown, NSW 2050, Australia
e-mail: ronald.trent@sydney.edu.au

S.A. Schneider, J.M.T. Brás (eds.), *Movement Disorder Genetics*,
DOI 10.1007/978-3-319-17223-1_21

Introduction

During the early 2000s, a handful of laboratories started to sell DNA genetic tests directly to the public. In the case of DNA genetic testing for *medical* purposes, there was no requirement for a medical practitioner to order the test or receive its report. The Internet was crucial in delivering this service as it allowed the customer to access DTC advertising. The customer would then decide what DNA genetic test to purchase. As the industry evolved, the customer would be offered a panel of tests for a range of health issues from predisposition to cancer to less serious conditions such as the restless leg syndrome. Since third parties including medical practitioners were excluded, it was claimed the DTC route would provide greater security particularly for privacy. DTC DNA genetic testing was feasible because specimens containing DNA could be easily transported by mail.

The mechanics of DTC medical DNA genetic testing are relatively simple. A customer decides what test to order or more likely a battery of tests advertised over the Internet. Forms are filled including consent, and a payment is made. A kit arrives in the mail or by courier and will allow DNA to be collected from saliva or a buccal scraping. The collection kit with customer DNA is returned to the company. The customer receives a copy of the results or can access them from the Internet. In some cases, the DTC genetic testing laboratory provides links to genetic counseling services which can also be purchased DTC.

Justification

Some reasons given to justify the use of DTC *medical* DNA genetic testing included (1) Empowering individuals to access genetic information to improve health and well-being and (2) Facilitating rapid diagnosis of disorders when healthcare resources are in short supply [1].

There were also counterarguments put forward raising serious concerns about DTC *medical* DNA testing service (Table 21.1). The ongoing debates led to a number of recommendations being formulated (Table 1 in [2]) while in Germany some types of DTC *medical* DNA genetic testing were banned [3].

DTC companies introduced innovative advertising strategies. For example, they made effective use of social media to facilitate connections with "genetically" similar friends. One company hosted a celebrity "spit" party to highlight this new type of testing. In 2008, *Time* magazine announced that the DTC DNA genetic test was the invention of the year [2]. Public interest in knowing about genetic discoveries and the potential for estimating health risk was considered significant, for example, ~75 % in one survey said they would be prepared to pay for this type of testing [2]. Apart from the media hype touting new genetic discoveries, there were optimistic estimates of the potential size of the DTC DNA testing market with one in 2007 predicting it would generate >$730 million annually with a 20 % growth rate.

Table 21.1 Concerns about DTC medical DNA genetic testing [1, 2]

Providing the individual with greater *autonomy* is a worthwhile goal although it is relevant to all aspects of clinical medicine, not only genetics. To say that genetics is *different* because genes somehow represent a more personal part of the individual is misleading as geneticists have tried to avoid this view with its implications for genetic determinism and stigmatization. There is little doubt that genetics, particularly in relationship to DNA and genetics, is complex, but whether it is different is arguable.
Making a *decision* on what tests are clinically useful is not easy with genetic DNA tests. Even more of an issue would be how to *interpret the results,* some of which will require considerable expertise which is unlikely to be possible without access to expert opinion including genetic counseling.
DTC DNA testing is a *commercial venture,* and so members of the community may be disadvantaged by not having access to these tests because of costs, availability of the Internet, or understanding what is for sale.
Evidence that results provided would lead to useful clinical interventions or decision-making is uncertain.
Protection for the individual, particularly in relation to privacy, may be compromised with DTC DNA testing conducted in overseas laboratories.
The *consequences* of DTC DNA testing on the individual (and family members) remain unknown including the potential for false-positive and false-negative results. The effects on the healthcare system should be considered.
DTC *advertising* can be misleading if the product sold appeared to have direct relevance to health and well-being, yet the accompanying disclaimer focused on the product as information which should not be used for medical decision-making.

Subsequent predictions were more realistic although commercially viable such as the market in 2010 was worth ~$10–$20 million annually [2].

Medical Research

The DTC industry took advantage of the public's interest in medical research to link DTC testing services with opportunities to allow the same DNA sample to be added to a DNA research bank. Justification was given as a way to obtain the large cohorts required for genetic research studies. Nevertheless, even with consent, there remained concerns such as (1) How did oversight or community expectations for medical research compare between different jurisdictions as samples to DTC laboratories came from multiple sources including offshore ones? This was particularly important for privacy. (2) What happened if the DTC DNA testing laboratory was sold or went into receivership? This became reality when the Icelandic company deCODE got into financial difficulties in 2009 and filed for bankruptcy. Apart from providing a DTC DNA testing service, deCODE had a very valuable commercial asset in its DNA biobank of 140,000 specimens linked to medical records [4]. At the time, there was concern that the DNA and medical information resource might be sold to pay creditors. Eventually, deCODE was sold, its DTC service discontinued, and the DNA biobank preserved for ongoing research.

Sales Product

DTC DNA testing services provided a range of services for (1) medical (health-related) disorders, (2) recreational purposes, (3) identification of human traits, and (4) forensic or legal testing. The *medical* testing services have been the subject of much debate and are the topic of this chapter. The other products particularly those for recreational purposes including family tracing (genealogy) and DNA testing to select better diets (nutrigenetics) or skin products (dermatogenetics) are much less controversial as *caveat emptor* applies like other commercial transactions. Debate continues on the ethical and societal implications of DNA genetic testing for human traits such as the prediction of athletic performance particularly in children, or identifying fetal sex during pregnancy for family balancing [2].

A key question with DTC DNA genetic testing is what actually is being sold? When viewing the companies' Internet sites, the "average" reader might assume that medical-type DNA genetic tests are being advertised and so provide a result that could be used in personalized healthcare. Based on the result, some interventions would be possible leading to better health and well-being. Alternatively, when reading the various product disclaimers on the same Internet sites, the product for sale is described as "information" provided for this purpose alone.

Legally, there is some leeway in terms of what can be claimed in advertising. For example, saying that "product X is the best available" may not be entirely true, but in contemporary marketing, it might be reasonable to expect the "average" person will take this with a degree of cynicism and buy or not buy the product with this in mind. At worse, the person will lose money. On the other hand, the same flexibility may be problematic with health issues where the consequences for error are more significant.

Oversight

Some regulatory bodies struggled when it came to dealing with the somewhat vague concept of "information" because their governing Acts referred to more tangible products such as medical devices, drugs, and so on. Nevertheless, the claim that only "information" was being sold was criticized on ethical grounds if information was not guaranteed to have scientific relevance and/or even of being correct, unless these facts were clearly known at the time of purchase or consent.

It is important to distinguish DTC DNA genetic testing provided *locally,* i.e., by laboratories within the same regulatory or legal jurisdiction as the customer. In these circumstances the customer has a better understanding of and access to the relevant consumer protection laws including those relating to privacy. Should something go wrong, the customer can seek legal redress. In contrast, DTC offered in different jurisdictions particularly *offshore* laboratories places the customer at a significant disadvantage when things go wrong. Some might say the customer has little if any legal protection unless he or she understands the legal environment that the

DTC testing company operates in and/or can afford to take legal action in that jurisdiction. Most DTC DNA testing providers are located within the USA [5].

Measuring the Clinical Value of a DNA Genetic Test

For a medical DNA genetic test (and any type of clinical investigational test), a number of criteria should be assessed before the test becomes a component of clinical care. The evaluative process can be demanding and time consuming but necessary to provide the evidence for decision-making. The same rigor is not required for DNA tests discovered as part of research activities as these tests are subject to ongoing scrutiny such as peer review. With accumulation of sufficient data, their clinical value would become apparent, at which time they could be discarded or moved into the more regulated clinical service. Various parameters listed below are used to assess the clinical value of laboratory tests. For genetic tests, there is also consideration of the ethical, legal, and social implications (ELSI).

Clinical Utility

An acceptable medical test should have clinical utility, i.e., the test should provide information from which health-related decisions/interventions can be made, and health-related risks should not occur as a consequence of the testing [6, 7]. Measuring clinical utility in mainstream medical practice is not always easy.

Some DTC product disclosure brochures are ambiguous when it comes to clinical utility. For example, one company's Terms and Conditions for genetic *predisposition* testing states, *(i) All materials and products ....are provided for informational and educational purposes only. (ii) I agree not to hold ......liable for any damages caused as a result of the use of the information or products contained herein, and (iii) The purpose of the molecular genetic test is to ascertain if I, my child or an individual for ....are carrying mutation(s) predisposing to or causing the specific diseases or conditions covered in the ordered test* [8].

In the above disclaimer, the consumer has conflicting information. First, the product is described as *genetic predisposition testing*. To a geneticist, this terminology means the DNA genetic test will provide information in the form of a risk estimate that in the future, a particular disease or trait will develop (or it will not develop) based on changes detected in a gene. So the product for sale seems to be a DNA genetic test providing information for medical decision-making as is further implied in part (iii) of the company's disclaimer.

However, the disclaimer also states that the DNA genetic test is for *informational and educational purposes only*, which implies the product should not be used for medical decision-making. This ambiguity could be resolved with "truth in advertising" although, like the laboratory test, it would be difficult to regulate when it was provided through the Internet particularly offshore locations.

5' - **atg**aaggccttcgagtccctcaagtccttcCAGCAGCAGCAGCAG

CAGCAGCAGCAGCAGCAGCAGCAGCAGCAGCAG

caacagccgccaCCGCCGCCGCCGCCGCCGcctcctcagcttcctcagccg

ccgccg - 3'

≥ 40	• Will develop Huntington disease
≤ 26	• Normal - no progression to Huntington disease
27–39	• Might develop Huntington disease at an older age • Offspring might be at risk if repeats increase in size

Fig. 21.1 Huntington's disease (HD) DNA genetic testing. Although testing for a rare genetic disorder, the HD test is technically straightforward as it measures CAG repeat numbers located at the 5′ end of *HHT*. The start of the gene is depicted as an atg which is followed by a variable number of CAG repeats (capitalized). The interpretation of the result is unequivocal for normal or abnormal while results in the so-called intermediate range 27–39 require more care in understanding clinical significance for the person being tested and family members. This DNA test illustrates two different purposes for the same test. The *diagnostic* test is used to confirm that an individual presenting with a neurological disorder such as dementia or a movement disorder like chorea has HD. ELSI for this test is less of an issue as the patient has an existing medical problem and the test is simply confirming a clinical suspicion. In contrast, the same DNA test can be used to assess risk in family members and so becomes a *predictive* DNA test. ELSI is more significant because *asymptomatic* individuals are now tested. Whether the result comes back positive or negative has widespread implications for all, including risks to offspring and the possibility of not being able to access life (and in some jurisdictions health) insurance

Clinical Validity

This measure describes the accuracy with which a test identifies a particular clinical condition [6]. For a number of DNA genetic tests for Mendelian-type genetic disorders such as Huntington's disease (HD), the result is very accurate at detecting those with this disorder (sensitivity) or excluding those without the disorder (specificity). The DNA test itself measures the number of CAG repeats associated with the *HTT* gene. Those with ≥40 repeats have or will get this autosomal dominant disorder because the penetrance is 100 %. There is now sufficient clinical experience to allow reasonable interpretations to be made for different CAG repeat numbers (Fig. 21.1). Setting aside important considerations like the pre- and post-test genetic counseling requirements and ELSI associated with the HD predictive test, the clinical validity for this test is high even if offered DTC. In contrast, the clinical validity for more complex genetic disorders will be poor as illustrated below under Genetics to Genomics.

Analytic Validity

This describes the technical ability of the DNA testing laboratory to carry out the test accurately. As shown in one study, analytic validity was not an issue in DTC DNA testing [9]. This can be attributed to the sophisticated analytic platforms now available for testing, many of which are automated. It is likely most laboratories that have undergone appropriate accreditation will be able to carry out DNA genetic testing satisfactorily. Therefore, the customer, when selecting a DTC DNA testing service, should know something of the accreditation standards, and this is more likely to be possible if the test is ordered from a local laboratory rather than an offshore one. The DTC company example quoted earlier is accredited to the international standard ISO 17025 [8]. However, in some jurisdictions such as Australia, this standard is not acceptable for *medical* DNA testing, and a higher one ISO 15189 is required [10].

Analytic validity is directed to the laboratory component of the test. However, there is an equally important second component to any DNA genetic test, and that is the *result* and what it means in the context of that individual's health. As shown in the same publication which confirmed satisfactory performance for analytic validity in two USA-based DTC DNA testing companies, the *interpretation* of some laboratory results by these companies was poor since they reported different risks - both high and low for the same genetic disorder in the same customer [9]!

Ethical, Legal, and Social Implications (ELSI)

Another measure for the value of a DNA genetic test is its ELSI. Although more difficult to evaluate, ELSI should be considered particularly for DNA tests associated with significant risk [7]. For DTC DNA genetic testing, the following ELSI are relevant [2, 5, 7]: (1) Marketing, especially truth in advertising and consumer trust, (2) Psychosocial impact on the customer (and potentially family members), (3) Implications for the healthcare system, and (4) Privacy.

One complexity when considering the ELSI component of a DNA genetic test is the understanding that the *same test* can be used for *different purposes*. Therefore, potential advantages, disadvantages, and risks need to be considered for each test *and* the purpose of that test. Table 3.7 in reference [7] provides a classification of DNA genetic tests based on purpose. Further information may also be found in Chap. 10 in this book. Examples of three different tests follow to highlight considerations around ELSI.

First is the DNA *diagnostic* test, which would be relatively low risk from the ELSI perspective. In this scenario, the medical practitioner is dealing with a patient who has certain signs and/or symptoms consistent with an established clinical problem. The diagnostic DNA test forms part of the medical workup to identify the clinical problem. Even if the wrong DNA test is selected or the result of the DNA test is incorrect, it is likely the medical practitioner will, in the course of time, repeat the test or query its result because it will be inconsistent with the clinical phenotype. This type of follow-up is not likely in the DTC approach.

The second example is the *predictive* DNA test, which lies at the other end of the risk spectrum because it is looking into the future and assessing risk. The accuracy of this prediction may not be straightforward as it can be influenced by other genetic and/or environmental factors involved in pathogenesis. As well as accuracy, there is always the possibility of error with any laboratory test, and this should be discussed in the pretest counseling. Errors with predictive DNA tests (ordered by the medical practitioner or DTC) are particularly problematic because the patient is asymptomatic and so errors may not become apparent for years, by which time the patient and relatives will have made important life decisions based on incorrect DNA test information.

A third type of test offered DTC is based on *research* findings that may or may not have been confirmed. Internationally, there is strong interest in expediting the translation of medical research into clinical practice. While praiseworthy, this goal is problematic if research discoveries are used for clinical decision-making before sufficient evidence accumulates. The overlapping of research into clinical care is evident in the DTC industry which frequently promises the latest findings. One DTC DNA testing company advertised its medical testing products as (1) Established research reports (earlier described by the company as *Clinical reports*) and (2) preliminary research reports [7].

Genetics to Genomics

The evaluation of DNA *genetic* tests is demanding even when single or few genes are involved. Not surprisingly, the evaluation of *genomic* tests to assess many or all human genes is particularly problematic. With few exceptions, traditional DNA genetic testing services do not offer DNA *genomic* tests for clinical decision-making in the complex genetic disorders since there is some way to go before they can be shown to have clinical utility and validity, i.e., these tests still represent research in progress. Nevertheless, DTC companies are offering genomic tests as shown by a complex disorder such as type 2 diabetes (T2D) suspected to have many disease-causing genes as well as environmental contributors [7].

One of the first high-profile genomics-based tests was publicly announced in 2007, when James Watson of Watson and Crick fame allowed his whole genome sequence (WGS) (minus a few genes with neuropsychiatric relevance) to be published for all to see. Subsequently, the cost for a WGS dropped dramatically from the estimated $1 million for Watson's WGS to a few thousand dollars today. The era of looking for multiple changes in many or all human genes had started. The DTC DNA genetic testing industry was quick to move in this direction, promising, for a relatively small amount of money, that a comprehensive profile for various genetic risk factors could be provided.

DTC genomic testing is usually carried out with a large panel of DNA polymorphisms called SNPs (single-nucleotide polymorphisms). For this analysis, it is necessary to have population-based data, e.g., the SNP profile for thousands of individuals with T2D versus the SNP profile for a similar number without T2D. The SNP profile for the individual who has purchased the DTC test is then compared with the population data, and from this, a relative or absolute risk is calculated. Reference [9] shows how these calculations are made.

There are a number of problems using SNP markers for DTC DNA testing in a complex genetic disorder like T2D: (1) The DNA test does not take into consideration environmental factors associated with this disorder, (2) An assumption is made that population-based data from research studies can be directly compared with an individual's profile to generate a personal risk, (3) Important variables might not have been adequately controlled in the original research study including how a phenotype was defined and/or the possibility of population stratification based on ethnicity [7].

Finally, customers and health professionals (medical practitioners and genetic counselors) may not be familiar with the way risk is calculated. For example, a change in risk from the population-based 1 % to a customer's 1.6 % might look impressive since it represents a 60 % increase. But to the individual, this risk can be meaningless. One study showed only around 7 % health professionals who had specialized in genetics were comfortable with the interpretation of DTC DNA genetic testing [11].

Models of Care with DNA Genetic Testing

Traditional Approach

The medical DNA genetic test has been available since the mid-1970s, and medical practitioners can order these tests for different clinical indications as described earlier. Although arguably outdated, the traditional model of care places the medical practitioner in the central role to discuss with the patient the options for DNA genetic testing and then working with the testing laboratory to have the test undertaken. The medical practitioner gets the result and explains its significance to the patient.

This model is criticized by those in the DTC industry because (1) it can be seen to be paternalistic, (2) it takes away autonomy from the individual, and (3) genetics is "special" since data generated are particularly sensitive. However, the later view is not necessarily correct as genetic information is generally considered to be no different to other types of medical information although it can be more complex (Table 21.1) [12].

The three steps involved in having a DNA genetic test are summarized below. Each requires input from an expert. This helps to ensure the consent is informed so that appropriate decisions can be made. Should anything go wrong, someone can be held accountable.

Step 1 is to select the right test for the right clinical circumstance. In some cases, this will not be difficult, but in others, it is a challenge particularly when the customer is offered a panel of DNA tests. These considerations *before* ordering a DNA genetic test are important but difficult unless there is access to a professional who preferably has some knowledge of the individual's relevant medical and family history.

Step 2 involves the assessment of risk for a DNA genetic test. Two questions are needed at this stage. Can the laboratory deliver the test advertised? Will the result(s) cause more harm than good for the customer (and family members)? For the former, the customer will need to have some knowledge of the laboratory's performance and accreditation status. For the latter, ELSI will depend on the test ordered and its purpose.

Duty of care and confidentiality are key requirements in the patient/medical practitioner relationship. However, they are challenging with genetic testing involving germline (inherited) DNA because results might have significance for family members particularly when testing for serious genetic disorders when another issue (duty to warn) arises. This dilemma can be exemplified with the HD model discussed earlier. A person being tested for this serious neurodegenerative disorder and shown to have a positive result means other members of the family (siblings and offspring) are now at 50 % chance of getting HD. In this circumstance, does the medical practitioner have a duty of care or a duty to warn the relatives? How can this risk be conveyed to family members without infringing their privacy, assuming that the family members want to know? There have been some legal cases in the USA starting to explore this aspect of the patient/family/medical practitioner relationships in genetic practice. The courts have confirmed the medical practitioner has a duty of care to family members although they differ in the requirements for duty to warn (Table 21.2).

Some jurisdictions have attempted to resolve the complex issue around privacy and duty of care/duty to warn in predictive DNA testing for serious genetic disorders. One model allows exemptions in the privacy laws so the medical practitioner can disclose DNA test results to relatives in certain circumstances [14]. These aspects of ELSI remain work in progress. They are not addressed when DNA genetic testing is delivered DTC.

Step 3 What does the result mean? The degree of difficulty in understanding the DTC result is a spectrum from a relatively straightforward yes-or-no-type result, for example, the patient has or does not have sickle cell disease because the one DNA mutation causing this disorder is or is not present to the other extreme where the understanding of risk or the significance of a change in the DNA sequence will require expert input. At times, the expert will have to admit that a firm conclusion cannot be made as shown by new terminology emerging to describe changes in the DNA sequence that cannot be classified as causative or noncausative of disease.

Table 21.2 Case studies on the *duty to warn* relatives of risk following DNA genetic testing [13]

Case	Circumstances	Court ruling
Pate v Threlkel 1995	Appellant filed a suit against a medical practitioner who had treated her mother for an autosomal dominant form of genetic thyroid cancer but had not warned the appellant she was at risk. Subsequently, the appellant developed thyroid cancer which she claimed could have been avoided had she been warned.	It was sufficient for the medical practitioner to advise the mother to inform her daughter (appellant) in terms of his duty to warn.
Safer v Estate of Pack 1996	The appellant sued the estate of the medical practitioner who had treated her father 30 years earlier for an autosomal dominant form of genetic colon cancer. She claimed after developing colon cancer that she would have avoided this treatable cancer if she had been warned when her father had been treated.	In a different decision, the court stated that it was insufficient for the medical practitioner to ask the father to tell his daughter. He should have taken "reasonable steps" to ensure that immediate family members were warned.
Molloy v Meier 2004	A child had the fragile X form of mental retardation, but this information did not reach the biological parents. Ten years later, the mother had another child with fragile X. She sued the medical practitioners who had cared for her first child for not warning her of this risk.	The court ruled that a medical practitioner had a duty to warn biological parents of risks for genetic disorders even though the patient was an affected child and not the parents.

These are called VUS (variant of unknown significance). In a disorder like breast cancer, the frequency of VUS findings in genes like *BRCA1* and *BRCA2* is around 15 % of results [15].

DTC DNA Testing as a Model of Care

An alternative and to some extent attractive model of care has been developed through DTC DNA testing. Attractive because it places the consumer in the driving seat and builds on the public interest in the Internet as exemplified by the rise in online shopping. A bonus is the ease of buying the DNA test in the comfort of the home compared to the more complex and expensive practice or hospital environment. Examples of some tests offered DTC are found in Table 21.3 with comments on the potential usefulness of these products.

A leading USA-based DTC DNA genetic testing company is 23AndMe [16]. A little over a year ago, it was offering a wide range of DNA genetic tests covering >200 medical conditions and traits including T2D, arthritis, cancer (breast, prostate, and colon), heart and bone diseases, Parkinson's disease, Crohn's and Coeliac diseases, and many others – all for a special price of $99! Today, it is only selling ancestry DNA genetic tests until it has satisfied a number of concerns from the USA's FDA (Food and Drug Administration) [17].

Table 21.3 Examples of DTC DNA genetic testing

Testing for	Comment
Medical testing	There are a whole range of tests sold DTC that are linked to medical conditions. Particularly concerning are those involving serious disorders such as cancer. Whether it is acceptable that these tests can be advertised as simply providing "information" will become more evident when the current FDA review and a class action are concluded.
Recreational testing	An example would be genealogy with many having a strong interest in tracing their ancestry. Although there are DNA genetic markers like SNPs that are found in particular ethnic groups, it would be expecting a lot of a DTC DNA genetic test to identify distant relatives as is claimed in some advertisements. Other types of recreational testing involve the use of DNA genetic markers to identify optimal diets for well-being or products to improve skin aging.
Testing for traits	A test widely advertised DTC looks at athletic ability based on a number of research studies showing genes contribute to this trait. The same studies also acknowledge that the elite athlete phenotype is complex with important genetic (often multiple) and environmental factors playing a role. These interactions are not taken into consideration by having a single genetic test so the information provided would be limited. It is particularly concerning when these tests are ordered on children as it is not clear what the results will mean to the children's long-term development or involvement in sport.
Forensic or legal testing	The usual test ordered here would be paternity testing although some DTC services are advertising for infidelity testing which assays various objects for DNA from third parties. Another relationship test would involve immigration disputes where proving a blood relationship might prove beneficial. How useful these DNA tests are in the legal process will depend on whether the laboratory has obtained the appropriate court accreditation. Chain of custody would need to be proven, and this might be difficult in the DTC context.

Like most of the regulatory agencies, the FDA maintained a low-key approach to DTC DNA testing despite adverse reports and publicity (Table 21.4). Two US states, New York and Maryland, had made it difficult for their residents to access health-related DNA DTC tests [20]. So the regulatory landscape was confusing until the FDA took action in late 2013 to demand resolution of some issues that it had highlighted earlier to 23andMe. The FDA put a hold on that company's DTC medical DNA testing service until these were addressed. In early 2014, the 23andMe company published an update on its website explaining that it was working with the FDA to resolve these issues and until then it was no longer providing a medical testing service [21]. In Feb 2015 the FDA gave approval for 23 and Me to market one DNA genetic test DTC. This was to detect carriers for the rare genetic disorder Bloom syndrome. www.fda.gov/NewsEvents/Newsroom/PressAnnouncements/ucm435003.htm

A further development in 2013 was the class action lawsuit filed in California alleging that 23andMe (1) falsely and misleadingly advertises their saliva collection kit/personal genomic service as providing health reports on 240+ conditions and traits, drug response, and carrier status among other things when there is no analytical or clinical validation for the personal genomic service for its advertised uses, (2) uses the information it collects from the DNA tests consumers pay to take to

Table 21.4 Adverse reports and publicity involving DTC DNA genetic testing [2, 18, 19]

Report/incident	Findings
2006 US Government Accountability Office (GAO) report looked at nutrigenetic applications of DTC DNA testing with the GAO sending samples to four testing laboratories that had advertised through the Internet. Fourteen samples of DNA purporting to represent 14 adult males and females were referred although in reality 12 of the samples had come from a 9-month-old female and 2 from a 48-year-old male.	The GAO received different DTC DNA testing results for these samples. In some cases, companies offered to sell the customer expensive supplements that had been made based on his or her DNA results. The GAO expressed concern that different fictitious adults seemed to be getting different advice (yet the DNA came from the same person). When supplements were analyzed, they contained various vitamins that could also be found in cheaper generic products.
A second GAO study in 2010 was broader and targeted some of the large companies that had been advertising a range of products including what appeared to be DNA testing for medical purposes.	The GAO's conclusions were sobering; for example, it stated that *10 of the 15 companies we investigated engaged in some form of fraudulent, deceptive, or otherwise questionable marketing practices.*
There was further adverse publicity in 2010 when the 23andMe company had to apologize for 96 incorrect results because DNA samples had been inserted in the wrong orientation when tested.	This incident also showed that the company was not actually doing the test but referring DNA samples to another laboratory which would have made it difficult for customers to access the accreditation status of the testing laboratory.

generate databases and statistical information that it then markets to other sources and the scientific community in general even though the test results are meaningless, and (3) despite 23andMe's failure to receive marketing authorization or approval from the FDA, the defendant has slowly increased its list of indications for the personal genomic service and initiated new marketing campaigns including TV advertisements in violation of the Federal Food, Drug, and Cosmetic Act [22]. This legal challenge is underway in the USA and will influence the future direction of the DTC DNA testing industry.

Genetic Counseling

The importance of genetic counseling as an adjunct to DNA genetic testing has always been accepted. Who gives this counseling and how intensive it needs to be will ultimately depend on the seriousness of the underlying disorder *and* the type of DNA genetic test ordered. For example, DNA testing for genetic predisposition to breast cancer should be accompanied by intensive and professional counseling because the genetics of this disorder are complex, and even mutations found within known causative genes may demonstrate variable penetrance, e.g., 40–70 % depending on the mutation found as well as other risk factors such as the population being tested [7]. Options for intervention involve major surgery such as prophylactic mastectomy. Thus, the patient must have all the relevant information including accurate risk estimations so appropriate decision-making becomes possible.

In response to criticism that consumers have no support or counseling, some companies formed partnerships with DTC genetic counseling services accessible by phone or through the Internet. Some of these are located overseas so there are limitations on knowing how good they are or having access to the courts should problems arise.

Evolution of DTC DNA Genetic and Genomic Testing

Uptake and Growth

Debate about the DTC DNA testing industry has been difficult because it is not known how many members of the public are buying this product. One study estimated ~20,000–30,000 customers had purchased tests from the three largest companies in 2009 (23andMe, Navigenics and deCODEme) [23]. If correct, then the impact of DTC DNA testing on the healthcare system needing to deal with the consequences might not be that significant [2]. A preliminary report in 2011 suggested that there were no short-term changes in psychological health, diet, exercise, or the use of screening tests following DTC testing [24].

At its peak, there were around 30 DTC DNA testing companies in operation. The numbers and their products were closely monitored by the USA-based Genetics & Public Policy Center, which periodically updated a table and published it on its website [25]. This table listed the companies offering this service and their products. The latest version in 2011 changed format as it subdivided tests into those DTC and those "DTC" but ordered by a medical practitioner. Thus, as the industry evolved, there was a move back to include the medical practitioner at least to order the test.

As mentioned earlier, a number of national committees responded to the developments in DTC DNA genetic testing and proposed guidelines including codes of conduct on how this new model for medical DNA testing might be regulated. Although laudable and perhaps the only way forward given the regulatory complexity particularly with overseas-based laboratories, many of these recommendations were voluntary and did not identify the means by which they might be enforced or acted on should there be problems [26].

Future

If the legal and regulatory environment continues to toughen, the move to include medical practitioners will increase. In this way, companies can continue DTC advertising and the profits from testing while the responsibility for ordering and interpreting reports shifts to the medical practitioner. It would be important, if this trend continued, for the relevant colleges or associations to develop policies on this new model of care.

Some insight into what the DTC DNA testing industry might look like in the future is provided by the USA-based company KNOME. Originally, this company offered a WGS to the few who could afford it [27]. Subsequently, the company evolved from a DNA *testing* service to a DNA *interpretation* service which allows customers to bring along their WGS and obtain a regular update on any new findings that had emerged of relevance to the customer's DNA profile [28]. Commercially, this made sense as it was likely that when WGS became a routine test, it might only be needed once per lifetime as germline DNA would not change. However, the re-examination of the sequence data is potentially a lifetime activity as more information became available or the individual develops or becomes at risk for new disorders allowing a genetic component or cause to be sought in the WGS.

It is likely that different permutations of the DTC model will continue to emerge to provide an alternative product competing with or even replacing the more traditional approach to DNA genetic testing. In parallel with this, it would be necessary to ensure measures of the tests' clinical value including ELSI are taken on by the industry.

References

1. European Academies Science Advisory Council 2012. Direct to Consumer genetic testing. www.easac.eu/fileadmin/PDF_s/reports_statements/Easac_12_DTCGT-Lay_Web.pdf. Accessed 1 Sept 2014.
2. Caulfield T, McGuire AL. Direct-to-consumer genetic testing: perceptions, problems, and policy responses. Annu Rev Med. 2012;63:23–33.
3. Borry P, van Hellemondt E, Sprumont D, et al. Legislation on direct-to-consumer genetic testing in seven European countries. Eur J Hum Genet. 2012;20:715–21.
4. Rojahn SY. Biotech Amgen to buy genetics pioneer DeCode. 2012. www.technologyreview.com/view/508591/biotech-amgen-to-buy-genetics-pioneer-decode/. Accessed 1 Sept 2014.
5. Critchley C, Nicol D, Otlowski M, Chalmers D. Public reaction to direct-to-consumer online genetic tests: comparing attitudes, trust and intentions across commercial and conventional providers. Public Underst Sci, published online Feb 19 2014.
6. Burke W. Genetic tests: clinical validity and clinical utility. 2014. http://onlinelibrary.wiley.com/doi/10.1002/0471142905.hg0915s81/pdf. Accessed 1 Sept 2014.
7. Trent RJ. Molecular medicine: genomics to personalized healthcare. 4th ed. Amsterdam: Elsevier; 2012.
8. easyDNA – terms and conditions for genetic predisposition test. www.easydna.ie/genetic-predisposition-dna-testing/terms-and-conditions.html. Accessed 1 Sept 2014.
9. Ng PC, Murray SS, Levy S, Venter JC. An agenda for personalized medicine. Nature. 2009;461:724–6.
10. Guidance for the implementation of a medical laboratory accreditation system. 2012. http://ilac.org/publications-and-resources/ilac-documents/guidance-series/ Accessed 1 April 2015.
11. Brett GR, Metcalfe SA, Amor DJ, Halliday J. An exploration of genetic health professionals' experience with direct-to-consumer genetic testing in their clinical practice. Eur J Hum Genet. 2012;20:825–30.

12. Evans JP, Burke W. Genetic exceptionalism. Too much of a good thing? Genet Med. 2008;10:500–1.
13. Offit K, Groeger E, Turner S, Wadsworth EA, Weiser MA. The "duty to warn" a patient's family members about hereditary disease risks. JAMA. 2004;292:1469–73.
14. Use and disclosure of genetic information to a patient's genetic relatives under Section 95AA of the Privacy Act. 1988. (Cth). www.nhmrc.gov.au/guidelines/publications/pr3. Accessed 1 Sept 2014.
15. Moghadasi S, Hofland N, Wouts JN, Hogervorst FBL, Wijnen JT, Vreeswijk MPG, van Asperen CJ. Variants of uncertain significance in BRCA1 and BRCA2 assessment of in silico analysis and a proposal for communication in genetic counselling. J Med Genet. 2013;50: 74–9.
16. 23AndMe – leading DTC DNA genetic testing company in USA. www.23andme.com/. Accessed 1 Sept 2014.
17. PHG information on: FDA desist letter to 23andMe. www.phgfoundation.org/news/15045/. Accessed 1 Sept 2014.
18. United States Government Accountability Office 2006 report. Nutrigenetic testing: tests purchased from four web sites mislead consumers. www.gao.gov/new.items/d06977t.pdf. Accessed 1 Sept 2014.
19. United States Government Accountability Office 2010 report: direct-to-consumer genetic tests: misleading test results are further complicated by deceptive marketing and other questionable practices. www.gao.gov/new.items/d10847t.pdf. Accessed 1 Sept 2014.
20. NY and MD limits on 23andMe. www.legalgenealogist.com/blog/2012/12/23/ny-and-md-limits-on-23andme/. Accessed 1 Sept 2014.
21. An FDA update for 23andMe customers. http://blog.23andme.com/news/an-fda-update-for-23andme-customers/. Accessed 1 Sept 2014.
22. Wagner JK. Troubles keep coming for 23andMe. Genomics law report. 2013. www.genomicslawreport.com/index.php/2013/12/05/troubles-keep-coming-for-23andme/. Accessed 1 Sept 2014.
23. Wright CF, Gregory-Jones S. Size of the direct-to-consumer genomic testing market. Genet Med. 2010;12:594.
24. Bloss CS, Schork NJ, Topol EJ. Effect of direct-to-consumer genomewide profiling to assess disease risk. N Engl J Med. 2011;364:524–34.
25. List of 2011 DTC companies alphabetically and by disease category. www.dnapolicy.org/news.release.php?action=detail&pressrelease_id=145. Accessed 1 Sept 2014.
26. Anonymous editorial. New guidelines for genetic tests are welcome but insufficient. Lancet. 2010; 376:488.
27. Harmon A. Gene map becomes a luxury item. www.nytimes.com/2008/03/04/health/research/04geno.html?_r=0&pagewanted=print. Accessed 1 Sept 2014.
28. KNOME. www.knome.com/. Accessed 1 Sept 2014.

Part III
Ethical and Legal Aspects of Genetic Testing in the Clinical and Research Setting

Chapter 22
Current Ethical Issues Related to the Implementation of Whole-Exome and Whole-Genome Sequencing

Pascal Borry, Davit Chokoshvili, Emilia Niemiec, Louiza Kalokairinou, Danya F. Vears, and Heidi Carmen Howard

Abstract We have briefly discussed herein four of the many aspects that raise concerns in the context of implementation of whole-exome and whole-genome sequencing (mainly) in the clinical realm. Namely, we addressed issues surrounding: (1) the duty to hunt for variants known to have a health impact, (2) such "hunting" or opportunistic screening in children, (3) challenges to the consent process, and (4) the commercialization of genetic testing direct to consumer.

Keywords Whole-exome sequencing (WES) • Whole-genome sequencing (WGS) • Genomic variants • Genetic testing • Opportunistic screening • Hereditary diseases • Informed consent • Direct-to-consumer (DTC) genetic testing • Undiagnosed genetic conditions

---

P. Borry, PhD (✉) • D. Chokoshvili, MA, MSc • L. Kalokairinou, LLM, MSc
Department of Public Health and Primary Care, KU Leuven, Leuven 3000, Belgium
e-mail: pascal.borry@med.kuleuven.be

E. Niemiec, MSc
Erasmus Mundus Joint International Doctoral Fellow in Law, Science and Technology, Brussels, Belgium

Department of Law, University of Turin, Italy

Centre for Ethics and Law in the Life Sciences, Leibniz University, Hannover, Germany

D.F. Vears, BS, MS
School of Population and Global Health, Centre for Health Equity, University of Melbourne, Parkville, VIC 3052, Australia

H.C. Howard, PhD
Department of Public Health and Caring Sciences, Centre for Research Ethics and Bioethic, Uppsala University, Uppsala SE-751 22, Sweden

S.A. Schneider, J.M.T. Brás (eds.), *Movement Disorder Genetics*,
DOI 10.1007/978-3-319-17223-1_22

Introduction

The Human Genome Project, a global collaborative effort aimed at sequencing the entire human genome, cost over $2.7 billion and took more than 10 years to complete. The first draft of the human genome was published in 2001 [1]. Since then, rapid advancements in *next-generation* sequencing technologies (NGS, i.e., new high-throughput and massively parallel DNA-sequencing technologies) have led to a drastic decrease in both the price and time needed for genome sequencing. As of 2014, the National Human Genome Research Institute estimates the average cost of whole-genome sequencing (WGS) at approximately $4,000–5,000 [2], while the time required for this (without interpretation of variants) has been reduced to several days [3]. For over a decade now, the target price of $1,000 per genome has been discussed, and recently some companies have announced having reached this goal, or of being very close to it [4]. Moreover, whole-exome sequencing (WES), which analyzes only 1 % of the genome, the protein-coding sections [5], entails lower costs, and for now appears to be preferred in the clinical diagnostic setting [6].

The decreasing cost and time of sequencing have led to the expectation that WES/WGS will become commonplace in medical practice, including diagnostics, as well as in population screening [7, 8]. In the past few years, both WES and WGS have been successfully used to identify causative mutations in some highly selected patients with rare or undiagnosed diseases of genetic origin [7, 9–12]. Although the relatively high costs of WES/WGS currently preclude large-scale adoption of genome sequencing in the clinical setting, it has been suggested that rapidly diminishing sequencing costs may soon make the techniques cost-effective in a broader range of clinical cases such as personalized diagnosis and personalized drug therapy. Moreover, some have predicted that sequencing technologies will also be applied in public health programs, such as newborn screening programs [13].

Despite the potential promises of WES/WGS in clinical practice, a number of challenges have been identified with regard to the potential implementation of sequencing technologies in health care. Firstly, even though the analytic validity of WES/WGS has improved dramatically, current sequencing techniques remain imperfect. For example, a recent study reported that, depending on the sequencing platform used, WGS failed to sufficiently cover from 10 to 19 % of inherited disease genes of interest [5, 14]. Imperfect analytic validity of WGS is worrisome, since given the large scale of the human genome (>3 billion base pairs), even a very small percentage of erroneous results would translate into a high number of incorrect variants in absolute terms [12].

Secondly, owing to the present limited understanding of the human genome, many variants currently identified through WES/WGS are unclassified; that is to say that they are variants of unknown significance, and their potential effect or impact on an individual's health is has yet to be determined [7]. Indeed, debates have been ongoing regarding to what extent such findings should be reported to patients. Although unknown or unclassified variants may be valuable for research purposes, in the healthcare setting, they might offer little benefit to the individual patient as long as their true meaning has not been correctly understood. Furthermore, a large number of genetic variants, when combined with other genetic variants or environmental factors, may be suspected of playing a role in an individual's predisposition to multifactorial conditions, such as cancer, diabetes, and cardiovascular diseases. However, the predictive value of such results may be low [8]. Although this is not specific to the technique of WGS/WES, given the large amounts of data generated with these approaches, one could predict that there will be more of these variants found with uncertain meaning. Moreover, the use of WES/WGS may reveal variants unrelated to the primary indication for sequencing (i.e., unsolicited or incidental findings) and lead to the question of which findings should be communicated to patients [7], how, and by whom [15]. This issue becomes even more knotty when the individual tested is a child, and findings may be relevant only later in life or may be predominantly informative (at the time of testing) for family members (but not necessarily for the child being tested).

Thirdly, the amount and variety of information obtained through WES/WGS have important implications for information provision and counseling to the patients undergoing the procedure. Due to the complexity of the procedure – including technical aspects of WES/WGS, diagnostic value, likelihood of unsolicited/incidental findings, and implications of the test results for other family members – pretest counseling involving the informed consent procedure could drastically increase the time of the counseling process [16, 17]. Such counseling sessions should, ideally, clearly distinguish among the types of expected results in order to facilitate an informed decision by the patient [18]. Notably, post-test counseling may be equally time-consuming, especially if the patient chooses to receive extensive information on incidental findings [7]. Furthermore, additional counseling and consent sessions may be required in those cases where either the patient's biological sample or data derived through WES/WGS are to be retained for future research purposes.

Evidently, there are several concerns with respect to the implementation of WGS/WES; herein, we outline four important ethical challenges to the implementation of these approaches in clinical care (and the related commercial context). To begin with, the issues related to unsolicited findings and opportunistic screening in WES/WGS will be discussed: first in more general terms and secondly with respect to a pediatric population. Next, problems with informed consent will be covered. Finally, ethical issues regarding direct-to-consumer genetic testing will be considered.

Unsolicited Findings and the Duty to Hunt

As alluded to above, the increasing use of high-throughput technologies and approaches in genomics, both in the research and clinical contexts, has increased stakeholders' focus on the topic of unsolicited findings. Unsolicited findings have also been referred to as incidental findings, unsolicited variants, unanticipated results, secondary variants, unexpected or off-target results, unsought results, or unrelated findings [19], as well as non-incidental secondary findings, serendipitous, or iatrogenic findings [20]. The exact meaning of each term as well as their merits has, to some extent, been debated and could, arguably, be even further discussed [19, 21, 22]. However, for the purpose of this chapter, we will use the term unsolicited finding to mean a result found during research or clinical testing that is beyond the aims of the study or the original reason to conduct clinical testing.

Although unsolicited findings are not specific to genomics, the phenomenon is viewed as needing particular attention given the fact that we can now generate unprecedentedly large quantities of sequencing data in a very short time and therefore have access to a lot of information, whether or not it is related to the initial question posed [23]. Many authors have discussed whether or how unsolicited results should be returned to patients in the clinic [24] or to research participants in a research study [25]. Although there remains a lot of discussion regarding details, there appears to be a consensus taking shape: should a clinician or researcher discover a medically actionable variant with established health impact, this information should be returned to patients/participants [26, 27]. For example, the European Society of Human Genetics recommends "If the detection of an unsolicited genetic variant is indicative of serious health problems (either in the person tested or his or her close relatives) that allow for treatment or prevention, in principle, a health-care professional should report such genetic variants" [18]. This being said, the details regarding which variants have utility or impact and the criteria needed to make these decisions are still being debated [23].

Closely related to this topic is the notion of the "duty to hunt" for genomic variants that may have a health impact for patients; that is to say, when performing WES/WGS, do physicians and/or researchers have a duty to actively search the sequence data for variants known to have a health impact but that are not necessarily related to the indication for performing the sequencing in the first place? Although some authors have referred to the findings obtained through this "hunt" as incidental findings [20], others have commented that such intentional "hunting" or searching could not be described as "incidental," at least not in the "usual sense of the term" and have described the phenomenon as "opportunistic screening" [28, 29]. The discussion regarding the return of results, including the duty to hunt, differs somewhat depending on the context, clinical, or research [30]; herein, we focus on the issue of the duty to hunt in the clinical context.

Perhaps, the most well-known stance supporting a duty to hunt in the clinical context comes from the American College of Medical Genetics and Genomics (ACMG) which, in the first half of 2013, published recommendations supporting "that laboratories performing clinical sequencing seek and report mutations of the specified classes or types in the genes listed here. This evaluation and reporting should be performed for all clinical germline (constitutional) exome and genome sequencing, including the "normal" of tumor-normal subtractive analyses in all subjects, irrespective of age but excluding fetal samples" [20]. The ACMG provided a list of 56 genes associated with 24 inherited conditions that should be screened whenever a patient (of any age) is offered sequencing. The list was developed based on what the ACMG called a "consensus-driven assessment of clinical validity and utility" and focuses on conditions with relatively high penetrance and for which an intervention may be possible. Importantly, the list does not include conditions that are already part of newborn screening. The initial recommendations proposed that patients could not refuse the testing of these 56 genes without also forfeiting the access to WES/WGS. However, in the face of criticisms concerning the lack of support for patient autonomy, shared decision-making, and for patients' right "not to know" [28, 31, 32], the ACMG changed their stance on this point the following year [33]. The rationale for opportunistic screening is based mainly on the medical benefit for patients and their families, where the identification of a genetic risk could allow for the early adoption of prevention or treatment measures. Furthermore, it is based on the fiduciary duty of clinicians and laboratory personnel to prevent harm. It should be noted, however, that these recommendations are not meant for sequencing done in the context of preconception, prenatal, or newborn sequencing, nor do they apply to the sequencing of healthy children and adults [20].

A number of concerns have been raised in reaction to these recommendations, including a lack of evidence for establishing the list of genes and the lack of information about frequencies of variants in healthy or not-at-risk populations [28]. Such a lack of information could subsequently lead to erroneous classifications of variants as pathogenic, which could cause needless anxiety and cause patients to seek inappropriate and costly follow-up medical procedures [34]. The fact that important stakeholders, such as members of the public and primary care physicians, were absent from the discussion [32] has also been mentioned as a weakness. Of major concern is also the potentially extremely high costs in terms of time, resources, effort, and money to conduct such screening [32]. Furthermore, there has been criticism regarding the screening of children in this context, especially for adult-onset disorders (see below).

Although other professional associations' and policy groups' guidelines have mentioned opportunistic screening, they have not outright recommended it [29, 35]. Moreover, the European Society of Human Genetics' guidelines on the use of WGS in health care advise that approaches such as targeting and filtering be used employed to reduce the chances of even encountering unsolicited findings: "When in the clinical setting either targeted sequencing or analysis of genome data is possible, it is preferable to use a targeted approach first in order to avoid unsolicited findings or findings that cannot be interpreted. Filtering should limit the analysis to specific (sets of) genes. Known genetic variants with limited or no clinical utility should be filtered out (if possible neither analyzed nor reported)" [18]. Although only indirectly addressed within the context of the management of incidental findings in the clinical context, the Presidential Commission for the Study of Bioethical Issues recommends that "Medical educators, both in the classroom and clinic, should continue to cultivate 'diagnostic elegance' and 'therapeutic parsimony' amongst practitioners—ordering and conducting only tests and interventions necessary for addressing health concerns related to their patient" [36].

In conclusion, currently, there is no general agreement regarding whether clinicians who use WGS or WES for diagnostic purposes also have a duty to hunt for other variants with health impacts. There is, however, a large consensus that much more evidence is needed [20, 28, 34] regarding opportunistic screening and its potential impact on the healthcare system and on patients. Even the ACMG recognizes that "there are insufficient data on penetrance and clinical utility to fully support these recommendations, and we encourage the creation of an ongoing process for updating these recommendations at least annually as further data are collected" [20].

Opportunistic Screening in Children

As previously mentioned, the introduction of WES/WGS in the clinic may revolutionize the potential for finding the (molecular) diagnosis of genetic conditions, including movement disorders. Although this may confer benefits in terms of reducing the diagnostic odyssey, and/or improving patient management [7] as well as revealing potential risks for relatives, it also raises ethical issues in relation to genetic testing in children.

Consider this scenario: *8-year-old Jack is referred to your clinic for investigation of the genetic cause of his progressive ataxia. His parents, who are considering having a second child, are keen to find out the genetic basis of his condition in order to avoid having a second affected child. Given there are several candidate genes, you decide whole-genome sequencing will be most cost-effective. Following testing, you receive the laboratory report which reveals the genetic cause for Jack's progressive ataxia, as well as a result unrelated to diagnosing the ataxia – that he carries a variant in BRCA1. This variant is expected to be pathogenic and therefore has health implications for Jack, one of his parents, and potentially their extended family members.*

As described in the previous section, the use of WES/WGS raises the question as to whether laboratories should limit their reporting of results only to the findings that are relevant to the clinical question at stake or to "hunt" for other variants known to have a health impact. The previously mentioned ACMG guidelines, which recommend the active search of a selected group of genes, including those for conditions with adult onset, have led to a heated debate regarding whether these recommendations should also apply to children. The ACMG states that "masking or tailoring the reporting of such information according to the age of the patient could place an unrealistic burden upon laboratories facing increasing volumes of clinical sequencing. The Working Group also felt that the ethical concerns about providing children with genetic risk information about adult-onset diseases were outweighed by the potential benefit to the future health of the child and the child's parent of discovering an incidental finding where intervention might be possible. Therefore, the Working Group recommended that recommendations for seeking and reporting incidental findings not be limited by the age of the person being sequenced" [20].

These recommendations appear to be in stark contrast to previous recommendations for predictive testing in children as well as to a set of guidelines which were jointly released by the American Academy of Pediatrics (AAP) and the ACMG in 2013 [37, 38]. The AAP/ACMG guidelines recommend that children should generally not receive genetic testing for adult-onset disorders, particularly where no treatment is available [37, 38]. It should be noted, however, that the contextual background of testing differs somewhat for each set of guidelines. The AAP/ACMG guidelines are generally situated in a clinical setting where parents may request predictive testing for their child for an adult-onset condition that is already known in the family [37, 38]; no particular strategy or tool for testing is mentioned nor do they mention a situation of opportunistic screening. The ACMG guidelines, on the other hand, relate specifically to a situation such as Jack's, described above, where WES/WGS is used as a diagnostic approach [20].

This contextual difference translates to two important distinctions between the WES/WGS diagnostic approach from the standard predictive testing context [39]. First, the nature of the tools or approach used for diagnostic purposes in Jack's case means that the sequence data is already available for the "hunt" rather than a specific test being performed only for the reason of testing an adult-onset condition. Second, the genetic predisposition Jack carries for BRCA1 may not have been identified previously in the family, and reporting of the variant could, therefore, potentially lead to early detection of risk and implementation of screening for both Jack in the future and also for relatives. These are the primary drivers of the ACMG's recommendations for reporting these variants [20].

Although the reporting of results from opportunistic screening might result in health benefits for the children or their family, we must also consider the potential (harmful) impact when one of these variants is identified in a child and disclosed to the family. Standard genetic guidelines for predictive testing in children often indicate that when there is no medical benefit from performing predictive testing, then it is in the child's best interests to postpone testing until the child is able to make an autonomous decision [37, 38, 40–42]. That being said, the AAP/ACMG guidelines also leave some room for alternate routes when they state that "…after careful genetic counseling, it may be ethically acceptable to proceed with predictive genetic testing to resolve disabling parental anxiety or to support life-planning decisions that parents sincerely believe to be in the child's best interest" [38]. One of the challenges in the context of genetic testing is that there are many different views regarding exactly what constitutes as being in the child's best interests [43].

One way of determining what is in the child's best interests might be to assess the harms of reporting and not reporting the results from opportunistic screening (or unsolicited findings). Some authors have proposed that the harms of reporting such results in children are limited to the imposition of undesired genetic information on the child and their family [44]. They argue that this is outweighed by the potential harm of removing family members' opportunities to avoid illness through screening [44]. Although genetic guidelines generally recommend against providing predictive testing in young children, few studies have investigated the psychological impact of testing [40–42, 45]. There is, therefore, little in the way of evidence to suggest that identification of an unsolicited finding (or results from opportunistic screening) predisposing a child to a genetic condition would cause psychological harm. However, lack of evidence does not equate to evidence of a lack of harm, and therefore, additional empirical studies to investigate this are required.

The ACMG has taken a more family-based approach to what is in the child's best interests. They argue that identification of these pathogenic variants in children benefits the child, first by providing them with important information about their future health risks and, second, through the potential health benefits to their parents should they be detected prior to displaying symptoms of the genetic condition for which a mutation was detected. Therefore, the ACMG believes that the ethical concerns are outweighed by the "potential benefit to the future health of the child and the child's parents" [20]. For this reason, their follow-up recommendations indicated that it could be viewed as unethical if laboratories do not report these unsolicited findings, because they are failing to allow parents to act in their child's best interests and avoid preventable harm [44, 46]. This is in line with literature acknowledging that parents are best placed to consider all the factors that impact on their family and should therefore be allowed to make decisions in a way that takes the family's best interests into account [47]. This being said, whether parents will be sufficiently informed regarding the unsolicited information they might receive in order to make decisions on behalf of their children and their broader family is unclear.

One should consider what else is at stake for the child if we report the results of opportunistic screening (or unsolicited results). A commonly stated argument against predictive testing in children is that, as well as removing their right to privacy (regarding their genetic result), it impinges on their future autonomy, specifically the child's ability to make his/her own decisions about whether they want to know their genetic status when they are older [42]. This concept has been referred to as "the child's right to an open future" and rests on the notion that genetic testing would narrow the child's future options [48, 49]. Likewise, when the results of opportunistic screening are reported to the clinician and subsequently to Jack's parents and Jack, we are removing the child's right not to know whether he has a *BRCA1* mutation. From this perspective, preservation of the child's future autonomy would involve either not conducting the screening at all for adult-onset disorders or, in the case of a truly "stumbled upon" incidental finding, to not report it to the clinician. Alternatively, the result could be reported to the clinician and held in trust until the child is able to make an autonomous decision. However, one might also view that by disclosing the results of opportunistic screening to the family, we are in fact broadening the options available to Jack and his family by providing them with opportunities for further screening and preventative care.

Debate continues as to whether laboratories should "hunt for" and report back results for a preset list of genes when WES/WGS is conducted in the clinical setting in children or whether reporting should be restricted to findings relevant to the quest for a diagnosis. Ultimately, it depends on the importance one places on the preservation of the child's right not to know information about their genetic risks compared to the potential health benefits for the family. Given that once information is known, it cannot be "unknown," perhaps the initial premise should be to remain cautious until more evidence is amassed regarding the impact of returning results to children for adult-onset disorders and limit reporting to the original clinical question and, in doing so, promote the child's future autonomy.

Informed Consent for WES and WGS in Diagnostics

Informed consent in clinical practice functions as a permission given for the performance of a medical procedure by a capacitated patient to whom the information about the procedure has been given, who understands it fully, and voluntarily consents to it. Informed consent has been integrated in most jurisdictions as a legal requirement and supported ethically as ultimate respect for the autonomy of individuals and their right to self-determination [17]. It has been argued that in order to obtain genuine informed consent, the information about the procedure (or in this context the genetic test) presented to a patient should be accurate, relevant, and understandable, and the patient should have the opportunity to freely withdraw consent [17, 50]. Yet, obtaining valid and adequate informed consent for some medical procedures poses challenges such as those related to proper communication of the information and its comprehension, which is particularly relevant for informed consent for genetic testing. The fact that clinical genetic testing is usually offered with both pre- and post-test genetic counseling is an indication of how important and potentially complex communication can be in this context. Herein, we offer a list of issues that should be considered when planning for the informed consent procedure for WES/WGS.

Indeed, the implementation of WES and WGS adds further challenges and amplifies those already existing related to the informed consent procedure for "traditional" genetic tests. This is primarily caused by the vast amount of complex information that may be extracted from whole-exome or whole-genome sequence data. This information varies with respect to the clinical significance and predictive value, which may influence the individual's desire to obtain particular results [51]. Related to this, the potential for unsolicited findings is of particular concern in the informed consent process. Among others, they raise a question about the categories or types of genetic variants (i.e., those with high penetrance or clinical utility or health impact) that should be retrieved from a whole-genome sequence [18, 20] and what should be reported to patients. Even if sequencing is targeted and filters are applied to WES/WGS with the aim of obtaining only findings relevant to the medical indication in question, unsolicited findings may nevertheless appear in the process of sequence analysis and interpretation. Although unsolicited findings exceed the initial scope of the test, they may be clinically actionable, which poses questions about the obligation to disclose them [36]. Additionally, the significance of sequencing data may change with time as our understanding of variants progresses through genomics research. Therefore, the storage of the data should be considered as well as the possibility of reanalyzing and reinterpreting data in the light of new scientific findings and whether the patient agrees to be recontacted for this information (or for any incidental finding). Furthermore, in the case where clinical whole-genome sequencing is coupled with research, this subject, including the issue of data sharing, should be discussed during the informed consent process [52]. Finally, as with other genetic tests, some of the outcomes of WES/WGS for hereditary diseases concern not only the patient but also the relatives or future offspring; thus, this introduces the dilemma of potential obligation to disclose some information to family members [25]. Additional difficulties appear in case of WES/WGS offered for children, whose "right not to know" regarding health prospects should be retained as much as possible [51] in the case of testing for adult-onset conditions. All of the issues outlined above make the process of designing appropriate informed consent procedures in the context of WES/WGS particularly challenging. It is crucial to communicate with the patient regarding these factors and, in particular, to communicate the meaning and implications of the different types of expected findings in an understandable way that would allow truly informed decision-making.

Given these challenges, many societies and experts have attempted to face or overcome the difficulties of informed consent in this new context of WES/WGS. Ayuso et al. specifically analyzed publications and guidelines concerning or related to informed consent for WGS in the clinical context [53]. The authors found a relatively high level of consistency among the guidelines and proposed a minimum list of information that should be provided to the patient, which are the management of incidental findings, the scope, a description indicating the kind of information to be obtained, the possible benefits and risks, the availability of alternative tests, the voluntary nature of the test, the possibility of refusal, the future use of the data, and the confidentiality of the outcomes. Pretest counseling has been underlined by the authors of the abovementioned publication as well as by other experts in various recommendations as a crucial element of informed consent [53]. Pretest counseling should prevent informed consent from being reduced to the mere signing of a document. It should be ensured through dialogue that the patient truly understands the information provided and is competent to make a choice. Fulfilling these requirements in the context of WES/WGS will demand time-consuming counseling sessions provided by properly trained professionals [55].

Various authors have also suggested new strategies of informed consent that may minimize information overload by introducing clinically relevant categories of diseases and traits, layers of indispensable and additional information, and informational and decisional phases of consent that require it to be stretched in time [56–59]. Dynamic models of consent, where the use of information technology interfaces places patients at the center of the decision-making process and allows them to be more engaged over the entire time span of use of their sample/information, may also help to ease the challenges of consent for WGS/WES [60]. These different strategies may facilitate the counseling and informed decision-making of the patient regarding the type of test they want to consent to and categories of results that will be returned.

Concluding, informed consent is just one of the elements related to the ethical issues around WES/WGS. Its adequacy may not resolve the other ethical issues related to data handling and return of results; however, efforts should be made to implement the proposed recommendations and new strategies of informed consent for WES/WGS into clinical practice. Thereafter, studies may be conducted toward optimizing informed consent procedures so that it may fulfill its functions more adequately.

Genetic Testing Beyond the Clinic: Commercialization of Genetic Tests

Although not, strictly speaking, a part of the realm of "clinical" genetics per se, direct-to-consumer (DTC) genetic testing, in many ways, brushes up to the activities of clinical genetics (e.g., some of the types of tests being offered and the inclusion of healthcare professionals in the process). Furthermore, as a relatively new phenomenon, which has sparked a great deal of debate in the last years, we chose to address these activities and their ethical dimensions herein. Unlike the previous sections, however, we do not confine the discussion only to WES/WGS and the companies offering these services DTC, as these are fairly recent, and the ethical issues surrounding companies offering genome-wide testing are very similar to those offering WES/WGS. Furthermore, it is important to note that all three previous topics discussed are relevant concerns, albeit with some variations, for companies offering WES/WGS DTC.

For more than a decade now, several for-profit companies have been commercializing genetic tests through the Internet, often without involving a healthcare professional in their services [61]. Such tests are advertised directly to the public, and consumers may order and receive the tests themselves, or through a healthcare provider [62]. The majority of direct-to-consumer (DTC) genetic testing companies are based in the USA, although the number of companies established in Europe and Asia is also growing [63]. The DTC genetic testing market comprises a very heterogeneous spectrum of companies and products, while its size is still unspecified [64].

Currently, a wide variety of genetic tests is available DTC, including tests for recreational purposes, such as athletic performance and ancestry tests and tests for health-related purposes such as tests for multifactorial or monogenic disorders, test for carrier status, and nutrigenomics and pharmacogenomics tests. While in previous years the most comprehensive testing was offered mostly by companies genotyping hundreds of thousands to millions of SNPs, more recently companies are now also offering whole-genome and whole-exome sequencing directly to the public.

Specifically for conditions under the umbrella of movement disorders, various consumers might be able to find tests DTC, including tests for susceptibility to Parkinson's disease [65], Tourette syndrome [66], and restless legs syndrome [67], as well as carrier tests for ataxia-telangiectasia (ATM) [68] and rare diseases such as myoclonus dystonia (DYT11) and Rett syndrome (MECP2) [68]. In the past, some companies have also offered susceptibility tests for essential tremor, tardive dyskinesia, and progressive supranuclear palsy [69]. Indeed, DTC genetic tests on offer are frequently subject to changes, as the DTC genetic testing market is a particularly dynamic field.

Supporters of DTC genetic testing claim that such tests promote genetic education of consumers, empower them to improve their health by making their own healthcare decisions, and enhance their autonomy [70]. In addition, given that DTC genetic testing may potentially enable consumers to control who has access to their test results, this type of testing is considered, by some, to protect privacy of genetic information toward employers and insurance companies [71].

Nevertheless, DTC genetic testing has also been subject to a lot of criticism over the past years, and concerns have been raised by several authors and professional organizations regarding the potential risks stemming from such tests. One of the main concerns regarding this type of testing has to do with the uncertain clinical validity and utility of many of the tests offered DTC. When it comes to susceptibility testing for common complex disorders, such as Parkinson's disease, where the development of the disorder is usually the result of several genetic mutations acting in combination with other nongenetic factors [72], the predictive value of individual genetic variants remains low [72], and the commercialization of such tests is often considered to be premature [73]. The clinical utility of such tests is also questionable in many cases, since the test results are often not clinically actionable, and the health advice provided along with them is usually generic [74]. When thinking of rare monogenetic disorders, some concerns also exist about the extent to which the pathogenicity of variants is known, as well as penetrance and expressivity, especially in healthy populations, which have traditionally not been studied for such disorders. Moreover, when using WES/WGS, the problems of reporting (or not) variants of unknown significance remain.

In addition, it has been claimed that without genetic counseling and individualized supervision from a healthcare professional, consumers are more likely to misinterpret the test results and potentially take inappropriate healthcare actions or experience unnecessary anxiety [71]. The importance of medical supervision and pre- and post-test genetic counseling in the context of genetic testing for movement disorders is often underlined, since the test results are, in many cases, inconclusive, and their interpretation requires a high level of expertise in genetics [75, 76]. Furthermore, in light of the limited clinical interventions available for disorders like Parkinson's disease, performing the appropriate test for the appropriate person is particularly important, in order to avoid unnecessary distress and redundant visits to healthcare professionals [75]. It is important, therefore, that this type of testing is performed in the context of genetic counseling and that it is based on an informed decision of the patient [75]. Despite the fact that lately, many DTC genetic testing companies tend to involve healthcare professionals in their services, various concerns remain. Including a medical prescription on paper for genetic tests is not a guarantee of an adequate informed consent procedure and pretest counseling. In most cases, any physician seems to be allowed to order genetic tests regardless of whether he/she has adequate training to do so. Finally, some healthcare professionals may be employed or otherwise collaborating or linked with some companies, raising doubts about their impartiality [62].

Several professional organizations, genetic societies, and bioethics committees have addressed concerns related to DTC genetic testing, stressing in guidelines and recommendations the importance of medical supervision, genetic counseling, and informed consent and ensuring the quality of the tests [72, 77, 78]. Nevertheless, the effective regulation of this field remains a challenge, since the regulatory landscape both in Europe and the USA is rather fragmented and complex, leaving some important gaps [63]. Furthermore, the idea of a "one size fits all" regulation for all types of tests (e.g., ancestry, health related, etc.) may not be the most coherent approach. Finally, enforcement of national legislation may be problematic, given the global character of this industry which operates mostly through the Internet [79].

Conclusion

We have briefly discussed herein four of the many aspects that raise concerns in the context of implementation of whole-exome and whole-genome sequencing (mainly) in the clinical realm. Namely, we addressed issues surrounding (1) the duty to hunt for variants known to have a health impact, (2) such "hunting" or opportunistic screening in children, (3) challenges to the consent process, and (4) the commercialization of genetic testing direct to consumer. Indeed, none of these are new issues per se, but each issue when brought into the context of WES/WGS has new particularities and appears to be exacerbated by these high-throughput approaches. Furthermore, it is clear that the ethical and procedural frameworks previously created to deal with these aspects for "traditional" clinical genetic testing (i.e., where one or few genetic tests were performed usually sequentially) are, at best being challenged by the use of WES/WGS, and at worse, completely inept to properly manage these areas and concerns.

It is evident that, overall, more evidence is needed in order to pave the route to responsibly manage the implementation of WES/WGS in clinical care. Regarding the return of incidental findings and/or opportunistic screening, it will be important to closely study centers and pilot projects that currently offer these services to patients and to study the impact on patients. Additionally, with respect to programs for opportunistic screening, like that proposed by the ACMG, evidence is needed regarding the penetrance and mutagenicity of the 56 genes in healthy populations. Evidence is also needed specifically regarding the return of results for children, especially for adult-onset disorders. Are children negatively impacted by such information? Is there a benefit to them knowing? With respect to the ACMG guidelines, there is also a need to discuss and reconcile the discrepancies between traditional guidelines that suggest no testing in children for adult-onset disorders unless action can be taken to reduce the chances of developing the disorder. This discussion should also address the fact that DTC genetic testing companies can, and do, test children for adult-onset disorders. Regarding consent, new models and procedures of consent need to be carefully planned to integrate all the aspects and information needed to obtain proper informed consent in the context of WES/WGS. These then need to be tested on patient populations and the impact on patients measured. Finally, the DTC offer of genetic testing should continue to be monitored, as this group of actors has tended to offer services that go well beyond what we have been used to in the traditional clinical context.

References

1. Lander ES, Linton LM, Birren B, Nusbaum C, Zody MC, Baldwin J, et al. Initial sequencing and analysis of the human genome. Nature. 2001;409(6822):860–921.
2. Wetterstrand KA. DNA sequencing costs: data from the NHGRI Genome Sequencing Program (GSP). http://www.genome.gov/sequencingcosts/. Accessed 21 Aug 2014.
3. Middha S, Baheti S, Hart SN, Kocher JP. From days to hours: reporting clinically actionable variants from whole genome sequencing. PLoS One. 2014;9(2):e86803.
4. Hayden EC. Is the $1,000 genome for real. Nature News; 2014.
5. Feero WG. Clinical application of whole-genome sequencing: proceed with care. JAMA. 2014;311(10):1017–9.
6. Biesecker LG, Shianna KV, Mullikin JC. Exome sequencing: the expert view. Genome Biol. 2011;12(9):128.
7. Taber KAJ, Dickinson BD, Wilson M. The promise and challenges of next-generation genome sequencing for clinical care. JAMA. 2014;174(2):275–80.
8. Howard HC, Swinnen E, Douw K, Vondeling H, Cassiman JJ, Cambon-Thomsen A, et al. The ethical introduction of genome-based information and technologies into public health. Public Health Genomics. 2013;16(3):100–9.
9. Ashley EA, Butte AJ, Wheeler MT, Chen R, Klein TE, Dewey FE, et al. Clinical assessment incorporating a personal genome. Lancet. 2010;375(9725):1525–35.
10. Need AC, Shashi V, Hitomi Y, Schoch K, Shianna KV, McDonald MT, et al. Clinical application of exome sequencing in undiagnosed genetic conditions. J Med Genet. 2012;49(6):353–61.
11. Worthey E, Bick D, Dimmock D, Shimoyama M, Veith R, Kowalski G, et al. Clinical diagnostic whole genome sequencing in a paediatric population: experience from our WGS genetics clinic. BMC Proceedings. 2012;6(Suppl 6):O11.
12. Linderman MD, Brandt T, Edelmann L, Jabado O, Kasai Y, Kornreich R, et al. Analytical validation of whole exome and whole genome sequencing for clinical applications. BMC Med Genomics. 2014;7(1):20.
13. Goldenberg AJ, Sharp RR. The ethical hazards and programmatic challenges of genomic newborn screening. JAMA. 2012;307(5):461–2.
14. Dewey FE, Grove ME, Pan C, Goldstein BA, Bernstein JA, Chaib H, et al. Clinical interpretation and implications of whole-genome sequencing. JAMA. 2014;311(10):1035–45.
15. Pyeritz RE. The coming explosion in genetic testing – is there a duty to recontact. N Engl J Med. 2011;365(15):1367–9.
16. Williams J, Faucett A, Smith-Packard B, Wagner M, Williams M. An assessment of time involved in pre-test case review and counseling for a whole genome sequencing clinical research program. J Genet Couns. 2014;23(4):516–21.
17. Council of Europe. Convention for the protection of human rights and dignity of the human being with regard to the application of biology and medicine: convention on human rights and biomedicine. 1997. http://conventions.coe.int/Treaty/en/Treaties/Html/164.htm. Accessed 6 April 2015
18. van El CG, Cornel MC, Borry P, Hastings RJ, Fellmann F, Hodgson SV, et al. Whole-genome sequencing in health care. Eur J Hum Genet. 2013;21:S1–5.
19. Christenhusz GM, Devriendt K, Dierickx K. Secondary variants – in defense of a more fitting term in the incidental findings debate. Eur J Hum Genet. 2014;21(12):1331–4.
20. Green RC, Berg JS, Grody WW, Kalia SS, Korf BR, Martin CL, et al. ACMG recommendations for reporting of incidental findings in clinical exome and genome sequencing. Genet Med. 2013;15(7):565–74.
21. Crawford G, Fenwick A, Lucassen A. A more fitting term in the incidental findings debate: one term does not fit all situations. Eur J Hum Genet. 2014;22(8):957.
22. Parens E, Appelbaum P, Chung W. Incidental findings in the era of whole genome sequencing? Hastings Cent Rep. 2013;43(4):16–9.

23. Burke W, Trinidad SB, Clayton EW. Seeking genomic knowledge: the case for clinical restraint. Hastings Law J. 2013;64(6):1650.
24. Berg JS, Amendola LM, Eng C, Van Allen E, Gray SW, Wagle N, et al. Processes and preliminary outputs for identification of actionable genes as incidental findings in genomic sequence data in the Clinical Sequencing Exploratory Research Consortium. Genet Med. 2013;15(11):860–7.
25. Caulfield T, McGuire AL, Cho M, Buchanan JA, Burgess MM, Danilczyk U, et al. Research ethics recommendations for whole-genome research: consensus statement. PLoS Biol. 2008;6(3):e73.
26. Jarvik GP, Amendola LM, Berg JS, Brothers K, Clayton EW, Chung W, et al. Return of genomic results to research participants: the floor, the ceiling, and the choices in between. Am J Hum Genet. 2014;94(6):818–26.
27. McGuire AL, Lupski JR. Personal genome research: what should the participant be told? Trends Genet. 2010;26(5):199–201.
28. Burke W, Antommaria AHM, Bennett R, Botkin J, Clayton EW, Henderson GE, et al. Recommendations for returning genomic incidental findings? We need to talk! Genet Med. 2013;15(11):854–9.
29. PGH Foundation. Managing incidental and pertinent findings from WGS in the 100,000 Genome project. Cambridge (UK): PHG Foundation; 2013.
30. Burke W, Evans BJ, Jarvik GP. Return of results: ethical and legal distinctions between research and clinical care. Wiley Online Library. Am J Med Genet Part C Semin Med Genet. 2014;166C:105–11.
31. Vayena E, Tasioulas J. Genetic incidental findings: autonomy regained? Genet Med. 2013;15(11):868–70.
32. Ross LF, Rothstein MA, Clayton EW. Mandatory extended searches in all genome sequencing:"incidental findings," patient autonomy, and shared decision making. JAMA. 2013;310(4):367–8.
33. Conley J. ACMG backs down a bit. Genomics law report. 2014. http://www.genomicslawreport.com/index.php/2014/04/07/acmg-backs-down-a-bit/. Accessed 12 Aug 2014.
34. Klitzman R, Buquez B, Appelbaum PS, Fyer A, Chung WK. Processes and factors involved in decisions regarding return of incidental genomic findings in research. Genet Med. 2013;16:311–17.
35. Middleton A, Patch C, Wiggins J, Barnes K, Crawford G, Benjamin C, et al. Position statement on opportunistic genomic screening from the Association of Genetic Nurses and Counsellors (UK and Ireland). Eur J Hum Genet. 2014;22(8):955–6.
36. Presidential Commission for the Study of Bioethical Issues. Anticipate and communicate: ethical management of incidental secondary findings in the clinical, research and direct-to-consumer context. Washington: Presidential Commission for the Study of Bioethical Issues; 2013.
37. Ross LF, Saal HM, David KL, Anderson RR, American Academy of Pediatrics. Technical report: ethical and policy issues in genetic testing and screening of children. Genet Med. 2013;15(3):234–45.
38. Fallat ME, Katz AL, Mercurio MR, Moon MR, Okun AL, Webb SA, et al. Ethical and policy issues in genetic testing and screening of children. Pediatrics. 2013;131(3):620–2.
39. Clayton EW, McCullough LB, Biesecker LG, Joffe S, Ross LF, Wolf SM, et al. Addressing the ethical challenges in genetic testing and sequencing of children. Am J Bioeth. 2014;14(3):3–9.
40. Borry P, Stultiens L, Nys H, Cassiman JJ, Dierickx K. Presymptomatic and predictive genetic testing in minors: a systematic review of guidelines and position papers. Clin Genet. 2006;70(5):374–81.
41. Wilfond BS, Pelias MZ, Knoppers BM, Reilly PR, Wertz DC, Billings P, et al. Points to consider-ethical, legal, and psychosocial implications of genetic testing in children and adolescents. Chicago: University of Chicago Press; 1995.
42. Clarke A. The genetic testing of children. Working Party of the Clinical Genetics Society (UK). J Med Genet. 1994;31(10):785.

43. McDougall RJ, Notini L. Overriding parents' medical decisions for their children: a systematic review of normative literature. J Med Ethics. 2014;40(7):448–52.
44. McGuire AL, Joffe S, Koenig BA, Biesecker BB, McCullough LB, Blumenthal-Barby JS, et al. Point-counterpoint. Ethics and genomic incidental findings. Science (New York, NY). 2013;340(6136):1047–8.
45. Mand C, Gillam L, Duncan RE, Delatycki MB. "It was the missing piece": adolescent experiences of predictive genetic testing for adult-onset conditions. Genet Med. 2013;15(8):643–9.
46. American College of Medical Genetics and Genomics. Incidental findings in clinical genomics: a clarification. Genet Med. 2013;15(8):664–6.
47. Schoeman F. Parental discretion and children's rights: background and implications for medical decision-making. J Med Philos. 1985;10(1):45–62.
48. Davis DS. Genetic dilemmas and the child's right to an open future. Rutgers Law J. 1997;28:549.
49. Feinberg J. A child's right to an open future. In: Aiken W, LaFollete H, editors. Whose child? Parental rights, parental authority and state power. Totowa: Rowman and Littlefield; 1980. p. 124–53.
50. O'Neill O. Some limits of informed consent. J Med Ethics. 2003;29(1):4–7.
51. Pinxten W, Howard HC. Ethical issues raised by whole genome sequencing. Best Pract Res Clin Gastroenterol. 2014;28(2):269–79.
52. McGuire AL, Beskow LM. Informed consent in genomics and genetic research. Annu Rev Genomics Hum Genet. 2010;11:361.
53. Ayuso C, Millán JM, Mancheño M, Dal-Ré R. Informed consent for whole-genome sequencing studies in the clinical setting. Proposed recommendations on essential content and process. Eur J Hum Genet. 2013;21(10):1054–9.
54. Council of Europe. Additional protocol to the convention on human rights and biomedicine, concerning genetic testing for health purposes. 2008. http://conventions.coe.int/Treaty/en/Treaties/Html/203.htm Accessed 6 April 2015
55. Bick D, Dimmock D. Whole exome and whole genome sequencing. Curr Opin Pediatr. 2011;23(6):594–600.
56. Berg JS, Khoury MJ, Evans JP. Deploying whole genome sequencing in clinical practice and public health: meeting the challenge one bin at a time. Genet Med. 2011;13(6):499–504.
57. Bunnik EM, Janssens ACJW, Schermer MH. Informed consent in direct-to-consumer personal genome testing: the outline of a model between specific and generic consent. Bioethics. 2014;28(7):343–51.
58. Bunnik EM, Janssens ACJ, Schermer MH. A tiered-layered-staged model for informed consent in personal genome testing. Eur J Hum Genet. 2012;21(6):596–601.
59. Bradbury AR, Patrick-Miller L, Domchek S. Multiplex genetic testing: reconsidering utility and informed consent in the era of next-generation sequencing. Genet Med. 2015;17(2):97–8.
60. Kaye J, Whitley EA, Lund D, Morrison M, Teare H, Melham K. Dynamic consent: a patient interface for twenty-first century research networks. Eur J Hum Genet. 2014;23:141–6.
61. Borry P, Cornel MC, Howard HC. Where are you going, where have you been: a recent history of the direct-to-consumer genetic testing market. J Community Genet. 2010;1(3):101–6.
62. Howard HC, Borry P. Is there a doctor in the house? J Community Genet. 2012;3(2):105–12.
63. Hogarth S, Javitt G, Melzer D. The current landscape for direct-to-consumer genetic testing: legal, ethical, and policy issues. Annu Rev Genomics Hum Genet. 2008;9:161–82.
64. Wright CF, Gregory-Jones S. Size of the direct-to-consumer genomic testing market. Genet Med. 2010;12(9):594.
65. Pathway genomics. 2014. https://www.pathway.com/dna-reports/health-conditions-dna-insight. Accessed 1 Sept 2014.
66. Ilumina. 2014. http://res.illumina.com/documents/products/gene_lists/gene_list_trugenome_predisposition_screen.pdf. Accessed 9 Sept 2014.
67. Gene planet. 2014. http://www.geneplanet.com/genetic-analysis/list-of-analyses.html/. Accessed 9 Sept 2014.
68. Gentle. 2014. https://results.gentlelabs.com/categories. Accessed 1 Sept 2014.

69. Genetics and Public Policy Center. 2011. http://www.dnapolicy.org/resources/DTCAug2011byDiseasecategory.pdf. Accessed 1 Sept 2014.
70. Marietta C, McGuire AL. Currents in contemporary ethics. J Law Med Ethics. 2009;37(2):369–74.
71. McBride CM, Wade CH, Kaphingst KA. Consumers' views of direct-to-consumer genetic information. Annu Rev Genomics Hum Genet. 2010;11:427–46.
72. ter Meulen V, Boccia S, Cornel M, Delpech M, De Paepe A, Estivill X, et al. "Direct-to-consumer genetic testing for health-related purposes in the European Union." EASAC Policy Report 18, 2012.
73. Becker F, van El CG, Ibarreta D, Zika E, Hogarth S, Borry P, et al. Genetic testing and common disorders in a public health framework: how to assess relevance and possibilities. Eur J Hum Genet. 2011;19:S6–44.
74. Borry P, Henneman L. Debating the clinical utility of direct-to-consumer genetic testing for addiction susceptibility. Addiction. 2012;107(12):2076–7.
75. Klein C, Westenberger A. Genetics of Parkinson's disease. Cold Spring Harb Perspect Med. 2012;2(1):a008888.
76. Schneider SA, Klein C. What is the role of genetic testing in movement disorders practice? Curr Neurol Neurosci Rep. 2011;11(4):351–61.
77. European Society of Human Genetics. Statement of the ESHG on direct-to-consumer genetic testing for health-related purposes. Eur J Hum Genet. 2010;18(12):1271.
78. Human Genetics Commission. "A common framework of principles for direct-to-consumer genetic testing services." London: Human Genetics Commission, 2010.
79. Hauskeller C. Direct to consumer genetic testing. BMJ. 2011;342.

Chapter 23
Implications for Health and Life Insurances and Other Legal Aspects of Genetic Testing

Ida Ngueng Feze, Shahad Salman, and Yann Joly

Abstract Scientific breakthroughs have fostered the development of new genomic tools, which are generating an unprecedented amount of genetic data. This information has been a catalyst in the transition towards personalized medicine by rapidly becoming integrated to the health care and the research settings but also through the use of direct-to-consumer genetic services. Despite the wealth of perceived benefits in improved diagnosis, treatments, and preventive measures, concerns continue to be raised about the use of genetic information for nontherapeutic purposes and genetic discrimination in the context of insurance. As various neurologists and researchers in movement disorder genetics are increasingly being solicited to assist patients to deal with these concerns, they are confronted with the changing landscape of ethical and legal issues and facing a need for additional knowledge and resources about the implications that genetics may have on the insurability of patients and their family members.

Keywords Direct-to-consumer • Duty to disclose • Family history • Genetic discrimination • Genetic testing • Insurance • Movement disorders

Introduction

As research progresses, scientific breakthroughs in genetics and related fields and the developments of new genomic tools such as next-generation sequencing or genome-wide association studies have generated an unprecedented amount of genetic information. This important volume of genetic data has been a catalyst force for the transition towards personalized medicine, thereby contributing to further our understanding of the nature and causes of diseases, improving current tools, and developing new instruments to prevent, screen, and treat diseases [15, 42, 68, 92]. This information has also been facilitating the prediction of risks for future diseases,

I. Ngueng Feze, BA, JD, LLM • S. Salman, LLB, JD, LLM • Y. Joly, DCL (PhD) (✉)
Faculty of Medicine, Department of Human Genetics, Centre of Genomics and Policy, McGill University, Montreal H3A 0G1, Canada
e-mail: yann.joly@mcgill.ca

S.A. Schneider, J.M.T. Brás (eds.), *Movement Disorder Genetics*,
DOI 10.1007/978-3-319-17223-1_23

providing valuable information to patients for their reproductive decision-making and assisting in the development, selection, and dosing of newer, improved, or alternative medications [20, 54, 68, 106].

There are currently more than 1,500 single and multifactorial conditions that can be genetically tested, with most developments concerning common diseases [20]. Among those, some genetic tests are capable of detecting gene mutations responsible for a number of late-onset neurodegenerative conditions and can even be used to predict the future health status of individuals at risk before they develop a condition [43]. With proper translation into practice, the data derived from recent developments may potentially have further significant implications in the context of neurogenetics research and thereby foster an accelerated availability of newer neuropreventive, neuroprotective, neurorestorative, and gene-specific diagnostic instruments and treatments [56, 103].

Despite these perceived benefits, the use of genetic information by third parties outside of the clinical or research context has been at the heart of an ongoing ethical and legal debate for the past three decades, since the publication of the first report by Billings et al. in the late 1980s [7, 27, 49]. With the unprecedented amount of genetic data being generated and its increasing availability, concerns have brought further attention to the potential occurrence of "genetic discrimination." Genetic discrimination is the possibility that genetic information used for nontherapeutic purposes may serve to discriminate against an individual or a segment of the population based on their genetic makeup, thereby preventing them from accessing important social goods such as insurance, employment, or housing.

Patients have expressed concerns that their genetic information may be used by insurers to discriminate them or their family members and have consequently declined recommended clinical genetic testing or participation in genomic research [4, 34, 39, 55]. Reports on the fear of genetic discrimination have emerged internationally [34, 80, 90, 93, 95, 115]. Instances of discriminatory practices against individuals tested for or with a family history of Huntington's disease (Huntington) have been widely documented [10, 24, 51, 64]. This may also explain, in part, why the number of individuals undertaking presymptomatic genetic testing for Huntington has remained low [78]. Similar reports of perceived discrimination or fear thereof have also been noted with patients at risk for Alzheimer's disease [24, 61, 117] and other autosomal dominant adult-onset neuromuscular disorders [12]. Genetic information derived from genetic tests capable of indicating or predicting a major neurological disorder or a susceptibility to a neurological disorder has been considered highly sensitive so to require specific written consent from patients to prevent potential violation of confidentiality and protect privacy [30]. In this context, given the highly invasive nature of these types of disorders, genetic test results may be a significant source of additional psychosocial harm due to knowledge of diagnosis, carrier status, or the risk for potential stigmatization or discrimination [43, 104]. However, aside from few well-known highly penetrant, adult-onset monogenic conditions, data supporting a systemic discriminatory use of genetic information in life insurance and other forms of personal insurance (except for health insurance) has been scarce or difficult to interpret [51].

The fear of genetic discrimination is a complex, multifaceted ethical, psychosocial, and legal phenomenon that health professionals are increasingly being called to address. For example, genetic counselors have been recommended to address matters concerning personal insurance with their patients [98]. The incidence and fear of genetic discrimination may create significant barriers to clinical care and genetic research. This can potentially compromise the prospect of a fair and equitable delivery of personalized medicine, if selected individuals are excluded from these benefits due to genetic discrimination.

This chapter presents an overview of some of the issues and practical considerations that health professionals in the context of movement disorders may encounter or take into account when being called to address concerns or incidents related to genetics and personal insurance.

Context

Concepts and Definitions

Genetic information may be derived and given differing considerations and values depending on a country's particular sociocultural and legal context. Consequently, defining genetic information has also proven to be a challenging task for health professionals, researchers, and policymakers alike as it may result in definitions being too narrow and restrictive or too broad [99]. For instance, the *Genetic Information Nondiscrimination Act* (GINA) adopted in the United States defines genetic information broadly as information about an individual's genetic tests, the genetic tests of family members, or the occurrence of a disease in family members of an individual [32]. The relevance of genetic information for insurance underwriting may also be influenced by the context from which the information is derived, including family history, DNA test, and genetic test results derived in the context of clinical care, research, or through the use of direct-to-consumer (DTC) Internet services [100]. These sources of genetic data have varying degrees of reliability. For example, genetic information obtained in the context of research may not meet analytical validity, clinical validity, and utility or raise substantial ethical or legal issues [23, 59]. DTC genetic services also seem to suffer from the same lack of validity or raise additional ethical questions [14, 25, 45, 114].

It has been apprehended that genetic information could be used outside of the therapeutic context to discriminate against individuals. This has been commonly referred to as genetic discrimination, which may be defined as the differential treatment of an individual on the basis of her/his genetic makeup [94]. Genetic discrimination has also been defined differently based on a social, ethical, legal, cultural, or scholarly context or perspective [51]. In the legal context, for example, differential treatment is referred to as "legal-illegal (illicit) discrimination" [89]. It is important to note here that genetic discrimination in the context of personal insurance is not necessarily illegal as the use of questions related to health, family history, or genetic information may be permitted by national laws in some countries [58, 66]. Moreover, from the perspectives of insurers, "rational actuarial discrimination" or the differential treatment of individuals based on their health risks is considered an integral part of the underwriting process through which insurability (the eligibility to insurance coverage) and premium amounts are established [73, 86]. Given that such treatment must also be justified by actuarial data applied objectively and consistently [2], it could be argued that not integrating genetic data may in itself constitute or result in actuarial inaccuracies or improper discrimination [50]. Insurers claim that preventing them from requesting or accessing such information, when available to patients, may result in adverse selection and could potentially threaten the viability of the insurance market.

Essentially, adverse selection occurs when companies incur higher costs than anticipated due to an important number of high-risk applicants purchasing insurance without disclosing their risk information or when insurers have the information but are not able to require that such applicants pay higher premiums [35, 67]. In spite of the concerns raised by the industry, multiple reports have demonstrated that preventing insurers from having access to genetic data has or will have no significant economic impact on the insurance market [44, 71, 72].

Differential treatments based on genetic information may potentially expose patients to stressful situations including being found ineligible for insurance coverage, required to pay higher premium amount, or presented with exclusionary clauses in their insurance contracts. Genetic discrimination, real, perceived, or anticipated, may also constitute an additional source of anxiety and psychosocial harms for patients and their family members [11, 12, 31, 80]. The risk of being exposed to genetic discrimination may affect patients differently depending on their insurance needs and presence of siblings or children but also according to the type of insurance they presently have or seek (life, health, disability, etc.) and the type of plan concerned (life term, specific term, etc.) [94]. Ultimately, when confronted with issues of genetics and personal insurance, patients and sometimes family members at risk will turn to health professionals for assistance on how to cope, deal with, or avoid genetic discrimination.

Strategies Addressing Patients' Concerns about Genetic Discrimination

Due to numerous concerns about the potential impact that genetic test results and pharmacogenetics testing may have on their patient's insurability, health professionals have proposed a variety of coping strategies aimed at assisting patients with concerns, fears, or incidence of genetic discrimination. These include paying out of pocket rather than billing the insurer for genetic testing or undergoing anonymous genetic testing [74, 94, 116]. Given the significant number of those strategies, this section will review three main approaches from which ethical and legal issues may arise: advising patients to secure insurance coverage before testing, withholding information from third parties, and the issues that health professionals may face when patients ask them about genetic profiles obtained through the use of DTC genetic services.

It is important to note that strategies aimed to avoid genetic discrimination or alleviate patients' concerns will be most relevant in countries where no laws, policies, or voluntary agreements exist to prevent or prohibit genetic discrimination. These strategies may nevertheless be of relevance in countries such as the United States, where specific legal protections against genetic discrimination are limited to a particular insurance type or context.

Securing Insurance Before Undergoing Genetic Testing

A frequent suggestion made by health professionals to patients concerned with how genetic testing may impact their insurability is to secure all insurance needs especially life, disability, and long-term care before undergoing genetic testing [35, 52, 57, 94]. This strategy has been used to assist patients concerned about potential genetic discrimination or negative impacts on their insurability or that of their family members to avoid negative differential treatments. Nonetheless, studies on insurance application forms have revealed that insurers routinely ask applicants about test results, their visits to health professionals, and advice received about certain diseases, including recommendations to undergo genetic testing, pending testing, and even testing being contemplated [70, 75, 76, 84]. In fact, as genetic information has been increasingly more available, insurance application forms have started to include questions that are more "searching" notably by seeking information about the test that the applicant has been recommended to undergo and visits that the applicant has made to other health professionals aside from physicians (this may include genetic counselors or geneticists). This new line of questioning from insurers may be used to deter applicants from purchasing insurance before test results are available or, when applicable, to prevent applicants from escaping their duty to disclose test results [87, 88].

Patients advised to secure insurance needs before undergoing genetic testing may have to declare on insurance proposition forms that they have been advised to undergo such test, thereby potentially defeating the anticipated aim of the strategy. These types of questions have been criticized for their intrusiveness and the potential conflict they may create by deterring patients from seeking valuable medical advice for fear of having to declare it on an insurance application form and seeing their insurability being negatively impacted [70, 84]. In fact, the Council of Europe has expressed its opposition to questions that are too vague and that may result in insurance applicants disclosing more than what would be needed for insurance underwriting purposes [22]. As we will see in greater detail in our section discussing the duty to disclose, the legal framework has an important impact on what insurers can ask and whether they are allowed to collect genetic information depending on applicable laws and policies.

Thus, health professionals should be cognizant, when advising patients to secure insurance needs before testing, that patients may be required to disclose to the insurer that they have been recommended to undergo genetic testing as insurance questionnaires ought to be answered truthfully.

Withholding Information from Insurers

Electronic health records have been increasingly used by clinicians to ensure that patients receive the full benefits that personalized medicine has to offer and to facilitate a more efficient collection, documentation, and interpretation of genetic information for clinical decision-making, disease risk assessment and diagnosis, drug therapy, and dose selection [85]. With this standardization of data collection, issues surrounding the use of, security of, and access to genetic information and family history have remained a concern for patients and health professionals alike, notably in the apprehension of genetic discrimination [102]. Genetic data is often kept separate from other clinical data and is therefore most frequently sent to clinicians in separate narrative reports requiring a manual search for information outside the electronic health record [111]. Since information entered into electronic health medical records is virtually impossible to remove, patients and their support groups have been requesting physicians and other health professionals to exclude genetic information from the medical record and/or to use "shadow charts" (parallel medical charts not integrated in the patient's medical record) [12, 57, 94]. Responding to patients' concerns as well as their own, health professionals have used different approaches to withhold information from third parties including voluntarily excluding information from medical records, keeping separate files, or even encoding information using broad generic terms rather than specific diagnoses [33]. These practices have also raised additional ethical questions including the scope and significance of the genetic information being excluded (e.g., whether family member's genetic test results and risks be excluded), how such exclusion should be done, whether it should be documented, and whether insurers should be informed that data has been excluded from the medical record [57].

While excluding information from the health record may seem to address concerns of privacy and fear of genetic discrimination, it also poses some medical risks for the patient and exposes health professionals to ethical and legal sanctions. Indeed, for movement disorders such as myotonic dystrophy or other rare conditions, if a patient is treated by another physician who does not have access to the information excluded from the medical record, this withholding may lead to clinicians potentially missing a diagnosis, ordering unnecessary tests, or even jeopardizing the patient's treatment in case of an emergency situation [29, 57]. By excluding or disguising information in the medical records, health professionals may be reinforcing the fear that genetic test results are indeed a cause for discrimination. This directly undermines the principle function of the medical record, which is to serve as a vehicle for continued care for patients [57]. Moreover, disguising or excluding genetic information from the medical record may also have some dire repercussions for health professionals as such conduct raises some ethical and professional issues as well as potential legal liability depending on institutional protocols and local laws [28, 57]. The risk for professional and legal sanctions may cause some physicians to insist on documenting medical results and refuse patients' requests that genetic information be omitted from their medical records [57]. In turn, such potential refusal may lead patients to turn to DTC genetic services.

Impact of Genetic Profiles from Direct-to-Consumer Testing

The democratization of scientific knowledge to the general public has seen the recent sprawling of companies offering low-cost, DTC genetic testing via the Internet [103]. These services include testing for movement disorders that are not currently offered in some national health services [8]. For instance, the company 23andMe offers a variety of tests (carrier status or disease risk) for disorders including restless leg syndrome, Tourette syndrome, essential tremor, tardive dyskinesia, and Parkinson disease [104]. Regulatory pressures to regulate these new services have called for the requirement that physicians be more involved [19]. The widespread availability of DTC services has also brought awareness about genetics among specialist physicians outside of primary care providers [81].

As DTC companies are directing patients to seek assistance from their healthcare providers to discuss their genetic profile, physicians, genetic counselors, or even neurologists and other health professionals may have a responsibility to discuss this information with their patients [96]. However, a significant number of health professionals have reported lacking sufficient knowledge about genetics, genetic testing, genetic counseling, and whole-genome scanning and do not feel prepared to answer patients' questions about DTC genetic testing [36, 38, 96, 108]. Moreover, it should be remembered that the vast majority of DTC results currently available do not meet the threshold of analytical validity, clinical validity, and utility. In this context, interpreting or filtering the actionable results from the rest of the data will be challenging even for experts [104, 112].

While adequate training and additional resources will be required to properly evaluate the validity and relevance of genetic profiles obtained from DTC genetic testing, health professionals should advise patients that obtaining such information may also have an impact on their insurability. In fact, these DTC genetic profiles may not only have an impact on a patient's ability to obtain personal insurance but may also have implications for the insurability of other family members [77]. Genetic information, even when obtained in the context of DTC genetic services, may be considered part of family history, which is taken into consideration when assessing an application's health risk through insurance underwriting (for more details, see infra Section "The Impact of Family History Versus Genetic Test Results" on the implications of family history).

Points to Consider when Addressing Concerns About Genetics and Personal Insurance

In light of the genetic discrimination debate, some countries have adopted a variety of laws and policies to prevent insurers from having access to genetic information, while others have preferred to maintain the status quo by not adopting any legislation specific to genetic discrimination [49]. Issues about genetics and personal insurance are thus specific to the national legal context where health professionals practice. Consequently, physicians and healthcare providers in general should have a good understanding of current applicable national and regional legal protections and of their limitations.

Introduction to the Applicable Legal Frameworks and Principles

Countries have adopted a plethora of laws and various strategies to address genetic discrimination that fall into five main approaches: human rights, prohibitive, limitative, moratorium, and status quo [101]. On the international and regional levels, different institutions such as the Council of Europe have adopted human rights norms including genetic characteristics as an unlawful ground of discrimination [21]. At the national level, for instance, countries such as France, Belgium, Germany, and Norway have adopted laws that prohibit or limit insurers' access or use of genetic information [105]. In the United States, a similar restrictive approach has also been adopted but only in health insurance and employment, not applicable to life, disability, or critical illness types of coverage [32]. Other countries, such as Sweden, have opted for legislation aiming to limit the use of genetic information by insurers only for insurance policies beyond a certain value provided in the legislation, thereby following a limitative or a "fair limits" approach [49, 109]. Other countries have also implemented alternative or mixed approaches. The United Kingdom provided an alternative to legislation by implementing voluntary agreements (i.e., moratoria and concordat) between the government and the insurance industry limiting the use of genetic data in insurance underwriting [90]. Lastly, some countries, such as Canada and Australia, have maintained a legal status quo and chose not to adopt any specific legislation addressing genetic discrimination, as they presently consider genetic information like any other type of medical data and rely on general nondiscrimination and privacy mechanisms to address potential issues [49].

In sum, countries have opted for different legislative or policy options to prohibit or mitigate the consequences of the use of genetic information by insurers. However, limited data or legal cases are available in these countries to assess the effectiveness of the different avenues they have adopted [101]. Meanwhile, health professionals need accurate and up-to-date information about their local legal context in order to provide patients with adequate help and understand the available alternatives that can guide their patients through the fear of genetic discrimination, especially in countries that have maintained a status quo approach and have not provided specific protections.

Understanding the Local Legal Context

Legal protections and policies are unique to the jurisdiction where the health professional is located. A lack of knowledge about genetic discrimination and applicable legal protections may have an impact on physicians' perspective and attitude towards genetic discrimination and willingness to refer patients for genetic testing [27, 46]. Therefore, it is important that physicians be familiar with current local legislation in their country (and/or state) in order to be in a position to explain and discuss them with patients considering genetic testing. Relevant points include information about current legal protections against genetic discrimination and their limitations and the uncertainty related to other applicable protections (privacy laws or human rights instruments) that have not yet been tested or could become problematic in the near future [94, 98, 110]. Voluntary policies adopted by the insurance industry may also be relevant to such discussions [26]. In Canada, where no specific anti-genetic discrimination laws exist, the insurance industry has adopted a policy not to require insurance applicants to undergo genetic testing. However, the applicants are still required to disclose the results of any genetic test already undertaken at the time of the conclusion of the contract [16]. In the United Kingdom, the industry has adopted a voluntary moratorium not to use genetic information for insurance policies under a certain value; this agreement has been sanctioned by the government [49, 101].

Local laws may have a direct impact on patients' rights but also on physicians' ethical and legal duties. For instance, the *Code of Medical Ethics of the American Medical Association* states that physicians may have to maintain separate files for genetic testing results in order to ensure that such results are not sent to health insurance companies and, that in such cases, the insurer should be notified that some data have been withheld [3]. Engaging in practices that depart from the code of ethics may trigger sanctions of varying degrees from institutional or professional disciplinary actions to legal liability (malpractice) depending on the local legal context [57]. This is especially relevant when patients concerned by genetic discrimination request that information be withheld from insurers or from medical records.

Nongenetic health specialists are often less knowledgeable about legal protections in place in their country or state, but even genetic health professionals have also been reported to lack knowledge of applicable protection and their limitations [46, 60]. For example, in the United States, despite the major debate surrounding genetic discrimination and the adoption of GINA, many health professionals still lack basic knowledge about the enactment, content, and limits of the legislation [91]. This denotes the need for further continued training and additional resources and tools for all professionals as well as patients [96]. Incomplete, inaccurate, or misleading information may have significant consequences for patients, especially in jurisdictions where patients are required to disclose certain information to insurers.

Patients and Research Participants' Duty to Disclose Information to Insurers

Generally, the duty to disclose requires that patients applying for insurance provide all relevant information known to them at the time of the application to the insurer in order for the latter to provide coverage amount based on a fair assessment of the applicant's risk. When applicable, this duty has been expressed in a similar manner in different jurisdictions. For example, in Canada, provincial insurance laws have similar requirements that an insurance applicant ought to disclose all the facts known to him which are likely to materially influence an insurer's decision to cover the health risk [47, 97]. In Australia, the *Insurance Contracts Act* requires "to disclose to the insurer every matter that you know, or could reasonably be expected to know, that is relevant to the insurer's decision…" [48]. The disclosure process is facilitated by the insurance proposition form but is not limited to this document as applicants may have to share additional information through other means such as conversations with the insurance representative. Additionally, applicants who have knowledge concerning health risk not specifically asked about on an application form may nevertheless be required to disclose it to the insurer.

Health professionals have often had difficulties translating the full extent of this obligation to their patients. For example, some patients have been told not to disclose test results or that they could lie on application forms, while others were reminded that lying on insurance forms may be considered fraudulent behavior [4, 94].

Patients who fail to comply with their insurance disclosure obligation may see their life insurance contract annulled by the courts at the request of the insurer. Some may argue that there is room to debate about whether genetic information can be deemed relevant for insurance underwriting [35, 57]. While it may well be the case, particularly for genetic information obtained from genetic research or DTC genetic services, in the context of clinical genetic testing for monogenic conditions such as Huntington, the relevance of the genetic results for underwriting could be more easily argued. However, from an ethical standpoint, barring access to a vulnerable population group (individuals at risk of developing Huntington) from the pool of insurable individuals is problematic given the increasingly important social role played by insurance in contemporary society.

An illustration of a contract cancelation due to a failure to disclose genetic information has been seen in the Province of Quebec, Canada, in the case of *Audet c. Industrielle-Alliance* [5]. In this matter, Mr. Tremblay was identified as a mutation gene carrier for Steinert's disease (myotonic dystrophy type 1) in 1980. Upon learning of his carrier status and in light of the fact that his father and brother had both been affected by the disease, Mr. Tremblay and his wife decided not to have any children for fear they could transmit the gene. When he went to purchase a life insurance policy 7 years later, Mr. Tremblay failed to disclose his carrier status to the insurance broker and negatively responded to a question on the insurance application form asking whether he had any physical or mental anomalies. A year later, Mr. Tremblay passed away in a car accident, and the payment of the insurance benefits became the object of a court dispute about whether fraud or a failure to disclose had rendered the contract null and void. The Court sided with the insurer in a brief opinion that considered the following facts: Mr. Tremblay failed to disclose his carrier status, was already symptomatic when he applied for insurance, and had personal knowledge of the particularities of the disease having two affected family members. The court estimated that these elements were sufficient to amount to a failure on Mr. Tremblay's part to meet the requirements of the duty to disclose. While this is the only case in Canada attesting of the annulment of an insurance contract on such basis, this case also provides some indication as to how neurological diseases were considered by insurers at the time. Indeed, during this trial, two insurers declared that if they had had knowledge of his carrier status for Steinert's disease or the fact that he was affected by the disease at the time of the application, he would have been denied coverage or imposed a premium higher by at least 300 %.

Genetic testing was also at the center of a more recent Canadian case involving, Ms. Adacsi, a surviving guest at a house that caught fire, killing three persons. In the matter of *Adacsi* v *Amin*, when Ms. Adacsi requested that her injuries and inability to return to work be compensated under the house owner's insurance for damages, genetic testing became at issue. Given Ms. Adacsi's family history of Huntington, the insurer requested that she submit to a genetic test to determine the appropriate amount of damages that should be paid. Upon her refusal to submit to the test, the courts held that it was in fact proper for an insurer to require a beneficiary to submit to a genetic test when her health status is in direct relation with the amount of damages to be paid. Ms. Adacsi appealed the judgment requiring her to undergo genetic testing. When confirming the previous decision to require her to undergo testing, the appellate court judge noted that while the genetic test could not determine whether her symptoms could be attributed to Huntington rather than the fire, it would nevertheless indicate whether Huntington could be ruled out as a possible contributor [1]. Ms Adacsi's appeal of this later decision was not entertained by the Supreme Court of Canada. This case also illustrates how issues of genetics can manifest in a variety of ways and may involve different types of insurance products.

These two cases are vivid examples of the importance of genetic information in insurance processes. The *Audet* case particularly illustrates how the duty to disclose is related to the personal knowledge that the applicant has when applying for insurance (this may also be the case at the time of renewal depending on the insurance contract). So while some patients may turn to DTC services in order to avoid having their genetic profile included in their medical record, obtaining genetic information that way may nevertheless place them at risk to be required to disclose such genetic information on some insurance forms [19, 84, 115]. Indeed, studies have demonstrated that insurers use broad open-ended questions that may require the disclosure of genetic information obtained outside of clinical care (which could include DTC test results) [70, 84]. These types of questions are aimed at soliciting a broad disclosure of information.

Knowledge of genomic information may also bring unwanted ethical dilemmas about sharing such information with family members and other relatives not genetically related (i.e., spouse, dependents) as such information may also have an impact on their health and insurability [19]. For example, insurance forms may also assess the health risks of additional individuals included on the request for coverage such as a spouse or dependents who are not genetically related to the applicant [84]. Thus, a spouse who learns of a genetic risk may be required to disclose it to his/her spouse when they apply for insurance or when being added to an existing policy. In this respect, the duty to disclose may constitute an important barrier to the sharing of information among family members, especially in cases such as Huntington where incidence of insurance discrimination has been widely documented [9, 24, 51, 63]. These concerns may require that health professionals, such as neurologists, adapt their clinical interaction. From an approach traditionally exclusively focused on the individual patient, they should adopt a broader perspective to improve family communication by viewing the family and not just the patient as the unit of care in the context of genetics [82].

The local legal context provides the framework for the ongoing provision of genetic services in compliance with patients' and health professionals' rights and obligations. The growing interest and utilization of personalized medicine by clinicians outside the field of genetics will be accompanied by more discussions concerning the socio-ethical issues related to genetics and personal insurance [46]. Hence, health professionals ought to be cautious when discussing patients' legal rights and obligations as providing them with imprecise, inaccurate, or incomplete information could have some legal repercussions on their insurance contract and could even result in their policy being canceled.

Ultimately, when in doubt, genetic counselors have suggested seeking advice from other health professionals (physician-geneticists, experienced genetic counselors, or ethics committee) or refer patients to other professionals, such as insurance broker when patients have additional questions or concerns [12, 79]. While referring patients to seek assistance from insurance brokers may enable them to obtain and compare insurance information, they should be reminded that brokers represent the insurer's interests. Alternatively, concerned patients may also be referred to seek the advice of an attorney even if this option may be costly.

It is primordial that health professionals have reliable and up-to-date information in order to comprehend and address their patients' concerns. This requires that appropriate, practical resource tools on genetic and insurance are developed and made available to all stakeholders. Without the availability of such toolbox, health professionals will face a number of challenges trying to stay abreast of relevant applicable legal developments in their country, and the anxiety of patients and their family members may not be effectively reduced. Equipped with the proper tools, health professionals will be in a position to ensure that patients seeking genetic services are made aware of their duty to disclose, the available legal protections and remedies, as well as the potential limitations of the laws. This will avoid legal imbroglio and uncertainties that could make patients and research participants more anxious towards genetic testing.

Before and Beyond Genetic Testing: Other Implications of Genetics and Personal Insurance

The Fear of Genetic Discrimination

The fear of genetic discrimination is an important psychosocial factor that must be taken into consideration by health professionals being called to assist patients concerned about genetics and personal insurance [113]. This fear has been well documented in various reports attesting that it causes patients to decline clinically recommended testing or participation in genomic research or even lead them to undergo testing anonymously [4, 6, 34, 40, 41, 53]. The fear of genetic discrimination may not be related only to the actual incidence of discrimination. Media such as television, radio, magazines, and newspapers have the ability to influence the public's perception of the benefits or risks associated with genetics [18]. For example, the phenomenon called "genohype" captures the potential that media have to distort the risks and benefits of genetic research and create inflated public perceptions, which has been suggested to have an impact on the public's ability to participate in policy discussions or to utilize genetic services [13]. The fear of genetic discrimination may also stem from the narratives of past incidents being shared and passed on in families or communities. For example, in the Netherlands where a moratorium has been in place since the early 1990s and where test results from medical examination do not have to be disclosed in order to acquire life or disability insurance below a certain value [100], a recent study attested that these narratives of past incidents of discrimination may play a part in the persistence of the fear of discrimination [31]. Genetic counselors have often had to inform patients about the actual documented incidence of discrimination, which is usually rather low, to alleviate their anxiety [94].

When addressing issues of genetics and personal insurance, perceptions and knowledge of health professionals may also play an important role in evaluating the risk of discrimination or referring patients for genetic testing, which may either reassure or further underline patients' concerns. Nongenetics clinicians may have a gap in knowledge compared to genetics practitioners, and their practice could be influenced by their perception of genetic discrimination and their knowledge of legislative protections and published cases of insurance discrimination [46]. For example, primary care providers and other non-cancer professionals who had limited knowledge of legislative protection estimate the risk of genetic discrimination to be high in comparison with health professionals within the genetics field who are knowledgeable about these issues [27, 69, 83]. Health professionals therefore need access to proper training and appropriate tools about the incidence of genetic discrimination in their country in order to be able to more efficiently evaluate patients' fear and provide them with up-to-date, accessible information.

The fear of genetic discrimination, or concerns about genetic testing, may also create additional anxiety and psychosocial harms [103]. It is thus important that health professionals have an understanding of how the fear of genetic discrimination may affect their patients from a practical perspective as well as an emotional stand [20]. This psychological assessment may even require the assistance of other health professionals such as psychologists [12, 43, 79].

The Impact of Family History Versus Genetic Test Results

While patients may focus their attention on the potential negative impacts that genetic testing may have on their insurability, they are often not aware that family history may be even more informative when estimating health risks for insurance underwriting purposes. For example, personal and family medical history information can be used to determine whether an individual/family has an average, modest, or increased health risk for a range of specific conditions or diseases (i.e., Huntington) [98, 103]. In fact, insurers consider detailed family history as an important source of genetic information which, in some cases, may constitute a more accurate prediction of future health than the results of many current genetic tests, and most of their actuarial models are derived from family history rather than genetic test results [37, 62, 107]. Hence, a genetic test may therefore be used to confirm health risks already underlined by family history disclosed in the patient's insurance application questionnaire. This is especially relevant in the context of neurodegenerative disorders where genetic test results are often inconclusive [103]. Certain countries that have adopted legislation restricting insurers' access to genetic test results continue to allow insurers to ask questions about family history in their insurance forms [65]. This underlines the legal, ethical, and practical challenges of attempting to segregate genetic information from other types of medical data [84]. Indeed, this challenge resides in the combination of several intricate elements: first, all medical information (including family history) may be considered to be in part related to genetics; second, suggesting that genetic information should require additional protection may lead to foster genetic exceptionalism (the notion that genetic information should be treated differently from other medical data) [99]; and third, considering a protection solely based on genetic information would be unfair to patients or persons with health risks related to family history or environmental factors rather than genetic information. Moreover, little is actually known as to how family history is being integrated in insurance underwriting processes in light of recent genomic developments in treatments, tools, and preventive measures. Experts have proposed that actuarial risk stratification models integrate genetic data from population biobank projects with other medical data (e.g., clinical trials and cohort studies) in order to refine and update current risk assessment models [50].

Conclusion

The current genomic era has seen unprecedented advances in the quantity and quality of genetic information being generated. These recent discoveries are expected to have a more significant impact in the context of movement disorders (beyond the few late-onset, highly penetrant monogenic conditions such as Huntington) in the years to come. As genomic profiling and genetic information are integrated in health records and routine care, it is inevitable that a growing number of health professionals including physicians outside the field of genetics, genetic counselors, or even neurologists be requested to assist with the interpretation of genetic information and genetic profiles as well as its potential implications on patients' insurability [46, 17, 19].

This chapter has provided an overview of some of the main ethical and legal issues that nongenetics health professionals may be faced with or have to consider when patients call upon them for assistance with concerns about genetic discrimination and personal insurance. First, the weakness of strategies commonly used to cope with or avoid discrimination based on genetic information such as advising patients to secure insurance before genetic testing or withholding information from third parties or medical records has been highlighted as they may no longer afford the benefits anticipated. Indeed, in the context where insurers are not barred from requesting genetic information, questionnaires have become much more searching, and information-withholding techniques may have significant detrimental impact on patients' care. In addition, the growing use of DTC genetic services has engaged health professionals outside of the field of genetics to deal with the clinical utility and validity of genomic profiles obtained in such context. Second, the availability of basic resources on the occurrence of genetic discrimination and the local legal context is paramount to ensure that health professionals and patients receive accurate and complete information about existing applicable legal protections and their limitations. These resource tools should also include information about available nonlegal alternatives, such as seeking additional guidance from an ethics committee or referring patients to other specialists (i.e., insurance broker, genetic counselor, or attorney). Patients should be made aware of the potentially more significant impact that other medical data such as family history may have on their insurability. Thus, the intricate expansion of genomics in the context of movement disorders will require, as with other areas of personalized medicine, the availability of professional training and well-conceived resource tools to prepare health professionals, physicians and neurologists in particular, to meet the multifaceted challenges of genetics and personal insurance.

Acknowledgment The authors would like to thank Laura Crimi at the Centre of Genomics and Policy for her valuable assistance in the preparation of this book chapter.

References

1. Adasci v Amin (Alberta). 2013 ABCA 315. 2013.
2. American Academy of Actuaries. Risk classification in voluntary life insurance. Issue Brief. Washington D.C: Spring; 1997. p. 1–4.
3. American Medical Association Code of medical ethics, Opinion 2.135 Insurance companies and genetic information. From http://www.ama-assn.org/ama/pub/physician-resources/medical-ethics/code-medical-ethics.page. Accessed 20 July 2014.

4. Armstrong K, Weber B, FitzGerald G, Hershey J, Pauly M, Lemaire J, Subramanian K, Asch D. Life insurance and breast cancer risk assessment: adverse selection, genetic testing decisions, and discrimination. Am J Med Genet. 2003;120A:359–64.
5. Audet v. Industrielle-Alliance (Quebec).. [1990] R.R.A. 500 (C.S.). 1990.
6. Baruch S, Hudson KL. Civilian and military genetics: non-discrimination policy in a post-GINA world. Am J Hum Genet. 2008;83(4):435–44.
7. Billings P, Khon M, De Cuevas M, Beckwith J, Alper J, Natowicz M. Discrimination as a consequence of genetic testing. Am J Hum Genet. 1992;50(3):476–82.
8. Boddington P. The ethics and regulation of direct-to-consumer genetic testing. Genome Medicine. 2009;1(7):71.
9. Bombard Y, Veenstra G, Friedman JM, Creighton S, Currie L, Paulsen JS, Bottorff JL, Hayden MR, Group TCR-HCR. Perceptions of genetic discrimination among people at risk for Huntington's disease: a cross sectional survey. BMJ. 2009;338:b2175.
10. Bombard Y, Palin J, Friedman JM, Veenstra G, Creighton S, Bottorff JL, Hayden MR, The Canadian Respond-HD Collaborative Research Group. Beyond the patient: the broader impact of genetic discrimination among individuals at risk of Huntington disease. Am J Med Genet. 2012;159B:217–26.
11. Bombard Y, Penziner E, Suchowersky O, Guttman M, Paulsen JS, Bottorff JL, Hayden MR. Engagement with genetic discrimination: concerns and experiences in the context of Huntington Disease. Eur J Hum Genet. 2008;16:279–89.
12. Bower MA, McCarthy Veach P, Bartels DM, LeRoy BS. A survey of genetic counselors' strategies for addressing ethical and professional challenges in practice. J Genet Couns. 2002;11(3):77–101.
13. Bubela T, Caulfield T. Do the print media "hype" genetic research? A comparison of newspaper stories and peer-reviewed research papers. Can Med Assoc J. 2004;170(9):1399–407.
14. Bunnick E, Schermer M, Janssens AC. Personal genome testing: test characteristics to clarify the. BMC Med Ethics. 2011;12:11.
15. Burke W, Psatsy B. Personalized medicine in the era of genomics. JAMA J Am Med Assoc. 2007;298:1682–4.
16. Canadian Life and Health Association Inc. CLHIA position statement on genetic testing. CLHIA. 2010. Online: http://www.clhia.ca/domino/html/clhia/clhia_lp4w_lnd_webstation.nsf/resources/Guidelines/$file/Genetic_Testing_CLHIA_Industry_Position_2010.pdf.
17. Cardinal G, Deschênes M. Surveying the population biobankers. In: Knoppers BM, editor. Populations and genetics – legal and socio-ethical perspectives. Leiden: Martinus Nijhoff Publishers; 2003. p. 37–94.
18. Caulfield T, Bubela T, Murdoch CJ. Myriad and the mass media: the covering of a gene patent controversy. Genet Med. 2007;9(12):850–5.
19. Chen DT, Sheperd LL. Advising patients about obtaining genomic profiles. Neurol Clin Pract. 2011;1(1):5–13.
20. Clifton JM, VanBeuge SS, Mladenka C, Wosnik KK. The genetic information nondiscrimination act 2008: what clinicians should understand. J Am Acad Nurse Pract. 2010;22(5):246–9.
21. Council of Europe. Convention for the protection of human rights and dignity of the human being with regards to the application of biology and medicine: convention on human rights and biomedicine. vol 4.IV.1997. Oviedo: Council of Europe. 1997. Available from http://conventions.coe.int/Treaty/en/Treaties/Html/164.htm. Last accessed 29 July 2014.
22. Council of Europe. Consultation document on predictivity, genetic testing and insurance. DH-BIO/INF (2012)1. 2012.
23. Dressler LG. Disclosure of research results from cancer genomic studies: state of the science. Clin Cancer Res. 2009;15:4270–6.
24. Erwin C, Williams JK, Juhl AR, Mengeling M, Mills JA, Bombard Y, Hayden MR, Quaid K, Shoulson I, Taylor S, Paulsen JS. Perception, experience, and response to genetic discrimination in Huntington disease: the International RESPOND-HD Study. Am J Med Genet. 2010;153B(5):1081–93.

25. European Society of Human Genetics. Statement of the ESHG on direct-to-consumer genetic testing for health-related purposes. Eur J Hum Genet. 2010;18(12):1272–3.
26. Investment and Financial Services Association Limited. Life insurance and genetic testing in Australia. Sydney: IFSA; 2002.
27. Freedman AN, Wideroff L, Olson L, Davis W, Klabunde C, Srinath KP, Reeve BB, Croyle RT, Ballard-Barbash R. US physicians' attitudes toward genetic testing for cancer susceptibility. Am J Med Genet. 2003;120A(1):63–71.
28. Freeman VG, Rathore SS, Weinfurt KP, Schulman KA, Sulmasy DP. Lying for patients: physicians deception of third-party payers. Arch Intern Med. 1999;159(19):2263–70.
29. Frucht SJ. Movement disorder emergencies: diagnosis and treatment. In: Current clinical neurology. 2nd ed. New York: Humana Press; 2013.
30. Gasser T, Bressman S, Dürr A, Hinggins J, Klockgether T, Myers RH. Molecular diagnostic of inherited movement disorders: movement disorders society task force on molecular diagnostic. Mov Disord. 2003;18(1):3–18.
31. Geelen E, Horstman K, Marcelis CL, Doevendans PA, Van Hoyweghen I. Unravelling fears of genetic discrimination: an exploratory study of Dutch HCM families in an era of genetic non-discrimination acts. Eur J Hum Genet. 2012;20:1018–23.
32. Genetic Information Nondiscrimination Act. United States. 2008.
33. Geppert CMA, Weiss RL. Protecting patient confidentiality in primary care. Semin Med Pract. 2000;3(1):7–14.
34. Godard B, Pratte A, Dumont M, Simard-Lebrun A, Simard J. Factors associated with an individual's decision to withdraw from genetic testing for breast and ovarian cancer susceptibility: implications for counseling. Genet Test. 2007;11(1):45–54.
35. Godard B, Raeburn S, Pembrey M, Bobrow M, Farndon P, Ayme S. Genetic information and testing in insurance and employment: technical, social and ethical issues. Eur J Hum Genet. 2003;11 Suppl 2:S123–42.
36. Greendale K, Pyeritz RE. Empowering primary care heath professional in medical genetics: how soon? How fast? how far? Am J Med Genet. 2001;106(3):223–32.
37. Guttmacher AE, Collins F, Carmona RH. The family history – more important than ever. New Engl J Med. 2004;351(22):2333–6.
38. Guttmacher AE, Jenkins J, Uhlmann WR. Genomic medicine: who will practice it? A call to arms. Am J Med Genet. 2001;106:216–22.
39. Hadley D, Jenkins J, Dimond E, Nakahara K, Grogan L, Liewehr D, Steinberg S, Kirsch I. Genetic testing in families with hereditary nonpolyposis colorectal cancer. Arch Intern Med. 2003;163(5):573–82.
40. Hall MA, McEwen JE, Barton JC, Walker AP, Howe EG, Reiss JA, Power TE, Ellis SD, Tucker DC, Harrison BW, McLaren GD, Ruggiero A, Thomson EJ. Concerns in a primary care population about genetic discrimination by insurers. Genet Med. 2005;7(5):311–6.
41. Hall MA, Rich SS. Genetic privacy laws and patients' fear of discrimination by health insurers: the view from genetic counselors. Am Soc Law Med Ethics. 2000;28:245–57.
42. Hamburg M, Collins F. The path to personalized medicine. New Engl J Med. 2010;363:301–4.
43. Hess PG, Preloran HM, Browner CH. Diagnostic genetic testing for fatal illness: the experience of patients with movement disorders. New Genet Soc. 2009;28(1):3–18.
44. Hoy M, Durnin M. The potential economic impact of a ban on the use of genetic information for life and health insurance. Ottawa: Office of the Privacy Commissioner of Canada; 2012.
45. Hudson K, Javitt G, Burke W, Byers P, ASHG Social Issues Committee. ASHG statement on direct-to-consumer genetic testing in the United States. Am J Hum Genet. 2007;81(3):635–7.
46. Huizenga CR, Lowstuter K, Banks KC, Lagos VI, Vandergon VO, Weitzel JN. Evolving perspectives on genetic discrimination in health insurance among health care providers. Fam Cancer. 2010;9(2):253–60.
47. Insurance Act. R.S.O. 1990, c. I-4. Ontario, Canada. 1990.
48. Insurance Contracts Act. 1984. http://www.austlii.edu.au/au/legis/cth/consol_act/ica1984220/s21.html, Australia.

49. Joly Y, Braker M, Le Huynh M. Genetic discrimination in private insurance: global perspectives. New Genet Soc. 2010;29(4):351–68.
50. Joly Y, Burton H, Knoppers BM, Ngueng Feze I, Dent T, Pashayan N, Chowdhury S, Foulkes W, Hall A, Hamet P, Kirwan N, Macdonald AS, Simard J, Van Hoyweghen I. Life insurance: genomic stratification and risk classification. Eur J Hum Genet. 2014;22:575–9.
51. Joly Y, Ngueng Feze I, Simard J. Genetic discrimination and life insurance: a systematic review of the evidence. BMC Med. 2013;11:25.
52. Keogh LA, Otlowski M. Life insurance and genetic test results: a mutation carrier's fight to achieve full cover. Med J Aust. 2013;199(5):263–6.
53. Keogh LA, van Vliet CM, Studdert DM, Maskiell JA, Macrae FA, St John DJ, Gaff CL, Young MA, Southey MC, Giles G, Rosenthal DA, Hopper JL, Jenkins MA. Is uptake of genetic testing for colorectal cancer influenced by knowledge of insurance implications? Med J Aust. 2009;191(5):255–8.
54. Kimmich O, Bradley D, Whelan R, Mulrooney N, Reilly RB, Hutchinson S, O'Riordan S, Hutchinson M. Sporadic adult onset primary torsion dystonia is a genetic disorder by the temporal discrimination test. Brain J Neurol. 2011;134(9):2656–63.
55. Kirkland SA, Raina PS, Wolfson C, Strople G, Kits O, Dukeshire S, Angus CL, Szala-Meneok K, Uniat J, Keshavarz H, Furlini L, Pelletier A. Exploring the acceptability and feasibility of conducting a large longitudinal population-based study in Canada. Can J Aging. 2009;28(3):231–42.
56. Klein C, Schlossmacher MG. The genetics of Parkinson disease: implications for neurological care. Nat Clin Pract Neurol. 2006;2(3):136–46.
57. Klitzman R. Exclusion of genetic information from the medical record: ethical and medical dilemmas. JAMA. 2010;304(10):1120–1.
58. Knoppers BM, Godard B, Joly Y. Life insurance and genetics: a comparative international overview. In: Rothstein MA, editor. Genetics and life insurance: medical underwriting and social policy. Cambridge: MIT Press; 2004. p. 173–94.
59. Knoppers BM, Joly Y, Simard J, Durocher F. The emergence of an ethical duty to disclose genetic research results: international perspectives. Eur J Hum Genet. 2006;14:1170–8.
60. Laedtke AL, O'Neill SM, Rubinstein W, Vogel KJ. Family physicians' awareness and knowledge of the genetic information non-discrimination act (GINA). J Genet Couns. 2012;21:345–52.
61. Lautenbach DM, Christensen KD, Sparks JA, Green RC. Communicating genetic risk information for common disorders in the era of genomic medicine. Annu Rev Genomics Hum Genet. 2013;14:491–513.
62. Lemaire J, Subramanian K, Armstrong K, Asch D. Pricing term insurance in the presence of a family history of breast or ovarian cancer. North Am Actuar J. 2000;4:75–87.
63. Lemke T. "A slap in the face". An exploratory study of genetic discrimination in Germany. Genomics Soc Policy. 2009;5(2):22–39.
64. Lemke T. Perspectives on genetic discrimination. New York: Routledge; 2013.
65. Lemmens T. Can insurance law accommodate the uncertainty associated with preliminary genetic information? Can Bar Rev. 2004;83:357–410.
66. Lemmens T, Joly Y, Knoppers BM. Genetic and life insurance: a comparative analysis. GenEdit. 2004;2(2):1–15.
67. Lemmens T, Pullman D, Rodal R. Revisiting genetic discrimination issues in 2010: policy options for Canada. Ottawa: GPS; 2010.
68. Lichtenberg FR. The effect of pharmaceutical innovation on longevity: patient level evidence from the 1996–2002 medical expenditure panel survey and linked mortality public-use files. Forum Health Econ Policy. 2013;16(1):1–33.
69. Lowstuter K, Sand S, Blazer KR, MacDonald DJ, Banks KC, Lee CA, Schwerin BU, Juarez M, Uman GC, Weitzel N. Influence of genetic discrimination perceptions and knowledge on cancer genetics referral practice among clinicians. Genet Med. 2008;10:691–8.
70. Lynch EL, Doherty RJ, Gaff CL, Macrae FA, Linderman GJ. "Cancer in the family" and genetic testing: implications for life insurance. Med J Aust. 2003;179:480–3.

71. Macdonald AS. The actuarial relevance of genetic information in the life and health insurance context. Ottawa: Office of the Privacy Commissioner; 2011.
72. Macdonald AS, Yu F. The impact of genetic information on the insurance industry: conclusion from the 'bottom-up' modeling programme. ASTIN Bullet J Int Actuarial Assoc. 2011;41(2):343–76.
73. Malpas PJ. Is genetic Information relevantly different from other kinds of non-genetic information in the life insurance context? J Med Ethics. 2007;34:548–51.
74. Matloff ET, Shappell H, Brierley K, Bernhardt BA, Mckinnon W, Peshkin BN. What would you do? Specialists' perspectives on cancer genetic testing, prophylactic surgery, and insurance discrimination. J Clin Oncol. 2000;18(12):2484–92.
75. McEwen JE, McCarthy C, Reilly PR. A survey of state insurance commissioners concerning genetic testing and life insurance. Am J Hum Genet. 1992;55:785–92.
76. McEwen JE, McCarthy K, Reilly PR. A survey of medical directors of life insurance companies concerning use of genetic testing and life insurance. Am J Hum Genet. 1993;55: 33–45.
77. National Health and Medical Research Council. Discussing direct-to-consumer genetic DNA testing with patients: a short guide for health professionals. 2013. Published online at https://www.nhmrc.gov.au/guidelines-publications/g7 (Last accessed April 1, 2015)
78. Meiser B, Dunn S. Psychological impact of genetic testing for Huntington's disease: an update of the literature. J Neurol Neurosurg Psychiatry. 2000;69:574–8.
79. Meyer J, Westera J. Life insurance and genetic testing for prostate cancer: what advice for patients? ANZ J Surger. 2012;82(4):194–5.
80. Morren M, Rijken M, Baanders A, Bensing J. Perceived genetic knowledge, attitudes towards genetic testing, and the relationship between these among patients with a chronic disease. Patient Educ Couns. 2007;65(2):197–204.
81. Mouchawar J, Hensley-Alford S, Laurion S, Ellis J, Kulchak-Rahm A, Finucane ML, Meenan R, Axell L, Pollack R, Ritzwoller D. Impact of direct-to-consumer advertising for hereditary breast cancer testing on genetic services at a managed care organization: naturally-occurring experiment. Genet Med. 2005;7(3):191–7.
82. Nance MA. Genetics and genetic counseling related issues. In: Frucht SJ, editor. Movement disorder emergencies: diagnosis and treatment, Current clinical neurology. 2nd ed. New York: Human Press; 2013. p. 375–84.
83. Nedelcu R, Blazer KR, Schwerin BU, Gambol P, Manthat P, Uman GC, Weitzel JN. Genetic discrimination: the clinician perspective. Clin Genet. 2004;66:311–7.
84. Ngueng Feze I, Joly Y. Can't always get what you want? Try an indirect route you just might get what you need: a study on access to genetic data by Canadian life insurers. Curr Pharmacogenomics Pers Med. 2014;12:56–64.
85. NHS. House of Lords Science and Technology Committee – second report on genomic medicine. London: National Health Services; 2009.
86. Nowland W. Human genetics. A rational view of insurance and genetic discrimination. Science. 2002;297(5579):195–6.
87. Otlowski M. Avoiding genetic testing and insurance: an exploration of the legality and ethics of precautionary measures in anticipation of unfavorable test outcomes. Monash Bioeth Rev. 2001;20:24–32.
88. Otlowski M. Genetic testing and insurance: the case for regulation. Agenda. 2002;9(4):335–54.
89. Otlowski M, Barlow-Stewart K, Taylor S, Stranger M, Trealoar S. Investigating genetic discrimination in the Australian life insurance sector: the use of genetic test results in underwriting, 1999–2003. J Law Med. 2007;14:367–96.
90. Otlowski M, Taylor S, Bombard Y. Genetic discrimination: international perspectives. Annu Rev Genomics Hum Genet. 2012;13:433–54.
91. Pamarti AK. Genetic information nondiscrimination act (GINA) and its affects on genetic counseling practice: a survey of genetic counselors. Brandeis University, http://bir.brandeis.edu/bitstream/handle/10192/24364/Pamarti_thesis_GINA%20survey.pdf?sequence=1. 2011.

92. Pasche B, Absher D. Whole-genome sequencing: a step closer to personalized medicine. JAMA J Am Med Assoc. 2011;305:1596–7.
93. Peterson E, Milliron K, Lewis K, Goold S, Merajver S. Health insurance and discrimination concerns and BRCA1/2 testing in a clinic population. Cancer Epidemiol Biomarkers Prev. 2007;11:79–87.
94. Pfeffer NL, McCarthy Veach P, LeRoy BS. An investigation of genetic counselors' discussions of genetic discrimination with cancer risk patients. J Genet Couns. 2003;12(5):419–38.
95. Phoenix Strategic Perspective Inc. Survey of Canadians on privacy-related issues. Ottawa: Office of the Privacy Commissioner of Canada; 2013
96. Powell KP, Cogswell WA, Christianson CA, Dave G, Verma A, Eubanks S, Henrich V. Primary care physicians' awareness, experience and opinions of direct-to-consumer genetic testing. J Genet Couns. 2011;21:113–26.
97. Quebec Civil Code, LRQ, c C-1991.
98. Riley B, Culver J, Skrzynia C, Senter L, Peters J, Costalas J, Callif-Daley F, Grumet S, Hunt K, Nagy R, McKinnon W, Petrucilli N, Bennett R, Trepanier A. Essential elements of genetic cancer risk assessment, counseling, and testing: updated recommendations of the national society of genetic counselors. J Genet Couns. 2012;21(2):151–61.
99. Rothstein MA. Why treating genetic information separately is a bad idea. Texas Rev Law Pol. 1999;4(1):33–7.
100. Rothstein MA, Joly Y. Genetic discrimination in life insurance: contemporary issues and approaches in the global economy. In: Atkinson P, Glasner P, Lock M, editors. The handbook of genetics and society: mapping the new genomic era. London: Routledge; 2009. p. 127–44.
101. Joly Y, Kim R, Salman S, Ngueng Feze I. The use of genetic information outside of the therapeutic or health research relationship: an international perspective. In: Quinn G, De Paor A, Blanck P, editors. Genetic discrimination: transatlantic perspectives on the case for a European level legal response. New York: Routledge; 2015.
102. Scheuner MT, De Vries H, Kim B, Meili RC, Olmstead SH, Teleki S. Are electronic health records ready for genomic medicine? Genet Med. 2009;11(7):510–7.
103. Schneider SA, Klein C. What is the role of genetic testing in movement disorders practice? Curr Neurol Neurosci Rep. 2011;11:351–61.
104. Schneider SA, Schneider UH, Klein C. Genetic testing for neurologic disorder. Semin Neurol. 2011;31(5):542–52.
105. Soini S. Genetic testing legislation in western Europe – a fluctuating regulatory target. J Community Genet. 2012;3(2):143–53.
106. Stefansson H, Rye DB, Hicks A, Petursson H, Ingason A, Thorgeirsson TE, Palsson S, Sigmundsson T, Sigurdsson A, Eiriksdottir I, Soebech E, Bliwise D, Beck J, Rosen A, Waddy S, Trotti L, Iranzo A, Thambisetty M, Hardarson GA, Kristjansson K, Gudmundsson L, Thorsteinsdottir U, Kong A, Gulcher JR, Gudbjartsson D, Stefansson K. A genetic risk factor for periodic limb movements in sleep. New Engl J Med. 2007;357:639–47.
107. Subramanian K, Lemaire J, Hershey J, Pauly M, Armstrong K, Asch D. Estimating adverse selection costs from genetic testing for breast and ovarian cancer: the case of life insurance. J Risk Insur. 1999;66:531–50.
108. Suther S, Goodson P. Barrier to the provision of genetic services by primary care physicians: a systematic review of the literature. Genet Med. 2003;5(2):70–6.
109. Sweden. The Genetic Integrity Act, no. 351. 2006.
110. Trepanier A, Ahrens M, McKinnon W, Peters J, Stopfer J, Grumet SC, Manley S, Culver JO, Acton R, Larsen-Haidle J, Correia LA, Bennett R, Pettersen B, Ferlita TD, Costalas JW, Hunt K, Donlon S, Skrzynia C, Farrell C, Callif-Daley F, Walsh Vockley C, National Society of Genetic Counselors. Genetic cancer risk assessment and counseling: recommendations of the national society of genetic counselors. J Genet Couns. 2004;13(2):83–114.
111. Ullman-Cullere MH, Mathew JP. Emerging landscape of genomics in the electronic health record for personalized medicine. Hum Mutat. 2011;32(5):512–6.
112. Van den Berg S, Shen Y, Jones SJM, Gibson WT. Genetic counseling in direct-to-consumer exome sequencing: a case report. J Genet Couns. 2014. doi:10.1007/s10897-014-9737-0.

113. Van Hoyweghen I, Horstman K. European practices of genetic information and insurance: lessons for the genetic information nondiscrimination act. JAMA. 2008;300(3):326–7.
114. Wade CH, Wilfond BS. Ethical and clinical practice considerations for genetic counselors related to direct-to-consumer marketing of genetic tests. Am J Med Genet. 2006;142C(4):284–92.
115. Wilde A, Meiser B, Mitchell P, Schofield P. Public interest in predictive genetic testing, including direct-to-consumer testing, for susceptibility to major depression: preliminary findings. Eur J Hum Genet. 2010;18:47–51.
116. Zgheib NK, Arawi T, Mahfouz R, Sabra R. Attitudes of health care professionals towards pharmacogenetic testing. Mol Diagn Ther. 2011;15(2):115–22.
117. Zick C, Mathews C, Roberts J, Cook-Deegan R, Pokorski R, Green RC. Genetic testing for Alzheimer's disease and its impact on insurance purchasing behavior. Health Aff. 2005;24:483–90.

Index

S.A. Schneider, J.M.T. Brás (eds.), *Movement Disorder Genetics*,
DOI 10.1007/978-3-319-17223-1

L

M

Q

R

S

T

Printed by Printforce, the Netherlands